ACUTE CORONARY SYNDROMES

A Companion to BRAUNWALD'S HEART DISEASE

ACUTE CORONARY SYNDROMES

A Companion to BRAUNWALD'S HEART DISEASE

EDITION 2

DAVID A. MORROW, MD, MPH

Director, Levine Cardiac Intensive Care Unit
Professor of Medicine
Harvard Medical School
Cardiovascular Medicine
Brigham and Women's Hospital
Boston, Massachusetts

ROBERT P. GIUGLIANO, MD, ScM

Senior Staff
Professor of Medicine
Harvard Medical School
Cardiovascular Medicine
Brigham and Women's Hospital
Boston, Massachusetts

ELSEVIER

Elsevier
1600 John F. Kennedy Blvd.
Ste 1800
Philadelphia, PA 19103-2899

ACUTE CORONARY SYNDROMES, SECOND EDITION ISBN: 978-0-443-11869-2

Senior Content Strategist: Melanie Tucker
Senior Content Development Specialist: Suddha Satwa Sen
Publishing Services Manager: Deepthi Unni
Project Manager: Nandhini Thanga Alagu
Design Direction: Renee Duenow

Printed in India
Last digit is the print number: 9 8 7 6 5 4 3 2 1

To Dr. Eugene Braunwald,
whose unwavering commitment to excellence
is the foundation for
Braunwald's Heart Disease
and each of its companions.

Contributors

Antonio Abbate, MD, PhD
Professor of Medicine
Department of Medicine
University of Virginia
Charlottesville, Virginia

Nandan S. Anavekar, MBBCh
Professor of Medicine
Cardiovascular Diseases and Radiology
Mayo Clinic
Rochester, Minnesota

Dominick J. Angiolillo, MD, PhD
Professor of Medicine
Cardiology
University of Florida
Jacksonville, Florida

Paul W. Armstrong, MD
Distinguished University Professor
Canadian VIGOUR Centre, Department of Medicine
University of Alberta
Edmonton, Alberta, Canada

Kevin R. Bainey, MD, MSc
Associate Professor of Medicine (Cardiology)
Director, Interventional Cardiology
Mazankowski Alberta Heart Institute
Faculty, Canadian VIGOUR Centre
University of Alberta
Edmonton, Alberta, Canada

David D. Berg, MD, MPH
Assistant Professor of Medicine
Cardiovascular Division
Brigham and Women's Hospital
Harvard Medical School
Boston, Massachusetts

Deepak L. Bhatt, MD, MPH, MBA
Director of Mount Sinai Fuster Heart Hospital
Mount Sinai Fuster Heart Hospital
Icahn School of Medicine at Mount Sinai
New York, New York
Dr. Valentin Fuster Professor of Cardiovascular Medicine (with Tenure)
Icahn School of Medicine at Mount Sinai
New York, New York

Erin A. Bohula May, MD, DPhil
Assistant Professor of Medicine
Cardiovascular Division
Brigham & Women's Hospital
Harvard Medical School
Boston, Massachusetts

Jason S. Bradfield, MD
Associate Professor of Medicine
UCLA Cardiac Arrhythmia Center
Ronald Reagan UCLA Medical Center
Los Angeles, California

Eugene Braunwald, MD, MD(Hon), ScD(Hon), FRCP
Distinguished Hersey Professor of Medicine
Harvard Medical School
Founding Chairman, TIMI Study Group
Brigham and Women's Hospital
Boston, Massachusetts

Jacob A. Burns, MD
Advanced Fellow in Cardiovascular Disease
Cardiovascular Division
Brigham and Women's Hospital
Boston, Massachusetts

Spencer Carter, MD
Assistant Professor
Cardiology
University of Utah
Salt Lake City, Utah

Noel C. Chan, MBBS, FRACP, FRCPA
Associate Professor of Medicine
McMaster University
Hamilton, Ontario, Canada

Derek P. Chew, MBBS, MPH, PhD, FRACP, FESC, FACC, FCSANZ
Professor of Cardiology
Victorian Heart Hospital
Melbourne, Victoria, Australia
Professor of Cardiology
Victorian Heart Institute
Victoria, Australia

Marco G. Del Buono, MD, PhD
Medical Doctor
Cardiology
Fondazione Policlinico Gemelli
Rome, Italy

Jeremiah P. Depta, MD, MPHS, MBA, FACC, FSCAI
Director, Advanced Valvular and Structural Heart Disease Program
Sands Constellation Heart Institute
Rochester General Hospital
Rochester, New York

Marcelo F. Di Carli, MD
Executive Director, Cardiovascular Imaging Program
Medicine and Radiology
Brigham and Women's Hospital
Boston, Massachusetts
Chief, Division of Nuclear Medicine and Molecular Imaging
Radiology
Brigham and Women's Hospital
Boston, Massachusetts

Sanjay Divakaran, MD, MPH
Associate Chief and Clinical Director
Division of Cardiovascular Medicine
Brigham and Women's Hospital
Boston, Massachusetts
Assistant Professor of Medicine
Harvard Medical School
Boston, Massachusetts

Anique Ducharme, MD, MSc
Director of the Heart Failure Clinic
Department of Medicine
Montreal Heart Institute
Montreal, Quebec, Canada
Professor of Medicine
University of Montreal
Montreal, Quebec, Canada

John W. Eikelboom, MBBS, MSc, FRACP, FRCPA, FRCPC
Senior Investigator
Professor of Medicine
Population Health Research Institute
McMaster University
Hamilton, Ontario, Canada

James C. Fang, MD
Professor of Medicine
Division of Cardiovascular Diseases
Executive Director, Cardiovascular Service Line
University of Utah Health Sciences
Salt Lake City, Utah
Chief, Cardiovascular Medicine
Internal Medicine
University of Utah
Salt Lake City, Utah

Francesco Franchi, MD
Associate Professor
Medicine—Division of Cardiology
University of Florida College of Medicine
Jacksonville, Florida

J. Michael Gaziano, MD, MPH
Director, MAVERIC
VA Boston Healthcare System
Boston, Massachusetts
Chief, Division of Aging
Brigham and Women's Hospital
Boston, Massachusetts

Thomas A. Gaziano, MD, MSC
Associate Professor of Medicine
Harvard Medical School
Boston, Massachusetts
Associate Physician
Cardiovascular Medicine
Brigham & Women's Hospital
Boston, Massachusetts

Robert P. Giugliano, MD, ScM
Senior Staff
Professor of Medicine
Harvard Medical School
Cardiovascular Medicine
Brigham and Women's Hospital
Boston, Massachusetts

Shaun G. Goodman, MD, MSc, FRCPC, FACC, FAHA, FESC, FCCS
Associate Head, Division of Cardiology
St. Michael's Hospital
Unity Health Toronto
Toronto, Ontario, Canada
Co-Director
Canadian VIGOUR Centre
University of Alberta
Edmonton, Alberta, Canada
Associate Director
Peter Munk Cardiac Centre Clinical Trials and Translation Unit
University Health Network
Toronto, Ontario, Canada

John D. Grizzard, MD
Associate Professor
Radiology and Cardiology
VCU Health Systems
Richmond, Virginia

Sharon L. Hale, BS
Research Scientist (Retired)
Huntington Medical Research Institutes
Pasadena, California

Timothy D. Henry, MD
Medical Director
The Carl and Edyth Lindner Center for Research and Education at The Christ Hospital
The Christ Hospital Health Network
Cincinnati, Ohio

Stefan James, MD, PhD
Professor of Cardiology
Scientific Director of Uppsala Clinical Research Center
Department of Medical Sciences
Uppsala, Sweden

Ik-Kyung Jang, MD, PhD
Allan and Gill Gray Professor of Medicine
Cardiology Division
Massachusetts General Hospital
Harvard Medical School
Boston, Massachusetts

Hayan Jouni, MD
Assistant Professor of Medicine
Cardiovascular Medicine
Mayo Clinic
Rochester, Minnesota

Julia Karady, MD, PhD, MPH
Instructor
Radiology Department
Massachusetts General Hospital
Boston, Massachusetts

Raymond J. Kim, MD
Professor
Medicine and Radiology
Duke University Medical Center
Durham, North Carolina
Director
Duke Cardiovascular Magnetic Resonance Center
Duke University Medical Center
Durham, North Carolina

Robert A. Kloner, MD, PhD
Chief Science Officer
Cardiovascular Research
Huntington Medical Research Institutes
Pasadena, California
Professor of Medicine (Clinical Scholar)
Medicine
Keck School of Medicine at University of Southern California
Los Angeles, California
Director and Chair of Cardiovascular Research Institute
Huntington Medical Research Institutes
Pasadena, California
Visiting Associate in Aerospace
Division of Engineering and Applied Science
California Institute of Technology
Pasadena, California

David C. Lange, MD
Medical Director of Structural Heart Interventions
Cardiology
Kaiser Santa Clara Medical Center
Santa Clara, California

Peter Libby, MD
Cardiovascular Specialist
Cardiovascular Medicine
Brigham and Women's Hospital/Harvard Medical School
Boston, Massachusetts

Varun Malik, MBBS, BMedSci, PhD
Clinical Senior Lecturer, Academic Cardiologist and Electrophysiologist
School of Medicine
University of Adelaide
Adelaide, South Australia, Australia

Yoshiyasu Minami, MD, PhD
Assistant Professor
Cardiovascular Medicine
Kitasato University School of Medicine
Sagamihara, Japan

Gilles Montalescot, MD, PhD
Professor
Cardiologie
Pitié-Salpêtrière hospital
Paris, France

David A. Morrow, MD, MPH
Director, Levine Cardiac Intensive Care Unit
Professor of Medicine
Harvard Medical School
Cardiovascular Medicine
Brigham and Women's Hospital
Boston, Massachusetts

Matthias Nahrendorf, MD, PhD
Professor
Department of Radiology
Massachusetts General Hospital
Harvard Medical School
Boston, Massachusetts

Daniel S. Ong, MD
Interventional Cardiologist
The Heart Hospital
Baylor Scott & White
Plano, Texas

Luis Ortega-Paz, MD, PhD
Assistant Professor
Cardiology/Internal Medicine
University of Florida College of Medicine-Jacksonville
Jacksonville, Florida

Michelle L. O'Donoghue, MD, MPH
McGillycuddy Logue Endowed Chair of Cardiovascular Medicine
Senior Investigator
TIMI Study Group
Cardiovascular Division
Brigham and Women's Hospital
Boston, Massachusetts
Associate Professor of Medicine
Harvard Medical School
Boston, Massachusetts

Siddharth M. Patel, MD, MPH
Associate Physician, Cardiovascular Division
Department of Medicine
Brigham and Women's Hospital
Harvard Medical School
Boston, Massachusetts

Sunil V. Rao, MD
Professor of Medicine
Cardiology
NYU Langone Health System
New York, New York

Louai Razzouk, MD, MPH
Assistant Professor of Medicine
Medicine
NYU Grossman School of Medicine
New York, New York

Harmony R. Reynolds, MD, FACC, FACP, FAHA
Associate Professor of Medicine
Medicine
NYU Grossman School of Medicine
New York, New York

Marc S. Sabatine, MD, MPH
Chairman
TIMI Study Group
Lewis Dexter, MD, Endowed Chair in Cardiovascular Medicine
Brigham and Women's Hospital
Boston, Massachusetts
Professor of Medicine
Harvard Medical School
Boston, Massachusetts

Benjamin M. Scirica, MD, MPH
Senior Investigator
TIMI Study Group
Cardiovascular Division
Brigham and Women's Hospital
Boston, Massachusetts
Professor of Medicine
Harvard Medical School
Boston, Massachusetts

Kalyanam Shivkumar, MD, PhD, FACC
Director, UCLA Cardiac Arrhythmia Center & EP Programs
Medicine & Radiology
UCLA Health System
Los Angeles, California
Professor of Medicine (Cardiology), Radiology and Bioengineering
University of California, Los Angeles
Los Angeles, California
Director & Chief, UCLA Cardiovascular & Interventional Porgrams
UCLA Health System
Los Angeles, California

Johanne Silvain, MD, PhD
Head of Department
Institut de Cardiologie
Pitié-Salpêtrière Hospital (AP-HP)
Paris, France
Professor of Cardiology
Cardiology
Sorbonne University Medecine
Paris, France
ACTION Group
Institut de Cardiologie
Paris, France

Peter R. Sinnaeve, MD, PhD
Professor
Department of Cardiovascular Medicine
University Hospitals Leuven, Leuven, Belgium

Nathaniel R. Smilowitz, MD, MS
Assistant Professor of Medicine
Division of Cardiology, Department of Medicine
NYU Langone Health
New York, New York

Filip K. Swirski, PhD
Professor
Cardiovascular Research Institute
Icahn School of Medicine at Mount Sinai
New York, New York

Jean-Claude Tardif, MD
Director Research Center
Montreal Heart Institute
Montreal, Quebec, Canada
Professor of Medicine
Université de Montréal
Montreal, Quebec, Canada

Rod S. Taylor, MSc, PhD
Professor
MRC/CSO Social and Public Health Sciences Unit & Robertson Centre for Biostatistics
School of Health and Well Being
University of Glasgow
Glasgow, United Kingdom

James E. Udelson, MD
Chief, Division of Cardiology
CardioVascular Center
Tufts Medical Center
Boston, Massachusetts

Frans J. Van de Werf, MD, PhD
Em Professor of Cardiology
CV Sciences
KU Leuven
Leuven, Vlaams Brabant, Belgium

Harvey D. White, MB ChB, DSc, FRACP, FACC, FESC, FAHA, FHKCC (Hon), FCSANZ (life member), FNZMA, FRSNZ
Cardiologist and Director of the Green Lane Cardiovascular Research Unit
Green Lane Cardiovascular Service
Health NZ—Te Whatu Ora
Te Toka Tumai
Auckland City Hospital
Auckland, New Zealand
Honorary Clinical Professor
Department of Medicine
University of Auckland
Auckland, New Zealand

Andrew T. Yan, MD
Professor of Medicine
Professor of Medical Imaging
University of Toronto
Toronto, Ontario, Canada

Mehmet Yildiz, MD
Cardiology Fellow
Department of Cardiology
The Christ Hospital Health Network, Heart and Vascular Institute
Cincinnati, Ohio

Michel Zeitouni, MD, PhD
Associate Professor
Department of Cardiology
Pitié Salpêtrière Hospital
Paris, France

Ann-Dorthe Olsen Zwisler, PhD
Cardiologist
Department of Cardiology
Odense University Hospital
Odense, Denmark
Professor preventive cardiology and palliative care
Danish Knowledge Centre for Rehabilitation and Palliative Care
Odense University Hospital
Odense, Denmark
Professor preventive cardiology and palliative care
Department of Clinical Research
University of Southern Denmark
Odense, Denmark

Foreword

Early in the 20th century, coronary artery disease was recognized as a serious condition, but the distinction between its two principal presentations, chronic stable angina pectoris and acute myocardial infarction, was not clear. By the 1920s, the separate clinical and pathologic manifestations of chronic angina pectoris and acute infarction had been established and their differences recognized. In the 1920s a syndrome intermediate between angina pectoris and acute myocardial infarction, the so-called "intermediate syndrome," later renamed *unstable angina,* was found to be quite common. By the 1960s, increasing attention was focused on the separation of patients with acute myocardial infarction into those who presented with ST segment elevation (STEMI) and non-ST-elevation myocardial infarction (NSTEMI). All three of these conditions—unstable angina, STEMI, and NSTEMI—were considered to make up the acute coronary syndrome (ACS). With the development of more sensitive biochemical markers of myocardial necrosis, especially the troponins, the distinction between unstable angina and NSTEMI has become blurred, and an increasing fraction of patients with the former condition have been shown to have myocardial necrosis (i.e., infarction). Thus it now appears that a large majority of patients with acute coronary syndrome actually have acute myocardial infarction.

Research on this condition has moved forward on many fronts. This text, masterfully edited by Robert Giugliano and David Morrow, experienced clinicians and investigators in this field, captures the major developments which include the many epidemiologic, clinical, pathophysiologic, and therapeutic advances in myocardial infarction. Among them are the prehospital assessment and care, the role of optical coherence tomography and of a variety of imaging techniques in the diagnosis and management of patients with STEMI who are unable to undergo immediate coronary arterial stenting; the optimal timing of revascularization in patients with NSTEMI; the individualization of antiplatelet therapy, the application of mechanical circulatory support for patients with cardiogenic shock, efforts to reverse myocardial infarction-induced ventricular remodeling, and how to manage patients without coronary obstruction.

The enormous worldwide frequency of ACS and its seriousness place this condition at the very "heart" of cardiology. Indeed, just about every practicing adult cardiologist—whether invasive or noninvasive, whether primarily office- or hospital-based, whether subspecializing in hypertension, heart failure, arrhythmias, prevention, or rehabilitation—encounters patients with this condition and should be acquainted with the important recent developments in diagnosis and management.

Cardiologists dealing with these patients as well as trainees and clinical investigators will be indebted to Drs. Giugliano and Morrow and their talented authors for providing this important new book. We are proud that it is a companion to *Heart Disease—A Textbook of Cardiovascular Medicine*.

Eugene Braunwald
Boston, Massachusetts
Robert O. Bonow
Chicago, Illinois
Douglas L. Mann
St. Louis, Missouri
Gordon F. Tomaselli
Baltimore, Maryland
Deepak L. Bhatt
New York, New York
Scott D. Solomon
Boston, Massachusetts
Peter Libby
Boston, Massachusetts

Preface

Cardiovascular disease remains the most common cause of death worldwide, with ischemic heart disease contributing to half of those deaths, driven primarily by deaths related to *Acute Coronary Syndrome* (ACS). This edition of *Acute Coronary Syndromes: A Companion to Braunwald's Heart Disease* aims to distill the most important general principles of management and capture the contemporary state of the art of clinical care as well as translational and clinical science impacting the management of ACS. This textbook should be valuable for clinical practitioners, medical trainees, and scientists with an interest in ischemic heart disease and its complications.

The contributors to this text have labored to produce a book that will serve equally well for comprehensive review and as a readily accessible clinical resource for the busy clinician, both as a traditional printed book and an interactive online text that is optimized for tablet and hand-held electronic reading.

The book is framed by the clinical course of care for the patient with ACS. After setting the stage with an overview and overarching classification, the subsequent six sections navigate through (1) initial clinical evaluation, risk assessment, and in-hospital management of ACS; (2) advanced imaging; (3) evaluation and treatment, including complications; (4) short- and long-term secondary prevention planning at hospital discharge; and (5) the evolving epidemiology and emerging pathobiological concepts. In these sections, internationally recognized leaders in their field have not only reviewed the current evidence and professional guidelines but also offered their own perspectives on "best practice" in areas where there is equipoise or controversy.

It remains a tremendous privilege and pleasure to work with the exceptional group of clinical experts, educators, and clinician-scientists who have contributed to this text, and we wish to thank each of them.

Robert P. Giugliano, MD, SM
David A. Morrow, MD, MPH
Boston, Massachusetts

Contents

Braunwald's Heart Disease Family of Books

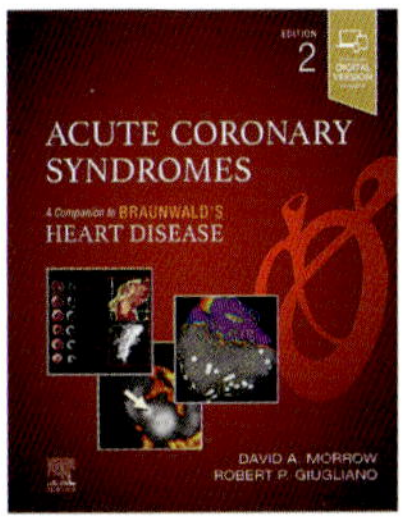

MORROW AND GIUGLIANO
Acute Coronary Syndromes

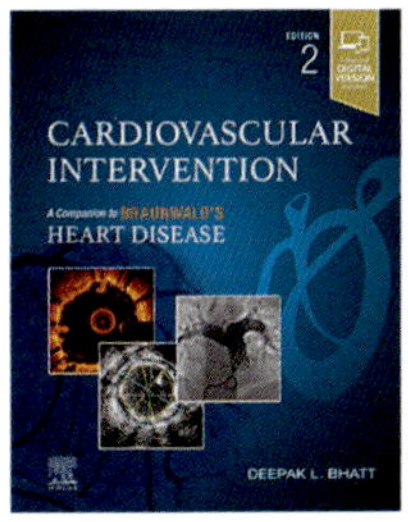

BHATT
Cardiovascular Intervention

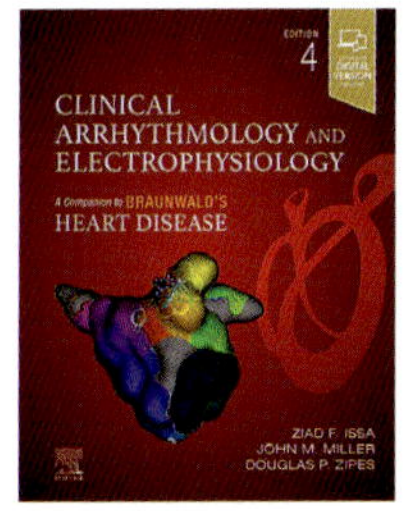

ISSA, MILLER, ZIPES
Clinical Arrhythmology and Electrophysiology

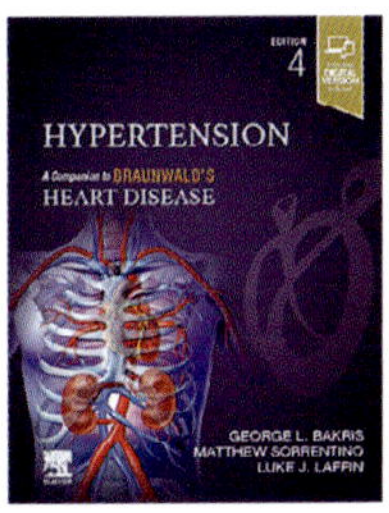

BAKRIS, SORRENTINO, AND LAFFIN
Hypertension

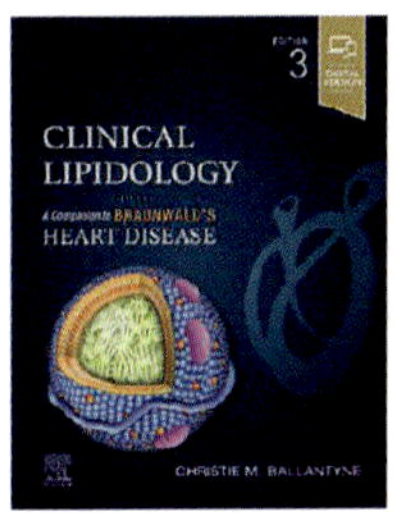

BALLANTYNE
Clinical Lipidology

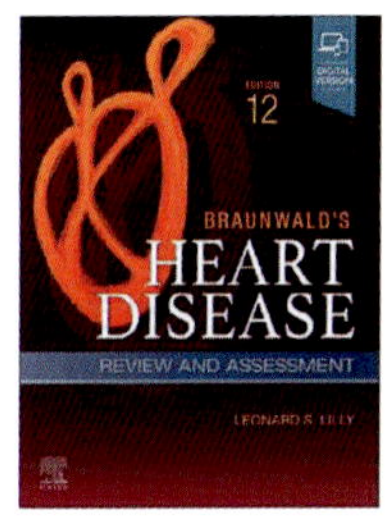

LILLY
Braunwald's Heart Disease Review and Assessment

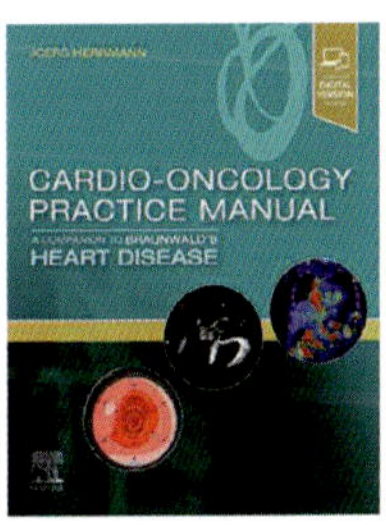

HERRMANN
Cardio-Oncology Practice Manual

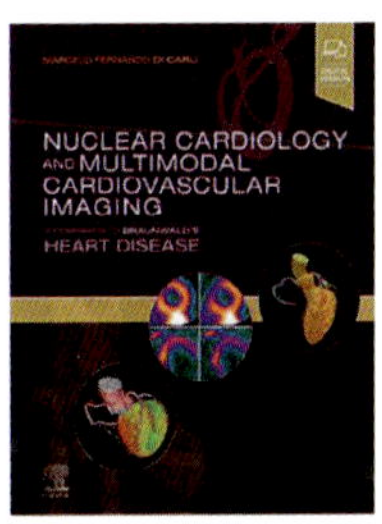

DI CARLI
Nuclear Cardiology and Multimodal Cardiovascular Imaging

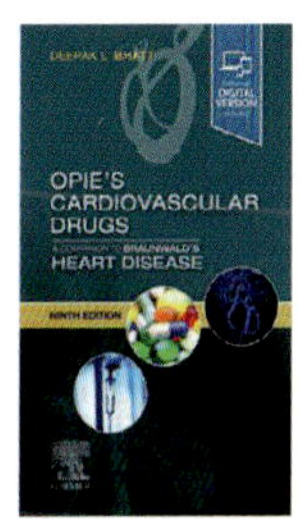

BHATT
Opie's Cardiovascular Drugs

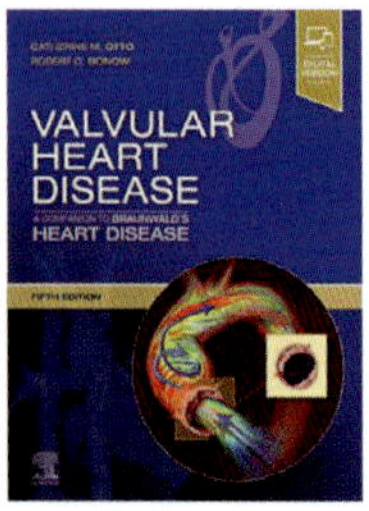

OTTO AND BONOW
Valvular Heart Disease

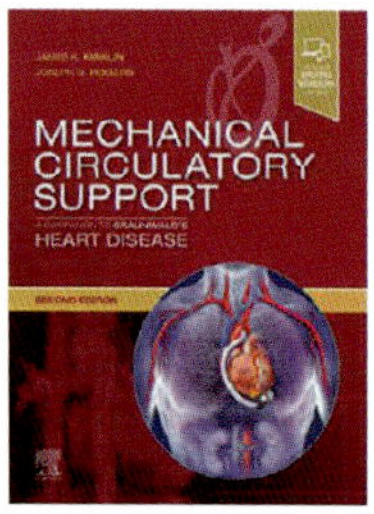

KIRKLIN AND ROGERS
Mechanical Circulatory Support

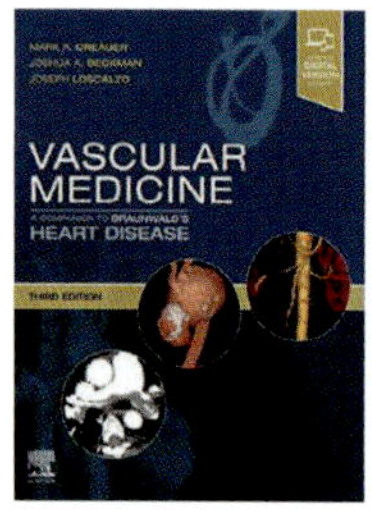

CREAGER
Vascular Medicine

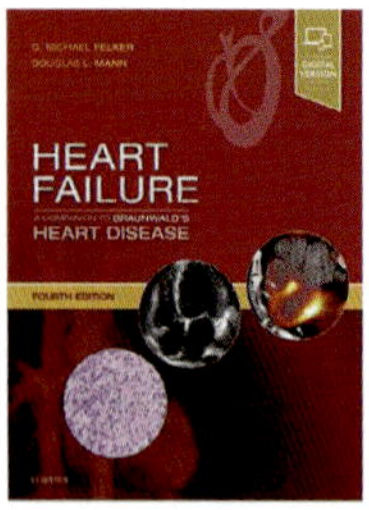

FELKER AND MANN
Heart Failure

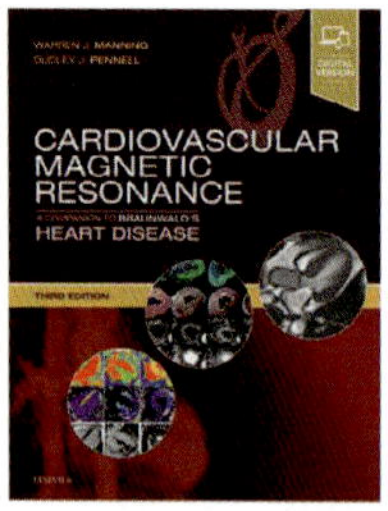

MANNING AND PENNELL
Cardiovascular Magnetic Resonance

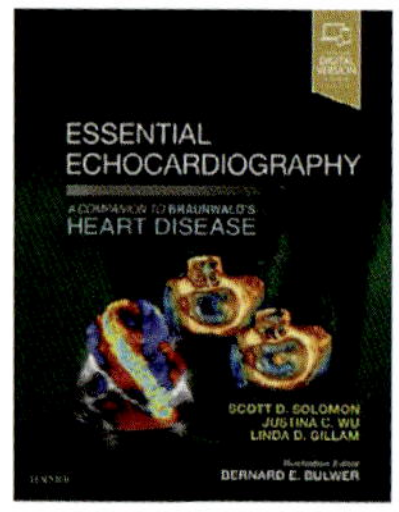

SOLOMON, WU, AND GILLAM
Essential Echocardiography

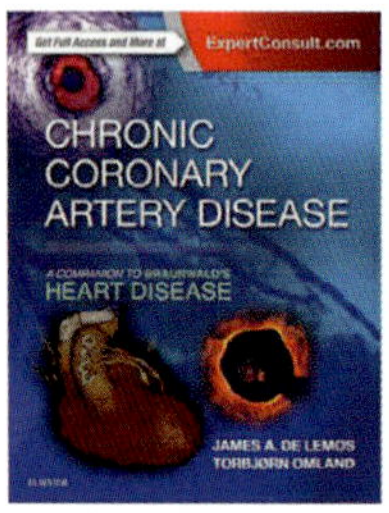

DE LEMOS AND OMLAND
Chronic Coronary Artery Disease

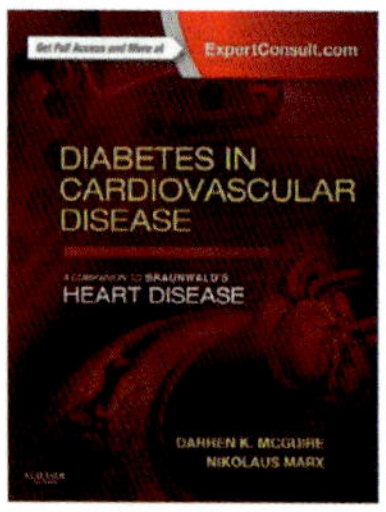

MCGUIRE AND MARX
Diabetes in Cardiovascular Disease

1 Overview of the Patient With Acute Coronary Syndrome

ROBERT P. GIUGLIANO

INTRODUCTION

Despite many advances since the initial description in 1912 by James Herrick of the clinical syndrome subsequently known as *myocardial infarction* (MI), *ischemic heart disease* (IHD) is the most common manifestation of *cardiovascular disease* (CVD). As of 2020, CVD remained the most common cause of death worldwide (19.1 million[1]), affecting >10% of the global adult population (see Chapter 31). IHD is estimated to cause half of the deaths attributed to CVD, driven primarily by deaths related to *acute coronary syndrome* (ACS) or its complications.[2]

TYPES OF ACUTE CORONARY SYNDROMES

By definition, ACS is characterized by the sudden onset of signs and symptoms of myocardial ischemia and carries the risk of early death, hence the need for immediate evaluation and hospitalization. ACS encompasses a spectrum of diseases (Fig. 1.1) that include acute MI and unstable angina (UA), the latter being defined as ACS without the evidence of myocardial necrosis by laboratory testing or ancillary testing (electrocardiography, imaging, pathology) (see Chapter 2). Acute MI is further subclassified at *ST-elevation MI* (STEMI) or *non-ST-elevation MI* (NSTEMI) based on the presence or absence of persistent (>20 minutes) elevation of the ST segments in two or more geographically contiguous leads on electrocardiography. It is important to recognize that many conditions may result in elevation of cardiac biomarkers (especially current-generation high-sensitivity cardiac-specific troponins) and that many of such elevations do not represent an MI (see Chapter 2). Thus, the diagnosis of MI requires additional clinical criteria indicative of myocardial ischemia (symptoms and/or other diagnostic findings on electrocardiogram or imaging studies, see Chapter 4) (Fig. 1.2), as well as consideration of alternative etiology for elevations in cardiac biomarkers that may be cardiovascular (e.g., pulmonary embolism, heart failure, myocarditis) or noncardiovascular (e.g., sepsis, renal failure) in origin.

BROAD OVERVIEW OF ACUTE CORONARY SYNDROME MANAGEMENT

Fortunately, continued developments in the fields of prevention, immediate coronary reperfusion see Chapters 8 and 9), and management of life-threatening complications of ACS (e.g., ventricular arrhythmias that can lead to cardiac arrest, [see Chapter 23], cardiogenic shock [see Chapter 21], mechanical complications [see Chapter 22], and thromboembolism) have lowered early mortality to <10% in hospitalized patients in developed countries.[3] Much of the reduction in early mortality in ACS can be attributed to advances in prehospital and emergency medical care and better coordination of initial triage and care between hospitals in care networks (List 1.1) (see Chapter 3).

Pillars of early hospital management include early recognition of ACS, considering invasive management in patients with STEMI (see Chapters 6, 8, 11) or high-risk NSTE-ACS (see Chapters 10 and 11), initiating antithrombotic therapy (see Chapters 12 and 13), appropriate use of coronary revascularization (percutaneous coronary intervention (PCI), see Chapters 8, 10–11, or coronary artery bypass graft surgery (CABG), see Chapter 10), use of further diagnostic investigations to risk stratify patients (see Chapters 4, 6, and 14–18), and early initiation of secondary prevention measures (Fig. 1.3) (see Chapter 29). Toward the end of hospitalization, all patients should be evaluated for cardiac rehabilitation (see Chapter 29) and measures to optimize a healthy lifestyle (diet, exercise, weight management, stress reduction, and evaluation of social determinants of health).

The scope of ACS covered in this textbook is wide and draws upon an international group of experts covering topics in ACS, including the initial evaluation (see Chapters 3–5) and risk stratification (see Chapter 6), initial treatment (see Chapters 7–13), in-hospital evaluation (see Chapters 14–18), complications (see Chapters 19–24), secondary prevention (see Chapters 25–30), epidemiology (see Chapter 31), and pathobiology (see Chapter 32). With the 2023 release of the European Society of Cardiology ACS Guideline[3], which includes 37 new recommendations (Table 1.1) and 18 revised recommendations (Table 1.2),

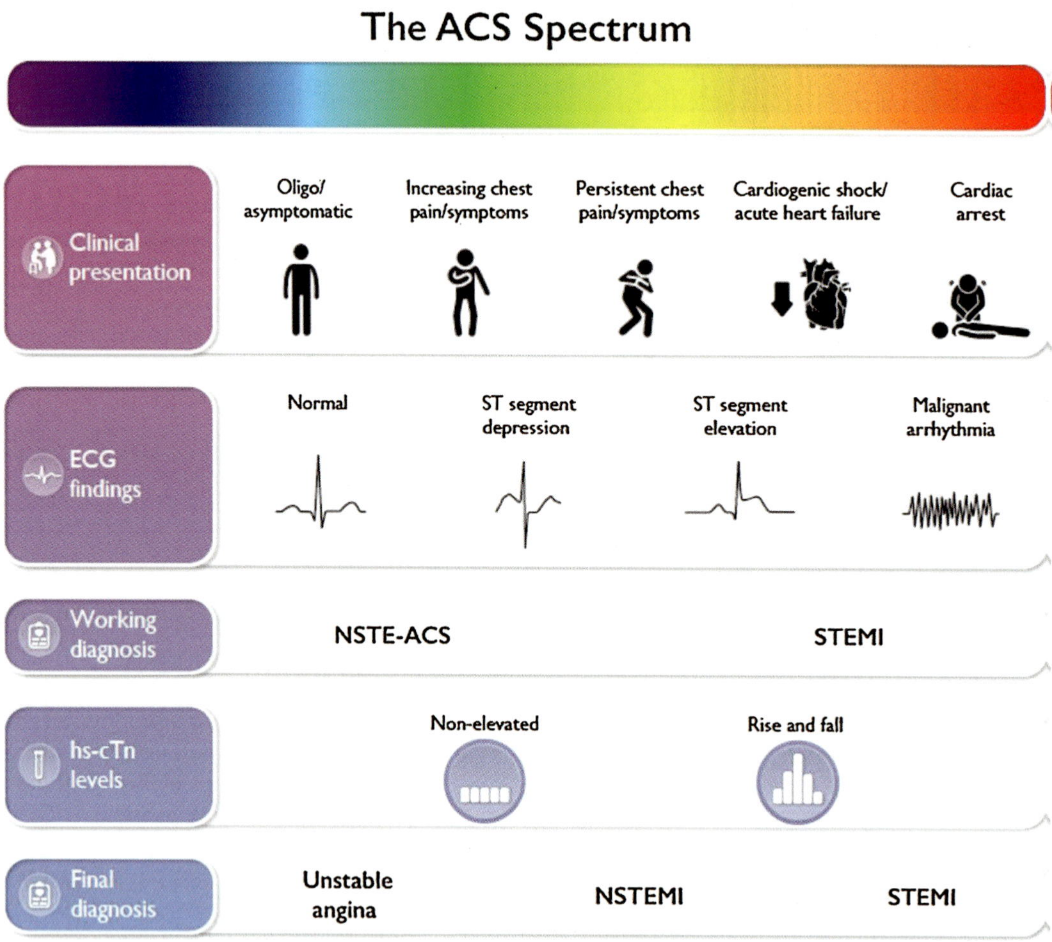

FIG. 1.1 The ACS spectrum. The spectrum of clinical presentations, electrocardiographic findings, and high-sensitivity cardiac troponin levels in patients with acute coronary syndrome. *ACS*, Acute coronary syndrome; *ECG*, electrocardiogram; *hs-cTn*, high-sensitivity cardiac troponin; *NSTE-ACS*, non-ST-elevation acute coronary syndrome; *NSTEMI*, non-ST-elevation myocardial infarction; *STEMI*, ST-elevation myocardial infarction. *(From Byrne RA, Rossello X, Coughlan JJ, et al. The 2023 ESC guidelines for the management of acute coronary syndromes. Eur Heart J. 2023;44(38):3720–3826. https://doi.org/10.1093/eurheartj/ehad191)*

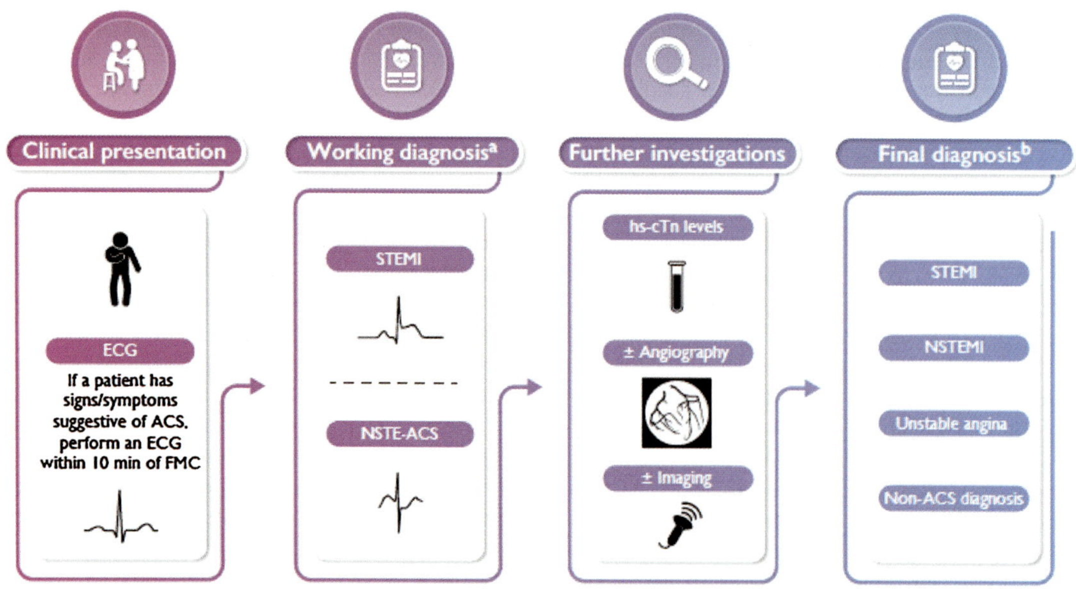

FIG. 1.2 Classification of patients presenting with suspected acute coronary syndrome: From a working to a final diagnosis. *ACS*, Acute coronary syndrome; *ECG*, electrocardiogram; *FMC*, first medical contact; *hs-cTn*, high-sensitivity cardiac troponin; *MI*, myocardial infarction; *NSTE-ACS*, non-ST-elevation acute coronary syndrome; *NSTEMI*, non-ST-elevation myocardial infarction; *STEMI*, ST-elevation myocardial infarction. [a]The working ACS diagnosis can be classified as STEMI or NSTE-ACS based on the available clinical information and ECG findings. This allows for initial triage and assessment. [b]The final diagnosis is based on symptoms, ECG, and troponin for the diagnosis of MI as well as the results of other tests (i.e., imaging and/or angiography) to facilitate understanding of the mechanism and subclassification of the type of MI. Patients initially assigned a working diagnosis of STEMI or NSTE-ACS may eventually receive a final non-ACS diagnosis. *(From Byrne RA, Rossello X, Coughlan JJ, et al. The 2023 ESC guidelines for the management of acute coronary syndromes. Eur Heart J. 2023;44(38):3720–3826. https://doi.org/10.1093/eurheartj/ehad191)*

LIST 1.1 Improvements in Pre-hospital and Emergency Care of ACS

Public Awareness of ACS

- Heart attack awareness programs supported by medical societies, hospitals, and governmental agencies to enhance awareness of ACS symptoms and promote early medical attention
- Educational efforts regarding the risks of heart disease in females and potential differences in symptoms compared to males (e.g., Go Red for Women)
- Community campaigns to educate the population (particularly less well-served groups such as those in deprived communities, ethnic minorities) on recognition of ischemic symptoms and preferential use of emergency medical services for patients with possible ACS symptoms
- Educational programs in schools, local communities, and regions to teach Basic Life Support (BLS)

Primary Care Providers/General Practitioners

- Education and training to permit delivery optimal prehospital care
- Up to date certification in BLS and awareness of on-site availability of defibrillators
- Establishing protocols to contact Emergency Medical Services (EMS) to minimize prehospital delays

Prehospital Logistics

- Education of "first responders" on the recognition of ischemic symptoms, initial patient assessment and BLS
- Expansion of pool of "first responders" who can provide an initial assessment and BLS
- Access to a 12-lead ECG for all medical and paramedical personnel caring for ACS patients
- Education of above personnel to identify persistent ST elevation or equivalent
- Equipping Emergency Medical Services with electrocardiograms, defibrillators, telemetry devices, and at least one person trained in advanced life support
- Protocol-driven decisions in the prehospital setting, including choice of target hospital, initial pharmacologic and nonpharmacologic therapies, and need for emergent coronary angiography, based on ECG-guided risk stratification

Healthcare Systems

- Development of multidisciplinary ACS treatment pathways to optimally triage patients, initiate early treatments, and minimize time to coronary reperfusion in STEMI
- Periodic review of time-to-treatment metrics as part of a program of continuous quality improvement

Organization of STEMI Treatment Networks

- Development of a regional reperfusion strategy to maximize the efficiency of care in networks between hospital with various levels of clinical services ("hub and spoke" model)
- In centers where the expected transfer time to a primary PCI center exceeds the maximal allowed delays, institution of protocols for rapid fibrinolysis for STEMI, followed by immediate transfer to a center with 24/7 PCI services
- Identification of PCI centers capable of 24/7 emergency invasive management and intensive care
- Identification of more advanced centers that offer cardiothoracic surgical services and advanced mechanical hemodynamic support

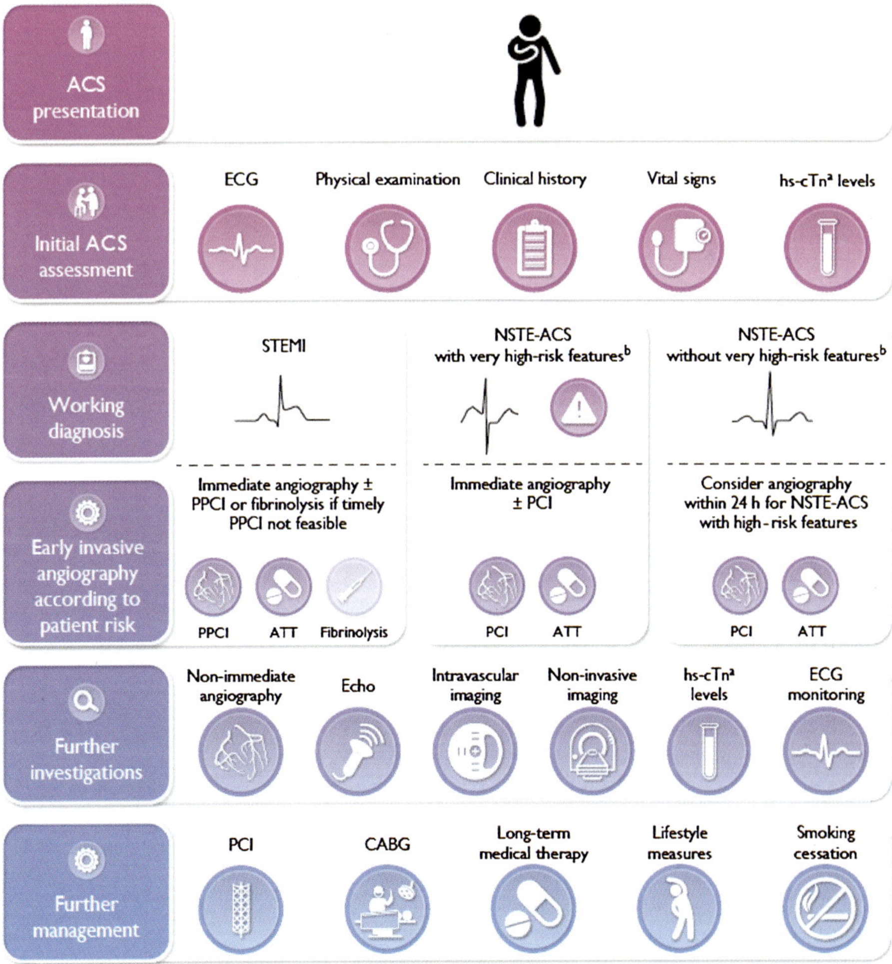

FIG. 1.3 Broad overview of ACS management. *ACS*, Acute coronary syndrome; *ATT*, antithrombotic therapy; *CABG*, coronary artery bypass grafting; *ECG*, electrocardiogram; *hs-cTn*, high-sensitivity cardiac troponin; *NSTE-ACS*, non-ST-elevation acute coronary syndrome; *PPCI*, primary percutaneous coronary intervention; *STEMI*, ST-elevation myocardial infarction. [a]Results of hs-cTn measurements are not required for the initial stratification of ACS and the initial emergency management (i.e., for patients with a working diagnosis of STEMI or very high-risk NSTE-ACS) should not be delayed based on this. [b]For patients with NSTE-ACS with very high-risk features, immediate angiography is recommended. For patients with NSTE-ACS with high-risk features, early invasive angiography (i.e., <24 h) should be considered and inpatient invasive angiography is recommended. *(From Byrne RA, Rossello X, Coughlan JJ, et al. The 2023 ESC guidelines for the management of acute coronary syndromes. Eur Heart J. 2023;44(38):3720–3826. https://doi.org/10.1093/eurheartj/ehad191)*

TABLE 1.1 New Recommendations in the 2023 ESC ACS Guideline

RECOMMENDATIONS	CLASS[a]	LEVEL[b]
Recommendations for antiplatelet and anticoagulant therapy in acute coronary syndrome		
If patients presenting with ACS stop DAPT to undergo coronary artery bypass grafting, it is recommended that they resume DAPT after surgery for at least 12 months.	I	C
In older ACS patients, especially if HBR, clopidogrel as the $P2Y_{12}$ receptor inhibitor may be considered.	IIb	B
Recommendations for alternative antithrombotic therapy regimens		
In patients who are event free after 3–6 months of DAPT and who are not high ischemic risk, single antiplatelet therapy (preferably with a $P2Y_{12}$ receptor inhibitor) should be considered.	IIa	A
$P2Y_{12}$ inhibitor monotherapy may be considered as an alternative to aspirin monotherapy for long-term treatment.	IIb	A
In HBR patients, aspirin or $P2Y_{12}$ receptor inhibitor monotherapy after 1 month of DAPT may be considered.	IIb	B
In patients requiring OAC, withdrawing antiplatelet therapy at 6 months while continuing OAC may be considered.	IIb	B
De-escalation of antiplatelet therapy in the first 30 days after an ACS event is not recommended.	III	B
Recommendations for cardiac arrest and out-of-hospital cardiac arrest		
Evaluation of neurological prognosis (no earlier than 72 h after admission) is recommended in all comatose survivors after cardiac arrest.	I	C
Transport of patients with out-of-hospital cardiac arrest to a cardiac arrest center according to local protocol should be considered.	IIa	C
Recommendations for technical aspects of invasive strategies		
In patients with spontaneous coronary artery dissection, PCI is recommended only for patients with symptoms and signs of ongoing myocardial ischemia, a large area of myocardium in jeopardy, and reduced antegrade flow.	I	C
Intravascular imaging should be considered to guide PCI.	IIa	A
Intravascular imaging (preferably optical coherence tomography) may be considered in patients with ambiguous culprit lesions.	IIb	C
Recommendations for multivessel disease in ACS patients presenting in cardiogenic shock		
Staged PCI of non-IRA should be considered.	IIa	C
Recommendations for multivessel disease in hemodynamically stable STEMI patients undergoing primary PCI		
It is recommended that PCI of the non-IRA is based on angiographic severity.	I	B
Invasive epicardial functional assessment of nonculprit segments of the IRA is not recommended during the index procedure.	III	C
Recommendations for acute coronary syndrome complications		
Implantation of a permanent pacemaker is recommended when high-degree AV block does not resolve within a waiting period of at least 5 days after MI.	I	C
Cardiac magnetic resonance imaging should be considered in patients with equivocal echocardiographic images or in cases of high clinical suspicion of LV thrombus.	IIa	C
Following an acute anterior MI, a contrast echocardiogram may be considered for the detection of LV thrombus if the apex is not well visualized on echocardiography.	IIb	C
In selected patients with high-degree AV block in the context of an anterior wall MI and acute heart failure, early device implantation (cardiac resynchronization therapy-defibrillator/pacemaker) may be considered.	IIb	C
In patients with recurrent life-threatening ventricular arrhythmias, sedation or general anesthesia to reduce sympathetic drive may be considered.	IIb	C
Recommendations for acute coronary syndrome comorbid conditions		
It is recommended to base the choice of long-term glucose-lowering treatment on the presence of comorbidities, including heart failure, chronic kidney disease, and obesity.	I	A
For frail, older patients with comorbidities, a holistic approach is recommended to individualize interventional and pharmacological treatments after careful evaluation of the risks and benefits.	I	B
An invasive strategy is recommended in cancer patients presenting with high-risk ACS with expected survival ≥6 months.	I	B
A temporary interruption of cancer therapy is recommended in patients in whom the cancer therapy is suspected to be a contributing cause of ACS.	I	C
A conservative noninvasive strategy should be considered in ACS patients with poor cancer prognosis (i.e., with expected life survival <6 months) and/or very high bleeding risk.	IIa	C
Aspirin is not recommended in cancer patients with a platelet count <10,000/UL.	III	C
Clopidogrel is not recommended in cancer patients with a platelet count <30,000/μL.	III	C
In ACS patients with cancer and <50,000/μL platelet count, prasugrel or ticagrelor are not recommended.	III	C
Recommendations for long-term management		
It is recommended to intensify lipid-lowering therapy during the index ACS hospitalization for patients who were on lipid-lowering therapy before admission.	I	C
Low-dose colchicine (0.5 mg once a day) may be considered, particularly if other risk factors are insufficiently controlled or if recurrent cardiovascular disease events occur under optimal therapy.	IIb	A
Combination therapy with a high-dose statin plus ezetimibe may be considered during index hospitalization.	IIb	B
Recommendations for patient perspectives in acute coronary syndrome care		
Patient-centered care is recommended by assessing and adhering to individual patient preferences, needs, and beliefs, ensuring that patient values are used to inform all clinical decisions.	I	B
It is recommended to include ACS patients in decision making (as much as their condition allows) and to inform them about the risk of adverse events, radiation exposure, and alternative options. Decision aids should be used to facilitate the discussion.	I	B
It is recommended to assess symptoms using methods that help patients to describe their experience.	I	C
Use of the "teach back" technique for decision support during the securing of informed consent should be considered.	IIa	B

RECOMMENDATIONS	CLASS[a]	LEVEL[b]
Patient discharge information should be provided in both written and verbal formats prior to discharge. Adequate preparation and education for patient discharge using the teach back technique and/or motivational interviewing, giving information in chunks and checking for understanding should be considered.	IIa	B
Assessment of mental well-being using a validated tool and onward psychological referral when appropriate should be considered.	IIa	B

[a]Class of recommendation.
[b]Level of evidence.
ACS, Acute coronary syndrome; *AV*, atrioventricular; *DAPT*, dual antiplatelet therapy; *HBR*, high bleeding risk; *IRA*, infarct-related artery; *LV*, left ventricular(cle); *MI*, myocardial infarction; *OAC*, oral anticoagulant/ation; *PCI*, percutaneous coronary intervention; *STEMI*, ST-elevation myocardial infarction.
From Byrne RA, Rossello X, Coughlan JJ, et al. The 2023 ESC guidelines for the management of acute coronary syndromes. *Eur Heart J*. 2023;44(38):3720–3826. https://doi.org/10.1093/eurheartj/ehad191

TABLE 1.2 Revised Recommendations in the 2023 ESC ACS Guideline

Recommendations for imaging for patients with suspected NSTE-ACS					
In patients with no recurrence of chest pain, normal ECG findings, and normal levels of cardiac troponin (preferably high sensitivity) but still with suspected ACS, a non-invasive stress test (preferably with imaging) for inducible ischemia or CCTA is recommended before deciding on an invasive approach.	I	B	In patients with suspected ACS, nonelevated (or uncertain) hs-cTn, no ECG changes and no recurrence of pain incorporating CCTA or a noninvasive stress imaging test as part of the initial workup should be considered.	IIa	A
Recommendations for timing of invasive strategy in NSTE-ACS					
An early invasive strategy within 24 h is recommended in patients with any of the following high-risk criteria: • Diagnosis of NSTEMI suggested by the diagnostic algorithm recommended in Section 3 • Dynamic or presumably new contiguous ST/T-segment changes suggesting ongoing ischemia • Transient ST-segment elevation • GRACE risk score >140.	I	A	An early invasive strategy within 24 h should be considered in patients with at least one of the following high-risk criteria: • Confirmed diagnosis of NSTEMI based on current recommended ESC hs-cTn algorithms • Dynamic ST-segment or T-wave changes • Transient ST-segment elevation • GRACE risk score >140	IIa	A
Recommendations for antiplatelet and anticoagulant therapy in STEMI					
A potent $P2Y_{12}$ inhibitor (prasugrel or ticagrelor), or clopidogrel if these are not available or are contraindicated, is recommended before (or at latest at the time of) PCI, and maintained over 12 months, unless there are contraindications such as excessive risk of bleeding.	I	A	Pretreatment with a $P2Y_{12}$ receptor inhibitor may be considered in patients undergoing a primary PCI strategy.	IIb	B
Recommendations for long-term antithrombotic therapy					
After stent implantation in patients undergoing a strategy of DAPT, stopping aspirin after 3–6 months should be considered, depending on the balance between the ischemic and bleeding risks.	IIa	A	In patients who are event-free after 3–6 months of DAPT and who are not high ischemic risk SAPT (preferably with a $P2Y_{12}$ receptor inhibitor) should be considered.	IIa	A
Recommendations for cardiac arrest and out-of-hospital cardiac arrest					
Delayed as opposed to immediate angiography should be considered among hemodynamically stable patients without ST-segment elevation successfully resuscitated after out-of-hospital cardiac arrest.	IIa	B	Routine immediate angiography after resuscitated cardiac arrest is not recommended in hemodynamically stable patients without persistent ST-segment elevation (or equivalents).	III	A
Targeted temperature management (also called therapeutic hypothermia), aiming for a constant temperature between 32°C and 36°C for at least 24 h, is indicated in patients who remain unconscious after resuscitation from cardiac arrest (of presumed cardiac cause).	I	B	Temperature control (i.e., continuous monitoring of core temperature and active prevention of fever [i.e., >37.7°C]) is recommended after either out-of-hospital or in-hospital cardiac arrest for adults who remain unresponsive after return of spontaneous circulation.	I	B
Recommendations for in-hospital management					
When echocardiography is suboptimal/inconclusive, an alternative imaging method (CMR preferably) should be considered.	IIa	C	When echocardiography is suboptimal/inconclusive, CMR imaging may be considered.	IIb	C
Recommendations for management of multivessel disease in hemodynamically stable STEMI patients undergoing primary PCI					
Routine revascularization of non-IRA lesions should be considered in STEMI patients with multivessel disease before hospital discharge.	IIa	A	Complete revascularization is recommended either during the index PCI procedure or within 45 days.	I	A
Recommendations for acute coronary syndrome comorbid conditions					
Glucose-lowering therapy should be considered in ACS patients with blood glucose >10 mmol/L (>180 mg/dL), with the target adapted to comorbidities, while episodes of hypoglycemia should be avoided.	IIa	B	Glucose-lowering therapy should be considered in patients with ACS with persistent hyperglycemia, while episodes of hypoglycemia should be avoided.	IIa	C

[a]Class of recommendation.
[b]Level of evidence.
ACS, Acute coronary syndrome; *CCTA*, coronary computed tomography angiography; *CMR*, cardiac magnetic resonance; *DAPT*, dual antiplatelet therapy; *ECG*, electrocardiography/gram; *ESC*, European Society of Cardiology; *GRACE*, Global Registry of Acute Coronary Events; *hs-cTn*, high-sensitivity cardiac troponin; *IRA*, infarct-related artery; *NSTE-ACS*, non-ST-Elevation acute coronary syndrome; *NSTEMI*, non-ST-elevation myocardial infarction; *PCI*, percutaneous coronary intervention; *SAPT*, single antiplatelet therapy; *STEMI*, ST-elevation myocardial infarction.
From Byrne RA, Rossello X, Coughlan JJ, et al. The 2023 ESC guidelines for the management of acute coronary syndromes. *Eur Heart J*. 2023;44(38):3720–3826. https://doi.org/10.1093/eurheartj/ehad191

LIST 1.2 Top 10 Recommendations from the ACC/AHA/SCAI PCI Guidelines

1. Treatment decisions regarding coronary revascularization in patients with coronary artery disease should be based on clinical indications, regardless of sex, race, or ethnicity because there is no evidence that some patients benefit less than others and efforts to reduce disparities of care are warranted.
2. In patients being considered for coronary revascularization for whom the optimal treatment strategy is unclear, a multidisciplinary Heart Team approach is recommended. Treatment decisions should be patient centered, incorporate patient preferences and goals, and include shared decision making.
3. For patients with significant left main disease, surgical revascularization is indicated to improve survival relative to that likely to be achieved with medical therapy. Percutaneous revascularization is a reasonable option to improve survival, compared with medical therapy, in selected patients with low to medium anatomic complexity of coronary artery disease and left main disease that is equally suitable for surgical or percutaneous revascularization.
4. Updated evidence from contemporary trials supplements older evidence with regard to the mortality benefit of revascularization in patients with stable ischemic heart disease, normal left ventricular ejection fraction, and triple-vessel coronary artery disease. Surgical revascularization may be reasonable for improving survival. The survival benefit with percutaneous revascularization is uncertain. Revascularization decisions are based on consideration of disease complexity, technical feasibility of treatment, and a Heart Team discussion.
5. The use of a radial artery as a surgical revascularization conduit is preferred versus the use of a saphenous vein conduit to bypass the second most important target vessel with significant stenosis after the left anterior descending coronary artery. Benefits include superior patency, reduced adverse cardiac events, and improved survival.
6. Radial artery access is recommended in patients undergoing percutaneous intervention who have acute coronary syndrome or stable ischemic heart disease to reduce bleeding and vascular complications compared with a femoral approach. Patients with acute coronary syndrome also benefit from a reduction in mortality rate with this approach.
7. A short duration of dual antiplatelet therapy after percutaneous revascularization in patients with stable ischemic heart disease is reasonable to reduce the risk of bleeding events. After consideration of recurrent ischemia and bleeding risks, select patients may safely transition to $P2Y_{12}$ inhibitor monotherapy and stop aspirin after 1 to 3 months of dual antiplatelet therapy.
8. Staged percutaneous intervention (while in hospital or after discharge) of a significantly stenosed nonculprit artery in patients presenting with an ST-segment-elevation myocardial infarction is recommended in select patients to improve outcomes. Percutaneous intervention of the nonculprit artery at the time of primary percutaneous coronary intervention is less clear and may be considered in stable patients with uncomplicated revascularization of the culprit artery, low-complexity nonculprit artery disease, and normal renal function. In contrast, percutaneous intervention of the nonculprit artery can be harmful in patients with cardiogenic shock.
9. Revascularization decisions in patients with diabetes and multivessel coronary artery disease are optimized by the use of a Heart Team approach. Patients with diabetes who have triple-vessel disease should undergo surgical revascularization; percutaneous coronary intervention may be considered if they are poor candidates for surgery.
10. Treatment decisions for patients undergoing surgical revascularization of coronary artery disease should include the calculation of a patient's surgical risk with the Society of Thoracic Surgeons score. The usefulness of the SYNTAX score calculation in treatment decisions is less clear because of the interobserver variability in its calculation and its absence of clinical variables.

From Lawton JS, Tamis-Holland JE, Bangalore S, et al. 2021 ACC/AHA/SCAI guideline for coronary artery revascularization. *J Am Coll Cardiol.* 2022;79(2):e21–e129.

and a list of top 10 recommendations from the 2021 ACC/AHA/SCAI Guideline for Coronary Artery Revascularization[4] (List 1.2), a detailed update on ACS is timely. The subsequent chapters also draw upon the latest information from recent guidelines and expert statements, landmark randomized clinical trials, and high-quality registries and mechanistic studies on various aspects of ACS.

REFERENCES

1. GBD Database [Internet]. IHME. [cited May 31, 2023]. Available from: http://www.healthdata.org/data-tools.
2. Byrne RA, Rossello X, Coughlan JJ, et al. The 2023 ESC guidelines for the management of acute coronary syndromes. *Eur Heart J.* 2023;44(38):3720–3826. https://doi.org/10.1093/eurheartj/ehad191.
3. Camacho X, Nedkoff L, Wright FL, et al. Relative contribution of trends in myocardial infarction event rates and case fatality to declines in mortality: an international comparative study of 1.95 million events in 80.4 million people in four countries. *Lancet Public Health.* 2022;7(3):e229–e239.
4. Lawton JS, Tamis-Holland JE, Bangalore S, et al. 2021 ACC/AHA/SCAI guideline for coronary artery revascularization. *J Am Coll Cardiol.* 2022;79(2):e21–e129.

2 Classification and Diagnosis of Acute Coronary Syndromes

DAVID A. MORROW AND EUGENE BRAUNWALD

INTRODUCTION

Until the beginning of 20th century, it was believed that coronary thrombosis was always immediately fatal. In 1910, two Ukrainian physicians described five patients with acute myocardial infarction (MI), in whom three were found to have coronary thrombosis at autopsy. In 1912, James Herrick articulated the first clear description in English of the clinical syndrome of acute MI in his landmark article, "Certain Clinical Features of Sudden Obstruction of the Coronary Arteries." Up to that time, although pathologists had made causal connections between thrombotic coronary occlusion and degenerative changes in the myocardium evident postmortem, a clinical syndrome of MI in surviving patients had not been described. The term acute coronary syndrome (ACS) which emerged more than 8 decades later is now used to denote any clinical presentation suggestive of acute myocardial ischemia caused by unstable ischemic heart disease. ACS encompasses both unstable angina (UA) and acute MI, in distinction from chronic stable angina and chronic coronary artery disease. In addition, some clinicians have adapted the use of ACS to imply acute coronary atherothrombosis, which is differentiated from ischemia caused by increased myocardial oxygen demand in the presence of stable coronary atherosclerotic lesions.

Over the past century, the classification of ACS, its epidemiology, and our understanding of its pathobiology have evolved considerably.[1–3] The epidemiology and natural history of ACS, the major cause of deaths due to atherosclerotic vascular disease, are reviewed in Chapter 31. The pathobiology of ACS is discussed in Chapter 32. Both a historical perspective and a summary of emerging concepts regarding mechanisms of myocardial ischemic injury and healing are provided in Chapter 32. Chapter 4 details burden of suspected ACS in emergency departments and the role of cardiac biomarkers of necrosis in the diagnosis of acute MI. In this chapter, we describe the evolution of the clinical classification of ACS, including UA, non–ST-elevation MI (NSTEMI), ST-elevation MI (STEMI), and the additional subclassification of the types of MI as defined in the section on Universal Definition of Myocardial Infarction. This chapter reflects our opinion that in the era of high-sensitivity assays for cardiac troponin (cTn), UA is a rare diagnostic entity.

SPECTRUM OF UNSTABLE ISCHEMIC HEART DISEASE

Stable ischemic heart disease (SIHD) is most commonly caused by atheromatous plaque that obstructs or gradually narrows one or more of the epicardial coronary arteries. Although the clinical manifestations of SIHD are variable, stable angina induced by increased effort, as classically described by Heberden in 1772, is typically the predominant symptom. UA is characterized by an accelerated pattern of increasing frequency and tempo of angina or angina at rest in the absence of MI. MI is defined by evidence of myocardial injury in a clinical setting consistent with acute myocardial ischemia. Because of the implications for treatment, including reperfusion therapy, MI is classified clinically into those cases in which the clinical presentation includes diagnostic ST-segment elevation on the 12-lead electrocardiogram (ECG) and those cases without ST-elevation at presentation, which are designated as NSTEMI (see section on Clinical Classification: Electrocardiography). Moreover, because of their indistinguishable clinical and electrocardiographic features (ST-segment depressions and T-wave inversion) and similar management, patients with UA and NSTEMI are commonly grouped together by the term non–ST-elevation ACS (NSTE-ACS) (Fig. 2.1).[4]

A nomenclature that incorporates the development of pathological Q waves (Q-wave MI) versus their absence (non–Q-wave MI) on the surface ECG is no longer deemed useful as part of initial management of acute MI; however, the presence of Q waves should be recognized as indicative of late presentation of a large MI. In addition to the categories already described, MI can be classified into various types, based on pathological, clinical, and prognostic differences, along with different treatment strategies (see section on Clinical Classification).

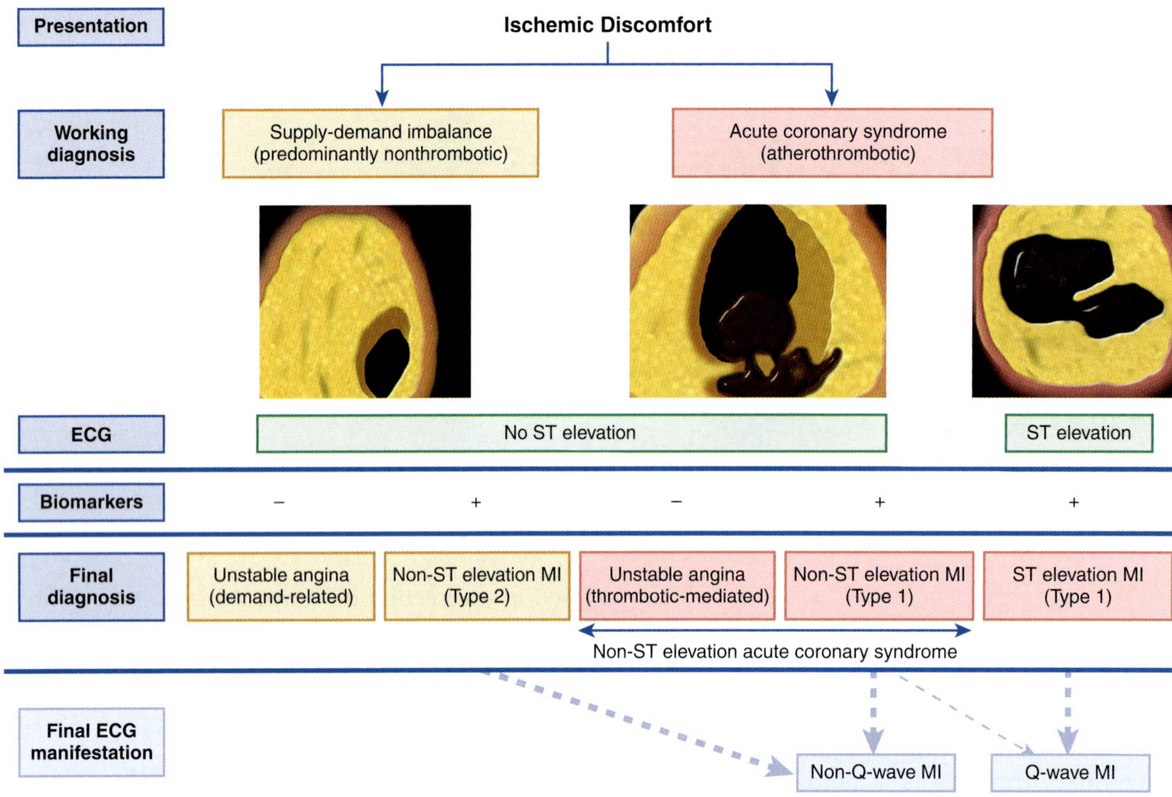

FIG. 2.1 Myocardial ischemia and infarction. Unstable ischemic syndromes may result from acute changes in either myocardial oxygen demand and/or supply. Predominantly nonthrombotically mediated events (*left side*) typically occur without ST-segment elevation but can result in myocardial infarction (MI) with elevated levels of cardiac biomarkers if the ischemia is sufficiently severe and prolonged (type 2 MI). Myocardial ischemia caused by acute coronary thrombosis (*right side*) may occur with or without ST-segment elevation. The distinction of whether MI has occurred is ultimately determined by the presence or absence of detectable elevation of circulating cardiac troponin. Non–Q-wave MI ultimately develops in most patients with non–ST-elevation MI (NSTEMI); Q-wave MI may develop in a few patients. MI that develops as the result of the atherothrombotic lesion of an acute coronary syndrome is classified as type I MI. *ECG*, Electrocardiography. *(From Scirica BM, Morrow DA. ST-elevation myocardial infarction: pathology, pathophysiology, and clinical features. In: Mann DL, Bhatt DL, Braunwald E, et al., eds. Braunwald's Heart Disease: A Textbook of Cardiovascular Medicine. 10th ed. Philadelphia, PA: Saunders; 2015.)*

Unstable Angina: A Historical Perspective

In the days of Herrick's original clinical description of MI; MI and angina were beginning to be recognized as manifestations of the same underlying disease process. Nevertheless, the conclusions by Ukrainian physicians Obrastzow and Straschesko that "the differential diagnosis of coronary thrombosis from angina pectoris is made by the presence of *status angiosus* with coronary thrombosis and its absence with isolated attacks of *angina pectoris*" reflected the prevailing view at the time that these two diagnoses were quite distinct. This distinction began to blur by 1937, when Sampson, Eliaser, and Feil, each described several patients with prolonged chest discomfort at rest that differed from stable angina and appeared sometimes to precede an acute MI. This pattern of symptoms was variously referred to as "pre-infarction angina" or "crescendo angina." In 1948, Wood proposed that this "intermediate coronary syndrome" between stable angina and MI was caused by "a coronary circulation insufficient to meet the full demands at rest yet sufficient to prevent MI." He recognized that, just as for acute MI, coronary thrombosis could be playing a role in this coronary insufficiency. Moreover, he observed that MI or death occurred in 12 of 25 patients with this intermediate coronary syndrome, whereas among 33 patients with the same syndrome whom he treated with oral anticoagulants, only three patients died or had an MI. It was nearly 25 years later, in 1971, Fowler and colleagues introduced the term "unstable angina."

At first, UA was considered to be quite rare, and as late as the 1950s, some experts even questioned its existence. Friedberg, in the leading cardiology textbook at the time, described these patients as "a motley group," which he recommended should be "best classified clinically as angina pectoris (more or less severe or prolonged) or as MI." Despite this debate, in the era predating the development of high-sensitivity assays for cTn, it appeared that UA was common. In 1991, the National Center for Health Statistics reported that UA was responsible for 570,000 hospitalizations annually in the United States, making UA one of the most common reasons for hospital admission.

In 1994, in the first published guidelines on its diagnosis and management, UA was defined as "a clinical syndrome falling between stable angina and MI." Three principal clinical presentations were considered to be typical of UA: (1) angina at rest; (2) new onset of severe exertional angina; and (3) distinct, often sudden, intensification of previously stable angina. Any one of these, in the absence of an acute MI (see section on Diagnosis of Myocardial Infarction), was the basis for a diagnosis of UA. UA could be further classified according to its severity, the clinical circumstances in which it occurred, and the presence or absence of electrocardiographic ST-segment deviations (Table 1.1).

TABLE 2.1 Original Braunwald Classification of Unstable Angina

		CLINICAL CIRCUMSTANCES		
		A	B	C
SEVERITY		DEVELOPS IN PRESENCE OF EXTRACARDIAC CONDITION THAT INTENSIFIES MYOCARDIAL ISCHEMIA (SECONDARY UA)	DEVELOPS IN THE ABSENCE OF EXTRACARDIAC CONDITION (PRIMARY UA)	DEVELOPS WITHIN 2 WEEKS AFTER ACUTE MYOCARDIAL INFARCTION (POSTINFARCTION UA)
I	New onset of severe angina or accelerated angina; no pain at rest	IA	IB	IC
II	Angina at rest within past month but not within preceding 48 h (angina at rest, subacute)	IIA	IIB	IIC
III	Angina at rest within 48 h (angina at rest, acute)	IIIA	IIIB Troponin negative IIIB Troponin Positive[a]	IIIC

[a]Now defined as myocardial infarction if cardiac troponin is more than the 99th percentile upper reference limit.
UA, Unstable angina.
From Braunwald E. Unstable angina—a classification. *Circulation*. 1989;80:410–414.

By the beginning of the 21st century, UA was firmly established as one possible manifestation of ACS; however, ambiguity had begun to creep into its definition. As an example, the World Health Organization revision of the definition of MI in 2008 to 2009 characterized UA as "new or worsening symptoms of ischemia (or changing symptom pattern) and ischemic ECG changes…with normal biomarkers," but noted that the "distinction between new angina, worsening angina, and unstable angina is notoriously difficult and based on a clinical assessment and a careful and full clinical history." At the same time, the increasing analytical sensitivity of assays for cTn decreased the proportion of patients with ACS with "normal biomarkers" (see section on Biomarkers of Myocyte Injury), resulting instead in the diagnosis of MI.[5] Although rates vary substantially across health care systems, the diagnosis of UA now constitutes <3% of diagnoses among patients with suspected ACS in some systems.[6] Nevertheless, despite this diminishing incidence, professional guidelines have preserved the category of UA for patients with high-risk coronary artery disease presenting with an unstable pattern of symptoms without biomarker evidence of myocardial injury meeting criteria for MI.[1,4]

Diagnosis of Myocardial Infarction

In 1971, the World Health Organization proposed that the diagnosis of MI required the presence of at least two of the following: (1) typical symptoms; (2) a typical ECG pattern involving the development of Q waves; and (3) an initial rise and subsequent fall in serum and/or plasma biomarkers of myocardial necrosis. Patients with similar clinical manifestations of myocardial ischemia as UA but who exhibited a typical pattern of a rise to abnormally elevated level(s) and subsequent fall in circulating biomarkers of necrosis were diagnosed with MI. Subsequently, the emergence of more sensitive and specific blood biomarkers of myocardial necrosis and precise imaging techniques prompted a reevaluation of this definition of MI. This effort resulted in an evolution of the definition of MI that placed greater emphasis on the detection of ischemic myocardial injury, either with sensitive biomarkers or with cardiac imaging.[1]

In 2000, the First Global MI Task Force, which was a collaborative joint committee of the European Society of Cardiology and the American College of Cardiology, articulated a new definition of MI that was founded on the principle that "any amount of myocardial necrosis caused by ischemia should be labeled as a [myocardial] infarct." In addition, this joint committee confirmed previous guidelines that established the 99th percentile in the distribution of cTn in an apparently healthy population as the upper reference limit (URL) for diagnosis of myocardial injury (see Chapter 4). The task force also recognized that as a consequence of this fundamental premise "an individual who was formerly diagnosed as having severe, stable, or UA pectoris might be diagnosed today with a small MI." These principles were refined by the Second Global MI Task Force in 2007, leading to the Universal Definition of Myocardial Infarction, which included a clinical classification of MI that placed emphasis on differentiating the various conditions that might lead to an MI (see the section on Clinical Classification of Myocardial Infarction). As well, recognition that in addition to myocyte necrosis, other causes of myocardial injury might result in the release of structural proteins from the myocardium, including normal turnover of myocardial cells, apoptosis, cellular release of cTn degradation products, increased cellular wall permeability, and the formation and release of membranous blebs. Subsequently, the 2012 Third Universal Definition of Myocardial Infarction responded to the development of even more sensitive assays for markers of such myocardial injury, and the 2019 Fourth Universal Definition of Myocardial Infarction further the developed the concept of nonischemic acute and chronic myocardial injury.[1]

The 2021 multisociety Guideline for the Evaluation and Diagnosis of Chest Pain recommends that patients who are suspected on clinical grounds of having ACS should undergo serial sampling for cTn; preferably with a high-sensitivity assay.[4] An MI, based on the Fourth Universal Definition of MI, is defined by a typical rise and/or fall of cTn, with at least one value above the assay's URL,

TABLE 2.2 Criteria for Acute Myocardial Infarction

The term acute myocardial infarction (MI) should be used when there is acute myocardial injury with clinical evidence of myocardial ischemia and with detection of a rise and/or fall of cTn values with at least one value above the 99th percentile of the upper reference limit (URL) and at least one of the following:

- Symptoms of ischemia
- New ischemic ECG changes
- Development of pathological Q waves
- Imaging evidence of new loss of viable myocardium or new regional wall motion abnormality in a pattern consistent with an ischemic etiology
- Identification of a coronary thrombus by angiography or autopsy (not for type 2 or 3 MIs)
- Pathological findings of an acute or a recent MI

- Coronary procedure-related MI
  Coronary procedure-related MI ≤48 h after the index procedure is arbitrarily defined by an elevation of cTn values >5 times for type 4a MI and >10 times for type 5 MI of the 99th percentile URL in patients with normal baseline values. Patients with elevated preprocedural cTn values, in whom the preprocedural cTn level is stable (≤20% variation) or falling must meet the criteria for a >5 or >10-fold increase and manifest a change from the baseline value of >20%. In addition, with at least one of the following:
  - New ischemic ECG changes (this criterion is related to type 4a MI only);
  - Development of new pathological Q waves;
  - Imaging evidence of loss of viable myocardium that is presumed to be new and in a pattern consistent with an ischemic etiology;
  - Angiographic findings consistent with a procedural flow-limiting complication such as coronary dissection, occlusion of a major epicardial artery or graft, side-branch occlusion-thrombus, disruption of collateral flow, or distal embolization.

From Thygesen K, Alpert JS, Jaffe AS, et al. Fourth universal definition of myocardial infarction. *J Am Coll Cardiol*. 2018;72:2231–2264.

accompanied by at least one other feature of ischemia (e.g., typical symptoms or ECG changes) (Table 2.2).[1]

Biomarkers of Myocyte Injury

First demonstrated with the myocardial band fraction of creatine kinase (CK-MB), and subsequently refined with cTn, patients with unstable ischemic symptoms and biomarker evidence of myocardial injury (i.e., NSTEMI or STEMI) are at significantly higher risk of death or recurrent ischemic events compared with patients presenting with UA, in whom, by definition, biomarkers of myocardial injury are not elevated.

Although, in the 1970s and 1980s, CK-MB was superior to previously available enzymes used as biomarkers of necrosis (total creatine kinase, aspartate aminotransferase, and alanine aminotransferase), it lacked optimal sensitivity and specificity. In 1987, Cummins and colleagues introduced an assay for cardiac-specific troponin I (cTnI), and shortly thereafter, Katus and colleagues developed an analogous assay for cardiac-specific troponin T (cTnT). Troponin I and T are components of the troponin regulatory complex that is bound to actin and modulate the interaction between actin and myosin in myocytes. In contrast to CK-MB, troponin I and T have cardiac isoforms (cTnI and cTnT) that are unique to cardiac myocytes and may be measured by assays that use monoclonal antibodies specific to epitopes of the cardiac form. Because of this greater tissue specificity, cTn allows the detection of a faint signal of release from cardiac myocytes against minimal background noise in the circulation and delivers considerably higher sensitivity and specificity than CK-MB. For example, in the TIMI 3 trial, 25% of the patients classified with UA, based on the absence of abnormally elevated concentrations of CK-MB, had cTnI ≥0.4 ng/mL ([400 ng/L], the cutpoint of a relatively insensitive assay from the mid-1990s), and therefore, should be reclassified as having had a NSTEMI. Thus, in retrospect, patients with UA made up a smaller percentage of patients with NSTE-ACS than had previously been believed.

Like the earlier classification of ACS patients based on CK-MB, this second wave of reclassification based on cTn also appeared to be clinically important. Among patients with normal CK-MB, patients with elevated cTn were at higher risk of adverse cardiac events than those without such elevations. In the TIMI 11B trial, we observed a sixfold increase in death or new MI in patients with normal CK-MB who had elevated cTnI compared with patients without such an elevation. The clinical relevance of such reclassification with cTn was reinforced by evidence that patients with ACS who had elevated cTn benefited more from newer therapies than patients in whom cTn was not detectable. These therapies included an early invasive strategy (Chapter 10), the addition of antiplatelet drugs (Chapter 13), and treatment with low-molecular-weight heparin rather than unfractionated heparin (Chapter 12).

Two critical trends in the clinical applications of cTn have since ushered in what we have viewed as a third wave of reclassification of ACS: (1) a move to lower diagnostic cutoffs for cTn and (2) progressive improvement in the analytical precision of assays for cTn that has further lowered diagnostic and prognostic decision limits.[2] At initial approval for clinical use, manufacturer-recommended cutpoints for cTn originated from comparative studies with CK-MB. However, this approach was flawed because the derived cutpoints were based on a comparison with a less sensitive test. For this reason, in 1999, laboratory professional guidelines recommended an additional lower cutpoint based on the distribution of cTn in a healthy reference population. This approach of defining an upper limit of normal at the 97.5th or 99th percentile of a reference population is the method used to establish cutpoints for many clinical laboratory tests. In 2000, cardiology and laboratory professional guidelines endorsed a single cutpoint for the diagnosis of MI at the 99th percentile URL for each assay. However, more than 20 years after the publication of the first Universal Definition of Myocardial Infarction, some laboratories have continued to report an inconclusive or suggestive range using two cTn cutpoints based on the outdated initial proposal from laboratory guidelines and some package inserts.[7] This practice is no longer consistent with present guidelines.[4]

The progressive improvement in analytical precision of assays for cTn during the past 25 years has driven both the limit of detection and the URL downward. This trend has resulted in an increasing proportion of patients with NSTE-ACS with a positive cTn result, and hence, a diagnosis of NSTEMI. In 1996, in the TIMI 3 trial, 25% of patients with UA had elevated cTnI (≥0.4 ng/mL). A decade later, in NSTE-ACS patients enrolled into the MERLIN-TIMI 36 trial, which used a widely available current-generation sensitive assay for cTnI (URL 0.04 ng/mL [40 ng/L]), we observed that 65% of patients with NSTE-ACS had a positive cTnI result, approximately 50%

of whom would not have been identified with CK-MB. Importantly, the subgroup of patients who had low-level elevations in cTnI that would not have been detected with the previous generation cTn assay turned out to be at similar heightened risk of death or recurrent ischemic events.

With yet another almost 2 decades of evolution, high-sensitivity assays with improved analytical precision have enabled limits of detection as low as 0.2 ng/L (0.0002 ng/mL) with consequent detection of cTn above the URL in 82% to 99% of patients with putative UA[8]; again, with data demonstrating a graded rise in the rate of adverse outcomes. Because they enable more rapid detection or exclusion of myocardial injury and offer superior risk assessment compared with prior generation assays, high-sensitivity assays are now preferred for diagnostic testing among patients with suspected ACS.[4] Clinically, there is a need to distinguish acute increases in cTn that occur due to MI from both acute nonischemic causes of myocardial injury and chronic, relatively stable, low-level concentrations that can exist in patients with SIHD or other structural heart diseases, but which are not indicative of ACS (see Chapter 4).[9]

CLASSICATION OF MYOCARDIAL INFARCTION

Pathological Description

The pathological diagnosis of MI requires evidence of myocardial cell death. Characteristic findings of myocyte necrosis include coagulation necrosis and contraction band necrosis, usually with patchy areas of myocytolysis at the periphery of the infarction. During the acute phase of MI, most of the myocyte loss occurs via coagulation necrosis, with ensuing inflammation, phagocytosis of necrotic myocytes, and repair eventuating into scar formation (see Chapter 32).

MI can be classified pathologically on gross examination as transmural, in which myocardial necrosis involves the full thickness (or nearly full thickness) of the ventricular wall and subendocardial (nontransmural) infarcts, in which the necrosis involves the subendocardium, the intramural myocardium, or both, without extending all the way through the ventricular wall to the epicardium (Fig. 2.2). Transmural infarction is more likely when coronary thrombosis is completely occlusive and is localized to the distribution of a single coronary artery. Subendocardial infarctions may result from severely narrowed, but still patent, coronary arteries or when significant collateral circulation to the infarcted region exists. Patchy subendocardial infarction may arise from reperfusion of an originally occlusive thrombus with restoration of blood flow before the wavefront of necrosis has extended from the subendocardium across the full thickness of the ventricular wall (see Chapter 20).

Clinical Classification

Electrocardiography

Abnormalities of the surface ECG during myocardial ischemia or infarction may include the PR segment, the QRS complex, the ST-segment, or the T wave. The earliest manifestation of myocardial ischemia is typically hyperacute T-wave amplitude followed by ST-segment changes. The loss of electromotive forces caused by myocardial necrosis leads to R-wave loss in the ECG territory of the MI. The development of Q waves is a result of delayed conduction through an ischemic area or conduction around an area of infarction, leading to recording potentials from the opposite ventricular wall. Criteria for Q waves consistent with previous MI are shown at the bottom of Table 2.3. Transient Q waves may be observed during an episode of acute ischemia or (rarely) during acute MI with successful reperfusion.

The term Q-wave infarction was often used synonymously with transmural infarction, whereas non–Q-wave infarctions were believed to be indicative of subendocardial infarctions. However, studies that used CMR imaging (Chapter 17) indicate that the development of Q waves on the ECG is influenced more by the size of the infarction than the extent of transmural involvement. Moreover, the classification of MI on the basis of Q waves has been supplanted by a focus on the presence or absence of initial ST-segment

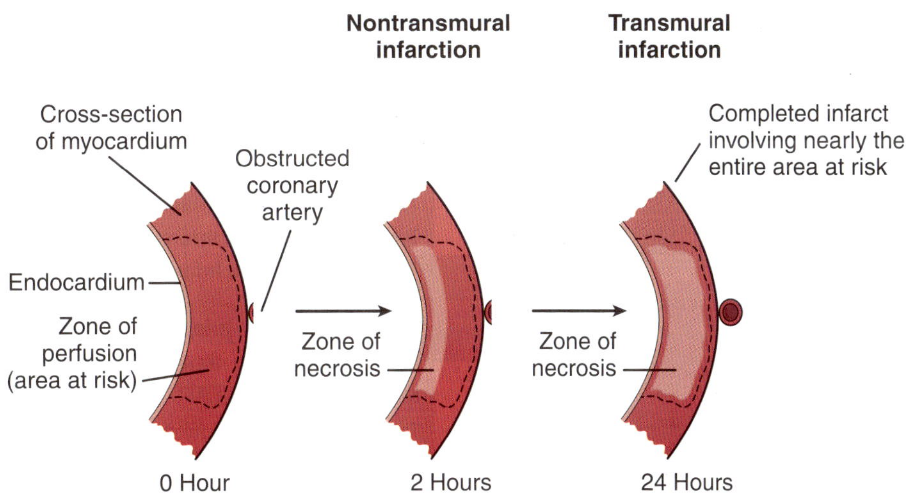

FIG. 2.2 The progression of myocardial necrosis after coronary artery occlusion. Necrosis begins in a small zone of the myocardium beneath the endocardial surface in the center of the ischemic zone. This entire region of myocardium (*dashed outline*) depends on the occluded vessel for perfusion and is the area at risk. A narrow zone of myocardium immediately beneath the endocardium is spared from necrosis because it can be oxygenated by diffusion from the ventricle. *(From Schoen FJ, Mitchell RN. The heart. In: Kumar V, Abbas AK, Aster JC, eds. Robbins and Cotran Pathologic Basis of Disease. 8th ed. Philadelphia, PA: Saunders; 2010.)*

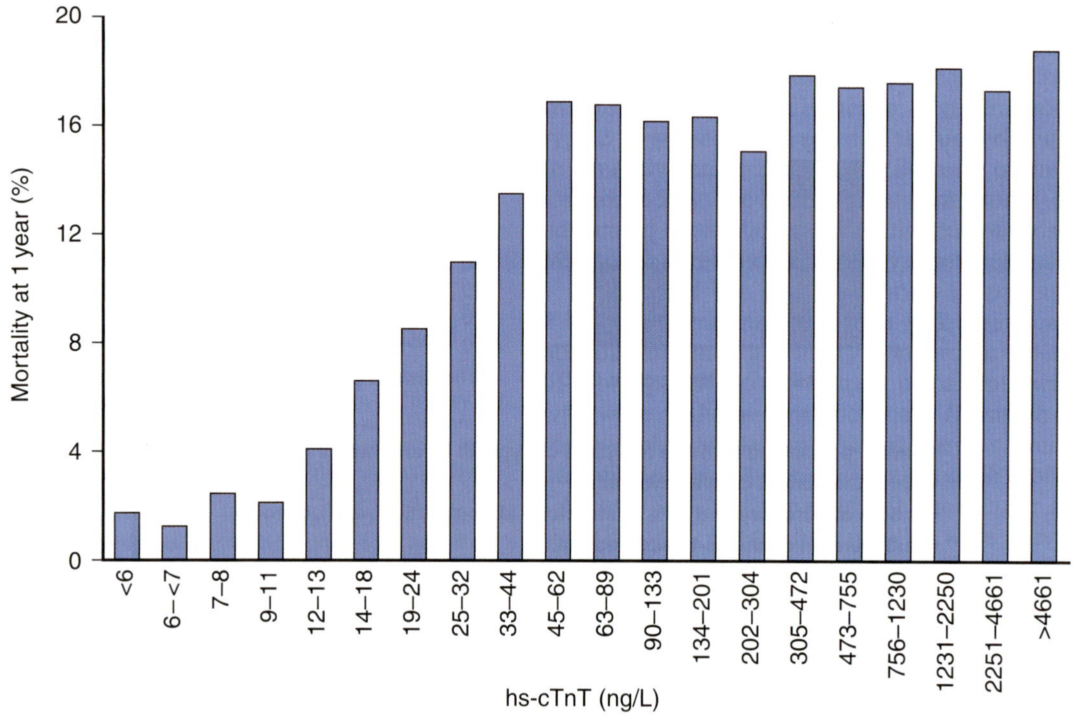

FIG. 2.8 Crude all-cause mortality at 1 year, stratified according to the level of maximal high-sensitivity cardiac troponin T (hs-cTnT), among 48,594 patients with suspected acute coronary syndrome followed in the SWEDEHEART registry. The risk began increasing at 12 to 13 ng/L of hsTnT (99th percentile upper reference limit = 14 ng/L). *(From Melki D, Lugnegård J, Alfredsson J, et al. Implications of introducing high-sensitivity cardiac troponin t into clinical practice data from the SWEDEHEART registry. J Am Coll Cardiol. 2015;65:1655–1664.)*

URL. Myocardial injury is the overarching category under which both ischemic and nonischemic causes can occur. Nonischemic myocardial injury should be distinguished from acute MI and should be further classified as either chronic or acute (see Fig. 4.8). Myocardial injury is considered acute if there is a rise and/or fall of cTn values.[1] It can be challenging to distinguish acute nonischemic myocardial injury from type 2 MI, in particular, with the latter being characterized as having clear evidence of myocardial ischemia as a cause. The presence of acute or chronic myocardial injury is associated with an adverse prognosis.[2] It is reasonable to pursue the cause of myocardial injury and tailor treatment to the inciting etiology. It is unknown whether, and should not be assumed that, antithrombotic therapies, and other therapies known to be beneficial for patients with type 1 MI, improve outcomes in patients with acute or chronic myocardial injury.

Classification by Myocardial Infarction Size

In addition to classification by MI type, the Universal Definition Classification System also has proposed categories of MI size based on the peak concentration of the cardiac biomarker (cTn preferred).[1] Data using both scintigraphy and cardiac magnetic resonance (CMR) suggest that peak cTn values correlate well with infarct size determined from imaging approaches. As for CK-MB, the correlation between cTn and MI size by CMR is less strong in NSTEMI than in STEMI. However, correlation ranges are good (0.80–0.93) and are better than the correlations reported for CK-MB. Clinicians should recognize that because of the improved sensitivity of cTn (compared with CK-MB) elevations relative to the URL differ between cTn and CK-MB in terms of the size of the infarct reflected (i.e., a twofold elevation of cTn reflects a substantially smaller amount of necrosis than a twofold elevation of CK-MB). The relative relationship between the two biomarkers will differ between each assay. As an approximation, in one comparative study of cTn and CK-MB based on prognosis rather than imaging of infarct size, a three-fold elevation of CK-MB was equivalent in frequency and 1-year mortality risk to a 60-fold elevation of cTn. As discussed in Chapter 6, the risk associated with elevation of cTn is, nonetheless, evident at even one- to twofold elevations above the URL in patients with a clinical syndrome consistent with myocardial ischemia (Fig. 2.8).

Myocardial Infarction in the Setting of Nonobstructive Coronary Arteries

Up to 20% (average approximately 6%) of participants in registries of patients with a clinical diagnosis of MI are found to have no evidence of obstructive epicardial coronary atherosclerosis at coronary angiography. Such patients with suspected MI with nonobstructive coronary arteries (MINOCA) are very difficult to discriminate from patients with nonischemic mechanisms of acute myocardial injury. See Chapter 28 for discussion of the epidemiology, diagnosis, and management of MINOCA.

SUMMARY

The terminology and epidemiology that describes unstable ischemic heart disease continue to evolve. Current nomenclature has shifted in focus toward alignment with discrete lines of clinical management. The term ACS captures the spectrum of unstable angina UA, NSTEMI, and STEMI. Although present guidelines remain silent on this issue, we favor reserving the term ACS for unstable ischemic syndromes of atherothrombotic causes to differentiate patients with acute thrombosis from the increasingly recognized, large group of patients with nonthrombotic, mostly demand-related ischemia and infarction (Fig. 2.1).

Initial classification of the patient with suspected ACS should be made based on the ECG to identify patients with STEMI who are candidates for immediate reperfusion therapy. Among patients with NSTE-ACS, the advent of more sensitive assays for cTn has shifted the epidemiology, such that the proportion of patients with NSTE-ACS who have demonstrable myocardial injury, and thus are classified as NSTEMI rather than UA, has steadily increased. In our view, when high-sensitivity assays for cTn are applied, it is an extremely small proportion of patients with unstable ischemic symptoms who do not manifest at least small amounts of myocardial injury, and for this reason, UA has become increasingly rare. Because the distinction between UA and NSTEMI has become highly dependent on the particular assay used for detecting cTn, the term UA has increasing ambiguity and means different things to different people. With this shift, the epidemiology of ACS has come full circle back to before the 1930s when two principal manifestations of symptomatic ischemic heart disease were recognized: SIHD and acute MI.

Because of an accompanying increase in the heterogeneity of patients with MI, it has become even more important to classify every MI. Equally important, MI must be distinguished from myocardial injury caused primarily by nonischemic causes, in which setting we advocate being descriptive for the purposes of clinical clarity (e.g., "myocardial injury caused by decompensated heart failure" or "myocardial injury caused by myocarditis.") The classification of MI based on the setting and suspected underlying pathology as captured by the Universal Definition of Myocardial Infarction classification system aids in defining rational pathways for treatment of the varied group of patients with MI encountered in clinical practice. A diagnosis of "acute MI" is no longer sufficient; instead, for example, a diagnosis of a "type 2 NSTEMI in the setting of uncontrolled hypertension" is substantially more useful for formulating a treatment plan and communicating with colleagues.

CLASSIC REFERENCES

Braunwald E, Morrow DA. Unstable angina: is it time for a requiem? *Circulation*. 2013;127:2452–2457.

Falk E, Nakano M, Bentzon JF, et al. Update on acute coronary syndromes: the pathologists' view. *Eur Heart J*. 2013;34:719–728.

Heberden W. *Commentaries on the History and Cure of Diseases*. London: Printed for T. Payne, Mews-Gate; 1802.

Herrick J. Certain clinical features of sudden obstruction of the coronary arteries. *Trans Am Assoc Physicians*. 1912;27:100–116.

Herrick JB. *A Short History of Cardiology*. Springfield, MA: Charles C. Thomas; 1942.

Levine SA. *Coronary Thrombosis: Its Various Clinical Features*. Baltimore: The Williams & Wilkins Company; 1929.

Nabel EG, Braunwald E. A tale of coronary artery disease and myocardial infarction. *N Engl J Med*. 2012;366:54–63.

Obrastzow WP, Straschesko ND. Zur Kenntnis der Thrombose der Koronararterien des Herzens. *Z Klin Med*. 1910;71:116–132.

REFERENCES

1. Thygesen K, Alpert JS, Jaffe AS, et al. Fourth universal definition of myocardial infarction (2018). *Eur Heart J*. 2019;40:237–269.
2. Morrow DA. The fourth universal definition of myocardial infarction and the emerging importance of myocardial injury. *Circulation*. 2020;141:172–175.
3. Libby P. Inflammation during the life cycle of the atherosclerotic plaque. *Cardiovasc Res*. 2021;117:2525–2536.
4. Gulati M, Levy PD, Mukherjee D, et al. 2021 AHA/ACC/ASE/CHEST/SAEM/SCCT/SCMR guideline for the evaluation and diagnosis of chest pain: a report of the American College of Cardiology/American Heart Association joint committee on clinical practice guidelines. *Circulation*. 2021;144:e368–e454.
5. Sandoval Y, Apple FS, Smith SW. High-sensitivity cardiac troponin assays and unstable angina. *Eur Heart J Acute Cardiovasc Care*. 2018;7:120–128.
6. Puelacher C, Gugala M, Adamson PD, et al. Incidence and outcomes of unstable angina compared with non-ST-elevation myocardial infarction. *Heart*. 2019;105:1423–1431.
7. Sandoval Y, Apple FS, Mahler SA, et al. High-sensitivity cardiac troponin and the 2021 AHA/ACC/ASE/CHEST/SAEM/SCCT/SCMR guidelines for the evaluation and diagnosis of acute chest pain. *Circulation*. 2022;146:569–581.
8. Bonaca MP, O'Malley RG, Murphy SA, et al. Prognostic performance of a high-sensitivity assay for cardiac troponin I after non-ST elevation acute coronary syndrome: analysis from MERLIN-TIMI 36. *Eur Heart J Acute Cardiovasc Care*. 2015;4:431–440.
9. Bulluck H, Paradies V, Barbato E, et al. Prognostically relevant periprocedural myocardial injury and infarction associated with percutaneous coronary interventions: a consensus document of the ESC working group on cellular biology of the heart and European Association of percutaneous cardiovascular interventions (EAPCI). *Eur Heart J*. 2021;42:2630–2642.
10. Sandoval Y, Jaffe AS. Type 2 myocardial infarction: JACC review topic of the week. *J Am Coll Cardiol*. 2019;73:1846–1860.
11. Raphael CE, Roger VL, Sandoval Y, et al. incidence, trends, and outcomes of type 2 myocardial infarction in a community cohort. *Circulation*. 2020;141:454–463.
12. Bularga A, Hung J, Daghem M, et al. Coronary artery and cardiac disease in patients with type 2 myocardial infarction: a prospective cohort study. *Circulation*. 2022;145:1188–1200.
13. Bergmark BA, Morrow DA. Cardiac troponin elevation after elective PCI: adding infarct to major injury. *Eur Heart J*. 2021;42:335–338.
14. Ueki Y, Otsuka T, Bar S, et al. Frequency and outcomes of periprocedural MI in patients with chronic coronary syndromes undergoing PCI. *J Am Coll Cardiol*. 2022;79:513–526.

SECTION II INITIAL EVALUATION & RISK STRATIFICATION

3 Prehospital Assessment and Systems of Care

MEHMET YILDIZ, DAVID C. LANGE, AND TIMOTHY D. HENRY

ABBREVIATIONS

ACS: Acute coronary syndrome
CCL: Cardiac catheterization laboratory
COVID-19: Coronavirus disease 2019
CPR: Cardiopulmonary resuscitation
D2B: Door-to-balloon
DIDO: Door-in-door-out
ED: Emergency department
EMS: Emergency medical service
FMC2D: First medical contact to device
OHCA: Out-of-hospital cardiac arrest
PHECG: Prehospital 12-lead electrocardiogram
PPCI: Primary percutaneous coronary interventions≤
PHCCLA: Prehospital cardiac catheterization laboratory activation
STEMI: ST-elevation myocardial infarction

INTRODUCTION

Nearly 750,000 Americans experience ST-elevation myocardial infarction (STEMI) annually in the United States (see Chapter 31). Decades ago, many of these patients did not receive appropriate timely treatment for this life-threatening condition; however, care for STEMI patients has evolved dramatically over the past 30 years. The 1990s was a period of rapid evolution in STEMI care, from fibrinolytic therapy to coronary angiography with balloon angioplasty, and subsequently, primary percutaneous coronary intervention (PPCI) with coronary stenting (see Chapter 8). However, it was not until the early 2000s that systems for delivery of care became a focus of attention. While invasive and noninvasive STEMI therapeutics have evolved, the development of local, regional, and national STEMI systems of care has drastically changed the approach to health care delivery for STEMI patients by providing timely access to PPCI.[1–4] The inception of these systems of care led to dramatic improvements in time to treatment in the 2000s (Fig. 3.1), albeit at a more steady pace after 2010, while mortality rates continued to decline (Fig. 3.2).[5,6] By the late 2020s, there were still approximately 10% of STEMI patients who did not receive any form of reperfusion therapy (PPCI or fibrinolysis).[2] Furthermore, of those who underwent PPCI, roughly 20% experienced delays in reperfusion for various reasons (Fig. 3.e1).[2] Finally, despite the overall rise in the utilization of PPCI among the general population, disparities in access to PPCI for at-risk health populations such as females, Black/African American, Hispanic White, rural communities, and individuals with lower socioeconomic status continue to exist (Fig. 3.3).[3,7]

Despite the gains that have been made in STEMI care in the past 2 decades, we still face challenges in delivering equitable and improved care. Implementation and proliferation of robust STEMI systems of care, supported by standardized protocols, can play a crucial role in closing the gap and providing optimal care for all patients, including the aforementioned underserved populations. For an effective STEMI system of care, it is essential to establish well-coordinated and comprehensive regional systems that incorporate the following key components: (1) prompt and comprehensive prehospital evaluation and triage,

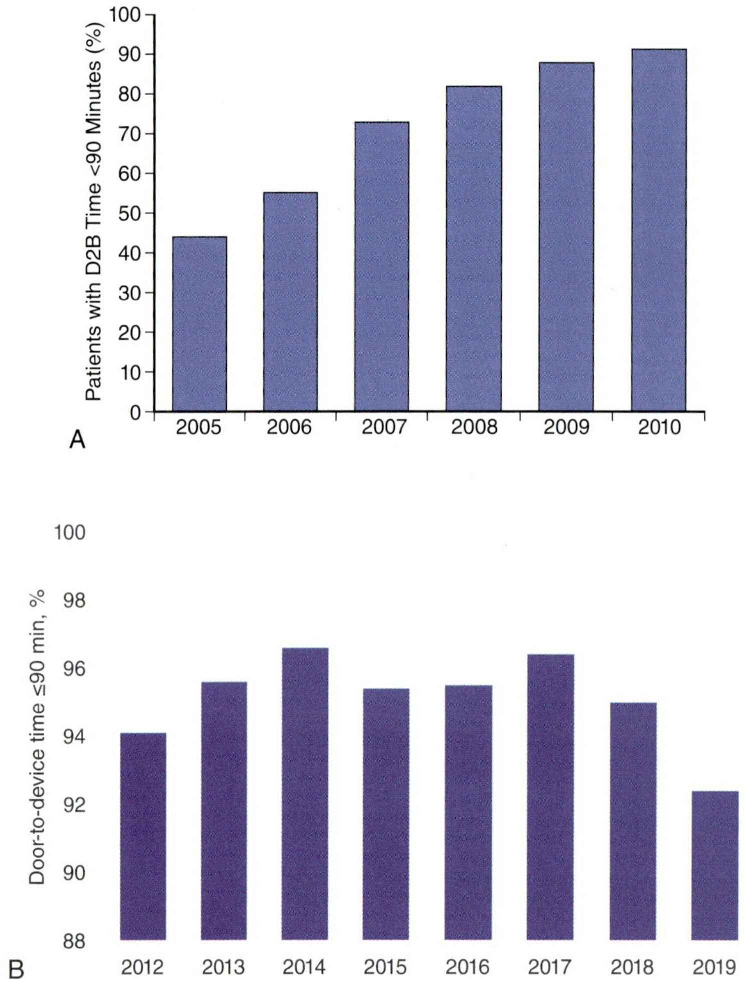

FIG. 3.1 (A) Trends in door-to-balloon (D2B) time among U.S. hospitals (2005–2010) showing marked improvement in the percentage of patients with D2B time of less than 90 minutes. (From Krumholz HM, Herrin J, Miller LE, et al. Improvements in door-to-balloon time in the United States, 2005 to 2010. *Circulation.* 2011;124:1038–1045.) (B) Trends in door-to-balloon (D2B) time among American Heart Association (AHA) Mission: Lifeline programs (2012–2020) showing a steady fluctuation in the percentage of patients with D2B time of less than 90 minutes. (Adapted from Jacobs AK, Ali MJ, Best PJ, et al. Systems of care for ST-segment-elevation myocardial infarction: a policy statement from the American Heart Association. *Circulation.* 2021;144(20):e310–e327.)

often conducted by emergency medical service (EMS); (2) designated hospitals and clinics as referral centers; and (3) regional tertiary care receiving centers equipped with the capability to perform PPCI, ideally with surgical support (Fig. 3.4). Collaboration and integration among these components are crucial for achieving optimal outcomes. Although these critical elements of triage, transportation, referral centers, and receiving centers are integral components of a STEMI system of care, no two STEMI systems are alike. Diversity in geography, politics, and sociodemographic across the United States and throughout the world results in a wide variety of STEMI systems, which are all directed toward the same goal—to increase access to timely reperfusion for STEMI by reducing delays in care.

In this chapter, we will explore the significant advancements in the STEMI systems over the past few decades; the significance of prehospital interventions in achieving timely reperfusion; the transformation of STEMI systems in both the United States and across the globe; the essential components of an ideal STEMI system of care from diagnosis to reperfusion; the challenges associated with delivering equitable and timely care in STEMI systems; and the future prospects of STEMI systems of care.

PREHOSPITAL EVALUATION

Evolution of Emergency Medical Services

The first United States Civilian Ambulance service was formed in 1865 in Cincinnati, Ohio. It comprised local hospital interns who drove a horse-drawn carriage (Fig. 3.e2). The first "rescue squad," designed to deliver basic first aid to civilians was formed in the late 1920s in Roanoke, Virginia. However, there were few advances in EMS until the late 1960s. In 1966, the National Academy of Sciences published a statement that many deaths in the United States were preventable and could be reduced through community education, safety standards, and prehospital coordination. This recognition, along with advances in the field of cardiopulmonary resuscitation (CPR) and management of out-of-hospital cardiac arrest (OHCA), served as the impetus for the first state-wide EMS system

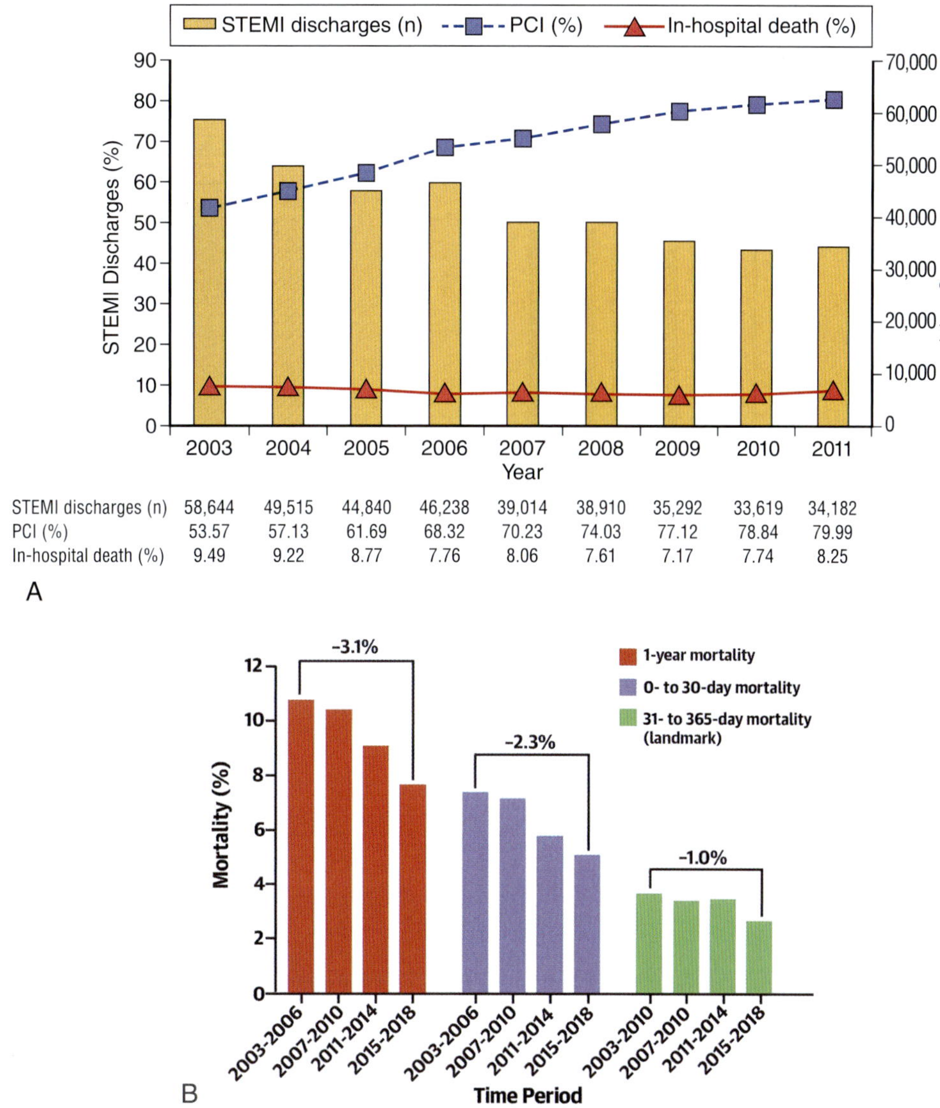

	2003	2004	2005	2006	2007	2008	2009	2010	2011
STEMI discharges (n)	58,644	49,515	44,840	46,238	39,014	38,910	35,292	33,619	34,182
PCI (%)	53.57	57.13	61.69	68.32	70.23	74.03	77.12	78.84	79.99
In-hospital death (%)	9.49	9.22	8.77	7.76	8.06	7.61	7.17	7.74	8.25

FIG. 3.2 (A) Trends in U.S. ST-elevation myocardial infarction (STEMI) care from 2003 to 2011 showing the use of primary PCI increased to 80% with decreasing mortality. PCI, percutaneous coronary intervention. (From Shah RU, Henry TD, Rutten-Ramos S, et al. Increasing percutaneous coronary interventions for ST-segment elevation myocardial infarction in the United States. *J Am Coll Cardiol Intv*. 2015;8:139–146.) (B) Improvements in short- and long-term mortality rates among ST-elevation myocardial infarction (STEMI) patients treated with primary percutaneous coronary intervention (PPCI) between 2003 and 2018 in Western Denmark Heart Registry. (From Thrane PG, et al. Trends in mortality following ST-segment elevation myocardial infarction treated with primary percutaneous coronary intervention: 2003–2018. *J Am Coll Cardiol*. 2023 in press.)

in Maryland, thanks in large part to the efforts of R. Adams Cowley. In 1968, St. Vincent's Hospital in New York City built the nation's first mobile coronary care unit, staffed initially with physicians and later by paramedics. This unit was the first to evaluate and triage patients with cardiac complaints and included a portable, battery-powered cardiac monitor and defibrillator, as well as supplies for intravenous access, mobile oxygen, and medications. From here, the modern-day EMS system was born. Today, EMS providers in the United States care for close to 30 million patients per year. The incorporation of various vehicles, including ambulance vans, helicopters, and airplanes, has allowed for rapid mobilization and transportation of patients over great distances in short periods of time.

With the development of formal EMS systems throughout the country, the framework was in place to build complex regional systems of care for a variety of medical conditions. The first systems of care were designed for trauma patients and acute cardiovascular emergencies, such as STEMI, stroke, and OHCA. The integration of EMS and the incorporation of the prehospital phase for acute coronary syndrome (ACS) evaluation and diagnosis are integral components of any regionalized STEMI system of care. EMS providers and other first responders have four primary responsibilities: (1) prehospital evaluation; (2) treatment; (3) triage; and (4) transfer (Fig. 3.5).

Prehospital Systems

The prehospital evaluation should consist of a focused history and physical examination, including a complete assessment of vital signs and a prehospital 12-lead electrocardiogram (PHECG). Early STEMI diagnosis based on the

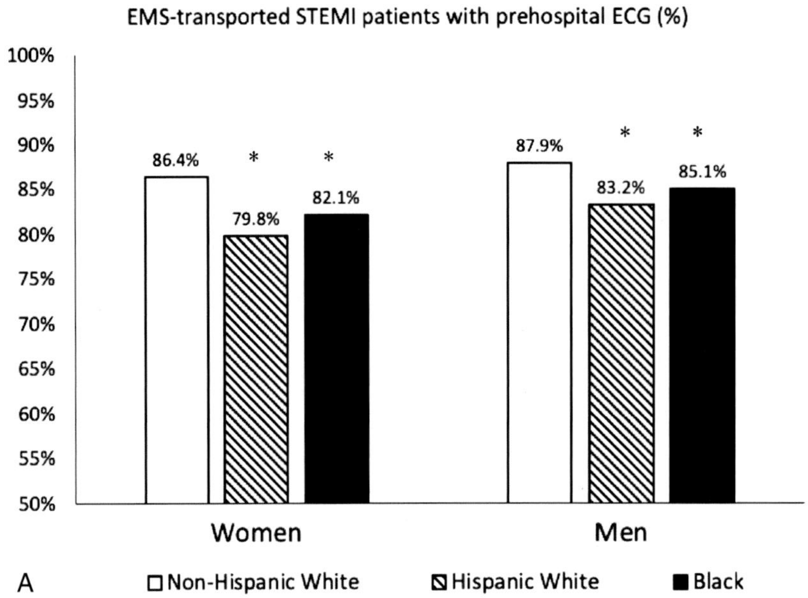

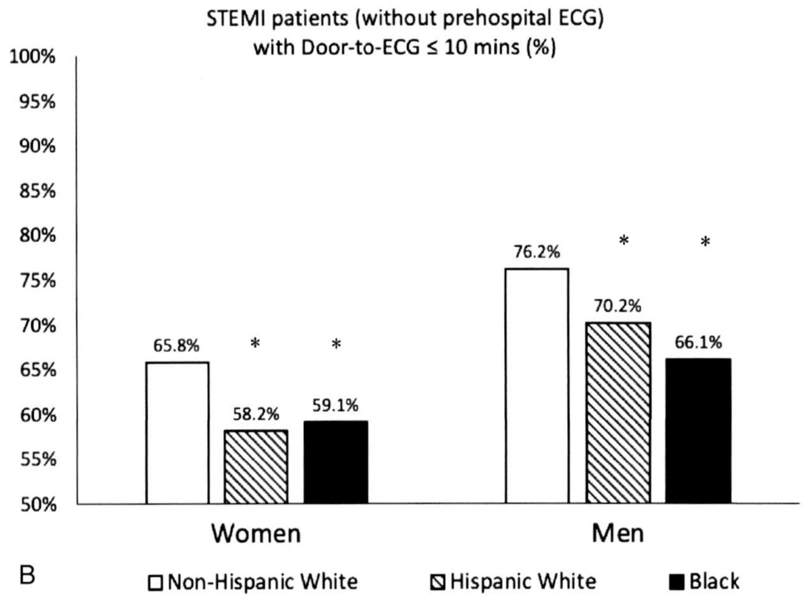

FIG. 3.3 (A) Hispanic White and Black/African American patients with ST-elevation myocardial infarction (STEMI) were less likely to achieve door-to-device goals of less than 90 minutes compared with Non-Hispanic White patients. (From Osho A, Fernandes MF, Poudel R, et al. Race-based differences in ST-elevation myocardial infarction (STEMI) process metrics and mortality from 2015–2021: an analysis of 178,062 patients from the American Heart Association get with the guidelines-coronary artery disease (GWTG-CAD) registry. *Circulation*. 2023;148(3):229–240.) (B) Hispanic White and Black/African American patients with ST-elevation myocardial infarction (STEMI) were less likely to achieve door-to-device goals of less than 90 minutes compared with Non-Hispanic White patients. (From Osho A, Fernandes MF, Poudel R, et al. Race-based differences in ST-elevation myocardial infarction (STEMI) process metrics and mortality from 2015–2021: an analysis of 178,062 patients from the American Heart Association get with the guidelines-coronary artery disease (GWTG-CAD). *Circulation*. 2023; 148(3):229–240.)

PHECG facilitates early reperfusion. While the door-to-balloon (D2B) time is widely recognized as an important metric for favorable survival, it is equally essential to focus on the time from the first medical contact to device (FMC2D), which includes the prehospital phase, in order to minimize total ischemic time. Systems that demonstrate the shortest D2B and FMC2D times are typically those that have implemented prehospital STEMI diagnosis along with the prehospital cardiac catheterization laboratory activation (PHCCLA). This strategy requires a multidisciplinary team approach in which either the emergency department (ED) physician or specially trained EMS providers are able to activate the cardiac catheterization laboratory (CCL) without cardiology consultation. Nevertheless, there are several factors that can impede the rapid recognition of STEMI, PHCCLA, and timely transfer to the nearest PPCI center. First, STEMI constitutes a small proportion of the total patients experiencing chest pain who are transported by EMS. Second, there is insufficient availability of PHECG capabilities in many EMS systems, particularly volunteer systems in rural areas. Third, certain geographical regions and STEMI systems mandate transport of suspected STEMI patients to the nearest hospital or clinic facility regardless of their PPCI capabilities or eligibility for fibrinolysis. Finally, the existence of different EMS regions in the United States (hospital-based, fire station-based, and

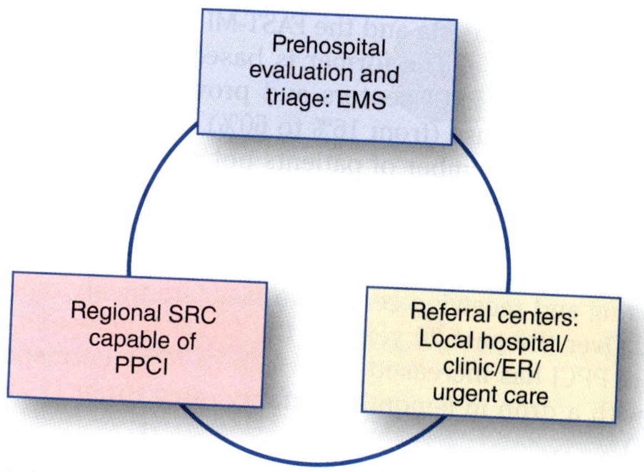

FIG. 3.4 Components of a successful system-of-care for ST-elevation myocardial infarction (STEMI). *EMS*, Emergency medical services; *ER*, emergency room; *PPCI*, primary percutaneous coronary intervention; *SRC*, STEMI-receiving center.

private third-party) introduces regional and geographical complexity and heterogeneity in the delivery of STEMI care. Due to these factors and more, PHCCLA is observed in less than half of the patients with STEMI who are transported by EMS.[8,9]

Conversely, there may be various reasons that may result in the cancellation of CCL activations (Fig. 3.6).[10] The issue of inappropriate CCL activation poses a significant challenge, as it can result in staff burnout, confusion for families and patients, and unnecessary resource utilization. Moreover, in such instances, an emerging data suggests that the absence of CCL activation or its cancellation for patients presenting with STEMI is associated with increased mortality risk compared to where CCL is appropriately preactivated.[11] To enhance timely reperfusion, it is essential to prioritize direct transfer to CCL, bypassing ED where appropriate, as this approach may also improve survival.[12] Overall, in order to enhance STEMI systems of care in the prehospital course, the American Heart Association (AHA)'s Mission: Lifeline Program introduced PreAct program to guide paramedics, in coordination with the ED staff, to acquire and interpret PHECG and subsequently activate CCL in the field, allowing for direct transfer to the CCL while bypassing the ED in appropriate clinical situations (Fig. 3.7).[13] Nevertheless, direct to the CCL may not always be a feasible option. In certain circumstances where initial evaluation/admission in the ED is warranted, such as when there is uncertainty in the diagnosis of STEMI, when the patient's mental state prevents them from providing consent, or when a do-not-resuscitate order is in place (see Chapter 8).

Integrated Emergency Medical Systems

Although the transport time to a specialized PPCI center is a "fixed" and largely nonmodifiable delay in care delivery, an integrated EMS system that incorporates PHCCLA allows for "parallel processing," where CCL staff can prepare to receive the STEMI patient to the CCL immediately upon arrival to the hospital. This type of process efficiency can be achieved only through an integrated system for STEMI care that incorporates the acquisition and interpretation of PHECG for early diagnosis, initial stabilization, expedited triage with prenotification, and predetermined transport destinations. Integrated EMS with well-designed standardized protocols is not only an absolute need for an efficient transport from the field to the PPCI center, but also for transporting patients from referring centers to receiving centers with minimal delay.

A more uniform evolution toward integrated STEMI care has been impeded by a lack of funding, diverging incentives, a lack of coordinated objectives and standardized protocols, and at times, competing strategies. The AHA recommends providing training and certification for EMS staff to acquire and interpret 12-lead ECGs in patients experiencing ischemic symptoms, to implement STEMI care pathways that empower EMS staff to PHCCLA, and support EMS agencies with trained staff, funding, research opportunities, and internal quality improvement programs.[5] Nonetheless, in many regions, particularly those without a state-regulated certificate of need requirements, there was a proliferation of new CCL for the provision of PPCI in centers without regard for PCI volume or surgical backup (Fig. 3.e3). Conversely, other regions have developed integrated EMS systems that focus on prehospital diagnosis, triage, and transfer to an established center of excellence proficient in both primary and elective PCI. Although the expansion of PPCI centers can improve access to care, more efficient use of existing PPCI centers through EMS integration has been proven to be a more cost-effective strategy. Recently, sophisticated modeling techniques have been used to compare the relative efficacy and/or cost of these competing strategies for the care of STEMI patients. Importantly, a strategy focused on EMS integration, prehospital diagnosis, triage, and transportation with more effective use of existing PPCI centers was found to be more effective and less costly than a strategy of creating new PCI centers facilities (Fig. 3.e4).

SYSTEMS OF CARE IN PRACTICE

STEMI Systems of Care: The European Experience

The rapid restoration of normal coronary blood flow, via pharmacological and/or mechanical recanalization of an occluded coronary artery, limits the extent of myocardial necrosis and reduces the mortality of patients who present with STEMI. PPCI has demonstrated more frequent, complete, and durable coronary reperfusion in both observational studies and randomized controlled clinical trials compared with fibrinolytics. For these reasons, PPCI is the preferred revascularization modality as long as an experienced operator can provide it in a timely manner (Fig. 3.8).[4] On the basis of these principles, the first randomized controlled trials, which compared long-distance transport to PPCI centers with fibrinolysis performed at local hospitals, were performed in Europe in the early 2000s. Overall, these studies demonstrated that transferring patients with STEMI to the PPCI center could be both safe and effective in the context of transfer-related delays

between 2008 and 2012, there was a significant increase in the proportion of patients receiving PPCI, both for direct presenters and transferred patients. The use of fibrinolytics decreased during the same period. Additionally, the utilization of PHECG increased, and various time-to-treatment metrics showed improvement. However, despite the improvements in quality metrics, the overall in-hospital mortality rates did not decrease, which was attributed to increased rates of cardiac arrest, Killip Class IV presentations, and cardiogenic shock during the study period. When excluding patients with cardiac arrest, adjusted in-hospital mortality rates did improve (from 5.3% to 3.7%) (Fig. 3.11).[1]

Despite the promising improvements, many hospitals still did not meet the recommended time goals, as outlined in the guidelines. To further enhance STEMI care, the AHA partnered with the Duke Clinical Research Institute to design the AHA Mission: Lifeline STEMI Systems Accelerator projects. Between 2012 and 2014, the first phase of the project, Accelator-1, involved 484 hospitals and 1253 EMS agencies in 16 regions. While there was a modest improvement in the proportion of STEMI patients meeting the guideline-recommended time goals for FMC2D (from 59% to 61% for direct presenters and from 38% to 50% for transferred patients), in-hospital mortality risks did not improve during the study period. However, it was observed that not all regions had implemented the necessary processes to enable EMS providers to obtain PHECGs, activate CCL, and bypass the ED. To address this, the project implemented full-time regional coordinators and conducted the follow-up Accelerator-2 study between 2015 and 2017, involving 12 metropolitan regions across the United States with 132 PPCI centers and 946 EMS agencies. Significant improvements were reported in achieving the guideline-recommended goals of FMC2D time (from 67% to 74% for direct presenters). In-hospital mortality and heart failure rates also significantly declined during the study period (from 4.4% to 2.3% and from 7.4% to 5%, respectively) (Fig. 3.12).[17]

Apart from the Accelerator projects, the initial trend of improved treatment times between 2008 and 2012 slowed down and remained relatively steady between 2012 and 2019.[5] In the most recent analysis using the AHA Mission: Lifeline data from 2018 to 2021, which included over 110,000 STEMI activations at 648 hospitals, the favorable trend in time to reperfusion goals continued. However, approximately 20% of patients who received PPCI experienced delays, with the proportion of delays increasing over time. Importantly, adjusted in-hospital mortality rates were lower for patients treated within the guideline-recommended time goals (OR, 0.40 [95% CI, 0.36–0.44]) for FMC2D within 90 minutes, OR, 0.51 [0.32–0.78] for DIDO within 30 minutes, and OR, 0.44 [0.26–0.71) for FMC2D within 120 minutes).[2]

Professional Society Guidelines

In the past decade, the successes in Minnesota, California, and North Carolina have been replicated across the United States. The AHA Mission: Lifeline and the ACC D2B Alliance have played crucial roles in the growth and expansion of STEMI systems of care and have contributed to a change in the ACC/AHA Guidelines for STEMI patients. Current guidelines give a class I, level of evidence B recommendation that "all communities should create and maintain a regional system of STEMI care." The same level of recommendation is given for performance of a 12-lead ECG by EMS personnel. Furthermore, regional STEMI systems models have stimulated the application of new systems of care models for other cardiovascular emergencies, including cardiogenic shock, OHCA, aortic dissection, and stroke.[18]

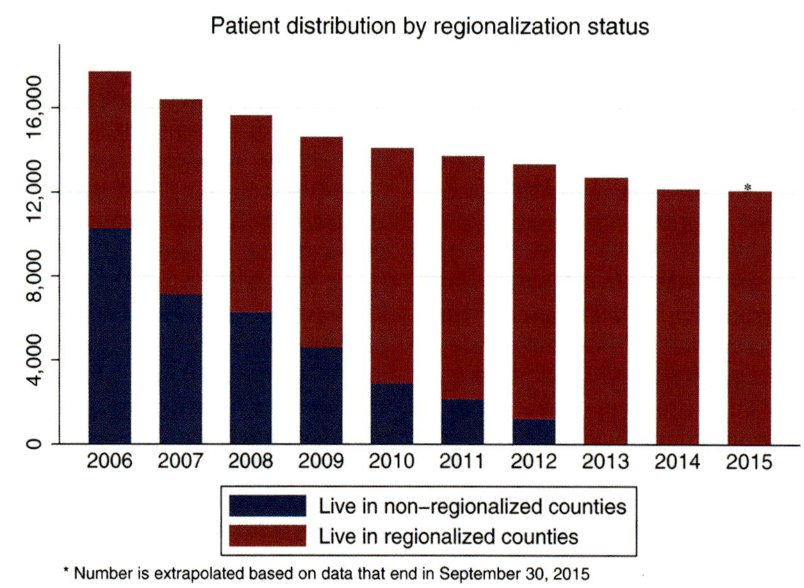

FIG. 3.10 Trends in regionalization in ST-elevation myocardial infarction (STEMI) care in the United States (2006–2015). (From Shen YC, Krumholz H, Hsia RY, et al. Association of cardiac care regionalization with access, treatment, and mortality among patients with ST-segment elevation myocardial infarction. *Circ Cardiovasc Qual Outcomes.* 2021;14(3):e007195.)

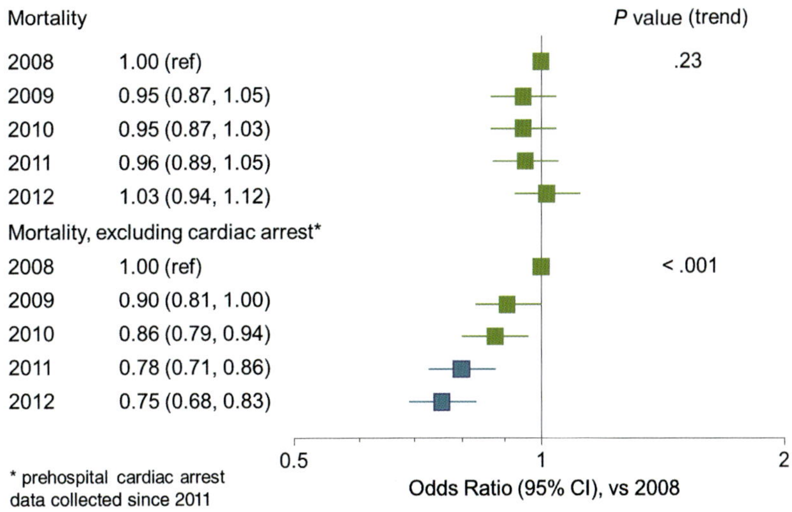

FIG. 3.11 In-hospital mortality risks in ST-elevation myocardial infarction (STEMI) in the United States (2008–2012). Marked improvement in in-hospital mortality risks only observed after excluding patients with cardiac arrest. (From Granger CB, Bates ER, Jollis JG, et al. Improving care of STEMI in the United States 2008 to 2012. *J Am Heart Assoc*. 2019;8(1):e008096.)

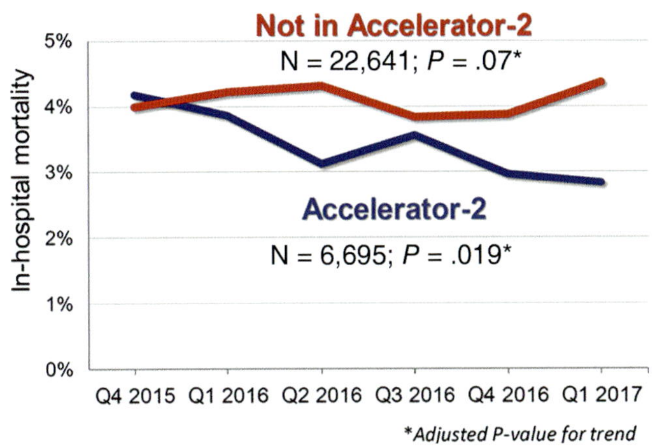

FIG. 3.12 Improvement in-hospital mortality risks by regionalization in Accelator-2 project. (From Jollis JG, Al-Khalidi HR, Roettig ML, et al. Impact of regionalization of ST-segment-elevation myocardial infarction care on treatment times and outcomes for emergency medical services-transported patients presenting to hospitals with percutaneous coronary intervention: mission: lifeline accelerator-2. *Circulation*. 2018;137(4):376–387.)

IDEAL SYSTEMS OF CARE NETWORK

There are certain key features that are common among successful systems of care. The success of any system is predicated upon the performance and the commitment of its individual members. This engagement includes the general public, integrated EMS, and STEMI referring and receiving centers.[5]

In the ideal system of care, the patients and community members would recognize the signs and symptoms of heart attack and appropriately respond immediately by calling EMS (via 911) rather than self-transport/walk-in. Moreover, automated external defibrillators should be available in public places and should be intuitive enough to be used by both lay people and medical professionals. If appropriate, the public would recognize the need for and would initiate CPR when applicable. These objectives can only be achieved through community outreach and education campaigns at local and national levels.

The ideal integrated EMS would have standardized "point-of-entry" protocols that clearly delineate which patients should be transported to the nearest referral hospital and which patients should be transported to the nearest receiving hospital. This decision making would be based, in part, on the acquisition, interpretation, and transmission of the PHECG. Successful implementation of such protocols is dependent not just on the acquisition of the PHECG, but also on the accurate interpretation followed by appropriate PHCCLA. This goal can be accomplished by a computer algorithm with or without EMS overread or by transmission to the receiving center. Systems must be activated in a timely and uniform fashion; a single phone call or page should alert all pertinent members of the system and should provide any pertinent updates on the patient's condition and status. These protocols are ideally created through the joint efforts of EMS personnel, ED physicians, cardiologists, hospital administrators, and staff. They should be supported by the payers and administrators within the system. In systems where PPCI is not available at all or in a timely fashion, the use of fibrinolytics as reperfusion therapy should be included as an alternative in the protocol (see Chapter 8).

The ideal referring hospitals should also have standardized point-of-entry protocols that clearly delineate which patients should be transferred to a referral center based on patient-specific risk criteria, indications, and contraindications to alternative therapies and the proximity to the nearest receiving center. Furthermore, these centers should have integrated plans for the return of patients to their local community hospitals and care centers for pre- and postdischarge follow-up care. The referral centers should have mechanisms that promote efficient transfer of data (medical records, study results, and so on) to the receiving centers for purposes of continuity of care and to avoid redundancies in the system. Referral and receiving centers should have standardized protocols in place to ensure the efficient delivery of evidenced-based therapies for all patients, while minimizing variability in the delivery of care and achieving the goals of DIDO time of less than 30 minutes and FMC2D of less than 120 minutes.

Finally, the ideal receiving center must have the facilities, expertise, equipment, and training to administer definitive therapy for each acute cardiovascular condition. These centers should meet minimal performance guidelines and should be involved in ongoing assessment and quality improvement efforts. These receiving centers should also have mechanisms to promote efficient transfer of data (medical records, study results, and so on) back to the referral centers to promote continuity of care and avoid redundancies in the system. They should also follow standardized protocols to minimize variability in the delivery of evidenced-based care and should clearly and consistently promote bidirectional feedback between the various members of the system. Moreover, they should also participate in national databases to contribute toward enhancing the quality and performance measures in STEMI care.

In addition to these individual components, the ideal system of care should have common features that are applicable to all members and components of the system itself. First, all members of the system must share a sense of teamwork and singular common purpose—to provide the highest quality care in the timeliest fashion possible. To do this, system members must share a mutual respect for each individual player and must understand that for the system to succeed, each member plays a critical role. Every member of the team is crucial, and improvements to the system require input and leadership at every level. The need for education, training, and retraining cannot be underestimated because of the large number of people involved and ongoing changes in both personnel and new data. Standardized protocols and order sets designed by use of guideline-based therapies ensure that the highest percentage of eligible patients receive the highest quality care. However, the same system needs to allow flexibility to address the individual needs of patients and physicians. All parties within the system would ideally be involved in ongoing data collection and research for quality assurance and improvement purposes. Feedback is a key component; this could include the transporting paramedics observing an angiogram, the interventional cardiologist calling the ED physician immediately following the procedure, and communication the following day among the system coordinators, EMS, and ED managers. The primary cardiologist should communicate with the primary care physician as well. Monthly, quarterly, and yearly quality reports provide ongoing and system-wide quality improvement. Financial and moral support from hospital administration is essential, and if missing, can create a major stumbling block. Perhaps the most important link in the chain is a passionate leader at every level.

Systems of Care: Success and Advantages

The advantages to a "systems of care" approach include increased access to tertiary care for patients with complex, high-risk conditions (Table 3.1). This access decreases the number of "eligible but untreated" patients in a wide geographic region. Standardized protocols within systems of care improve time to treatment, including FMC2D time,

TABLE 3.1 Advantages and Successes of ST-Elevation Myocardial Infarction Systems of Care

Improve access to tertiary care facilities
Decrease the number of "eligible, but untreated" patients
Shorter time-to-treatment through standardized protocols
Improved patient outcomes, including all-cause mortality, cardiovascular mortality, reinfarction, stroke, and length of hospitalization

From American Heart Association: Mission: Lifeline, 2015. http://www.heart.org/HEARTORG/HealthcareResearch/MissionLifelineHomePage/LearnAboutMissionLifeline/STEMI-Systems-of-Care_UCM_439065_SubHomePage.jsp.

while also providing clear communication and expectations for patients based on their point-of-entry. Furthermore, systems of care have consistently shown improvements in important outcomes, including all-cause mortality, cardiovascular mortality, re-infarction, stroke, and length of hospitalization. STEMI systems are now being implemented throughout the world with consistently positive results.

SYSTEMS OF CARE: CURRENT CHALLENGES, GAPS, AND BARRIERS

Systems Delays

Even in highly successful systems of care for STEMI patients with standardized transfer protocols, delays in reperfusion can still occur, with the DIDO time at referral hospitals being a significant challenge and a target for improvement. A study analyzing over 14,000 STEMI patients between 2007 and 2010 found that the median DIDO time was 68 minutes, and only approximately 11% of patients had a DIDO time under 30 minutes, with longer DIDO times being associated with increased mortality (Fig. 3.e11). This challenge persists in more recent years as a follow-up study of over 114,000 STEMI patients between 2018 and 2021 revealed that only 17% of patients requiring interhospital transfer were treated within the recommended 120 minutes.[2] Most transferred patients experienced the DIDO time over 30 minutes at the referring hospital, and the median time from symptom onset to PPCI was 240 minutes for transferred patients. Furthermore, achieving the target times of less than 30 minutes for DIDO and less than 120 minutes for FMC2D was associated with a significant reduction in in-hospital mortality risks by 49% and 56%, respectively.[2]

Delays within the health care system vary in duration and their impact on patient outcomes, as highlighted by Miedema et al., in their study involving 2034 STEMI patients transferred for PPCI. The most common delays occurred at the referral hospital, primarily due to transportation and delays in the ED. The longest delays were associated with initial ECGs that did not provide a definitive diagnosis and diagnostic uncertainties. However, the delays that had a significant clinical impact were related to cardiac arrest and cardiogenic shock. In many cases, cardiac arrest and/or shock were the cause of the delay rather than a consequence of it (Fig. 3.13). Notably, in the Get With The Guidelines–Coronary Artery Disease registry, 20% of patients undergoing PPCI were found to have

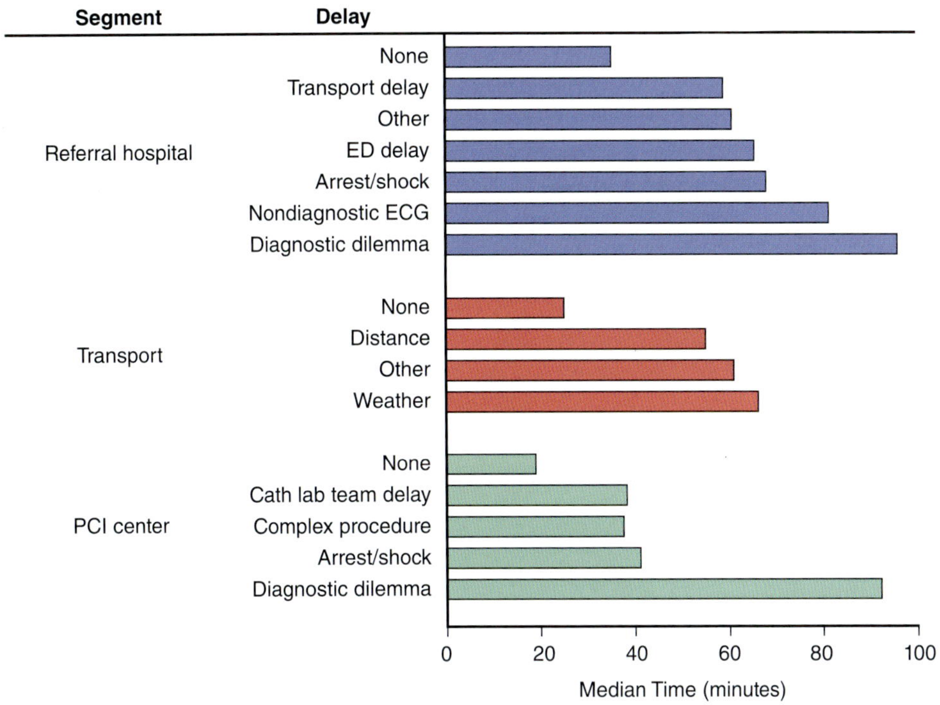

FIG. 3.13 Median times for individual delays at each of the three treatment segments. *ED*, Emergency department; *ECG*, electrocardiogram; *PCI*, percutaneous coronary intervention. (From Miedema MD, Newell MC, Duval S, et al. Causes of delay and associated mortality in patients transferred with ST-elevation myocardial infarction. *Circulation*. 2011;124:1636–1644.)

hospital-specific reasons for delays, including cardiac arrest and intubation needs, as well as other factors such as difficulty crossing the culprit lesion.[2] In 2020, due to the Coronavirus 2019 (COVID-19) pandemic, the need for additional personal protective equipment was added as a reason for delay.[2] Additionally, nonmodifiable delays unrelated to the health care system can contribute to extended transport time such as adverse weather conditions or long geographic distances. Finally, specific patient characteristics including older age or female sex, and atypical presentations such as the absence of chest pain have been identified as reasons for delay.[19]

In order to reduce variability and enhance the efficiency in interhospital transfer times, the AHA Mission: Lifeline Program developed strategies, named STAT TRANSFER program, consisting of policies promoting standardized transport from the field to STEMI receiving hospital, minimizing delays in ambulance arrival and initiation of transfer, ensuring uninterrupted ambulance coverage, meeting time goals at referring hospitals, selecting the appropriate receiving hospital, and tracking process performance (Figs. 3.e12 and 3.e13).[20]

Pharmaco-Invasive Strategy

While mechanical reperfusion is superior to pharmacological reperfusion in improving myocardial salvage and survival, it is crucial to note that its impact is time-dependent, emphasizing the importance of early PPCI (within 120 minutes of FMC) rather than late PPCI (see Chapter 8). Several large registries supported the use of a pharmaco-invasive strategy for expected delays. The French registry demonstrated that the pharmaco-invasive strategy was comparable to early PPCI (FMC2D ≤120 minutes) but superior to late PPCI (FMC2D >120 minutes) in terms of 5-year survival (HR 1.51 (1.13–2.02)).[21] Similarly, the Australian registry reported a higher 3-year mortality risk in patients undergoing late PPCI compared to those treated with the pharmaco-invasive approach (20.2% vs. 6.2%).[22] In parallel, MHI, in their Level 1 MI program, showed no difference in short-term mortality or bleeding risk between patients treated with half-dose fibrinolytic at referral centers (≥60 miles away from the PPCI center) compared to those with presented directly to the PPCI center. In line with these findings, the 2021 ACC/AHA/Society for Cardiovascular Angiography and Interventions (SCAI) Guideline for Coronary Artery Revascularization recommended fibrinolytic therapy if the anticipated FMC2D is over 120 minutes, followed by transfer to the PPCI center for routine coronary angiography within 3 to 24 hours (Class 2A), and considering rescue PCI (Class 1) if there is failed perfusion with fibrinolytic.[4]

Resources for Staffing, Research, and Quality Improvement

Maintaining adequate staffing requires a great deal of person-power, in addition to large financial overhead to operate these systems of care. Reimbursement is a common challenge because many different hospitals and providers may take care of a single patient during their stay within a system of care. Participation in research and quality improvement measures takes time, effort, and financial backing. Perhaps this accounts for the current gaps in knowledge regarding cost-effectiveness and certain outcome measures. Incomplete data collection and inadequate exchange of information are ongoing issues for many systems of care. Underreporting of outcomes and "scrubbing" data do little to enhance our understanding of patient outcomes. Multiple isolated medical record systems, both electronic and handwritten, are often forced to interact with one another within a given system of care.

Public Policy and Consideration of the Need

Public policy and oversight are another arena that provides unique challenges to each system of care. Regional transportation systems need to be developed in many areas of the country, and ongoing clarification on what constitutes an acceptable "receiving" center and "referring" center is needed. Public education and community outreach are necessary to teach patients and community members to recognize the signs and symptoms of a cardiac emergency and appropriately respond by activating EMS (via 911) immediately. Accurate mapping and denotation of receiving centers and referral centers are necessary to identify regions in need of more robust systems of care. This effort would also allow for new partnerships and would facilitate linking these hospitals into a more cohesive system of care. Furthermore, delineation of daytime PPCI centers and 24-hour PPCI centers is critical to reduce confusion and facilitate patient triage in a timely fashion.

COVID-19 Pandemic

The COVID-19 pandemic, caused by SARS-CoV-2, had a significant global impact on cardiovascular system through both direct and indirect mechanisms.[23,24] While there were initial concerns about COVID-19-related thrombosis leading to STEMI, large national studies reported STEMI rates of less than 1% among COVID-19 patients.[2,25] Moreover, the pandemic indirectly affected overall STEMI care, with a decrease in activation rates and an increase in complications and mortality rates.[24] The pandemic also had a deleterious effect on STEMI systems of care, leading to longer ischemic times, delays in treatment, and a preference for fibrinolytic therapy over PPCI to minimize the risk of virus spread. Up to 6% of the delay in reperfusion in 2020 was due to the need for additional personal protective equipment for suspected/confirmed COVID-19 infection. Thankfully, the incidence of these PPE-related delays has decreased to approximately 1% through the course of the pandemic.[2]

In order to alleviate the consequences on the STEMI systems of care, the AHA: Mission Lifeline emphasized several important recommendations: (1) continue to practice acquiring rapid PHECG, followed by timely interpretation and prompt notification of the findings; (2) immediately activate the CCL in cases of diagnostic ST elevation; (3) avoid any delays in PPCI while waiting for COVID-19 test results; and (4) prioritize PPCI as the preferred reperfusion strategy while reserving fibrinolytic therapy for those with anticipated time to reperfusion more than 120 minutes.[26] Similarly, a consensus statement from SCAI, ACC, and the American College of Emergency Physicians (ACEP) emphasized the adherence to PPCI as a reperfusion strategy while protecting CCL staff with necessary personal protective equipment.[27] Although the COVID-19 public health emergency ended in May 2023, it is crucial to learn from this experience and adapt STEMI systems of care locally and nationally to protect quality metrics and ensure timely mechanical reperfusion in STEMI patients during any future global health crisis.

Other Issues: In-Hospital ST-Elevation Myocardial Infarction, High-Risk ST-Elevation Myocardial Infarction, and False Activations

In-hospital STEMI has distinct characteristics and outcomes compared to out-of-hospital STEMI. Patients with in-hospital STEMI experience longer time-to-treatment (76 minutes vs. 66 minutes, Fig. 3.e14), more comorbidities, less typical symptoms, lower rates of PPCI, and increased risk of bleeding complications and in-hospital mortality.[28] National societies currently lack standardized clinical definitions and protocols for in-hospital STEMI. Three key areas that contribute to delays in in-hospital STEMI care are delays in ECG acquisition, interpretation, and activation of existing STEMI systems of care. To improve patient care, it is crucial to establish a hospital-wide approach to promptly obtain ECGs in patients showing signs and symptoms of ischemia, implement processes for immediate ECG review and interpretation, and establish a formal in-hospital STEMI activation protocol (Fig. 3.e15). Implementation of in-hospital STEMI quality improvement programs has shown significant reductions in symptom-to-first device activation times (by 72%) and increased rates of diagnostic cardiac catheterization (by 100%) and PPCI (by 73%).

A significant proportion of STEMI patients present with cardiogenic shock and/or OHCA, comprising approximately 8% and 11% of cases, respectively, and these conditions are associated with unfavorable outcomes including a roughly doubling of the risk of mortality when both conditions exist on presentation (see Chapter 21).[29,30] Timely reperfusion with PPCI, along with guideline-directed antithrombotic and supportive pharmacological and mechanical circulatory support, is crucial to improve outcomes in such life-threatening conditions. However, delays in reperfusion are commonly observed in these patient populations.[2] National initiatives, such as the AHA Mission: Lifeline STEMI Accelerator project conducted from 2012 to 2014, including these high-risk patients.[30] Despite quality improvement efforts, patients with STEMI and cardiogenic shock were still less likely to achieve the recommended reperfusion time compared to those without cardiogenic shock (37% vs. 54% for direct presenters and 44% vs. 47% for transferred patients).[30] In addition, in-hospital mortality rates remained high, even among patients who met the recommended time frame to the device for both direct presenters and transferred patients (20.4% and 19.8%, respectively). Higher mortality rates were observed when the recommended FMC2D was exceeded (39.1% and 35.1%, respectively). Conversely, there were somewhat more promising results for STEMI patients with OHCA during the same study period, with higher rates of PHECG acquisition (from 53.9% to 61.9%), an increased proportion of direct transfers to PPCI centers (from 74.7% to 83.6%), and improved achievement of the recommended goal of reperfusion within 90 minutes (from 34.5% to 41.8%). Nonetheless, efforts should continue at both local and national levels to improve the metrics and achieve the recommended goals of timely reperfusion and favorable outcomes in high-risk STEMI patients with cardiogenic shock and/or OHCA.

Finally, false or inappropriate activations have become a very challenging issue, with rates of inappropriate activations from 10% to as high as 40%, depending on definitions and regions. Reasons for false activations vary and include abnormal repolarization, nondiagnostic ECG, pericarditis, left bundle branch block, left ventricular hypertrophy, and previous MI, among others. Clinical predictors and outcomes for this emerging population have not been well characterized, and solutions for minimizing the false-positive rates without increasing the rates of missed STEMIs are complex at best. Refining these systems to improve the specificity of our STEMI selection process without sacrificing sensitivity is one of the greatest challenges that STEMI systems face.

FUTURE DIRECTIONS AND STRATEGIES FOR IMPROVEMENT

The advent of complex regional STEMI systems is a major achievement that has helped to improve the quality of cardiovascular care. Looking forward, ideally, the entire U.S. population will have locally designed regional systems not only to provide timely access to PPCI for all STEMI patients, but also to care for all acute cardiovascular emergencies. This lofty goal is not only possible but within our grasp in the next decade. We envision these same systems providing similar care, including standardized protocols and transfer plans, for all acute cardiovascular emergencies, including OHCA, aortic dissection, pulmonary embolism, stroke, abdominal aortic aneurysms, and non–ST-elevation ACS. With an added emphasis on data collection and monitoring, we are optimistic that we will identify new targets for improvement in care and clinical outcomes. In addition, this expansion would enable the growth of large registry databases, such as the ACTION-Get With the Guidelines and Cath-PCI registries. Advances in technology and migration toward electronic medical record systems should allow for further integration of medical information, more comprehensive data, and more transparent communication among providers, patients, and families. Further streamlining of processes including giving all EMS providers access to PHECG systems might allow for further reduction in FMC2D times. Finally, there are obvious areas for improvement that can be targeted, particularly with regard to in-hospital STEMIs and false activations. To quote Albert Einstein, "We cannot solve our problems with the same thinking we used when we created them." With novel approaches and further refinements to our current systems of care, we no doubt can solve the many challenges that we face today and look forward to the next set of challenges that might follow.

CLASSIC REFERENCES

Diercks DB, Kontos MC, Chen AY, et al. Utilization and impact of pre-hospital electrocardiograms for patients with acute ST-segment elevation myocardial infarction. *J Am Coll Cardiol*. 2009;53:161–166. https://doi.org/10.1016/j.jacc.2008.09.030.

Garberich RF, Traverse JH, Claussen MT, et al. ST-elevation myocardial infarction diagnosed after hospital admission. *Circulation*. 2014;129:1225–1232. https://doi.org/10.1161/CIRCULATIONAHA.113.005568.

Henry TD, Sharkey SW, Burke MN, et al. A regional system to provide timely access to percutaneous coronary intervention for ST-elevation myocardial infarction. *Circulation*. 2007;116:721–728. https://doi.org/10.1161/CIRCULATIONAHA.107.694141.

Jacobs AK, Antman EM, Faxon DP, Gregory T, Solis P. Development of systems of care for ST elevation myocardial infarction patients. *Circulation*. 2007;116:217–230. https://doi.org/10.1161/CIRCULATIONAHA.107.184043.

Jollis JG, Granger CB, Henry TD, et al. Systems of care for ST-segment–elevation myocardial infarction: a report from the American Heart Association's mission: lifeline. *Circ Cardiovasc Qual Outcomes*. 2012;5:423–428. https://doi.org/10.1161/CIRCOUTCOMES.111.964668.

Langabeer JR, Henry TD, Kereiakes DJ, et al. Growth in percutaneous coronary intervention capacity relative to population and disease prevalence. *J Am Heart Assoc*. 2013;2:e000370. https://doi.org/10.1161/JAHA.113.000370.

Larson DM, Duval S, Sharkey SW, et al. Safety and efficacy of a pharmaco-invasive reperfusion strategy in rural ST-elevation myocardial infarction patients with expected delays due to long-distance transfers. *Eur Heart J*. 2012;33:1232–1240. https://doi.org/10.1093/eurheartj/ehr403.

Larson DM, Menssen KM, Sharkey SW, et al. "False-Positive" cardiac catheterization laboratory activation among patients with suspected ST-segment elevation myocardial infarction. *JAMA*. 2007;298:2754. https://doi.org/10.1001/jama.298.23.2754.

Miedema MD, Newell MC, Duval S, et al. Causes of delay and associated mortality in patients transferred with ST-segment–elevation myocardial infarction. *Circulation*. 2011;124:1636–1644. https://doi.org/10.1161/CIRCULATIONAHA.111.033118.

O'Gara PT, Kushner FG, Ascheim DD, et al. 2013 ACCF/AHA guideline for the management of ST-elevation myocardial infarction. *Circulation*. 2013;127:e362–e425. https://doi.org/10.1161/CIR.0b013e3182742cf6.

REFERENCES

1. Granger CB, Bates ER, Jollis JG, et al. Improving care of STEMI in the United States 2008 to 2012. *J Am Heart Assoc*. 2019;8:e008096. https://doi.org/10.1161/JAHA.118.008096.
2. Jollis JG, Granger CB, Zègre-Hemsey JK, et al. Treatment time and in-hospital mortality among patients with ST-segment elevation myocardial infarction, 2018–2021. *JAMA*. 2022;328:2033. https://doi.org/10.1001/jama.2022.20149.
3. Ahuja KR, Saad AM, Nazir S, et al. Trends in clinical characteristics and outcomes in ST-elevation myocardial infarction hospitalizations in the United States, 2002–2016. *Curr Probl Cardiol*. 2022;47:101005. https://doi.org/10.1016/j.cpcardiol.2021.101005.
4. Lawton JS, Tamis-Holland JE, Bangalore S, et al. 2021 ACC/AHA/SCAI guideline for coronary artery revascularization: executive summary: a report of the American College of Cardiology/American Heart Association joint committee on clinical practice guidelines. *Circulation*. 2022;145:E4–E17. https://doi.org/10.1161/CIR.0000000000001039.
5. Jacobs AK, Ali MJ, Best PJ, et al. Systems of care for ST-segment–elevation myocardial infarction: a policy statement from the American Heart Association. *Circulation*. 2021;144:e310–e327. https://doi.org/10.1161/CIR.0000000000001025.
6. Thrane PG, Olesen KKW, Thim T, et al. 10-Year mortality after ST-segment elevation myocardial infarction compared to the general population. *J Am Coll Cardiol*. 2024;83(25):2615–2625. https://doi:10.1016/j.jacc.2024.04.025.
7. Osho A, Fernandes M, Poudel R, et al. Race-based differences in ST elevation myocardial infarction (STEMI) process metrics and mortality from 2015–2021: an analysis of 178,062 patients from the American Heart Association get with the guidelines-coronary artery disease (GWTG-CAD) registry. *Circulation*. 2023;148(3):229–240.
8. Shavadia JS, Roe MT, Chen AY, et al. Association between cardiac catheterization laboratory pre-activation and reperfusion timing metrics and outcomes in patients with ST-segment elevation myocardial infarction undergoing primary percutaneous coronary intervention. *JACC Cardiovasc Interv*. 2018;11:1837–1847. https://doi.org/10.1016/j.jcin.2018.07.020.
9. Hudzik B, Budaj A, Gierlotka M, et al. Assessment of quality of care of patients with ST-segment elevation myocardial infarction. *Eur Heart J Acute Cardiovasc Care*. 2020;9:893–901. https://doi.org/10.1177/2048872619882360.
10. Lange DC, Conte S, Pappas-Block E, et al. Cancellation of the cardiac catheterization lab after activation for ST-segment–elevation myocardial infarction. *Circ Cardiovasc Qual Outcomes*. 2018;11:e004464. https://doi.org/10.1161/CIRCOUTCOMES.117.004464.
11. Faour A, Pahn R, Cherrett C, et al. Late outcomes of patients with prehospital ST-segment elevation and appropriate cardiac catheterization laboratory nonactivation. *J Am Heart Assoc*. 2022;11:e025602. https://doi.org/10.1161/JAHA.121.025602.
12. Meisel SR, Kleiner-Shochat M, Abu-Fanne R, et al. Direct admission of patients with ST-Segment–elevation myocardial infarction to the catheterization laboratory shortens pain-to-balloon and door-to-balloon time intervals but only the pain-to-balloon interval impacts short- and long-term mortality. *J Am Heart Assoc*. 2021;10:1–12. https://doi.org/10.1161/JAHA.120.018343.
13. Kontos MC, Gunderson MR, Zegre-Hemsey JK, et al. Prehospital activation of hospital resources (PreAct) ST-Segment–elevation myocardial infarction (STEMI): a standardized approach to prehospital activation and direct to the catheterization laboratory for STEMI recommendations from the American Heart Association's mission: lifeline program. *J Am Heart Assoc*. 2020;9:e011963. https://doi.org/10.1161/JAHA.119.011963.
14. Ibanez B, James S, Agewall S, et al. 2017 ESC guidelines for the management of acute myocardial infarction in patients presenting with ST-segment elevation. *Eur Heart J*. 2018;39:119–177. https://doi.org/10.1093/eurheartj/ehx393.

15. Pera VK, Larson DM, Sharkey SW, et al. New or presumed new left bundle branch block in patients with suspected ST-elevation myocardial infarction. *Eur Heart J Acute Cardiovasc Care*. 2018;7:208–217. https://doi.org/10.1177/2048872617691508.
16. Shen Y-C, Krumholz H, Hsia RY. Association of cardiac care regionalization with access, treatment, and mortality among patients with ST-segment elevation myocardial infarction. *Circ Cardiovasc Qual Outcomes*. 2021;14:E007195. https://doi.org/10.1161/CIRCOUTCOMES.120.007195.
17. Jollis JG, Al-Khalidi HR, Roettig ML, et al. Impact of regionalization of ST-segment–elevation myocardial infarction care on treatment times and outcomes for emergency medical services–transported patients presenting to hospitals with percutaneous coronary intervention. *Circulation*. 2018;137:376–387. https://doi.org/10.1161/CIRCULATIONAHA.117.032446.
18. Henry TD, Tomey MI, Tamis-Holland JE, et al. Invasive management of acute myocardial infarction complicated by cardiogenic shock: a scientific statement from the American Heart Association. *Circulation*. 2021;143:E815–E829. https://doi.org/10.1161/CIR.0000000000000959.
19. Yildiz M, Wade SR, Henry TD. STEMI care 2021: addressing the knowledge gaps. *Am Heart J Plus*. 2021;11:100044. https://doi.org/10.1016/j.ahjo.2021.100044.
20. French WJ, Gunderson M, Travis D, et al. Emergency interhospital transfer of patients with ST-Segment–elevation myocardial infarction: call 9-1-1—the American Heart Association mission: lifeline program. *J Am Heart Assoc*. 2022;11:26700. https://doi.org/10.1161/JAHA.122.026700.
21. Danchin N, Popovic B, Puymirat E, et al. Five-year outcomes following timely primary percutaneous intervention, late primary percutaneous intervention, or a pharmaco-invasive strategy in ST-segment elevation myocardial infarction: the FAST-MI programme. *Eur Heart J*. 2020;41:858–866. https://doi.org/10.1093/eurheartj/ehz665.
22. Jamal J, Idris H, Faour A, et al. Late outcomes of ST-elevation myocardial infarction treated by pharmaco-invasive or primary percutaneous coronary intervention. *Eur Heart J*. 2023;44:516–528. https://doi.org/10.1093/eurheartj/ehac661.
23. Nadarajah R, Wu J, Hurdus B, et al. The collateral damage of COVID-19 to cardiovascular services: a meta-analysis. *Eur Heart J*. 2022;43:3164–3178. https://doi.org/10.1093/eurheartj/ehac227.
24. Henry TD, Kereiakes DJ. The direct and indirect effects of the COVID-19 pandemic on cardiovascular disease throughout the world. *Eur Heart J*. 2022;43:1154–1156. https://doi.org/10.1093/eurheartj/ehab782.
25. Bhatt AS, Varshney AS, Goodrich EL, et al. Epidemiology and management of ST-segment–elevation myocardial infarction in patients with COVID-19: a report from the American Heart Association COVID-19 cardiovascular disease registry. *J Am Heart Assoc*. 2022;11:24451. https://doi.org/10.1161/JAHA.121.024451.
26. Jacobs AK, Ali M, Best PJ, et al. Temporary emergency guidance to STEMI systems of care during the COVID-19 pandemic. *Circulation*. 2020;142:199–202. https://doi.org/10.1161/CIRCULATIONAHA.120.048180.
27. Mahmud E, Dauerman HL, Welt FGP, et al. Management of acute myocardial infarction during the COVID-19 pandemic. *J Am Coll Cardiol*. 2020;76:1375–1384. https://doi.org/10.1016/j.jacc.2020.04.039.
28. Levine GN, Dai X, Henry TD, et al. In-hospital ST-segment elevation myocardial infarction. *JAMA Cardiol*. 2018;3:527. https://doi.org/10.1001/jamacardio.2017.5356.
29. Omer MA, Tyler JM, Henry TD, et al. Clinical characteristics and outcomes of STEMI patients with cardiogenic shock and cardiac arrest. *JACC Cardiovasc Interv*. 2020;13:1211–1219. https://doi.org/10.1016/j.jcin.2020.04.004.
30. Kochar A, Al-Khalidi HR, Hansen SM, et al. Delays in primary percutaneous coronary intervention in ST-segment elevation myocardial infarction patients presenting with cardiogenic shock. *JACC Cardiovasc Interv*. 2018;11:1824–1833. https://doi.org/10.1016/j.jcin.2018.06.030.

4 Clinical Approach to Suspected Acute Coronary Syndrome

DAVID A. MORROW

INTRODUCTION

Chest symptoms suspicious for acute coronary syndrome (ACS) are among the most common reasons for emergency evaluation, accounting for six to seven million or approximately 5% of all emergency department (ED) visits each year in the United States.[1] The initial assessment of nontraumatic chest discomfort is challenging because of the broad range of possible causes (Fig. 4.1). The primary aim of the ED assessment is to rapidly identify the minority of patients whose symptoms are the manifestation of a life-threatening condition that should not be missed and to initiate appropriate therapy. More than 60% of patients who present with chest symptoms suspicious for MI are hospitalized for further testing, and the remainder undergo additional investigation in the ED. However, in most series of unselected populations, only 5% to 15% are ultimately determined to have an ACS, and less than 10% are found to have other life-threatening cardiopulmonary conditions. Therefore, an efficient but effective evaluation of this population of patients that avoids the excessive use of testing and minimizes empiric treatment is important.

Pathways for the triage and management of patients with ST-segment elevation on the presenting electrocardiogram (ECG) are described in Chapter 8. In contrast, strategies for evaluating low-risk patients with a low probability of MI are discussed in Chapter 7. The present chapter provides a general framework for the clinical approach to the assessment of patients with an intermediate or high probability of MI. Risk factors for MI are discussed in Chapter 31. The use of cardiac troponin (cTn) and other biomarkers for risk assessment is considered in Chapter 6. Chapter 6 also provides an in-depth discussion of other clinical tools for risk stratification of the patient with established ACS. Diagnostic imaging in the ED is described in Chapter 5.

GOALS OF THE INITIAL ASSESSMENT OF SUSPECTED ACUTE CORONARY SYNDROME

The fundamental goals of the initial assessment of the patient with chest symptoms suspicious for myocardial ischemia are (1) to assess the probability that the symptoms are caused by underlying myocardial ischemia (diagnosis), and (2) to determine the probability of major cardiovascular complications if the cause of the patient's presentation is myocardial ischemia (risk stratification).[1] These two concurrent probabilistic assessments rely on the clinical history, the physical examination, ECG, and initial cardiac biomarkers, and are intertwined because each of these elements provides information that influences both the diagnostic and prognostic probabilities (see the section on Clinical Approach to the Patient). Together, these two probabilistic assessments guide subsequent diagnostic testing, including the use of invasive coronary angiography, triage, and the initiation of empiric medical therapies while the diagnosis is established (Fig. 4.2).

CAUSES OF CHEST DISCOMFORT

The characteristics of symptoms caused by myocardial ischemia are discussed in this section. The major alternative causes of chest discomfort are summarized in Table 4.1 and described briefly in this section. In general, the initial diagnostic assessment of patients with acute chest discomfort centers around three categories: (1) myocardial ischemia; (2) other cardiopulmonary causes (pericardial disease, aortic emergencies, and pulmonary conditions); and (3) noncardiopulmonary chest pain. High-risk conditions, other than acute MI, to be considered in the differential diagnosis include acute aortic syndrome, pulmonary embolism, tension pneumothorax, and pericarditis with tamponade.

(e.g., >10 minutes) after nitroglycerin points away from myocardial ischemia. Esophageal discomfort can also be relieved by nitroglycerin.

Associated Symptoms

Diaphoresis, dyspnea, nausea, fatigue, faintness, and belching can all accompany chest pain caused by myocardial ischemia, or may exist alone as ischemic equivalents, particularly in women and older adults. Dyspnea is not specific for myocardial ischemia, but the presence of dyspnea as a symptom is important because it points to a cardiopulmonary cause, and when it accompanies myocardial ischemia, is an indicator of a higher risk of fatal complications (see Chapter 6). Sudden onset of significant respiratory distress should prompt consideration of pulmonary embolism and spontaneous pneumothorax. Presentation with syncope or presyncope should raise consideration of hemodynamically significant pulmonary embolism or aortic dissection, as well as ischemic arrhythmias. Although nausea and vomiting suggest a gastrointestinal disorder, these symptoms may occur with an MI (more commonly inferior MI), and are presumably related to vagal reflexes or stimulation of ventricular receptors as part of the Bezold-Jarisch reflex.

Medical History and Review of Systems

The patient should be assessed for risk factors for coronary atherosclerosis and conditions that may predispose the patient to specific other processes that may cause chest discomfort. For example, a history of connective tissue diseases (e.g., Marfan disease) should heighten the clinician's suspicion for an acute aortic syndrome or spontaneous pneumothorax. Review of the medical history should also include surveying for conditions that might contribute to myocardial supply-demand mismatch. Emotional stressors can also be a trigger for ACS.

Physical Examination

The physical examination of patients with chest discomfort can provide indirect evidence for myocardial ischemia by identifying contributors to supply-demand mismatch, such as uncontrolled hypertension, or consequences of ischemia, such as heart failure. In addition, the examination may help to identify specific alternative causes (e.g., pneumothorax or pneumonia) and provide an overall assessment of the clinical stability of the patient (Table 4.2). However, because the physical examination may be normal in patients with unstable ischemic heart disease, an unremarkable physical examination does not reliably exclude ACS as a cause of chest discomfort.

General

Patients with acute ACS often appear anxious, uncomfortable, or diaphoretic. In patients with early complications of MI, cyanosis or pallor may also be evident. Patients who are massaging or clutching their chests may describe their pain with a clenched fist held against the sternum (the Levine sign, named after Dr. Samuel A. Levine). Tachycardia and hypotension in the setting of an ACS are indicative of important hemodynamic consequences of the ACS and should prompt consideration of emerging cardiogenic shock (see Chapter 21) because of impaired left ventricular function or mechanical complications (see Chapter 22). The presence of low-grade fever should not dissuade

TABLE 4.2 Physical Exam Findings in Patients With Chest Pain

CLINICAL SYNDROME	FINDINGS
Emergency	
ACS	Diaphoresis, tachypnea, tachycardia, hypotension, crackles, S3, MR murmur; examination may be normal in uncomplicated cases
PE	Tachycardia and dyspnea among 90% of patients; pain with inspiration
Aortic dissection	Connective tissue disorders (e.g., Marfan syndrome), extremity pulse differential (30% of patients, type A > B) Severe pain, abrupt onset + pulse differential + widened mediastinum on CXR >80% probability of dissection Frequency of syncope >10%, AR 40%–75% (type A)
Esophageal rupture	Emesis, subcutaneous emphysema, pneumothorax (20% patients), unilateral decreased or absent breath sounds
Other	
Noncoronary cardiac: AS, AR, HCM	AS: Characteristic systolic murmur, tardus or parvus carotid pulse AR: Diastolic murmur at right of sternum, rapid carotid upstroke HCM: Increased or displaced left ventricular impulse, prominent *a* wave in jugular venous pressure, systolic murmur
Pericarditis	Fever, pleuritic chest pain increased in supine position, friction rub
Myocarditis	Fever, heart failure, S3
Esophagitis, peptic ulcer disease, gall bladder disease	Epigastric tenderness Right upper quadrant tenderness, Murphy sign
Pneumonia	Fever, localized chest pain, may be pleuritic, friction rub may be present, regional dullness to percussion, egophony
Pneumothorax	Dyspnea and pain on inspiration, unilateral absence of breath sounds
Costochondritis, Tietze syndrome	Tenderness of costochondral joints
Herpes zoster	Pain in dermatomal distribution, triggered by touch; characteristic rash (unilateral and dermatomal distribution)

ACS, Acute coronary syndrome; AR, aortic regurgitation; AS, aortic stenosis; CXR, chest x-ray; HCM, hypertrophic cardiomyopathy; LR, likelihood ratio; MR, mitral regurgitation; PE, pulmonary embolism; and PUD, peptic ulcer disease.

From Writing Committee Members; Gulati M, Levy PD, et al. 2021 AHA/ACC/ASE/CHEST/SAEM/SCCT/SCMR guideline for the evaluation and diagnosis of chest pain: a report of the American College of Cardiology/American Heart Association joint committee on clinical practice guidelines. *J Am Coll Cardiol*. 2021;78:e187–e285.

consideration of MI as a diagnosis, because fevers may occur with acute infarction.

Cardiopulmonary

The jugular venous pulse is often normal in patients with acute ACS. Palpation of the chest may reveal a dyskinetic ventricle in patients with large infarctions or previous MI. Cardiac auscultation may reveal a third or, more commonly, a fourth heart sound, reflecting myocardial systolic or diastolic dysfunction. Murmurs of mitral regurgitation or a harsh murmur of a ventricular septal defect may indicate mechanical complications of MI (see Chapter 22). Murmurs may reveal underlying cardiac disorders that contribute to ischemia (e.g., aortic stenosis or hypertrophic cardiomyopathy). Pericardial friction rubs reflect pericardial inflammation that may occur in late presentations of MI. Findings of pulmonary edema on examination in patients with MI are a harbinger of very poor prognosis (see Chapter 6).

Vascular

Pulse deficits may reflect underlying chronic atherosclerosis, which increases the likelihood of coronary artery disease. However, findings of acute limb ischemia, including loss of the pulse and pallor, particularly in the upper extremities, should prompt consideration and immediate evaluation for aortic dissection. The presence of peripheral artery disease is also an indicator of a higher risk of poor cardiovascular outcomes in the short and long term.

Other Elements of the Examination

The remaining elements of the examination, including the abdominal examination and musculoskeletal evaluation, may reveal evidence for alternative causes of chest discomfort, and thus, are critical components of the evaluation, together with the cardiopulmonary and vascular examinations (Table 4.2). Localized swelling, redness, or marked tenderness of the costochondral and chondrosternal articulations may occur in patients with costochondritis. Pain on palpation of these joints is a useful clinical sign; however, deep palpation may elicit pain in the absence of costochondritis, and chest wall tenderness does not exclude myocardial ischemia.

Electrocardiography

The ECG is pivotal for identifying patients with ongoing ischemia and is valuable for risk stratification (see Fig. 6.5). Professional society guidelines recommend that the first ECG be obtained within 10 minutes of first medical contact (see Chapter 3), with the primary goal of identifying patients with ST-segment elevation diagnostic of STEMI. ST-segment depression and symmetric T-wave inversions at least 0.2 mV in depth are useful for detecting myocardial ischemia in the absence of STEMI and are also indicative of a higher risk of death or recurrent ischemia (see Chapter 6). Serial acquisition of ECGs (e.g., every 15–30 minutes) is recommended in the emergency evaluation of suspected ACS. In addition, an ECG with right-sided lead placement should be considered in patients with a clinical suspicion of ischemia, as well as a nondiagnostic standard 12-lead ECG. Despite the value of ECG, its sensitivity for ischemia is as low as 20% in some studies.[4]

The J-point is used to determine the magnitude of the ST-segment deviation. For diagnosis of STEMI, ST-segment elevation should be present in at least two anatomically related leads. Criteria for diagnostic ST-elevation are listed in Table 2.3. Occasionally, ST-segment shifts caused by myocardial ischemia may meet the criteria in only one lead, with elevation less than the required ST-deviation in a contiguous lead. The clinician should recognize that lesser degrees of ST-deviation or T-wave inversion do not exclude acute myocardial ischemia or evolving MI. ST-segment deviation can be dynamic in the setting of myocardial ischemia. This variability is the rationale for serial recordings of the ECG in patients with a high clinical suspicion of MI and an initially nondiagnostic ECG. Continuous computer-assisted 12-lead ECG recording and ST-segment monitoring may also be useful. An ECG should also be repeated for patients with recurrence of symptoms after an asymptomatic interval. The evolution of ST-T waveforms and development of Q waves, when present, assist the clinician in estimating the time from the onset of the event, identifying the infarct-related artery, and gauging the amount of myocardium at risk. Each of these elements is also useful for assessing prognosis (see Chapter 6). More profound ST-segment deviation or T-wave inversion involving multiple leads and vascular territories is associated with a worse prognosis. The ECG may also detect the onset of arrhythmias, or intraventricular and atrioventricular conduction delays, which are discussed in Chapter 23.

Abnormalities of the ST segment and T wave may occur in a variety of conditions other than MI, including pulmonary embolism, ventricular hypertrophy, acute and chronic pericarditis, myocarditis, electrolyte imbalance, and metabolic disorders. ST-deviation may also be present in patients with chronic conditions such as left ventricular hypertrophy, left bundle branch block, Brugada syndrome, stress cardiomyopathy, and early repolarization patterns. Hyperventilation occurring in patients with panic disorder can also lead to nonspecific ST- and T-wave abnormalities. Q waves may occur because of myocardial fibrosis and cardiomyopathy in the absence of coronary artery disease.

Cardiac Biomarkers

Laboratory testing in patients with chest symptoms suspicious for ACS focuses on the detection of myocardial injury and the diagnosis of MI (see Chapter 2). In some cases, biomarkers that reflect the underlying contributors (e.g., inflammation) or consequences of ischemia (e.g., increased wall stress and end-diastolic pressures) may be useful (see Chapter 6). Because the biomarker offers high sensitivity and specificity for myocardial tissue, cardiac troponin (cTnI or cTnT) is the preferred biomarker to detect or exclude myocardial injury. High-sensitivity assays for cTn are widely commercially available and are preferred over prior generation assays because they facilitate more rapid detection or exclusion of myocardial injury and increase overall diagnostic accuracy.[1] Creatine kinase-MB does not add to cTn for the diagnostic assessment of these patients

HEART Score		
History	Highly suspicious Moderately suspicious Slightly suspicious	2 1 0
ECG	Significant ST-depression Nonspecific abnormality Normal	2 1 0
Age	≥65 years >45–<65 years ≤45 years	2 1 0
Risk factors	≥3 risk factors 1–2 risk factors None	2 1 0
Troponin (serial)	≥3 x 99th percentile 1–<3 x 99th percentile ≤99th percentile	2 1 0
	TOTAL	
	Low risk: 0–3 **Not low risk:** ≥4	

North American Chest Pain Rule	
High-risk criteria	**Y/N**
Typical symptoms of ischemia	
ECG: acute ischemic changes	
Age ≥50 years	
Known coronary artery disease	
Troponin (serial) >99th percentile	
Low risk: All no **Not low risk:** Any yes	

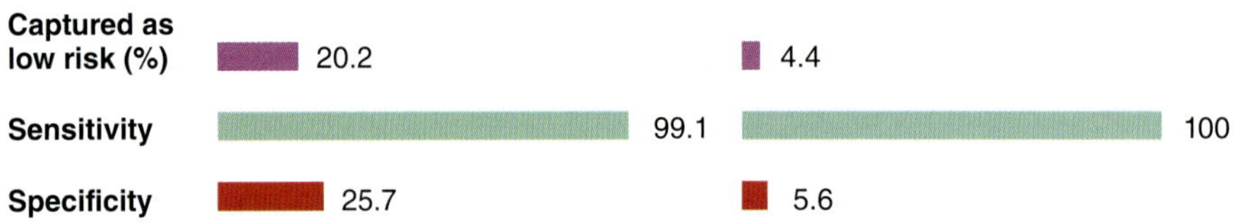

FIG. 4.6 Decision aids used in conjunction with serial measurement of cardiac troponin for evaluation of acute chest pain. *ECG*, Electrocardiography. (Data from Mahler SA, Miller CD, Hollander JE, et al. Identifying patients for early discharge: performance of decision rules among patients with acute chest pain. *Int J Cardiol.* 2013;168:795–802.)

and should not be used (Class 3:No benefit) for the assessment of suspected ACS.[1]

Professional society guidelines recommend using evidence-based clinical decision-pathways (CDPs) for the assessment of patients presenting with symptoms suspicious for ACS in order to classify their presentation as low-, intermediate-, or high-risk of a final diagnosis of ACS and short-term major cardiovascular events.[1] Most such CDPs incorporate cTn as a critical element (Fig. 4.6). An American College of Cardiology Expert Consensus Panel has provided an overview of how to apply a cTn-based CDP in clinical practice (Fig. 4.7).[5] For patients undergoing measurement of cTn for suspected ACS, serial cTn should be measured at presentation (time zero) and 1 to 3 hours for high-sensitivity assays and 3 to 6 hours later for conventional cTn assays. For patients with acute chest symptoms suspicious for ACS with onset at least 2–3 hours prior to ED arrival, a single high-sensitivity cTn value below an evidence-based decision limit (usually the limit of quantification) may be reasonable to exclude myocardial injury.[6] The use of cardiac biomarkers to identify low-risk patients with chest symptoms is discussed in additional detail in Chapter 7. Because the evidence-based decision-limits, level of detection, level of quantification, 99th percentile upper reference limit, analytical precision, and criteria for a significant delta are assay-specific and vary between cTn assays from different manufacturers, clinicians should be familiar with these analytical performance properties for the assay(s) that they use in their practice.[1,6] For patients with recurrent symptoms that are suspicious for ischemia, later serial measurements (e.g., 3 hours after symptom recurrence) should be considered in most cases. Moreover, in patients for whom the pretest probability of acute myocardial ischemia is particularly high, additional evaluation is warranted even if the initial cardiac biomarkers are not elevated above the 99th percentile URL. It is not necessary or advisable to measure cTn in patients without suspicion for ACS, unless it is being used for the specific purpose of risk stratification, such as in pulmonary embolism or heart failure.

Because of the higher negative predictive value of high-sensitivity assays for cTn, there is a tradeoff for detecting myocardial injury in a larger proportion of patients with non-ACS cardiopulmonary conditions than with the previous generations of assays. Because of this evolution in the analytical sensitivity, other aspects of the clinical evaluation are critical for the physician to formulate a probability that the symptoms represent ACS. In addition, the evaluation of serial values of cTn for evidence of a dynamic (rising and/or falling) pattern is important in discriminating acute causes of myocardial injury from chronic elevation caused by underlying structural heart disease, end-stage renal disease, or interfering antibodies (see Chapter 2).[4,7] Although it is sometimes challenging to diagnostically discriminate among these causes of myocardial injury, the finding of an elevated concentration of cTn is virtually always associated with a poorer prognosis; however, when it is the result of a chronic condition causing myocardial injury, the time course of that risk is over the long term and may warrant

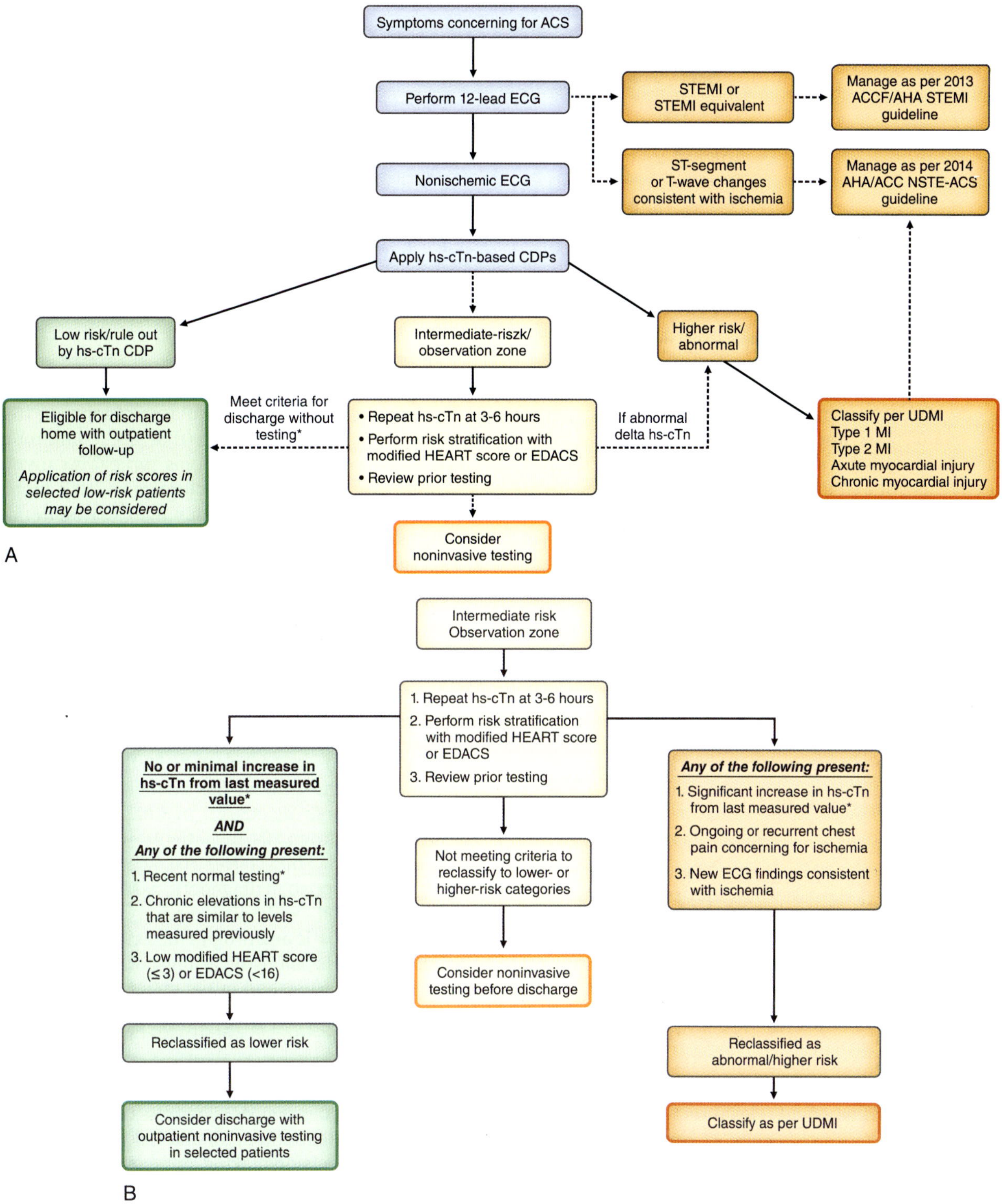

FIG. 4.7 Pathway for evaluation of suspected acute coronary syndrome using cardiac troponin-based clinical decision pathways. (A) Overall framework integrating cardiac troponin-based clinical decision pathways (CDPs). *Unchanged high-sensitivity troponin concentration (i.e., no or minimal change over serial measurements) with (1) recent normal testing (i.e., invasive or CT coronary angiogram <2 years ago or stress test <1 year ago); (2) symptoms inconsistent with possible ACS; (3) chronic elevations in hs-cTn that are unchanged compared with levels measured previously; or (4) a modified HEART score #3 or EDACS <16. ACC, American College Cardiology; ACS, acute coronary syndrome; AHA, American Heart Association; ECG, electrocardiogram; EDACS, emergency department assessment of chest pain score; HEART, history, ECG, age, risk factors, and troponin; hs-cTn, high-sensitivity cardiac troponin; MI, myocardial infarction; NSTE-ACS, non-ST-segment elevation acute coronary syndrome; STEMI, ST-segment elevation myocardial infarction; UDMI, universal definition of MI. (B) Algorithm for intermediate risk patients. *Evidence-based criteria do not exist to define change thresholds for hs-cTn at the 3- to 6-hour timepoint. Although a 20% relative change from the baseline measurement has been proposed to define significant change, this threshold lacks specificity at low hs-cTn values in part due to assay imprecision. Thus, at lower hs-cTn values near the sex-specific 99th percentile URL values, absolute changes should be used to define clinically-significant change, whereas at higher cTn values, a 20% relative change in values may be a more reasonable threshold. Clinical judgment is needed to interpret small fluctuations in hs-cTn values over serial measurements, as these small changes may reflect assay imprecision rather than acute cardiac injury. †Recent normal testing is considered an invasive or CT coronary angiogram <2 years without evidence of coronary plaque or a stress test <1 year without ischemia. (From Writing Committee; Kontos MC, de Lemos JA, et al. 2022 ACC expert consensus decision pathway on the evaluation and disposition of acute chest pain in the emergency department: a report of the American College of Cardiology solution set oversight committee. *J Am Coll Cardiol.* 2022;80:1925–1960.)

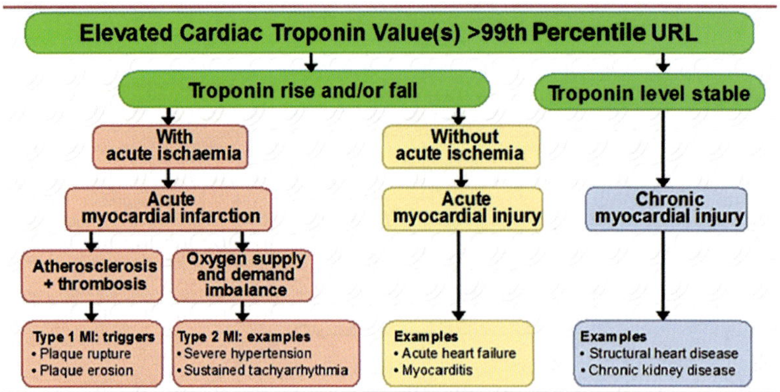

FIG. 4.8 Model for interpretation of myocardial injury and myocardial infarction. (From Thygesen K, Alpert JS, Jaffe AS, et al. Fourth universal definition of myocardial infarction. *J Am Coll Cardiol.* 2018;72:2231–2264.)

disease-modifying preventive therapies rather than acute invasive evaluations and interventions.[4,7] A structured approach to classifying myocardial injury is essential to the effective use of cTn for the evaluation of patients with suspected ACS (Fig. 4.8).[4]

Chest Radiography

The chest radiograph is often unremarkable in patients with ACS. When present, pulmonary edema is a poor prognostic indicator. The chest radiograph is useful for excluding other potential causes of chest symptoms. Specific findings include pulmonary parenchymal processes, widening of the mediastinum in some patients with aortic dissection, Hampton hump or Westermark sign in patients with pulmonary embolism, or pericardial calcification in chronic pericarditis.

Formulating a Clinical Probability of Acute Coronary Syndrome

Ultimately, the clinician must formulate a clinical impression of the probability that a patient's symptoms represent an ACS. In patients with ST-segment elevation that meet diagnostic criteria (see Table 2.3), the probability of ACS is extremely high, although up to 5% of such patients will end up having ACS excluded (see Chapter 2). Among patients without ST-segment elevation, establishing an initial diagnosis is more challenging. The clinician relies on the history, physical examination, and ECG with interpretation of cardiac biomarkers in that clinical context. Appropriate interpretation of cTn, which is a marker of myocardial injury that is not specific to ischemia, requires a "pretest" assessment of the likelihood that the patient's symptoms represent myocardial ischemia (Fig. 4.8). Clinical experience and sound judgment continue to play a critical role in the evaluation of patients with suspected ACS.

Because of the inherent challenges and high clinical stakes, multiple clinical algorithms have been developed to aid in decision-making during the assessment and triage of patients with chest pain suspicious for myocardial ischemia (see Fig. 4.6). Such decision aids are most commonly used to identify patients with low clinical probability of ACS who are candidates either for early provocative testing for ischemia or discharge from the ED (see Chapter 7). Elements that are common across these tools include (1) symptoms typical for myocardial ischemia, (2) known atherosclerosis or risk factors for atherosclerosis, including older age, (3) ischemic ECG abnormalities, and (4) elevated cTn. Reflecting their lack of specificity, the overall diagnostic performance of such decision aids is poor (area under the receiver-operating curve 0.55–0.65). However, the negative predictive performance of some such instruments is very high (>99%).[1] Nevertheless, no such decision aid (or single clinical factor) is sufficiently sensitive and well validated to use as a sole tool for clinical decisions.

Clinicians should differentiate between the diagnostic algorithms discussed previously in this chapter and in Chapter 7 and the clinical risk scores (e.g., the TIMI and GRACE risk scores discussed in Chapter 6) derived for assessment of prognosis in patients with an established diagnosis of ACS. These latter risk scores were not developed for the purpose of diagnostic assessment.

In conjunction with formulation of the previously described diagnostic and prognostic estimates, the clinician must also make decisions regarding additional testing, noninvasive and invasive, and initial empiric therapy. Because delay of treatment in patients with ACS is associated with adverse outcomes, timely initiation of therapy is a priority. As such, treatment, such as aspirin and an anticoagulant, is often initiated in patients with suspected ACS while diagnostic testing continues. Fig. 4.2 illustrates the interplay of the assessment of likelihood of MI and risk status with respect to therapeutic decision-making. For example, a patient with a low probability of ACS, but with a high-risk profile should the patient have unstable ischemic heart disease, may be treated similarly to a patient with a moderate probability of ACS who is at moderate risk of complications. Patients with a moderate or greater suspicion for ACS or who are at high risk, and in whom ACS has not been excluded, warrant initiation of treatment (see Fig. 4.2).

DECISIONS REGARDING ADDITIONAL TESTING

Invasive Coronary Evaluation

Patients with ST-segment elevation and a clinical presentation consistent with ischemia should undergo emergent

TABLE 4.3 Clinical Considerations for the Use of Non-invasive Testing for Coronary Artery Disease in Patients With Suspected Acute Coronary Syndrome

ISCHEMIA TEST MODALITY	STRENGTHS	LIMITATIONS	PATIENT CONSIDERATIONS FAVORING ITS USE
Exercise stress ECG	• Low cost • Wide availability • Assessment of exercise symptoms, capacity • No ionizing radiation	• Decreased accuracy compared with anatomical and stress-imaging tests • Requires interpretable ECG and ability to exercise sufficiently	• Rarely recommended as a stand-alone test due to frequent known CAD, inability to exercise, or significant arrhythmias
Stress echocardiography	• Wide availability • High diagnostic specificity • Assessment of ventricular and valvular function • No ionizing radiation	• Decreased sensitivity compared with anatomical and other stress-imaging tests • Dependent on good image quality • Requires dobutamine in patients unable to exercise	• Known good image quality and ability to exercise • Consider use of an ultrasound-enhancing agent to improve endocardial visualization • Known moderate or severe valvular disease
Stress/rest SPECT	• Wide availability • Relatively high diagnostic sensitivity • Assessment of ventricular function	• Increased artifacts resulting in nondiagnostic results and decreased diagnostic accuracy compared with stress/rest PET • Radiation exposure	• Known CAD or high CAC burden on chest • CT imaging • Preferred over stress echocardiography in patients who cannot exercise or who do not have significant bronchospastic disease
Stress/rest PET	• High diagnostic accuracy • Lower radiation exposure than SPECT • Measures myocardial blood flow and flow reserve • Assessment of ventricular function	• Limited availability • Relatively higher cost • Lack of exercise assessment	• Known CAD or high CAC burden on chest CT imaging • Preferred over SPECT due to higher diagnostic accuracy and lower rate of nondiagnostic test results
Stress CMR	• High diagnostic accuracy • Accurate assessment of chamber sizes, ventricular and valvular function • Diagnosis of prior infarction, scar, fibrosis • Measurement of myocardial blood flow and flow reserve is possible but not widely available currently • No ionizing radiation	• Limited availability • Relatively higher cost • Lack of exercise assessment • Long scan acquisition times • Claustrophobia • Often not immediately available to patients with pacemakers or ICDs • Contraindicated in patients with significant renal dysfunction	• Known CAD and/or cardiomyopathy • Elevated troponin not thought to be secondary to ACS • Known moderate or severe valvular disease • No significant renal dysfunction
Coronary CTA	• High diagnostic accuracy • Does not require exercise • Identifies nonobstructive CAD	• Radiation exposure • Lack of exercise assessment • Contraindicated in patients with significant renal dysfunction • Blooming artifacts when significant coronary calcification present • Atrial fibrillation or other arrhythmias • May require beta-blockade • Incidental noncardiac findings	• No known CAD • Absence of severe coronary calcification • Prior normal, mildly abnormal, or inconclusive stress test results • No known iodinated contrast medium allergy or significant renal dysfunction • Low likelihood of high-quality stress testing or lack of timely access

ACS, Acute coronary syndrome; *CAC,* coronary artery calcium; *CAD,* coronary artery disease; *CMR,* cardiovascular magnetic resonance; *CT,* computed tomography; *CTA,* computed tomography angiography; *ECG,* electrocardiogram; *ICD,* implantable cardioverter defibrillator; *PET,* positron emission tomography; *SPECT,* single-photon emission computed tomography.

From Writing Committee; Kontos MC, de Lemos JA, et al. 2022 ACC expert consensus decision pathway on the evaluation and disposition of acute chest pain in the emergency department: a report of the American College of Cardiology solution set oversight committee. *J Am Coll Cardiol.* 2022;80:1925–1960.

cardiac catheterization when available in a timely fashion in an experienced STEMI center (see Chapter 3 and Chapter 8). Decision-making regarding invasive coronary angiography in patients without diagnostic ST-segment elevation is discussed in Chapter 11. In general, patients with refractory symptoms or high-risk features should undergo coronary angiography for treatment if a diagnosis of ACS has been established or for completion of the diagnostic assessment when an alternative cause has not been identified. In patients at lower risk or in whom patient preferences or appropriateness for coronary angiography do not favor invasive evaluation, additional non-invasive assessment may be useful to establish the diagnosis and for risk assessment.

Non-invasive Testing for Ischemia

Exercise ECG with or without imaging has historically been used for completion of risk stratification in patients who have undergone an initial evaluation that has not revealed a specific cause of chest discomfort and has identified them as having a low, or in some cases intermediate, probability of ACS. However, although early exercise testing is safe in patients without high-risk findings after 8 to 12 hours of observation, professional society guidelines now recommend that in low-risk patients, urgent diagnostic testing for suspected coronary artery disease is *not* needed (see Chapter 7).[1] Rather, present guidelines for the evaluation of chest pain emphasize that it is patients who

In support of this notion, a study demonstrated high negative predictive value for cCTA among patients with NSTEACS. The VERDICT (Very Early Versus Deferred Invasive Evaluation Using Computerized Tomography in Patients with Acute Coronary Syndromes) trial studied 1023 patients randomized to early (within 12 hours) versus standard-timing (48–72 hours) of ICA. As an observational component of the trial, cCTA was performed prior to ICA in both groups. Independent of the randomization arm assignment, as well as patient and clinical characteristics, cCTA was demonstrated to have a high negative predictive value (90.0%, 95%CI: 86.8%–94.1%), though numerically somewhat lower than prior reports, to rule out significant CAD in patients with NSTEACS.[13] Compared to prior studies, the performance metrics of cCTA did not appear influenced by studying a higher-risk population; in fact, among the subgroup of patients with higher clinical risk (GRACE score >140) representing 74% of this population, the negative predictive value remained high (95.1%, 95%CI:87.8%–98.6%).

In a secondary analysis of the VERDICT trial, the prognostic value of cCTA-based risk assessment was compared to the gold standard ICA.[14] In a subset of 978 patients, the primary endpoint (composite of all-cause death non-fatal recurrent MI, hospitalization for refractory myocardial ischemia, and heart failure) occurred in 21.3% over a median of 4.2 years of follow-up. Obstructive CAD identified by cCTA was associated with an increased risk for events when compared to those with nonobstructive CAD (HR: 1.74, 95%CI 1.22–2.49). The investigators describe a similar ability of cCTA to identify patients with obstructive disease when compared to ICA. These results are in line with the results of a meta-analysis pooling data of approximately 120,000 patients, in which the presence of ≥50% stenosis severity by cCTA was associated with worse outcomes compared to nonobstructive CAD, although the cCTA findings were not contrasted to ICA.

Smulders et al., randomized 207 patients who had ruled in for NSTEACS but were clinically stable to 1 of 3 evaluation strategies—cCTA, cardiac MRI or usual care expected to involve ICA in most patients, with the primary endpoint being referral to ICA and secondary endpoint being 1-year outcome, with the hypothesis that screening prior to ICA by these advanced noninvasive imaging modalities would reduce the need for ICA at no adverse expense to outcome.[15] Referral to ICA was reduced significantly in both the cCTA and CMR groups compared to usual care (66%, 87%, and 100%, respectively) with similar 1-year outcomes (though with wide confidence intervals given the small size of the trial). The efficiency of finding obstructive CAD at ICA was highest in the cCTA group.

Therefore, compelling data for safety and accuracy support a potentially more prominent role of cCTA imaging in the work up of higher risk patients with biomarker-proven NSTEACS, particularly in the role of a gatekeeper to ICA. However, attractive attributes of the clinical impact of cCTA imaging, such as reduced hospital stay and costs when compared to standard of care, demonstrated among lower risk patients with suspected ACS are not yet proven for this higher risk patient population and warrants further investigations.

CAD-RADS for Reporting Coronary Artery Disease in Acute Chest Pain

The Coronary Artery Disease Reporting and Data System (CAD-RADS) was first released in 2016 and was reiterated in 2022 with the purpose to establish standardized reporting of coronary CTA and to provide clinical management recommendations based on coronary CTA findings to improve communication between the referring and reporting physicians and to standardize care based on coronary CT findings.[16]

CAD-RADS reports the greatest degree stenosis on a per patient basis and suggests clinical management based on reported severity (Table 5.3). It categorizes stenosis into 6 possible categories ranging from CAD-RADS 0 (complete absence of coronary artery disease) to CAD-RADS 5 (total occlusion of at least one vessel), as well as allows classification for non-diagnostic evaluation (CAD-RADS N). It also allows for distinction between high and very high-risk CAD phenotype (CADRADS 4 A and B) by differentiating single vessel obstructive versus multivessel or left main stenosis. In the most recent iteration of CAD-RADS, there is distinction on management recommendations based on the extent of underlying CAD (P1 and P2 mild to moderate amount of plaque in 1 to 2 vessels versus P3 and P4 severe to extensive amount of plaque in 2 to 3 vessels). Further, modifiers are used to denote specific findings, including modifier I for ischemia, modifier S for stent in situ, modifier G for status post CABG and modifier HRP for two or more high-risk features (i.e., positive remodeling, napkin-ring sign, low attenuation plaque, and spotty calcification) (Fig. 5.3).

Beyond a clear value in standardizing reporting and care, CAD-RADS facilitates the standardization of cCTA reporting in clinical trials. In a recent analysis, the prognostic value of CAD-RADS was assessed among 1492 low- to intermediate-risk patients presenting to the ED with acute chest pain.[17] Authors reported 7% MACE rate over a median of 31.5-month follow-up period and concluded that CAD-RADS based prognostic assessment significantly improved risk estimation and conferred incremental prognostic value compared to CAC scoring, independent of traditional cardiovascular risk factors.

Advanced cCTA Assessment

Atheroma Characterization

When assessing coronary artery plaque anatomy, the standard practice is to report stenosis severity rooted in the standard nomenclature of the ICA diagnosis of CAD, which for many years has been based simply on luminal obstruction. However, an increasingly recognized advantage of cCTA is its ability to assess coronary plaque morphology and components. As recognized by invasive intravascular imaging studies, coronary plaque characterization beyond stenosis severity holds important prognostic information. cCTA derived qualitative plaque characteristics of plaque composition (i.e., calcified, noncalcified, and mixed plaque types, Fig. 5.4) and vulnerability, including positive remodeling, low attenuation plaque components, the napkin-ring sign and spotty calcification are associated with current

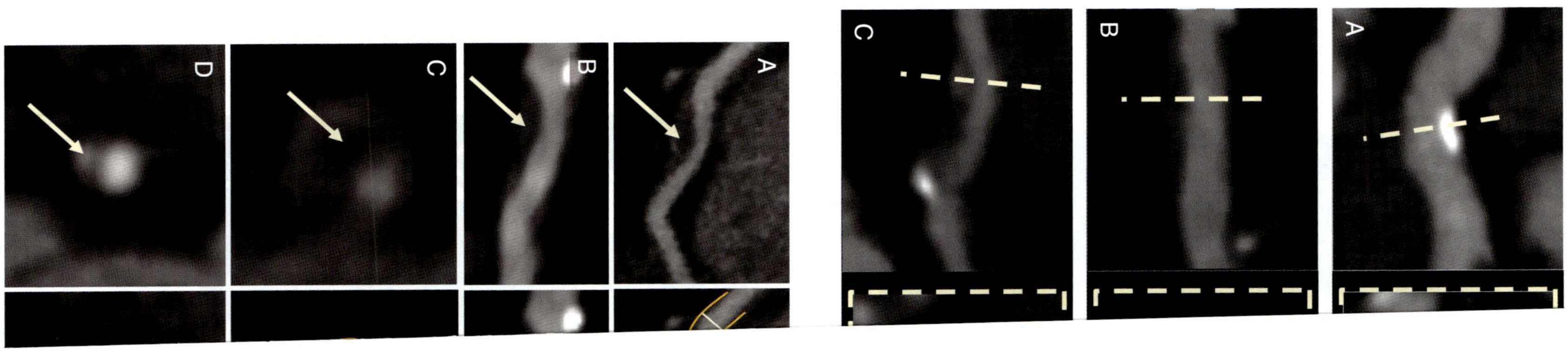

FIG. 5.5 High-risk plaque features as ca
represent the outer wall of the coronary
sent the luminal wall of the coronary arte
plaques. Panel A: Plaque with positive rem
plaque. The *blue circle* indicates the regi
Unit measurement. Panel C: Napkin-ring s
necrotic core. Panel D: Plaque with spotty
cates the spotty calcification. *ROI*, Region o

TABLE 5.3 Coronary Artery Disease Reporting and Data System for Patients Presenting with Acute Chest Pain

CATEGORY	DEGREE OF MAXIMAL CORONARY STENOSIS	INTERPRETATION	FURTHER CARDIAC INVESTIGATION	MANAGEMENT CONSIDERATION
CAD-RADS 0	0% (no plaque or stenosis)	ACS highly unlikely	No further evaluation of ACS is required. If Tn (+) consider other sources of increased troponin	Reassurance.
CAD-RADS 1	1%–24% (minimal stenosis or plaque with no stenosis)	ACS unlikely	No further evaluation of ACS is required. If Tn (+) consider other sources of increased troponin	Nonextensive CAD, i.e., P1 and P2 (1 or 2 vessel involvement): referral for outpatient follow-up for risk factor modification and preventive pharmacotherapy. Extensive disease, i.e., P3 and P4 (3 vessel with moderate to severe amount of CAD): referral for outpatient follow-up for aggressive risk factor modification and preventive pharmacotherapy.
CAD-RADS 2	25%–49% (Mild stenosis)	ACS less likely	No further evaluation of ACS is required. If clinical suspicion of ACS is high, Tn (+) or HRP features, consider hospital admission with cardiology consultation.	Non extensive CAD, i.e., P1 and P2 (1 or 2 vessel involvement): referral for outpatient follow-up for risk factor modification and preventive pharmacotherapy. Extensive disease i.e., P3 and P4 (3 vessel with moderate to severe amount of CAD): referral for outpatient follow-up for aggressive risk factor modification and preventive pharmacotherapy.
CAD-RADS 3	50%–69% (Moderate stenosis)	ACS possible	Consider hospital admission with cardiology consultation. Consider functional assessment, including FFR-CT, CTP, stress testing (ETT, stress echocardiogram, SPECT, PET, cardiac MRI).	Independent of CAD extent (i.e., P1, P2, P3, and P4) preventive management, including aggressive preventive pharmacotherapy. Other treatments, including anti-anginal therapies, should be considered per guideline-directed care. Consider revascularization if ischemia testing was positive (I+ modifier).
CAD-RADS 4A	70%––99% stenosis	ACS likely	Hospital admission with cardiology consultation. Consider ICA or functional assessment, including FFR-CT, CTP, stress testing (ETT, stress echocardiogram, SPECT, PET, cardiac MRI).	Independent of CAD extent (i.e., P1, P2, P3, and P4) preventive management, including aggressive preventive pharmacotherapy. Other treatments, including anti-anginal therapies and options for revascularization, should be considered per guideline-directed care.
CAD-RADS 4B	Left main ≥50% or 3 vessel obstructive (≥70%) disease	ACS likely		Independent of CAD extent (i.e., P1, P2, P3, and P4) preventive management, including aggressive preventive pharmacotherapy. Other treatments, including anti-anginal therapies and options for revascularization, should be considered per guideline-directed care.
CAD-RADS 5	100% (total occlusion)	ACS very likely	Hospital admission with cardiology consultation. Expedited ICA and revascularization if acute occlusion suspected (unless occlusion identifies to be chronic through CT imaging and clinical characteristics or patient history)	Independent of CAD extent preventive management, including aggressive preventive pharmacotherapy. Other treatments, including anti-anginal therapies and options for revascularization, should be considered per guideline-directed care.
CAD-RADS N	Non-diagnostic	ACS cannot be excluded	Additional or alternative evaluation for ACS is needed.	

ACS, Acute coronary syndrome; *CAD*, coronary artery disease; *CTP*, computed tomography perfusion; *ETT*, Exercise tolerance test; *FFR-CT*, CT base fractional flow reserve measurement; *HRP*, high-risk plaque; *MRI*, magnetic resonance imaging; *PET*, positron emission tomography; *SPECT*, single-photon emission positron tomography.
P1–4 refers to the extent of CAD in the coronary arteries (P1–2: mild to moderate amount of plaque in 1 to 2 vessels; P3–4: severe to extensive amount of plaque in 2 to 3 vessels).

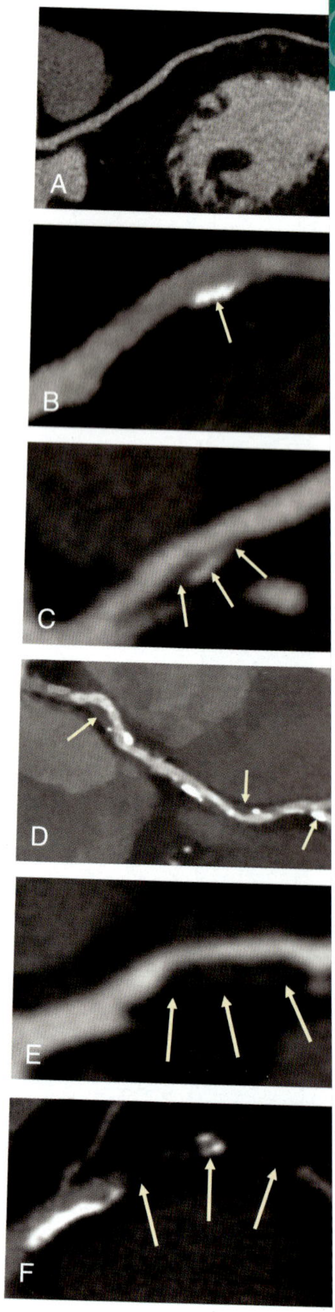

FIG. 5.3 Illustration of the assessme Artery Disease Reporting and Data Sys acute chest pain, which are based on th stenosis in coronary arteries with grea ter. Panel A: No plaque. Panel B: Plaq C: Plaque with mild stenosis. Panel D: Panel E: Obstructive plaque. Panel F: Oc

and future coronary events (Fig. of the ROMICAT II trial, vulnera associated with a 9-fold increas among low- to intermediate-risk acute chest pain independent of ical characteristics. Moreover, C plaques were better predictors o ventionally used in intravascular

While not yet widely reporte rapid development of more auto for cCTA images and the potential

6 Risk Stratification in Acute Coronary Syndromes

ANDREW T. YAN, DEREK P. CHEW, AND SHAUN G. GOODMAN

INTRODUCTION

Acute coronary syndrome (ACS), including unstable angina, non-ST-elevation myocardial infarction (NSTEMI), and ST-elevation myocardial infarction (STEMI) encompasses a disease spectrum with a variable prognosis (see Chapter 2). Multiple studies have consistently demonstrated a temporal trend toward improving clinical outcomes over the past decade, in association with the increasing use of pharmacological and interventional treatment in ACS.[1] However, a subset of high-risk patients still sustain a high rate of death and major adverse cardiovascular events, both in the short and long term. Effective risk stratification is essential to inform patients and families and to select the most appropriate treatment for the individual patient. Nevertheless, risk prediction at the bedside is challenging because it requires the simultaneous consideration of numerous interrelated prognostic factors.[2]

This chapter aims to provide an in-depth overview of *initial* risk stratification at the bedside among patients with a clinical diagnosis of ACS. Subsequent and further refinement of risk assessment in hospitals (invasive management and noninvasive imaging) will be the subject of other chapters (see Chapters 10 and 14). Herein, we will first discuss the clinical relevance of risk stratification and the rationale for accurate risk assessment in optimal ACS management. The prognostic utility of history, physical examination, electrocardiogram, and cardiac biomarkers will be reviewed. An integrated approach to ACS risk assessment using validated risk scores will be emphasized, together with some guiding principles for the interpretation of these risk assessment tools and recent randomized controlled trial data. Finally, we will identify some existing knowledge gaps and glimpse at future research directions to address them.

NEED FOR ACCURATE RISK STRATIFICATION

Patients with ACS may present along a continuum of severity, with short- and long-term risks governed by a complex interplay of underlying coronary artery disease, cardiac function, cardiovascular risk factors, and noncardiac comorbidities. While prompt reperfusion therapy is generally indicated for the vast majority of patients with STEMI, non-ST-elevation acute coronary syndrome (NSTE-ACS) is a more heterogeneous condition requiring a more tailored rather than "one size fits all" management. For example, both the TIMACS and VERDICT trials showed that early coronary angiography is more effective among high-risk NSTE-ACS patients with a GRACE risk score >140, as compared with the low and intermediate risk groups (P for interaction = .01 and .023, respectively).[3] Even for treatments with the same relative risk reduction (i.e., no treatment heterogeneity) regardless of baseline risk, a greater absolute risk reduction (hence a smaller number needed to treat) is expected among patients at the highest baseline risk, thereby helping to identify those patients who gain the most from intensive treatment. This paradigm has important implications on the cost effectiveness of treatment and timely access to care and can enhance the triage of ACS patients, especially in healthcare systems where resources are scarce and early invasive treatment may not be readily available. In addition, a larger absolute benefit of treatment may outweigh treatment or procedural risk, such that the treatment benefit:risk ratio may remain acceptable or even favorable for the individual patient (personalized medicine). Furthermore, risk assessment is needed to inform patients and families in weighing the competing risks and benefits of treatment options, thereby facilitating shared decision making that takes into consideration their own values and preferences (patient-centered

TABLE 6.1 Summary of Validated Risk Scores in Acute Coronary Syndromes

RISK SCORE	TIMI STEMI	TIMI UA/NSTEMI	GRACE[a]	PURSUIT	FRISC	OASIS	ACTION-GWTG	EMMACE
Derivation Dataset	Clinical Trial	Clinical Trial	Registry	Clinical Trial	Clinical Trial	Clinical Trial	Registry	Registry
Validation Dataset	Clinical Trial	Clinical Trial	Clinical Trial					
C-Statistic Development	0.779	Death or MI 0.66	Death 0.81 Death or MI 0.76	Death 0.814 Death or MI: 0.669	Death 0.77 Death or MI 0.70	CV Death, MI, Stroke 0.71	In-hospital death 0.88	30-day Death 0.79
C-Statistic Validation	0.746		Death 0.82					0.76
Components								
Demographic	Age, Weight	Age	Age	Age, Gender	Age	Age, Sex	Age	Age
Clinical History	DM, HTN, Angina	>3 risk factors, Known CAD, Prior ASA, Angina frequency		Angina Severity	Prior MI, diabetes	Prior MI/ Stroke		
Hemodynamic	HR, SBP, Killip Class		HR, SBP, Killip Class, Cardiac Arrest	Heart Failure			HR, SBP, Killip Class, Cardiac Arrest	HR, SBP
Cardiac	Anterior ST elevation/ LBBB	ST Changes	ST Changes	ST depression	ST depression		ST elevation	
Extra-cardiac			Creatinine				Creatinine	
Biomarkers		Myocardial Injury	Myocardial Injury		Myocardial injury Inflammatory	Myocardial Injury NT-proBNP, HBA1c	Myocardial injury	
Care	Delay >4 h							

[a]Mini-GRACE allows an estimate of risk when Killip class or creatinine are not known. GRACE 3.0 represents Machine machine-learning-based estimate of risk using the same variables.

From Haghbayan H, Gale CP, Chew DP, et al. Clinical risk prediction models for the prognosis and management of acute coronary syndromes. *Eur Heart J Qual Care Clin Outcomes*. 2021;7:222–228.

care).[4] Therefore, proper risk stratification is fundamental to the optimal management of ACS.

Despite the need to individualize ACS treatment according to risk, multiple studies have demonstrated a treatment-risk paradox in real-world practice, where high-risk patients are paradoxically managed more conservatively, with an associated worse outcome. While there might be a myriad of (potentially legitimate) reasons for this under-treatment (e.g., noncardiac comorbidities or patient preferences), data suggest that an under-recognition of the weight of various prognosticators by physicians may contribute to risk underestimation of ACS, when compared to objective clinical prediction models. While treating physicians may consider one or a few characteristics at a time, integrating multiple independent predictors of clinical outcomes simultaneously is challenging and only achievable via multivariable modeling.

DEMOGRAPHICS AND CLINICAL HISTORY

Age

Adults ≥75 years of age constitute approximately 30% to 40% of all ACS hospitalizations and account for the majority of ACS-related death. The higher age-related prevalence of risk factors and cumulative atherosclerotic burden leading to more extensive and complex coronary disease, compounded by geriatric syndromes, including multimorbidity and frailty, worsen the short- and long-term outcomes after ACS.[5] Aging is associated with declining kidney function, which in turn impacts ACS outcomes. Frailty confers significant prognostic value for mortality and morbidity in elderly ACS patients.[6] For example, the prevalence of frailty increases with age, and frailty is associated with higher mortality, longer length of stay, bleeding, and readmission after ACS.

Advanced age is the single powerful prognosticator in ACS and is incorporated in most common risk-prediction tools (Table 6.1; Figs. 6.1–6.3), including TIMI and GRACE risk scores. Its prognostic value is more pronounced in acute MI than in unstable angina. Notwithstanding, the importance of age tends to be underappreciated by clinicians using subjective global risk assessment. Moreover, among the more selected elderly patients in clinical trials, an early invasive strategy has been shown to reduce MI.[7] Thus, a systematic risk-assessment tool may mitigate this bias against chronological age.

Sex

As compared with men, women with ACS often present at an older age and have a higher burden of cardiovascular risk factors and comorbid conditions. Furthermore, women more often have less typical awareness of symptoms and seek medical attention later after symptom onset.[8] Registry data suggest that women more frequently had traditional risk factors but were less likely to receive

1. Find Points for Each Predictive Factor:

Killip Class	Points	SBP, mm Hg	Points	Heart Rate, Beats/min	Points	Age, y	Points	Creatinine Level, mg/dL	Points
I	0	≤80	58	≤50	0	≤30	0	0-0.39	1
II	20	80-99	53	50-69	3	30-39	8	0.40-0.79	4
III	39	100-119	43	70-89	9	40-49	25	0.80-1.19	7
IV	59	120-139	34	90-109	15	50-59	41	1.20-1.59	10
		140-159	24	110-149	24	60-69	58	1.60-1.99	13
		160-199	10	150-199	38	70-79	75	2.00-3.99	21
		≥200	0	≥200	46	80-89	91	>4.0	28
						≥90	100		

Other Risk Factors	Points
Cardiac Arrest at Admission	39
ST-Segment Deviation	28
Elevated Cardiac Enzyme Levels	14

2. Sum Points for All Predictive Factors:

Killip Class + SBP + Heart Rate + Age + Creatinine Level + Cardiac Arrest at Admission + ST-Segment Deviation + Elevated Cardiac Enzyme Levels = Total Points

3. Look Up Risk Corresponding to Total Points:

Total Points	≤60	70	80	90	100	110	120	130	140	150	160	170	180	190	200	210	220	230	240	≥250
Probability of In-Hospital Death, %	≤0.2	0.3	0.4	0.6	0.8	1.1	1.6	2.1	2.9	3.9	5.4	7.3	9.8	13	18	23	29	36	44	≥52

For example, a patient has Killip class II, SBP of 100 mm Hg, heart rate of 100 beats/min, is 65 years of age, has serum creatinine level of 1 mg/dL, did not have a cardiac arrest at admission but did have ST-segment deviation and elevated enzyme levels.

His score would be: 20 + 53 + 15 + 58 + 7 + 0 + 28 + 14 = 196

This person would have about a 16% risk of having an in-hospital death.

Similarly, a patient with Killip class I, SBP of 80 mm Hg, heart rate of 60 beats/min, is 55 years of age, has serum creatinine level of 0.4 mg/dL, and no risk factors would have the following score:

0 + 58 + 3 + 41 + 1 = 103, which gives approximately a 0.9% risk of having an in-hospital death.

FIG. 6.1 GRACE risk score for predicting in-hospital mortality. (From Granger CB, Goldberg RJ, Dabbous O, et al. Predictors of hospital mortality in the global registry of acute coronary events. *Arch Intern Med.* 2003;163(19):2345–2353.)

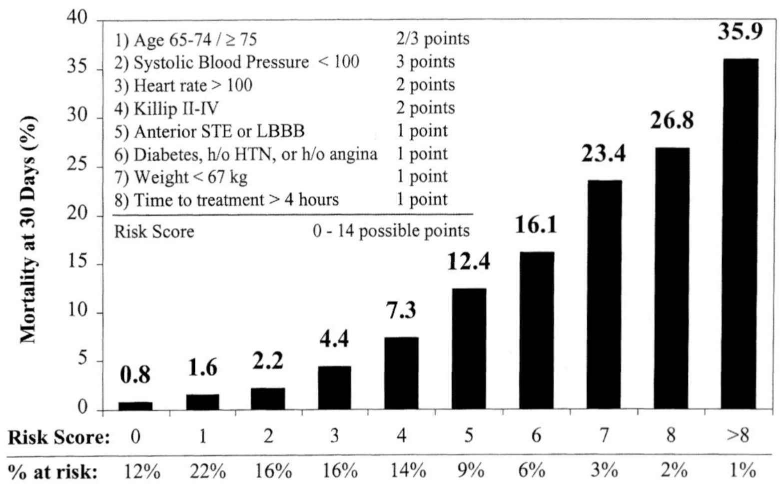

FIG. 6.2 TIMI risk score for ST-elevation myocardial infarction. (From Morrow DA, Antman EM, Charlesworth A, et al. TIMI risk score for ST-elevation myocardial infarction: a convenient, bedside, clinical score for risk assessment at presentation: an intravenous nPA for treatment of infarcting myocardium early II trial substudy. *Circulation.* 2000;102(17):2031–2037.)

evidence-based pharmacological and invasive therapies during hospitalization and upon discharge and referral to cardiac rehabilitation. This constellation of patient and system factors has been suggested to account for the sex differences in ACS outcomes. Women are also disproportionately represented among individuals with myocardial infarction with no obstructive coronary artery disease (MINOCA) and spontaneous coronary artery dissection. Moreover, there are limited and inconsistent data on their prognosis as compared to their counterparts with

Historical	Points
Age ≥65	1
≥3 CAD risk factors (FHx, HTN, ↑chol, DM, active smoker)	1
Known CAD (stenosis ≥50%)	1
ASA use in past 7 days	1
Presentation	
Recent (≤24 hour) severe angina	1
↑ Cardiac markers	1
ST deviation ≥0.05 mV	1
Risk Score = Total Points (0–7)	

Risk of cardiac events (%) by 14 days in TIMI 11B trial*		
Risk Score	**Death or MI**	**Death, MI, or Urgent Revascularization**
0/1	3	5
2	3	8
3	5	13
4	7	20
5	12	26
6/7	19	41

*Entry criteria: UA or NSTEMI defined as ischemic pain at rest within past 24 hours, with evidence of CAD (ST segment deviation or + biomarker).

FIG. 6.3 TIMI risk score for non-ST-elevation acute coronary syndrome. (From Antman EM, Cohen M, Bernink PJ, et al. The TIMI risk score for unstable angina/non-ST elevation MI: a method for prognostication and therapeutic decision making. *JAMA*. 2000;284(7):835–842.)

atherosclerotic disease.[9,10] Contemporary registries enrolling young patients with acute MI have demonstrated persistently worse outcomes in women compared with men, with higher rates of both coronary and noncardiac re-hospitalizations after index ACS.[11–13]

A pooled analysis of 11 randomized clinical trials that included 136,247 patients (28% women) showed that women are at higher unadjusted risk for death and adverse cardiovascular outcomes, but this increase in risk was substantially attenuated after controlling for other confounders. In a Canadian registry, the GRACE risk score was a validated predictor of mortality in both men and women with ACS.[14] Moreover, there was no significant interaction between sex and each GRACE risk score component, which implies that the prognostic value of these predictors (such as age, heart rate, blood pressure) is similar in both sexes.

Ethnicity

Multiple studies have reported racial disparities in ACS outcomes, which appear to be at least partly mediated by differences in both pharmacological and interventional treatment.[15] However, there is no consistent evidence that ethnicity is an independent predictor of outcome in ACS, after adjusting for cardiovascular risk factors and management.[16]

Diabetes

Approximately 20%–30% of ACS patients have diabetes, which is often associated with other cardiovascular risk factors and delay in presentation.[17,18] In a pooled analysis of 62,036 ACS patients from 11 TIMI trials, diabetes was an independent predictor of higher 30-day and 1-year mortality following STEMI and NSTE-ACS. ACS patients with diabetes are also at heightened risk for heart failure, cardiogenic shock, and acute kidney injury in hospitals. In a systematic review involving 304,253 ACS patients, higher HbA1c was a predictor for short-term mortality regardless of known or no known diabetes.[19] Furthermore, patients with acute MI have a high prevalence of newly discovered abnormal glucose tolerance, which is associated with higher risks of death and major adverse cardiovascular events.[20] A meta-analysis suggests that an early invasive strategy reduces nonfatal MI to a greater extent in diabetic than nondiabetic patients. Diabetes is also associated with more extensive and multivessel coronary artery disease that derives greater prognostic benefit from coronary bypass surgery as compared with percutaneous coronary intervention.

Chronic Kidney Disease

Chronic kidney disease is defined as kidney damage (as evidenced by albuminuria with an albumin-to-creatinine ratio >30 mg/g [3 mg/mmol]) and/or glomerular filtration rate <60 mL/min/1.73 m^2 that has been present for at least 3 months. Beyond its association with advanced age and traditional cardiovascular risk factors such as hypertension and insulin resistance/diabetes, chronic kidney disease accelerates atherosclerosis by promoting vascular calcification, inflammation, myocardial fibrosis, and hypertrophy.[21] In type 1 (acute) cardiorenal syndrome, acute kidney injury occurs in the setting of cardiogenic shock and heart failure complicating ACS.[22] Patients with chronic kidney disease are predisposed to both adverse cardiovascular and bleeding events. Baseline creatinine or creatinine clearance is a component of GRACE risk score and various bleeding risk scores including CRUSADE, ACUITY-HORIZONS, and ACTION-GWTG. Notably, these relationships are continuous, and even mild renal insufficiency is associated with an increased risk of death and adverse cardiovascular events after acute MI (Fig. 6.4). Assessment and monitoring of kidney function are crucial not only in initial risk stratification but also in the avoidance of bleeding through dose adjustment of antithrombotic therapies and contrast-induced nephropathy after a cardiac catheterization, which may result from iodinated contrast and aortic plaque microembolization.

In ACS patients, the Cockcroft-Gault equation for estimating GFR may be preferred because it exhibited better prediction for major adverse cardiovascular events, major bleeding, and all-cause mortality as compared with Modification of Diet in Renal Disease-4 equation and superior prediction for

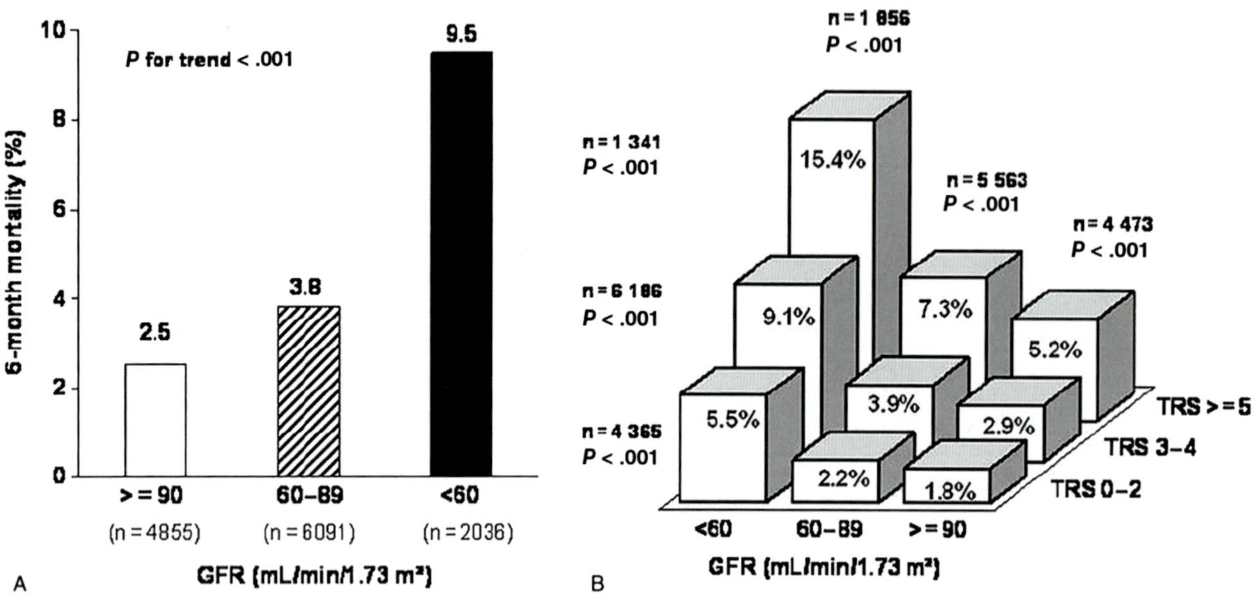

FIG. 6.4 Mortality at 6 months after acute coronary syndrome in relation to baseline glomerular filtration rate (GFR) (A) and stratified by GFR and TIMI risk score (B). (From Gibson CM, Dumaine RL, Gelfand EV et al. Association of glomerular filtration rate on presentation with subsequent mortality in non-ST-segment elevation acute coronary syndrome; observations in 13,307 patients in five TIMI trials. *Eur Heart J.* 2004;25(22):1998–2005.)

major bleeding as compared with Chronic Kidney Disease Epidemiology Collaboration (CKD-EPI) equation.[23]

Polyvascular Disease

Atherosclerosis is a multifactorial and systemic process. Polyvascular disease, defined as atherosclerosis affecting 2 or more arterial beds (coronary artery, cerebrovascular, peripheral artery disease), is present in about 13% of ACS patients and is likely underdiagnosed.[24] A positive correlation between the number of affected vascular beds and risks of MACEs and death in ACS patients has been described previously in multiple large registries and clinical trials. It is plausible that the worse outcome associated with polyvascular disease stems from the clustering of risk factors known to affect prognosis, including older age and diabetes, prior myocardial infarction, coronary artery bypass surgery, and chronic kidney disease. ACS patients with polyvascular have greater absolute risk reduction in cardiovascular events with further LDL-cholesterol lowering using PCSK9 inhibitor[25] and more intensive antithrombotic therapies.[26]

PHYSICAL EXAMINATION

A thorough physical examination is essential not only in the diagnosis but also prognostication of ACS. Vital signs on initial presentation carry substantial prognostic weight that may be under-recognized in clinical practice. Tachycardia and hypotension may herald cardiogenic shock, which is associated with a high mortality rate. Although hypertension is a cardiovascular risk factor that accelerates atherosclerosis in the long term, a higher blood pressure on acute presentation reflects more cardiac reserve and portends a better prognosis. For instance, the simple TIMI risk index calculated by heart rate x $(\text{age}/10)^2$/systolic blood pressure, has very good discrimination for 30-day mortality in both STEMI (c-statistic = 0.79) and NSTEMI (c-statistic = 0.73).

Acute decompensated heart failure in the setting of ACS is more common in older patients and those with hypertension, diabetes, pre-existing heart disease, and chronic kidney disease.[27] The incidence of acute heart failure complicating ACS range from 6% to >45% in registries, depending on the type of ACS and the definition of acute heart failure.[28] The combination of ACS and acute heart failure portends a dismal outlook. The Killip classification (class I to IV—based on the presence or absence of S3, rales, jugular venous distension, overt pulmonary edema, and cardiogenic shock), an indicator of the presence and severity of heart failure, is a strong predictor of mortality in acute STEMI. Although it was first described in patients with STEMI more than half a century ago, its independent prognostic value has been validated in a pooled analysis of clinical trials involving 26090 NSTE-ACS patients. Accordingly, heart rate, systolic blood pressure and Killip class are also powerful predictors in the GRACE risk score and TIMI risk score for STEMI (Figs. 6.1 and 6.2—note the number of points assigned to these predictor variables). Acute heart failure on ACS presentation is also associated with more frequent re-admissions, especially for heart failure.[28]

It is noteworthy that hypotension, heart failure, or cardiogenic shock may result from severe left ventricular dysfunction and/or a mechanical complication of acute MI, such as papillary muscle or ventricular free wall rupture (Chapter 22).[29] These extremely high-risk features warrant immediate investigations including echocardiography and specific treatment.

ELECTROCARDIOGRAM

Classification of ACS

Since its first description more than a century ago, the electrocardiogram (ECG) continues to provide important information about the presence, extent, and severity of myocardial ischemia.[30,31] Myocardial ischemia typically induces a shift of the ST-segment produced by the flow of currents that are generated by the voltage gradients across the boundary between the ischemic and nonischemic myocardium during the resting and plateau phases of the ventricular action potential, corresponding to the TQ and ST segments, respectively.[30] Thus, the ECG plays a key role in the initial evaluation, triage, and risk stratification of patients with symptoms compatible with an ACS. The ECG should therefore be acquired and interpreted promptly (i.e., target within 10 minutes) after first medical contact.[32] The Fourth Universal Definition of Myocardial Infarction (UDMI) notes the importance of then classifying MI according to the presence (or absence) of ST-segment deviation, notably diagnostic ST-segment elevation (STE) in 2 or more contiguous leads in the absence of a left bundle branch block (LBBB), designating an STEMI.[33] In addition to the standard 12-lead assessment, the use of additional right-sided precordial leads (V3R and V4R) in patients with inferior STEMI should be considered to identify concomitant right ventricular infarction.[34]

ST-Segment Versus Non-ST-Segment Elevation and Left Bundle Branch Block

STE in the corresponding clinical setting typically indicates transmural myocardial ischemia due to acute thrombotic occlusion of an epicardial coronary artery and is a class I indication for emergent reperfusion therapy by current guidelines. Prehospital ECGs reduce the time to diagnosis and treatment and can facilitate the triage of STEMI patients to hospitals with PCI capability (or to fibrinolysis if the former cannot be achieved) in a timely (e.g., <90 minutes from STEMI diagnosis) manner (see Chapter 3).

Up to one-third of patients with acute thrombotic occlusion of an epicardial coronary artery do not have initial STE meeting the thresholds set by the Fourth UDMI. This discordance may occur in the setting of small QRS complexes in the affected leads, especially in inferior STEMI, with myocardial protection due to preconditioning or residual collateral circulation. Guidelines recommend the use of additional posterior chest wall leads (i.e., V7–V9) to identify STE due to circumflex artery occlusion and repeated ECG recordings or monitoring of the ST segment to detect dynamic ECG changes, particularly if the initial ECG is nondiagnostic.[35] ST-segment depression in leads V1–V3 suggests myocardial ischemia (especially when the terminal T-wave is positive) with or without concomitant STE in V7–V9, and can be considered an STE "equivalent" identifying posterior MI.[30]

While the risk for adverse outcomes is initially (in-hospital and 30-day) higher with STEMI, it is recognized that NSTEACS (NSTEMI and unstable angina) patients experience higher rates of (re)-infarction, heart failure, and death by 6 months and beyond post-ACS.

New or presumed new LBBB has often been considered a STEMI equivalent; however, most cases of LBBB at the time of presentation are "not known to be old" simply because no prior ECG is available for comparison. Criteria for detecting acute ischemic ECG changes in LBBB, include STE ≥1 mm concordant with positive QRS complex, and use of the Sgarbossa criteria.[30,31,36] More recent guidelines note that new/presumed new LBBB at presentation is typically not caused by acute epicardial coronary occlusion, can confound STE analysis, and should not be considered diagnostic of STEMI-equivalent in isolation.

Although it has been suggested that the absolute sum of or the number of leads with STE correlates with the size of the ischemic area at risk, it should be noted that the various ECG leads record the vector of the global activation of the heart toward and away of the electrode and not "local" events. Thus, concomitant ischemia of opposing segments may result in "cancellation" of ST deviation in leads facing these segments.[30]

ST-Segment Deviation

Subendocardial ischemia may cause ST-segment depression (STD) in the ECG leads facing the involved zone.[30] STD is not only a qualitative marker that portends a worse prognosis than in ACS patients with a normal ECG, but also a quantitative marker of risk, as the number of leads with STD and the magnitude of STD (either within a single lead or as sum over all leads) are indicative of the extent of ischemia and correlate with prognosis.[37] For example, in the original derivation of the GRACE risk score for in-hospital mortality, STD (vs. no STD on ACS presentation) was associated with a >3-fold higher rate of death.[37] In a multivariable model incorporating other independent predictors for in-hospital mortality, including age, heart rate, systolic blood pressure and Killip class at presentation, initial serum creatinine and cardiac necrosis biomarker levels, and whether the patient experienced a cardiac arrest at hospital arrival, STD remained associated with a 2-3-fold increased odds for death. Similarly, in the GRACE risk score for postdischarge to 6 months, STD at presentation was independently associated with an approximately 1.5-fold increased odds for mortality.[37]

Diffuse STD (e.g., in ≥6 leads), often associated with inverted T waves and isolated STE in lead aVR (and/or V1) during episodes of chest pain has been described as a manifestation of diffuse subendocardial ischemia caused by left main-, left main equivalent-, or severe three vessel disease-related ischemia.[34,37] While the ECG may be normal or show only T-wave inversion (TWI) when the patient is asymptomatic, there appears to be an increased risk for developing cardiogenic shock and/or ventricular fibrillation; hence, early coronary angiography has been suggested for these patients.[34]

Q Waves and Other ECG Findings

Approximately 50% of patients presenting within 1 hour of onset of STEMI have Q waves in the leads with STE, especially in the anterior leads.[34] While these Q waves may reflect irreversible myocardial necrosis and portend a large infarction, some—potentially due to intense ischemia with a temporary loss of electrical activity in the region at risk ("myocardial concussion")—may be transient and do not necessarily represent irreversible damage. In contrast, in inferior STEMI, pre-existing Q waves may disappear during acute ischemia ("pulled up" by the injury current) and then reappear during reperfusion.

family member, is up-regulated in response to mechanical stress but only weakly correlated with NT-proBNP. It is also a marker of inflammation, fibrosis, and adverse myocardial remodeling. An ST2 assay has been approved by the FDA for prognostication in chronic heart failure, although its clinical role in ACS remains to be established. Several studies have shown its independent prognostic value in both STEMI and NSTEACS that may supplement risk scores. Copeptin, the c-terminal part of the prohormone of arginine vasopressin, is released from the neurohypophysis. Among ACS patients, copeptin predicted cardiovascular death and heart failure but not recurrent ischemic events. In a meta-analysis of 9090 patients with ACS, a neutrophil inflammatory marker myeloperoxidase (MPO) predicted mortality but not major adverse cardiovascular events.[70] Because Cystatin C is uniformly produced in all nucleated cells and filtered by glomeruli without secretion or resorption, it is deemed a better marker than the traditional measures of creatinine or eGFR in assessing kidney function. Cystatin C was associated with death and major adverse cardiovascular events in a meta-analysis,[71] and may offer additional prognostic information beyond eGFR and other cardiorenal markers.[72]

Numerous biomarkers have been studied and may complement each other for outcome prediction in ACS, and a multimarker approach appears promising. Nevertheless, there has been a paucity of data on head-to-head comparisons on their clinical utility and implications. A secondary analysis of the PLATO biomarker study evaluated cystatin-C, GDF-15, hsCRP, hs-cTnI, hs-cTnT, and NT-proBNP in 17095 ACS patients. NT-proBNP and GDF-15 were associated with death due to heart failure as well as arrhythmia and sudden cardiac death, while GDF-15 exhibited the strongest associations with other vascular or nonvascular mortality and possibly with fatal bleeding.[73] Whether and how these biomarkers can inform individualized management decisions (e.g., prevention of heart failure, avoidance of serious bleeding) deserve further investigation.[74]

While the prognostic importance of frailty is increasingly recognized,[6] its therapeutic implications remain to be elucidated. Because frail and multimorbid patients were under-represented in clinical trials that established the efficacy of early invasive strategy in ACS, caution is needed in extrapolating these results to vulnerable elderly patients. For example, a multicenter randomized trial of 167 elderly ACS patients with frailty failed to show any benefit of a routine invasive strategy on the number of days alive out of hospital or ischemic cardiac events.[75] As recommended in the AHA statement, the goals of care especially for elderly patients should extend beyond traditional cardiovascular outcomes, and incorporate patient-aligned goals and preferences to maximize quality-of-life outcomes such as symptoms and days out of hospital.[5] However, these patient-centered outcomes have not been the focus of existing validated risk scores.

Artificial intelligence and machine learning have already gained acceptance in many areas of clinical practice[76] and hold great promise not only in the early diagnosis but also in the prognostication and management of ACS.[77–79] GRACE risk score 3.0, which was re-developed by machine learning, contains identical predictor variables but is sex-specific and outperforms GRACE risk score 2.0 in terms of discrimination and calibration, leading to net re-classification in both men and women with NSTEACS.[53] Spatiotemporal multiomics studies are already yielding novel insight into the molecular and cellular underpinnings of ACS, accelerating target and biomarker discovery, and thereby paving the way for personalized medicine.[80]

Risk scores can now be readily embedded into electronic medical records which can efficiently handle vast amounts of real-time clinical data at both individual and population levels.[81] Such integration will expedite ongoing validation, re-calibration, and implementation of refined risk scores into contemporary practice. In an era of precision medicine and healthcare cost containment, the quality and cost effectiveness of objective risk-guided ACS care and patient satisfaction will likely top future research priorities.

CLASSIC REFERENCES

Antman EM, Cohen M, Bernink PJ, et al. The TIMI risk score for unstable angina/non-ST elevation MI: a method for prognostication and therapeutic decision making. *JAMA*. 2000;284(7):835–842. https://doi.org/10.1001/jama.284.7.835.

Bhatt DL, Peterson ED, Harrington RA, et al. Prior polyvascular disease: risk factor for adverse ischaemic outcomes in acute coronary syndromes. *Eur Heart J*. 2009;30(10):1195–1202. https://doi.org/10.1093/eurheartj/ehp099.

Donahoe SM, Stewart GC, McCabe CH, et al. Diabetes and mortality following acute coronary syndromes. *JAMA*. 2007;298(7):765–775. https://doi.org/10.1001/jama.298.7.765.

Franklin K, Goldberg RJ, Spencer F, et al. Implications of diabetes in patients with acute coronary syndromes. The global registry of acute coronary events. *Arch Intern Med*. 2004;164(13):1457–1463. https://doi.org/10.1001/archinte.164.13.1457.

Granger CB, Goldberg RJ, Dabbous O, et al. Predictors of hospital mortality in the global registry of acute coronary events. *Arch Intern Med*. 2003;163(19):2345–2353. https://doi.org/10.1001/archinte.163.19.2345.

Khot UN, Jia G, Moliterno DJ, et al. Prognostic importance of physical examination for heart failure in non-ST-elevation acute coronary syndromes: the enduring value of Killip classification. *JAMA*. 2003;290(16):2174–2181. https://doi.org/10.1001/jama.290.16.2174.

Mehta SR, Granger CB, Boden WE, et al. Early versus delayed invasive intervention in acute coronary syndromes. *N Engl J Med*. 2009;360(21):2165–2175. https://doi.org/10.1056/NEJMoa0807986.

Morrow DA, Antman EM, Charlesworth A, et al. TIMI risk score for ST-elevation myocardial infarction: a convenient, bedside, clinical score for risk assessment at presentation: an intravenous nPA for treatment of infarcting myocardium early II trial substudy. *Circulation*. 2000;102(17):2031–2037. https://doi.org/10.1161/01.cir.102.17.2031.

O'Donoghue ML, Vaidya A, Afsal R, et al. An invasive or conservative strategy in patients with diabetes mellitus and non-ST-segment elevation acute coronary syndromes: a collaborative meta-analysis of randomized trials. *J Am Coll Cardiol*. 2012;60(2):106–111. https://doi.org/10.1016/j.jacc.2012.02.059.

Yan AT, Yan RT, Huynh T, et al. Understanding physicians' risk stratification of acute coronary syndromes: insights from the Canadian ACS 2 registry. *Arch Intern Med*. 2009;169(4):372–378. https://doi.org/10.1001/archinternmed.2008.563.

REFERENCES

1. Hall M, Bebb OJ, Dondo TB, et al. Guideline-indicated treatments and diagnostics, GRACE risk score, and survival for non-ST elevation myocardial infarction. *Eur Heart J*. 2018;39(42):3798–3806.
2. Haghbayan H, Gale CP, Chew DP, et al. Clinical risk prediction models for the prognosis and management of acute coronary syndromes. *Eur Heart J Qual Care Clin Outcomes*. 2021;7(3):222–228.
3. Kofoed KF, Kelbaek H, Hansen PR, et al. Early versus standard care invasive examination and treatment of patients with non-ST-segment elevation acute coronary syndrome. *Circulation*. 2018;138(24):2741–2750.
4. Wilson TA, Hazlewood GS, Sajobi TT, et al. Preferences of patients with chronic kidney disease for invasive versus conservative treatment of acute coronary syndrome: a discrete choice experiment. *J Am Heart Assoc*. 2023;12(6):e028492.
5. Damluji AA, Forman DE, Wang TY, et al. Management of acute coronary syndrome in the older adult population: a scientific statement from the American Heart Association. *Circulation*. 2023;147(3):e32–e62.
6. Dou Q, Wang W, Wang H, et al. Prognostic value of frailty in elderly patients with acute coronary syndrome: a systematic review and meta-analysis. *BMC Geriatr*. 2019;19(1):222.
7. Kunadian V, Mossop H, Shields C, et al. Invasive Treatment Strategy for Older Patients with Myocardial Infarction. *N Engl J Med*. 2024;391(18):1673-1684. doi:10.1056/NEJMoa2407791.
8. van Oosterhout REM, de Boer AR, Maas A, Rutten FH, Bots ML, Peters SAE. Sex differences in symptom presentation in acute coronary syndromes: a systematic review and meta-analysis. *J Am Heart Assoc*. 2020;9(9):e014733.

9. Tamis-Holland JE, Jneid H, Reynolds HR, et al. Contemporary diagnosis and management of patients with myocardial infarction in the absence of obstructive coronary artery disease: a scientific statement from the American Heart Association. *Circulation.* 2019;139(18):e891–e908.
10. Hayes SN, Kim ESH, Saw J, et al. Spontaneous Coronary artery dissection: current state of the science: a scientific statement from the American Heart Association. *Circulation.* 2018;137(19):e523–e557.
11. Sawano M, Lu Y, Caraballo C, et al. Sex difference in outcomes of acute myocardial infarction in young patients. *J Am Coll Cardiol.* 2023;81(18):1797–1806.
12. DeFilippis EM, Collins BL, Singh A, et al. Women who experience a myocardial infarction at a young age have worse outcomes compared with men: the mass general brigham YOUNG-MI registry. *Eur Heart J.* 2020;41(42):4127–4137.
13. Gulati M, Holtzman JN, Kaur G. Increased rehospitalization in young women with acute myocardial infarction at 1 year: adding insult to infarct. *J Am Coll Cardiol.* 2023;81(18):1807–1809.
14. Gong IY, Goodman SG, Brieger D, et al. GRACE risk score: sex-based validity of in-hospital mortality prediction in Canadian patients with acute coronary syndrome. *Int J Cardiol.* 2017;244:24–29.
15. Jaiswal V, Hanif M, Ang SP, et al. Racial disparity among the clinical outcomes post-myocardial infarction patients: a systematic review and meta-analysis. *Curr Probl Cardiol.* 2023;48(4):101528.
16. Graham GN, Jones PG, Chan PS, Arnold SV, Krumholz HM, Spertus JA. Racial disparities in patient characteristics and survival after acute myocardial infarction. *JAMA Netw Open.* 2018;1(7):e184240.
17. Lettino M, Andell P, Zeymer U, et al. Diabetic patients with acute coronary syndromes in contemporary European registries: characteristics and outcomes. *Eur Heart J Cardiovasc Pharmacother.* 2017;3(4):198–213.
18. Schmitt VH, Hobohm L, Munzel T, Wenzel P, Gori T, Keller K. Impact of diabetes mellitus on mortality rates and outcomes in myocardial infarction. *Diabetes Metab.* 2021;47(4):101211.
19. Pan W, Lu H, Lian B, Liao P, Guo L, Zhang M. Prognostic value of HbA1c for in-hospital and short-term mortality in patients with acute coronary syndrome: a systematic review and meta-analysis. *Cardiovasc Diabetol.* 2019;18(1):169.
20. Laichuthai N, Abdul-Ghani M, Kosiborod M, Parksook WW, Kerr SJ, DeFronzo RA. Newly discovered abnormal glucose tolerance in patients with acute myocardial infarction and cardiovascular outcomes: a meta-analysis. *Diabetes Care.* 2020;43(8):1958–1966.
21. Jankowski J, Floege J, Fliser D, Bohm M, Marx N. Cardiovascular disease in chronic kidney disease: pathophysiological insights and therapeutic options. *Circulation.* 2021;143(11):1157–1172.
22. Rangaswami J, Bhalla V, Blair JEA, et al. Cardiorenal syndrome: classification, pathophysiology, diagnosis, and treatment strategies: a scientific statement from the American Heart Association. *Circulation.* 2019;139(16):e840–e878.
23. Rivera-Caravaca JM, Ruiz-Nodar JM, Tello-Montoliu A, et al. Disparities in the estimation of glomerular filtration rate according to cockcroft-gault, modification of diet in renal disease-4, and chronic kidney disease epidemiology collaboration equations and relation with outcomes in patients with acute coronary syndrome. *J Am Heart Assoc.* 2018;7(9):e008725.
24. Gutierrez JA, Aday AW, Patel MR, Jones WS. Polyvascular disease: reappraisal of the current clinical landscape. *Circ Cardiovasc Interv.* 2019;12(12):e007385.
25. Jukema JW, Szarek M, Zijlstra LE, et al. Alirocumab in patients with polyvascular disease and recent acute coronary syndrome: ODYSSEY OUTCOMES trial. *J Am Coll Cardiol.* 2019;74(9):1167–1176.
26. Weissler EH, Jones WS, Desormais I, et al. Polyvascular disease: a narrative review of current evidence and a consideration of the role of antithrombotic therapy. *Atherosclerosis.* 2020;315:10–17.
27. Harrington J, Jones WS, Udell JA, et al. Acute decompensated heart failure in the setting of acute coronary syndrome. *JACC Heart Fail.* 2022;10(6):404–414.
28. Harjola VP, Parissis J, Bauersachs J, et al. Acute coronary syndromes and acute heart failure: a diagnostic dilemma and high-risk combination. A statement from the acute heart failure committee of the heart failure association of the European Society of Cardiology. *Eur J Heart Fail.* 2020;22(8):1298–1314.
29. Samsky MD, Morrow DA, Proudfoot AG, Hochman JS, Thiele H, Rao SV. Cardiogenic shock after acute myocardial infarction: a review. *JAMA.* 2021;326(18):1840–1850.
30. Birnbaum Y, Rankinen J, Jneid H, Atar D, Nikus K. The role of ECG in the diagnosis and risk stratification of acute coronary syndromes: an old but indispensable tool. *Curr Cardiol Rep.* 2022;24(2):109–118.
31. Chong L, Chaitman BR. The year in review: electrocardiogram analysis and acute coronary syndromes. *Eur Heart J Acute Cardiovasc Care.* 2020;9(8):824–826.
32. Gulati M, Levy PD, Mukherjee D, et al. 2021 AHA/ACC/ASE/CHEST/SAEM/SCCT/SCMR guideline for the evaluation and diagnosis of chest pain: a report of the American College of Cardiology/American Heart Association joint committee on clinical practice guidelines. *Circulation.* 2021;144(22):e368–e454.
33. Thygesen K, Alpert JS, Jaffe AS, et al. Fourth universal definition of myocardial infarction (2018). *Circulation.* 2018;138(20):e618–e651.
34. Birnbaum Y, Rankinen J, Jneid H, Atar D, Nikus K. The role of ECG in the diagnosis and risk stratification of acute coronary syndromes: an old but indispensable tool. *Current Cardiology Reports.* 2022;24(2):109–118.
35. Gulati M, Levy PD, Mukherjee D, et al. 2021 AHA/ACC/ASE/CHEST/SAEM/SCCT/SCMR guideline for the evaluation and diagnosis of chest pain: a report of the American College of Cardiology/American Heart Association joint committee on clinical practice guidelines. *Circulation.* 2021;144(22):e368–e454.
36. Khawaja M, Thakker J, Kherallah R, Ye Y, Smith SW, Birnbaum Y. Diagnosis of occlusion myocardial infarction in patients with left bundle branch block and paced rhythms. *Curr Cardiol Rep.* 2021;23(12):187.
37. Collet J-P, Thiele H, Barbato E, et al. 2020 ESC guidelines for the management of acute coronary syndromes in patients presenting without persistent ST-segment elevation: the task force for the management of acute coronary syndromes in patients presenting without persistent ST-segment elevation of the European Society of Cardiology (ESC). *Eur Heart J.* 2020;42(14):1289–1367.
38. Wang A, Singh V, Duan Y, et al. Prognostic implications of ST-segment elevation in lead aVR in patients with acute coronary syndrome: a meta-analysis. *Ann Noninvasive Electrocardiol.* 2021;26(1):e12811.
39. Sandoval Y, Apple FS, Mahler SA, et al. High-sensitivity cardiac troponin and the 2021 AHA/ACC/ASE/CHEST/SAEM/SCCT/SCMR guidelines for the evaluation and diagnosis of acute chest pain. *Circulation.* 2022;146(7):569–581.
40. McCarthy C, Li S, Wang TY, et al. Implementation of high-sensitivity cardiac troponin assays in the United States. *J Am Coll Cardiol.* 2023;81(3):207–219.
41. Anand A, Lee KK, Chapman AR, et al. High-sensitivity cardiac troponin on presentation to rule out myocardial infarction: a stepped-wedge cluster randomized controlled trial. *Circulation.* 2021;143(23):2214–2224.
42. Neumann JT, Twerenbold R, Ojeda F, et al. Application of high-sensitivity troponin in suspected myocardial infarction. *N Engl J Med.* 2019;380(26):2529–2540.
43. Khullar N, Buckley AJ, O'Connor C, et al. Peak troponin T in STEMI: a predictor of all-cause mortality and left ventricular function. *Open Heart.* 2022;9(1):e001863.
44. Bagai A, Huang Z, Lokhnygina Y, et al. Magnitude of troponin elevation and long-term clinical outcomes in acute coronary syndrome patients treated with and without revascularization. *Circ Cardiovasc Interv.* 2015;8(6):e002314.
45. Coelho-Lima J, Georgiopoulos G, Ahmed J, et al. Prognostic value of admission high-sensitivity troponin in patients with ST-elevation myocardial infarction. *Heart.* 2021;107(23):1881–1888.
46. Eggers KM, Lindahl B. Prognostic biomarkers in acute coronary syndromes: risk stratification beyond cardiac troponins. *Curr Cardiol Rep.* 2017;19(4):29.
47. Mani P, Puri R, Schwartz GG, et al. Association of initial and serial C-reactive protein levels with adverse cardiovascular events and death after acute coronary syndrome: a secondary analysis of the VISTA-16 trial. *JAMA Cardiol.* 2019;4(4):314–320.
48. Lin XL, Sun HX, Li FQ, et al. Admission high-sensitivity C-reactive protein levels improve the Grace risk score prediction on in-hospital outcomes in acute myocardial infarction patients. *Clin Cardiol.* 2022;45(3):282–290.
49. Fan Z, Li Y, Ji H, Jian X. Prognostic utility of the combination of monocyte-to-lymphocyte ratio and neutrophil-to-lymphocyte ratio in patients with NSTEMI after primary percutaneous coronary intervention: a retrospective cohort study. *BMJ Open.* 2018;8(10):e023459.
50. Quan XQ, Wang RC, Zhang Q, Zhang CT, Sun L. The predictive value of lymphocyte-to-monocyte ratio in the prognosis of acute coronary syndrome patients: a systematic review and meta-analysis. *BMC Cardiovasc Disord.* 2020;20(1):338.
51. Chew DP, Juergens C, French J, et al. An examination of clinical intuition in risk assessment among acute coronary syndromes patients: observations from a prospective multi-center international observational registry. *Int J Cardiol.* 2014;171(2):209–216.
52. van der Sangen NMR, Azzahhafi J, Chan Pin Yin D, et al. External validation of the GRACE risk score and the risk-treatment paradox in patients with acute coronary syndrome. *Open Heart.* 2022;9(1):e001984.
53. Wenzl FA, Kraler S, Ambler G, et al. Sex-specific evaluation and redevelopment of the GRACE score in non-ST-segment elevation acute coronary syndromes in populations from the UK and Switzerland: a multinational analysis with external cohort validation. *Lancet.* 2022;400(10354):744–756.
54. Pencina MJ, D'Agostino RB, Sr Demler OV. Novel metrics for evaluating improvement in discrimination: net reclassification and integrated discrimination improvement for normal variables and nested models. *Stat Med.* 2012;31(2):101–113.
55. Thomas LE, O'Brien EC, Piccini JP, D'Agostino RB, Pencina MJ. Application of net reclassification index to non-nested and point-based risk prediction models: a review. *Eur Heart J.* 2019;40(23):1880–1887.
56. Antman EM, Cohen M, Bernink PJ, et al. The TIMI risk score for unstable angina/non-ST elevation MI: a method for prognostication and therapeutic decision making. *JAMA.* 2000;284(7):835–842.
57. Morrow DA, Antman EM, Charlesworth A, et al. TIMI risk score for ST-elevation myocardial infarction: a convenient, bedside, clinical score for risk assessment at presentation: an intravenous nPA for treatment of infarcting myocardium early II trial substudy. *Circulation.* 2000;102(17):2031–2037.
58. Fox KA, Dabbous OH, Goldberg RJ, et al. Prediction of risk of death and myocardial infarction in the six months after presentation with acute coronary syndrome: prospective multinational observational study (GRACE). *BMJ.* 2006;333(7578):1091.
59. Klingenberg R, Aghlmandi S, Raber L, et al. Improved risk stratification of patients with acute coronary syndromes using a combination of hsTnT, NT-proBNP and hsCRP with the GRACE score. *Eur Heart J Acute Cardiovasc Care.* 2018;7(2):129–138.
60. Batra G, Lindback J, Becker RC, et al. Biomarker-based prediction of recurrent ischemic events in patients with acute coronary syndromes. *J Am Coll Cardiol.* 2022;80(18):1735–1747.
61. Yeh RW, Secemsky EA, Kereiakes DJ, et al. Development and validation of a prediction rule for benefit and harm of dual antiplatelet therapy beyond 1 year after percutaneous coronary intervention. *JAMA.* 2016;315(16):1735–1749.
62. Costa F, van Klaveren D, James S, et al. Derivation and validation of the predicting bleeding complications in patients undergoing stent implantation and subsequent dual antiplatelet therapy (PRECISE-DAPT) score: a pooled analysis of individual-patient datasets from clinical trials. *Lancet.* 2017;389(10073):1025–1034.
63. Mehta SR, Granger CB, Boden WE, et al. Early versus delayed invasive intervention in acute coronary syndromes. *N Engl J Med.* 2009;360(21):2165–2175.
64. Everett CC, Fox KA, Reynolds C, et al. Evaluation of the impact of the GRACE risk score on the management and outcome of patients hospitalised with non-ST elevation acute coronary syndrome in the UK: protocol of the UKGRIS cluster-randomised registry-based trial. *BMJ Open.* 2019;9(9):e032165.

65. Chew DP, Hyun K, Morton E, et al. Objective risk assessment vs standard care for acute coronary syndromes: a randomized clinical trial. *JAMA Cardiol.* 2021;6(3):304–313.
66. Gale CP, Stocken DD, Aktaa S, et al. Effectiveness of GRACE risk score in patients admitted to hospital with non-ST elevation acute coronary syndrome (UKGRIS): parallel group cluster randomised controlled trial. *BMJ.* 2023;381:e073843.
67. Gullick J, Wu J, Chew D, et al. Objective risk assessment vs standard care for acute coronary syndromes-the Australian GRACE risk tool implementation study (AGRIS): a process evaluation. *BMC Health Serv Res.* 2022;22(1):380.
68. Chew DP, Scott IA, Cullen L, et al. National Heart Foundation of Australia and Cardiac Society of Australia and New Zealand: Australian clinical guidelines for the management of acute coronary syndromes 2016. *Med J Aust.* 2016;205(3):128–133.
69. Collet JP, Thiele H, Barbato E, et al. 2020 ESC guidelines for the management of acute coronary syndromes in patients presenting without persistent ST-segment elevation. *Eur Heart J.* 2021;42(14):1289–1367.
70. Kolodziej AR, Abo-Aly M, Elsawalhy E, Campbell C, Ziada KM, Abdel-Latif A. Prognostic role of elevated myeloperoxidase in patients with acute coronary syndrome: a systemic review and meta-analysis. *Mediators Inflamm.* 2019;2019:2872607.
71. Sun Y, Lu Q, Cheng B, Tao X. Prognostic value of cystatin C in patients with acute coronary syndrome: a systematic review and meta-analysis. *Eur J Clin Invest.* 2021;51(3):e13440.
72. Correa S, Morrow DA, Braunwald E, et al. Cystatin C for risk stratification in patients after an acute coronary syndrome. *J Am Heart Assoc.* 2018;7(20):e009077.
73. Lindholm D, James SK, Gabrysch K, et al. Association of multiple biomarkers with risk of all-cause and cause-specific mortality after acute coronary syndromes: a secondary analysis of the PLATO biomarker study. *JAMA Cardiol.* 2018;3(12):1160–1166.
74. Gaggin HK, Januzzi JL Jr. Moving the needle toward a more personalized means of patient care. *JAMA Cardiol.* 2018;3(12):1146–1148.
75. Sanchis J, Bueno H, Minana G, et al. Effect of routine invasive vs conservative strategy in older adults with frailty and non-ST-segment elevation acute myocardial infarction: a randomized clinical trial. *JAMA Intern Med.* 2023;183(5):407–415.
76. Haug CJ, Drazen JM. Artificial intelligence and machine learning in clinical medicine, 2023. *N Engl J Med.* 2023;388(13):1201–1208.
77. Wang H, Zu Q, Chen J, Yang Z, Ahmed MA. Application of Artificial intelligence in acute coronary syndrome: a brief literature review. *Adv Ther.* 2021;38(10):5078–5086.
78. Al-Zaiti S, Besomi L, Bouzid Z, et al. Machine learning-based prediction of acute coronary syndrome using only the pre-hospital 12-lead electrocardiogram. *Nat Commun.* 2020;11(1):3966.
79. Iannattone PA, Zhao X, VanHouten J, Garg A, Huynh T. Artificial intelligence for diagnosis of acute coronary syndromes: a meta-analysis of machine learning approaches. *Can J Cardiol.* 2020;36(4):577–583.
80. Schumacher D, Kramann R. Multiomic spatial mapping of myocardial infarction and implications for personalized therapy. *Arterioscler Thromb Vasc Biol.* 2023;43(2):192–202.
81. Harrington RA, Ohman EM. Risk stratification science goes to a new level. *JAMA Cardiol.* 2021;6(3):314–315.

7 Emergency Department Evaluation of the Lower-Risk Patient: Whom Can You Send Home?

BENJAMIN M. SCIRICA

INTRODUCTION

Of the more than 7 million visits to emergency departments (EDs) in the United States for chest pain or other potential ischemic symptoms, only a small minority will yield a diagnosis of acute coronary syndrome (ACS) (Fig. 7.1).[1] Identifying patients who can be discharged early, with minimal testing, while also ensuring that patients at high risk for cardiac events are appropriately triaged to receive more advanced evaluation and management remains one of the most common and challenging clinical scenarios that cardiologists, emergency medicine physicians, and primary care providers face daily.

Chest and abdominal pain are consistently the two most common symptoms prompting emergency room visits in the United States (see Chapter 4). However, the practice in the ED and inpatient evaluation of patients presenting with chest pain has evolved considerably. The two most important advances are the introduction of cardiac troponin assays (especially high-sensitivity assays) and more advanced imaging techniques, such as computed tomography coronary angiography.[1,2] Even though the rate of admission, transfer, or death has declined over the past decade, the burden of evaluating patients with chest pain in the ED and efforts to address the typically high rate of complications continue to create tremendous demands upon the health care system.

The clinical presentation of patients with suspected MI and the key considerations in the general approach to their evaluation are discussed in Chapter 4. The use of imaging is described in Chapter 5. This chapter reviews specific strategies and algorithms integrating each of the elements of clinical, laboratory, and imaging data to identify those patients for whom the probability that an ACS is the cause of their symptoms is deemed sufficiently low to "rule-out" ACS. An efficient approach to evaluating such "low-probability" patients should minimize the time until diagnosis, reduce the need for additional testing, and limit the duration of hospitalization while avoiding missing patients with ACS. For context, an acceptable "miss" rate for any strategy to exclude MI in patients presenting with chest pain must be less than 1%.

THE "LOW-PROBABILITY" VERSUS "LOW-RISK" ACS PATIENT

Before defining the specific population of patients who can be safely discharged from the ED, distinguishing between "low probability" and "low risk" is worthwhile because these two terms are often interchanged freely in discussing chest pain and ACS. In characterizing patients, it is often more appropriate to specify "low probability" for the presence of ACS rather than "low risk," which is most commonly employed in estimating the likelihood of subsequent cardiovascular events (see also Chapter 4 and Chapter 6). Risk stratification is critical in evaluating patients with documented ACS, and ACS risk scores incorporate many of the same clinical characteristics used for assessing the probability of ACS. However, the risk estimates and clinical implications in this patient population differ greatly from those in patients undergoing evaluation for suspected ischemic symptoms. For example, a patient may have a high probability of ACS and merit hospitalization but be at low or moderate risk for subsequent cardiovascular events (see Fig. 4.2). Risk stratification in patients with *documented* ACS is reviewed in detail in Chapter 6.

CONSIDERATIONS FOR DEFINING PROBABILITY AND RULING OUT ACUTE CORONARY SYNDROME

The initial evaluation of the patient with suspected ischemic symptoms integrates, at a minimum, the patient's comorbid conditions, history and presentation, and

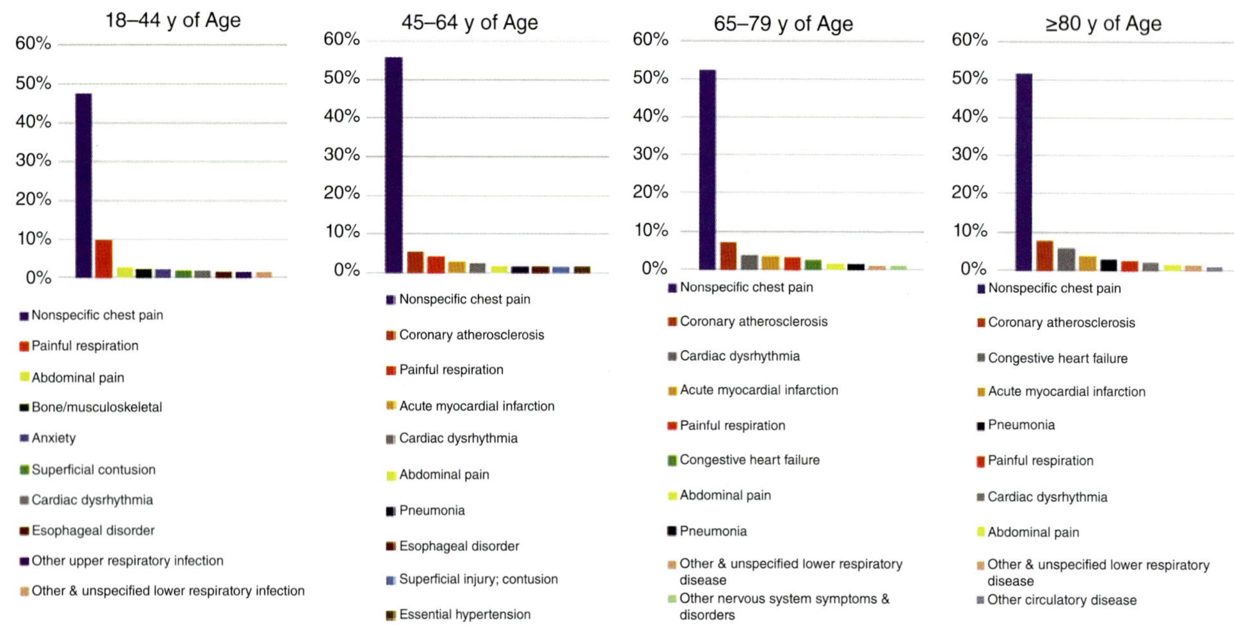

FIG. 7.1 Top 10 causes of chest pain in the ED based on age (weighted percentage). (From Gulati M, Levy PD, Mukherjee D, et al. 2021 AHA/ACC/ASE/CHEST/SAEM/SCCT/SCMR guideline for the evaluation and diagnosis of chest pain: a report of the American College of Cardiology/American Heart Association joint committee on clinical practice guidelines. *J Am Coll Cardiol.* 2021;78(22):e187–e285.)

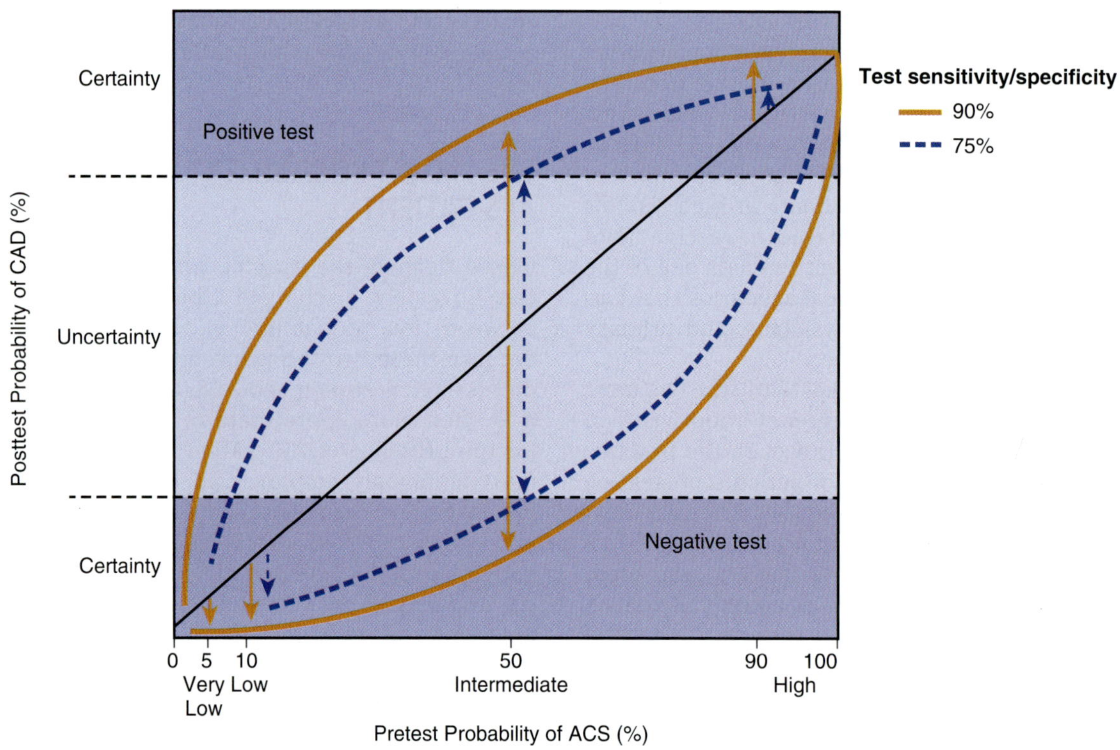

FIG. 7.2 The incremental value of a test to improve the diagnostic accuracy is dependent on the specific test characteristics (i.e., specificity and sensitivity) as well as the clinician's pre-test assessment, or probability, that the patient has the disease in question. The importance of the pre-test probability is illustrated in this figure and highlights that testing is most appropriate in patients with intermediate probability of the disease. For example, in a patient with an intermediate probability of ACS, a positive or negative test will move the post-test probability (*vertical axis*) quite dramatically, even if the test has a sensitivity/specificity of 75% (*dotted blue lines*) to an area of greater certainty. The diagnostic accuracy of any test improves wit higher sensitivity and specificity. It will move the post-test probability even further with 90% (*yellow lines*). Conversely, at the ends of the spectrum – low and high probability – the test will not meaningfully alter the post-test probability such that a positive test in a low probability patient is probably a false positive. *CAD*, Coronary artery disease. (Modified from Weustink AC, de Feyter PJ. The role of multi-slice computed tomography in stable angina management: a current perspective. *Neth Heart J.* 2011;19(7–8):336–343.)

electrocardiographic findings. Most patients, except those with the very lowest probability for ischemia, will also have at least one biomarker of myocyte necrosis (i.e., cTn) measured. The most challenging aspect of identifying patients with a low probability of ACS is the challenge in identifying a single "gold standard" test for ACS. Troponin assays are extremely sensitive for identifying myocardial injury but do not necessarily provide insight into the underlying cause (see Chapter 4). The diagnosis of MI is based on the clinical scenario, cTn results, and ultimately, medical judgment.[2]

Depending on clinical characteristics, electrocardiography findings, and biomarker results, most patients can be classified into groups of low, intermediate, or high probability of ACS. This first, immediate probability estimation is important because the value of all subsequent testing depends on the pretest probability of disease. Typically, additional testing is most useful in those patients with intermediate pretest probability (Fig. 7.2). Even a "negative" subsequent test would not be reassuring in patients with a high pretest probability because a higher-than-acceptable false-negative rate is likely. Conversely, in low-probability patients, a positive test result is much more likely to be a false-positive than to represent identifying a "true" ACS. It should be noted that some patients may have such a low probability of ACS that checking hsTn is not warranted.

In the initial evaluation of patients with suspected ischemia, it is often more important to "rule out" an unstable ischemic syndrome than to definitively "rule in" the diagnosis of ACS. In deciding whether a test is appropriate to rule out a disease, one must consider the underlying prevalence of the disease and the specificity of the test used to exclude the disease. For example, a computed tomography (CT) angiogram would be less helpful to exclude ACS in a patient with documented coronary disease. Similarly, measuring high-sensitivity cTn in a patient with end-stage renal disease and severe left ventricular hypertrophy will yield results that can be challenging to interpret.

Stable Versus Unstable Coronary Artery Disease

Another important distinction in evaluating patients with suspected ACS is the difference between stable coronary artery disease and an unstable coronary lesion precipitating ACS. Although known coronary artery disease increases the probability of developing ACS, stable coronary artery disease patients can present with nonischemic or even noncardiac causes of chest symptoms. Patients may have underlying asymptomatic coronary artery disease and present with symptomatic gastrointestinal reflux disease (GERD) symptoms. Thus, diagnosing coronary artery disease (e.g., with a "positive" stress test) does not equate to diagnosing ACS—a mistake commonly made in clinical practice and clinical investigation. The clinical scenario of presentation is essential to making the diagnosis of ACS.

High-Sensitivity Cardiac Troponin (hsTn)

As reviewed in Chapter 4, cTn is the gold standard for detecting myocardial injury. A cTn assay is considered to be a high-sensitivity assay if it detects a cTn concentration above the assay's limit-of-detection in at least 50% of healthy men and women with adequate precision (coefficient of variation at the 99th percentile ≤10%). hsTn assays are widely available in the United States and are recommended in most recent guidelines and position statements for evaluating patients with suspected ischemic chest pain.[3] Over the past decade, the more widespread use of hsTn has been the most important advancement in evaluating patients with suspected ACS and fundamentally altered the approach to evaluating acute chest pain.

Identifying the Low-Probability Patient

Although many different algorithms are available for defining a low probability for the presence of ACS, all classification strategies incorporate elements of history, physical examination, electrocardiogram, and cTn (see also Chapter 4).[1] Patients are considered to have a low probability for ACS if they do not have symptoms consistent with ischemia, including angina similar to previous angina or chest and left arm pain or discomfort (see Fig. 4.4). Low-probability patients tend to be younger and have fewer identifiable cardiovascular disease risk factors. On physical examination, the low-probability patient should be free of volume overload or extracardiac vascular disease manifestations. Patients are considered to be in the low-probability group if their ECG is normal with respect to ischemic changes or demonstrates, at most, T-wave flattening or inversions of less than 0.1 mV. Most importantly, initial levels of hsTn in a low-probability patient must not be elevated above established probabilistic cutpoints nor demonstrate dynamic changes.

Epidemiology of Low-Probability Patients

Most patients who present with chest pain have either a low or an intermediate probability for the presence of unstable coronary artery disease. It is difficult to accurately estimate the exact proportion of patients classified as low probability because of variable definitions across heterogeneous clinical studies and cohorts. With those caveats, 50%–60% of all patients presenting with acute chest pain appear to have a low probability of ACS.

CLINICAL DECISION PATHWAYS

Historically, patients presenting with suspected ischemic syndromes were given the classic diagnosis of "rule out MI" ("R/O MI"), which was actually a diagnostic strategy rather than a diagnosis. Before the introduction of cTn, a rule-out MI protocol would require serial (usually 3) ECGs and measurements of creatinine kinase (and MB fraction) separated by 6–8 hours given the release kinetics of creatinine kinase. Even then, the low sensitivity of non-cTn biomarkers meant that many patients required stress testing before safely being discharged. With the transition from CK-MB to earlier generation, non-high sensitive cTn assays, many clinical decision pathways (CDPs), sometimes called accelerated diagnostic protocols, were developed that required just two cTn measurements and shortened the interval between measurements to 2 and 6 hours, depending on the assay. hsTn introduced further modifications and improvements to the CDP framework as the newer assays are more sensitive and precise, allowing the detection of lower concentrations and earlier rises in circulating cTn than earlier-generation assays.

However, the goal of hsTn CDPs remains the same: Assign patients to 3 probability categories—low ("rule-out"), intermediate, or high ("rule-in") probability—which will determine patient disposition to, respectively, early discharge, need for more testing, or likely admission for ACS.

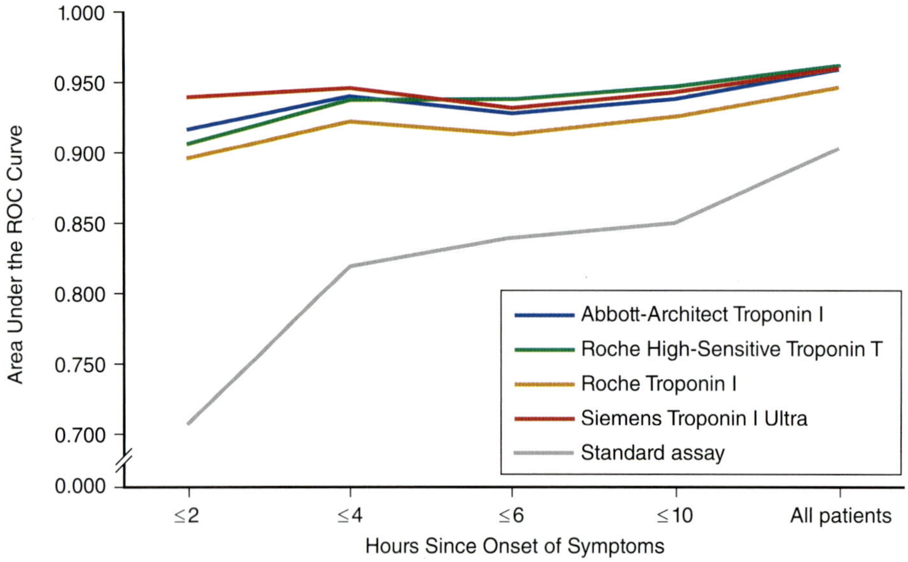

FIG. 7.3 Diagnostic accuracy of cardiac troponin assays at presentation according to time since onset of chest pain. The area under the receiver-operating-characteristic curve (AUC) is shown, according to the time since the onset of chest pain, for the four sensitive cardiac troponin assays and the standard assay performed on blood samples obtained at presentation for the diagnosis of acute myocardial infarction.

These protocols may be implemented in the ED, in dedicated chest pain units, and in inpatient wards. Current reimbursement in the United States rewards shorter hospital stays, with the goal of more patients discharged directly from the ED and limiting in-hospital stays to less than 24 hours. Thus, the metrics of a successful algorithm, in addition to ensuring a very low rate of missed ACS cases, include time until discharge and the need for subsequent testing.

hsTn Clinical Decision Pathways

The widespread implementation of more sensitive troponin assays significantly alters the approach to the patient with a low probability of ischemia. Multiple studies have now demonstrated that more sensitive assays for cTn can (1) detect myocardial damage at levels well below those for conventional assays, thus shifting the diagnosis of unstable angina to MI (see Chapter 2); and (2) identify necrosis earlier than older assays (Fig. 7.3). Thus, high-sensitivity assays for troponin (hsTn) further improve the ability to identify those patients with the lowest probability for ACS.[1,3–5] The concurrent increase in the proportion of patients without ACS who have elevated values of hsTn is discussed in Chapter 4. The gain in sensitivity for identifying myocardial necrosis (of any type) necessarily diminishes specificity for the diagnosis of ACS. Similarly, a nondetectable hsTn level increases the sensitivity for ruling out ACS, although at the price of identifying fewer patients in this low-probability category.

When used alone, hsTn assays have negative predictive values ranging from 92% to 100%. The diagnostic accuracy is lower when measured early after the onset of symptoms (less than 2 hours) but is still superior to that of conventional cTn assays. The variability in negative predictive values observed in different CDP studies is due to 1) differences in the study populations, 2) the timing of testing in relationship to symptoms, 3) the analytic properties of the assay, and most importantly, 4) the specific cutpoint used. For example, using a cutpoint of the lowest reporting limit (e.g., below 6 ng/L for the Roche hsTnT assay) gives a much higher negative predictive value than using the 99th percentile cutpoint (14 ng/L). The tradeoff of using the lower threshold is that fewer patients will be categorized as low probability.

However, a test with a negative predictive value of less than 99% typically is not acceptable for the early identification of patients who can be safely discharged from the ED after just one measurement. Therefore, most CDPs for chest pain incorporate two sequential cTn measurements.[1,6] Table 7.1 summarizes 4 different CDPs utilizing two serial hsTn assessments separated by 1 to 3 hours. The timing of the second assessment is key as the specific cutpoints for each CDP depend on samples being drawn at that particular time interval. In addition, each specific hsTn assay utilizes different cutpoints (both absolute and the change [i.e., "delta"]) for categorizing patients appropriately. (Fig. 7.4).

Overall, the performance of these 0/1 and 0/2 h CDPs is excellent and will "rule out" about 60%–65% of patients, "rule-in" approximately 15% for an MI, and assign 25%–30% to an indeterminate state. The efficacy, defined as the proportion of patients triaged with the CDP assigned as low probability and free death or MI at 30 days, is approximately 60% of patients with acute chest pain. A meta-analysis of CDPs found the sensitivities were all approximately 99% and NPV of approximately 99.5% for MI.[4]

Single Sample hsTn "Rule-out" Protocols

In certain circumstances, a single hsTn assessment is sufficient to exclude or "rule out" an ACS with high sensitivity and NPV. This approach, which greatly simplifies the evaluation of patients with chest pain, can only be utilized when the patient presents greater than 2 hours after the onset of chest discomfort. Even high-sensitivity assays may not detect circulating levels of cTn so soon after myocardial injury. As expected, this strategy will "rule-out" a smaller

TABLE 7.1 Clinical Decision Pathways With Hs-cTn

APPROACH	CRITERIA FOR RULE OUT	ADVANTAGES	DISADVANTAGES
0/3 h	Single hs-cTn <99th percentile URL if symptoms >6 h and now pain free OR If <6 h of symptoms, 0- and 3-h troponin less than the 99th percentile URL	• Uses 99th percentile URL cutoffs similar to conventional troponin, which is familiar to clinicians • Conceptually simpler • Validated	• Lower sensitivity and NPV, and fewer patients ruled out compared with other pathways
0/1-h rule out	Use baseline (0-h) and delta values at 1 h to assign patients to the rule-out, observation, or abnormal groups	• Takes advantage of better assay sensitivity and precision • Avoids inherent problems with 99th percentile URL value • Rules out a large proportion of patients	• Complex algorithm • Timing of blood draws very important • May miss late-presenting MI on the "flat" portion of a declining troponin trend
0/2-h rule out	Identical approach to 0/1-h rule out except delta assessed at 2 h	• Takes advantage of higher sensitivity and precision of assay • More practical for some centers that cannot routinely obtain 1-h samples • Better for early presenters than 0/1-h algorithm	• Longer time to rule out than 0/1-h algorithm • Equally complex as 0/1-h algorithm • May miss late-presenting MI on the "flat" portion of a declining troponin trend • Not validated in RCTs
High-STEACS	MI is ruled out if initial hs-cTnI <5 ng/L or hs-cTnT <6 ng/L (if >3 h from symptom onset) or if change from initial to 3-h hs-cTn is <3 ng/L and remains below sex-specific 99th percentile URL	• Takes advantage of better sensitivity and precision of assay • Safety and efficacy validated in randomized controlled trial • High rates of safe rule out • Uses sex-specific 99th percentile cutpoint	• Longer time to rule out for patients with initial hs-cTnI >5 ng/L or hs-cTnT ≥6 ng/L • Fewer patients discharged from ED than with 0/1- or 0/2-h algorithms

ED, Emergency department; *High-STEACS*, high-sensitivity troponin in the evaluation of patients with acute coronary syndrome; *hs-cTn*, high-sensitivity cardiac troponin; *hs-cTnI*, high-sensitivity cardiac troponin I; *hs-cTnT*, high-sensitivity cardiac troponin T; *LoQ*, limit of quantification; *MI*, myocardial infarction; *NPV*, negative predictive value; *RCT*, randomized controlled trial; *URL*, upper reference limit.

From Kontos MC, de Lemos JA, Deitelzweig SB, et al. 2022 ACC expert consensus decision pathway on the evaluation and disposition of acute chest pain in the emergency department: a report of the American College of Cardiology solution set oversight committee. *J Am Coll Cardiol*. 2022;80:1925–1960.

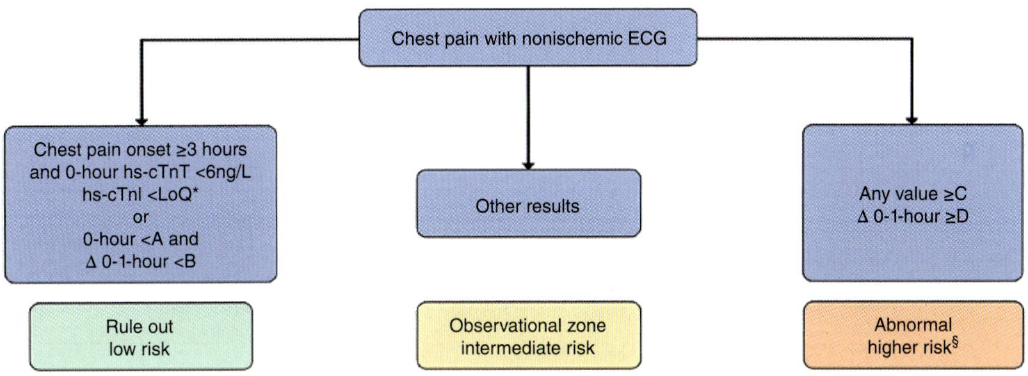

Assay	LoQ	A	B	C	D
Roche Elecys hs-cTnT	6	12	3	52	5
Abbott Architect hs-cTnI	4	5	2	52	6
Beckman Coulter Access hs-cTnI	3	5	4	50	15
Siemens ADVIA Centaur hs-cTnI	3	6	3	120	12
Siemens Atellica hs-cTnI	3	6	3	120	12
Siemens Dimension Vista hs-cTnI	3	5	2	107	19

FIG. 7.4 Modified European Society of Cardiology 0/1-hour CDP for ruling out MI. Note that variations of these rapid CDPs have been implemented in different centers, and modification of the algorithms shown may be considered based on local considerations. All values in the chart in are ng/L. *The LoQ may differ slightly from the 0-hour rule-out threshold tested in individual studies. Using a cutoff of <5 ng/L can also be considered instead of the LoQ for the 0-hour rule-out threshold for hs-cTnI assays. Additional evaluation should include at least one additional observation with hs-cTn measurement at 3–6 hours, with classification of myocardial injury into chronic myocardial injury, acute myocardial injury, type 1 MI, and type 2 MI, as per the Universal Definition of Myocardial Infarction. §Patients with acute MI should be managed according to standard practice guidelines. *CDP*, Clinical decision pathway; ECG, electrocardiogram; *hs-cTnI*, high-sensitivity cardiac troponin I; *hs-cTnT*, high-sensitivity cardiac troponin T; *LoQ*, limit of quantification; *MI*, myocardial infarction. (From Kontos MC, de Lemos JA, Deitelzweig SB, et al. 2022 ACC expert consensus decision pathway on the evaluation and disposition of acute chest pain in the emergency department: a report of the American College of Cardiology solution set oversight committee. *J Am Coll Cardiol*. 2022;80:1925–1960.)

proportion of patients than serial measurements (20%–60% of patients depending on the underlying rate of ACS); however, it still demonstrates consistent NPV greater than 99% across multiple studies.[7]

Intermediate Probability Patients

Patients not assigned initially as low probability (rule-out) or high probability (rule-in) using CDPs are binned as intermediate probability and require additional evaluation. In most clinical scenarios, the next step should be a third hsTn test at 3–6 hours from the initial sample. There is no evidence-based cutpoint for the 3–6 hours test; however, a reasonable threshold is a 20% change from the prior result. At lower levels near the sex-specific 99th percentile URL, absolute thresholds may be more appropriate than relative changes. As presented in Fig. 7.5, no or minimal change in hsTn from prior, together with any of several clinical features, including normal prior cardiac testing, known and stable hsTn elevation, or utilizing a clinical risk score can re-classify patients at a lower probability for consideration of early discharge. In contrast, a significant increase in hsTn, recurrent chest discomfort, or new ECG changes would signify high probability for ACS. Patients who remain at intermediate probability after the 3–6 hours hsTn measurement should be considered for additional noninvasive testing.

Before the introduction of hsTn, several CDPs incorporated clinical risk scores with biomarker data to improve the performance of CDPs. Two commonly used scores are the History, ECG, Age, Risk Factors, and Troponin (HEART) score or the ED Assessment of Chest Pain Score (EDACS) Table 7.2. With the introduction of hsTn, the HEART Score was updated to remove the troponin component. These scores can help triage patients in the intermediate zone after serial hsTn evaluations.

Given the high negative predictive value of many of the CDPs that utilize hsTn assays, the benefit of additional testing in low-probability patients is questionable. What additional test, for example, can improve on a negative predictive value of greater than 99%? However, for intermediate probability patients additional testing is reasonable.

Two categories of tests are available to confirm that the patient does not have ACS. Functional, or "provocative"

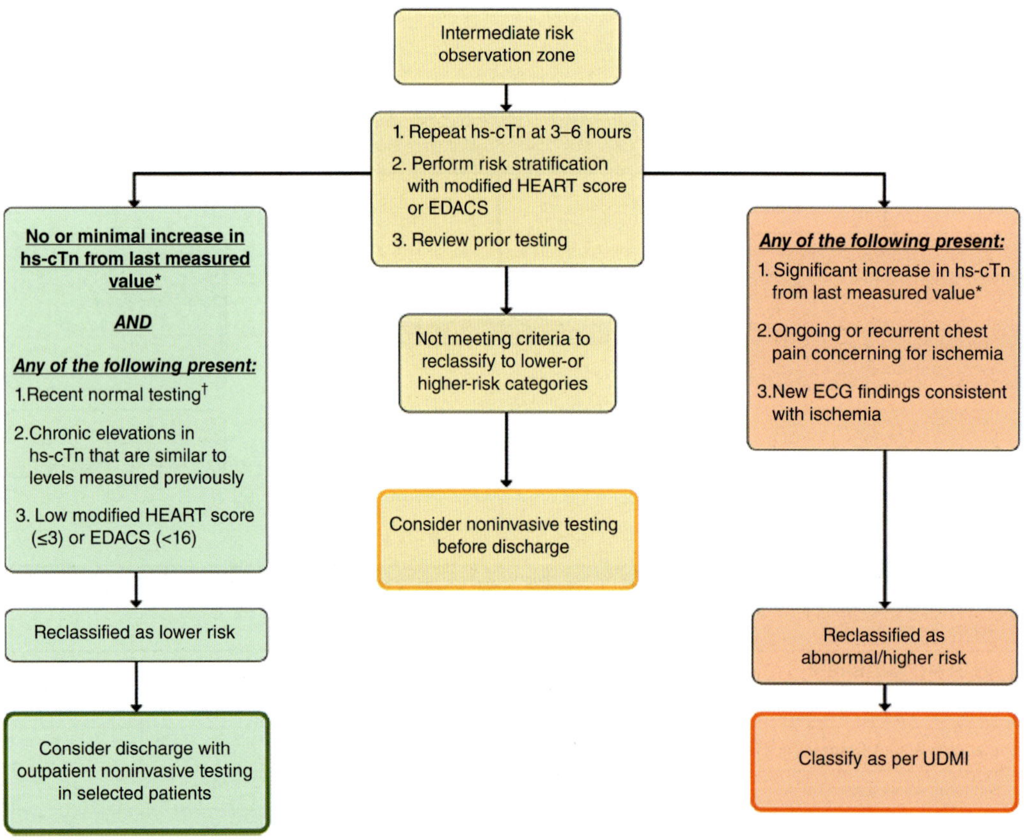

FIG. 7.5 Algorithm for intermediate-risk patients. *Evidence-based criteria do not exist to define change thresholds for hs-cTn at the 3- to 6-hour timepoint. Although a 20% relative change from the baseline measurement has been proposed to define significant change, this threshold lacks specificity at low hs-cTn values in part due to assay imprecision. Thus, at lower hs-cTn values near the sex-specific 99th percentile URL values, absolute changes should be used to define clinically significant change, whereas at higher troponin values, a 20% relative change in values may be a more reasonable threshold. Clinical judgment is needed to interpret small fluctuations in hs-cTn values over serial measurements, as these small changes may reflect assay imprecision rather than acute cardiac injury. †Recent normal testing is considered an invasive or CT coronary angiogram <2 years without evidence of coronary plaque or a stress test <1 year without ischemia. *ECG*, electrocardiogram; *EDACS*, Emergency Department Assessment of Chest Pain Score; *HEART*, History, ECG, Age, Risk Factors, and Troponin; *hs-cTn*, high-sensitivity cardiac troponin; *UDMI*, Universal Definition of Myocardial Infarction. (From Kontos MC, de Lemos JA, Deitelzweig SB, et al. 2022 ACC expert consensus decision pathway on the evaluation and disposition of acute chest pain in the emergency department: a report of the American College of Cardiology solution set oversight committee. *J Am Coll Cardiol.* 2022;80:1925–1960.)

TABLE 7.2 Modified HEART Scores and EDACS Data Components

HEART SCORE COMPONENTS LOW RISK: 0–3 POINTS; NON-LOW RISK: ≥4 POINTS		EDACS COMPONENTS LOW RISK: 0–15 POINTS; NON-LOW RISK: ≥16 POINTS	
History		Age, *y*	
High suspicion	2	18–45	2
Moderate suspicion	1	46–50	4
Low suspicion	0	51–55	6
Electrocardiogram		56–60	8
ST-segment deviation	2	61–65	10
Paced, LBBB, RBBB, or LVH	1	66–70	12
Normal or nonspecific changes	0	71–75	14
Age, y		76–80	16
>65	2	81–85	18
45–65	1	86+	20
<45	0	Male sex	6
Cardiac risk factors		Age 18–15 and either ≥3 cardiac risk factors or known CAD	4
≥3 or known CAD	2	Diaphoresis	3
1–2	1	Pain radiating to arm or shoulder	5
0	0	Pain worsened with inspiration	−4
		Pain reproduced by palpation	−6

CAD, Coronary artery disease; *EDACS*, emergency department assessment of chest pain; *HEART*, history, ECG, age, risk factors, and troponin; *LBBB*, left bundle branch block; *LVH*, left ventricular hypertrophy; *RBBB*, right bundle branch block.
From Kontos MC, de Lemos JA, Deitelzweig SB, et al. 2022 ACC expert consensus decision pathway on the evaluation and disposition of acute chest pain in the emergency department: a report of the American College of Cardiology solution set oversight committee. *J Am Coll Cardiol*. 2022;80:1925–1960.

testing, is a test to provoke ischemia. The exercise treadmill test (ETT), the classic functional test, is considered "positive" if it generates typical reproducible symptoms, ST-segment depression, or a drop in blood pressure. In a patient with unstable coronary syndrome, presumably with little ischemic reserve, one would expect the symptoms to begin at a low workload. Reconciling the diagnosis of an ACS with chest pain precipitated only in stage 4 of a standard Bruce protocol is challenging, and such chest pain is more likely to represent stable coronary disease in a patient with noncardiac symptoms at rest. A pharmacologic vasodilatory stress test poses a similar problem because it cannot identify "low-level" ischemia. Imaging studies, either myocardial perfusion imaging (MPI), echocardiography, or magnetic resonance imaging, typically improve the sensitivity and specificity of a standard ETT. Moreover, imaging should be used in patients with abnormal baseline ECG findings and those unable to exercise.

Of the functional tests, rest myocardial imaging, which uses either radiopharmaceutical labeling or echocardiography to identify ischemic areas at rest in patients with active pain, is the most intuitively rational test to exclude ACS (see Chapter 5). In studies of patients with acute chest pain rest MPI has a negative predictive value of 99% to 100%; in practice, however, mobilizing the resources to perform the test while the patient is experiencing chest pain is challenging. Moreover, most of the studies of rest MPI or echo for diagnostic evaluation of ACS were done before the widespread use of sensitive cTn assays.

The use of computed tomography angiography (CTA) as "anatomic" noninvasive testing is discussed in detail in Chapter 5. The completed studies of patients with suspected ischemic pain indicate that a CTA strategy significantly reduces the time to discharge from the ED but increases downstream testing, including invasive testing and radiation exposure. The absence of coronary atherosclerosis on CTA is reassuring in excluding a diagnosis of ACS; however, detecting a coronary lesion does not indicate whether it is the "culprit" lesion or just an asymptomatic stenosis unrelated to the presenting symptoms. Careful patient selection is critical to the utility of CTA in diagnosing ACS. The relative advantages and disadvantages of different testing modalities are presented in Table 7.3.

When Should Additional Noninvasive Testing Be Performed?

The argument for eliminating the subsequent testing after a hsTn CDP determines a patient to be low probability rests on the fact that if the pretest probability is low (in this case, less than 1%), then the value of an additional test, no matter how sensitive or specific, is minimal.

The results of noninvasive diagnostic testing are most likely to influence subsequent decisions when the pretest probability of ACS is in the intermediate range. If this patient's pretest probability of ACS was approximately 50%, an early positive stress test result would increase the likelihood of ischemia (posttest probability of approximately 85%), whereas a negative result on exercise testing dramatically reduces the likelihood (posttest probability less than 10%). By contrast, an abnormal result on exercise testing in a 35-year-old woman with noncardiac chest pain symptoms and normal ECG and biomarker levels (pretest probability of ACS of 1%) is likely to represent a false positive, prompting the use of unnecessary medications or invasive diagnostic testing; a negative result would support a low index of clinical suspicion for coronary heart disease (CHD). Therefore, noninvasive testing in such a low-risk patient would not be helpful (see Fig. 7.1).

Further supporting the concept of discharging patients with a low probability for the presence of ACS without any testing are the results of one of the CTA studies that measured hsTnT and found that in patients with undetectable hsTnT, the median calcium score was 0. Only 11%

TABLE 7.3 Clinical Considerations for the Use of Noninvasive Testing for Coronary Artery Disease

ISCHEMIA TEST MODALITY	STRENGTHS	LIMITATIONS	PATIENT CONSIDER ATIONS FAVORING ITS USE
Exercise stress ECG	• Low cost • Wide availability • Assessment of exercise symptoms, capacity • No ionizing radiation	• Decreased accuracy compared with anatomical and stress-imaging tests • Requires interpretable ECG and ability to exercise sufficiently	• Rarely recommended as a stand-alone test due to frequent known CAD, inability to exercise, or significant arrhythmias
Stress echocardiography	• Wide availability • High diagnostic specificity • Assessment of ventricular and valvular function • No ionizing radiation	• Decreased sensitivity compared with anatomical and other stress-imaging tests • Dependent on good image quality • Requires dobutamine in patients unable to exercise	• Known good image quality and ability to exercise • Consider use of an ultrasound-enhancing agent to improve endocardial visualization • Known moderate or severe valvular disease
Stress/rest SPECT	• Wide availability • Relatively high diagnostic sensitivity • Assessment of ventricular function	• Increased artifacts resulting in nondiagnostic results and decreased diagnostic accuracy compared with stress/rest PET • Radiation exposure	• Known CAD or high CAC burden on chest CT imaging • Preferred over stress echocardiography in patients who cannot exercise or who do not have significant bronchospastic disease
Stress/rest PET	• High diagnostic accuracy • Lower radiation exposure than • SPECT • Measures myocardial blood flow and flow reserve • Assessment of ventricular function	• Limited availability • Relatively higher cost • Lack of exercise assessment	• Known CAD or high CAC burden on chest CT imaging • Preferred over SPECT due to higher diagnostic accuracy and lower rate of nondiagnostic test results
Stress CMR	• High diagnostic accuracy • Accurate assessment of chamber sizes, ventricular and valvular function • Diagnosis of prior infarction, scar, fibrosis • Measurement of myocardial blood flow and flow reserve is possible but not widely available currently • No ionizing radiation	• Limited availability • Relatively higher cost • Lack of exercise assessment • Long scan acquisition times • Claustrophobia • Often not immediately available to patients with pacemakers or ICDs • Contraindicated in patients with significant renal dysfunction	• Known CAD and/or cardiomyopathy • Elevated troponin not thought to be secondary to ACS • Known moderate or severe valvular disease • No significant renal dysfunction
CTA	• High diagnostic accuracy • Does not require exercise • Identifies nonobstructive CAD	• Radiation exposure • Lack of exercise assessment • Contraindicated in patients with significant renal dysfunction • Blooming artifacts when significant coronary calcification present • Atrial fibrillation or other arrhythmias • May require beta-blockade • Incidental noncardiac findings	• No known CAD • Absence of severe coronary calcification • Prior normal, mildly abnormal, or inconclusive stress test results • No known iodinated contrast medium allergy or significant renal dysfunction • Low likelihood of high-quality stress testing or lack of timely access

ACS, Acute coronary syndrome; *CAC*, coronary artery calcium; *CAD*, coronary artery disease; *CMR*, cardiovascular magnetic resonance; *CT*, computed tomography; *CTA*, computed tomography angiography; *ECG*, electrocardiogram; *ICD*, implantable cardioverter defibrillator; *PET*, positron emission tomography; *SPECT*, single-photon emission computed tomography.

From Kontos MC, de Lemos JA, Deitelzweig SB, et al. 2022 ACC expert consensus decision pathway on the evaluation and disposition of acute chest pain in the emergency department: a report of the American College of Cardiology solution set oversight committee. *J Am Coll Cardiol*. 2022;80:1925–1960.

had evidence of any atherosclerosis, and none had stenosis greater than 50%. With the less sensitive conventional troponin assay, however, 12.5% of patients with an undetectable level of cTn had stenosis with greater than 70% occlusion.

Subsequent diagnostic testing still may play a role in the evaluation of "intermediate-probability" patients, many of whom will not require hospital admission but can be managed within the ED and/or in observation units, thereby preventing hospital admissions and additional health care costs.[8] In addition, as emphasized in the most recent guidelines, even intermediate-probability patients can be discharged home with planned outpatient testing within 72 hours.[1] The most challenging component of a discharge strategy before testing is establishing a system of care that ensures that the discharged patient will receive appropriate follow-up care. The critical link is the transfer of responsibility from the physician providing the initial care to the outpatient physician.

SUMMARY

Considering the number of patients presenting with suspected MI, the magnitude of associated health care resources, and the decades of research into ACS, the management and evaluation of patients with acute chest pain have remained very much an "art," still relying on clinical judgment. Moreover, entrenched practice patterns designed to prevent any missed cases of MI are slow to change in response to newer strategies that can identify a large population of patients who can be discharged home safely with the reassurance that they are at extremely low risk for subsequent ischemic events. Changing practice

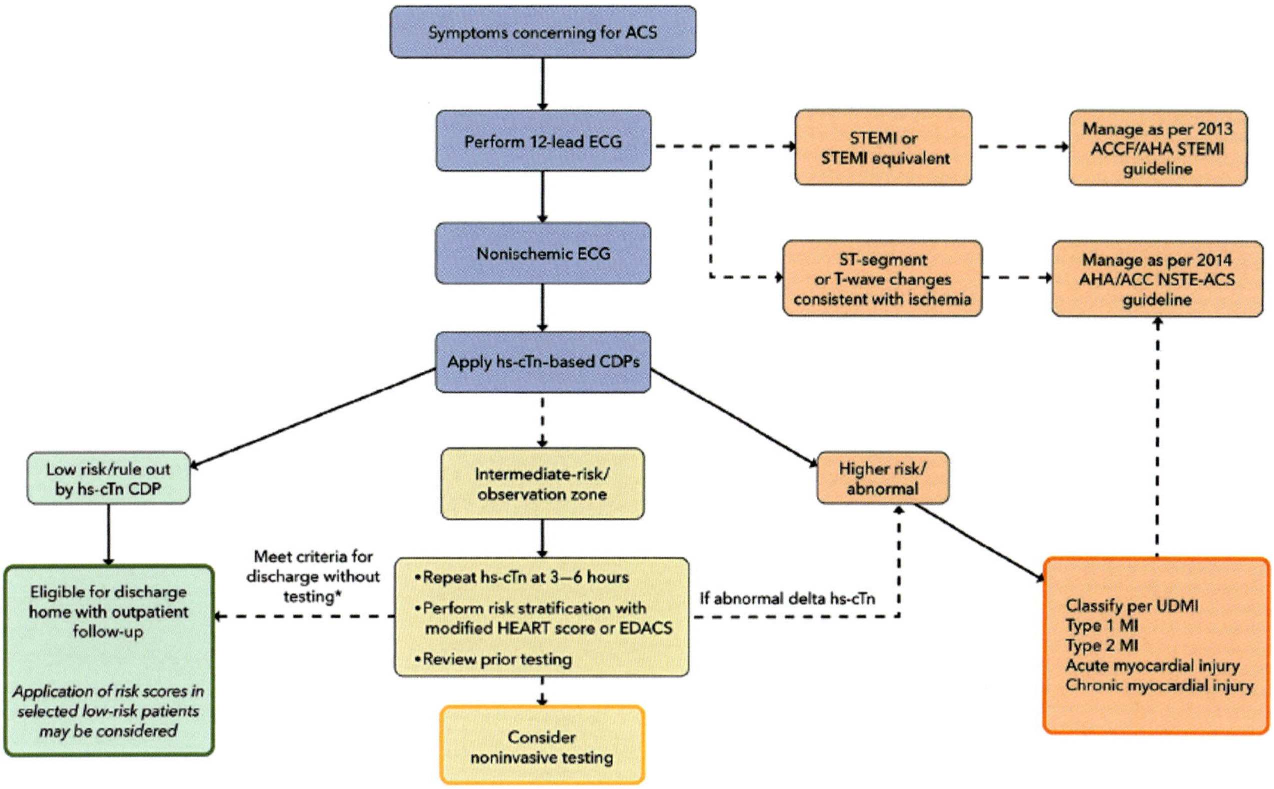

FIG. 7.6 Pathway summary graphic. *Unchanged high-sensitivity troponin concentration (i.e., no or minimal change over serial measurements) with (1) recent normal testing (i.e., invasive or CT coronary angiogram <2 years ago or stress test <1 year ago); (2) symptoms inconsistent with possible ACS; (3) chronic elevations in hs-cTn that are unchanged compared with levels measured previously; or (4) a modified HEART score <3 or EDACS <16. *ACC*, American College Cardiology; *ACS*, acute coronary syndrome; *AHA*, American Heart Association; *CDP*, clinical decision pathway; *ECG*, electrocardiogram; *EDACS*, Emergency Department Assessment of Chest Pain Score; *HEART*, History, ECG, Age, Risk Factors, and Troponin; *hs-cTn*, high-sensitivity cardiac troponin; *MI*, myocardial infarction; *NSTE-ACS*, non-ST-segment elevation acute coronary syndrome; *STEMI*, ST-segment elevation myocardial infarction; *UDMI*, Universal Definition of Myocardial Infarction. (From Kontos MC, de Lemos JA, Deitelzweig SB, et al. 2022 ACC expert consensus decision pathway on the evaluation and disposition of acute chest pain in the emergency department: a report of the American College of Cardiology solution set oversight committee. *J Am Coll Cardiol*. 2022;80:1925–1960.)

culture is challenging, especially one so intertwined with divergent incentives (e.g., the principle of beneficence, medicolegal issues, reimbursement rules). For example, only one-third of US hospitals were using hsTn assays by the end of 2021.[9] A collaborative, integrated approach (Fig. 7.6) that leverages ED, cardiology, and outpatient follow-up evaluation offers the greatest potential to expedite the investigation of chest pain, minimize unnecessary testing, and identify patients requiring urgent ACS management.

CLASSIC REFERENCES

Goldman L, Cook EF, Brand DA, et al. A computer protocol to predict myocardial infarction in emergency department patients with chest pain. *N Engl J Med*. 1988;318(13):797–803.

Reichlin T, Hochholzer W, Bassetti S, et al. Early diagnosis of myocardial infarction with sensitive cardiac troponin assays. *N Engl J Med*. 2009;361(9):858–867.

Keller T, Zeller T, Ojeda F, et al. Serial changes in highly sensitive troponin I assay and early diagnosis of myocardial infarction. *JAMA*. 2011;306(24):2684–2693.

Mahler SA, Riley RF, Hiestand BC, et al. The HEART pathway randomized trial: identifying emergency department patients with acute chest pain for early discharge. *Circ Cardiovasc Qual Outcomes*. 2015;8(2):195–203. https://doi.org/10.1161/CIRCOUTCOMES.114.001384.

Than MP, Pickering JW, Aldous SJ, et al. Effectiveness of EDACS versus ADAPT accelerated diagnostic pathways for chest pain: a pragmatic randomized controlled trial embedded within practice. *Ann Emerg Med*. 2016;68(1):93–102.e1. https://doi.org/10.1016/j.annemergmed.2016.01.001.

REFERENCES

1. Writing C, Kontos MC, de Lemos JA, et al. 2022 ACC expert consensus decision pathway on the evaluation and disposition of acute chest pain in the emergency department: a report of the American College of Cardiology solution set oversight committee. *J Am Coll Cardiol*. 2022;80(20):1925–1960. https://doi.org/10.1016/j.jacc.2022.08.750.
2. Writing Committee M, Gulati M, Levy PD, et al. 2021 AHA/ACC/ASE/CHEST/SAEM/SCCT/SCMR guideline for the evaluation and diagnosis of chest pain: a report of the American College of Cardiology/American Heart Association joint committee on clinical practice guidelines. *J Am Coll Cardiol*. 2021;78(22):e187–e285. https://doi.org/10.1016/j.jacc.2021.07.053.
3. Thygesen K, Alpert JS, Jaffe AS, et al. Fourth universal definition of myocardial infarction (2018). *J Am Coll Cardiol*. 2018;72(18):2231–2264. https://doi.org/10.1016/j.jacc.2018.08.1038.
4. Burgos LM, Trivi M, Costabel JP. Performance of the European Society of Cardiology 0/1-hour algorithm in the diagnosis of myocardial infarction with high-sensitivity cardiac troponin: systematic review and meta-analysis. *Eur Heart J Acute Cardiovasc Care*. 2021;10(3):279–286. https://doi.org/10.1177/2048872620935399.
5. Neumann JT, Twerenbold R, Ojeda F, et al. Application of high-sensitivity troponin in suspected myocardial infarction. *N Engl J Med*. 2019;380(26):2529–2540. https://doi.org/10.1056/NEJMoa1803377.
6. Anand A, Lee KK, Chapman AR, et al. High-sensitivity cardiac troponin on presentation to rule out myocardial infarction: a stepped-wedge cluster randomized controlled trial. *Circulation*. 2021;143(23):2214–2224. https://doi.org/10.1161/CIRCULATIONAHA.120.052380.
7. Jaffe AS, Body R, Mills NL, et al. Single troponin measurement to rule out myocardial infarction: JACC review topic of the week. *J Am Coll Cardiol*. 2023;82(1):60–69. https://doi.org/10.1016/j.jacc.2023.04.040.
8. Ganguli I, Cui J, Thakore N, et al. Downstream cascades of care following high-sensitivity troponin test implementation. *J Am Coll Cardiol*. 2021;77(25):3171–3179. https://doi.org/10.1016/j.jacc.2021.04.049.
9. McCarthy C, Li S, Wang TY, et al. Implementation of high-sensitivity cardiac troponin assays in the United States. *J Am Coll Cardiol*. 2023;81(3):207–219. https://doi.org/10.1016/j.jacc.2022.10.017.

8 Selection of Reperfusion Therapy and Transfer Strategies for Patients With STEMI

KEVIN R. BAINEY AND PAUL W. ARMSTRONG

INTRODUCTION

The evolution of acute reperfusion therapy for ST-elevation myocardial infarction (STEMI) continues to be influenced by new evidence emerging from randomized clinical trials. Of equal merit to these advances is their applicability and subsequent adherence to clinical guidelines in every day practice. Prompt recanalization of the infarct-related artery remains the cornerstone of reducing infarct size and improving morbidity and mortality. Renewed appreciation of the need to account for *total ischemic time* (time from sustained symptom onset to reperfusion) with focus on early recognition of symptoms and rapid initiation of treatment is paramount. The acknowledgment that early risk assessment informs diagnosis and guides utilization of appropriate contemporary pharmacologic and/or invasive strategies are key components of optimal patient-centered care. The continuing belief in some jurisdictions that primary percutaneous coronary intervention (PCI) is not only the preferred—but the only reperfusion strategy—is increasingly untenable as new quality assurance measures testify. Despite more than two decades of effort to facilitate timely access to primary PCI, contemporary metrics repeatedly demonstrate the inability to achieve prompt reperfusion with this strategy in a large fraction of STEMI patients requiring transfer to a PCI-capable hospital. Placing the large majority of STEMI patients worldwide in the context of their geographic location, access to timely and expert 24/7 primary PCI, transfer logistics, and the total elapsed ischemic time, not only unmasks the stark reality of global management challenges but also the attendant penalty patients suffer when reperfusion is delayed. For example, in the United States, it is estimated that 20% of the population lives more than 60 minutes away from a PCI-capable hospital which poses challenges to guideline-driven primary PCI time metrics. As outlined in Fig. 8.1, unforeseen obstacles can occur when aiming for timely primary PCI requiring transfer to a PCI-capable hospital from the ambulance or community site.

Accordingly, it is recognized that alternate reperfusion strategies need to be explored to reduce total ischemic time, particularly important in transfer patients. A pharmacoinvasive strategy of early fibrinolysis coupled with immediate transfer for routine coronary angiography has now emerged as a legitimate and effective alternative when timely primary PCI cannot be achieved.

The aim of this chapter is to provide insights regarding the selection of reperfusion strategies in STEMI patients whose initial medical contact is in an ambulance or a community hospital (non-PCI site) with planned transfer to a PCI-capable hospital. These recommendations will be based on four foundational and time-honored components embedded in the early evaluation of STEMI: (1) ***index STEMI risk***, (2) ***risk of pharmacoinvasive PCI***, (3) ***total ischemic time***, and (4) ***PCI-related delay***—the time required to reliably achieve expert primary PCI compared to the administration of fibrinolysis in the context of pharmacoinvasive PCI.

Four Tenants in Evaluating the Selection of Reperfusion Strategy for STEMI Patients Requiring Transfer to a PCI-Capable Hospital

A "one-size-fits-all" approach is inadequate to address the needs of patients with STEMI requiring transfer to a health care facility whether it be an ambulance or a community hospital. For that reason, application of evidence-based reperfusion choices to promote and sustain high-quality reperfusion, limit myocardial damage, prevent unfavorable left ventricular remodeling, and reduce mechanical complications of myocardial infarction is a key responsibility

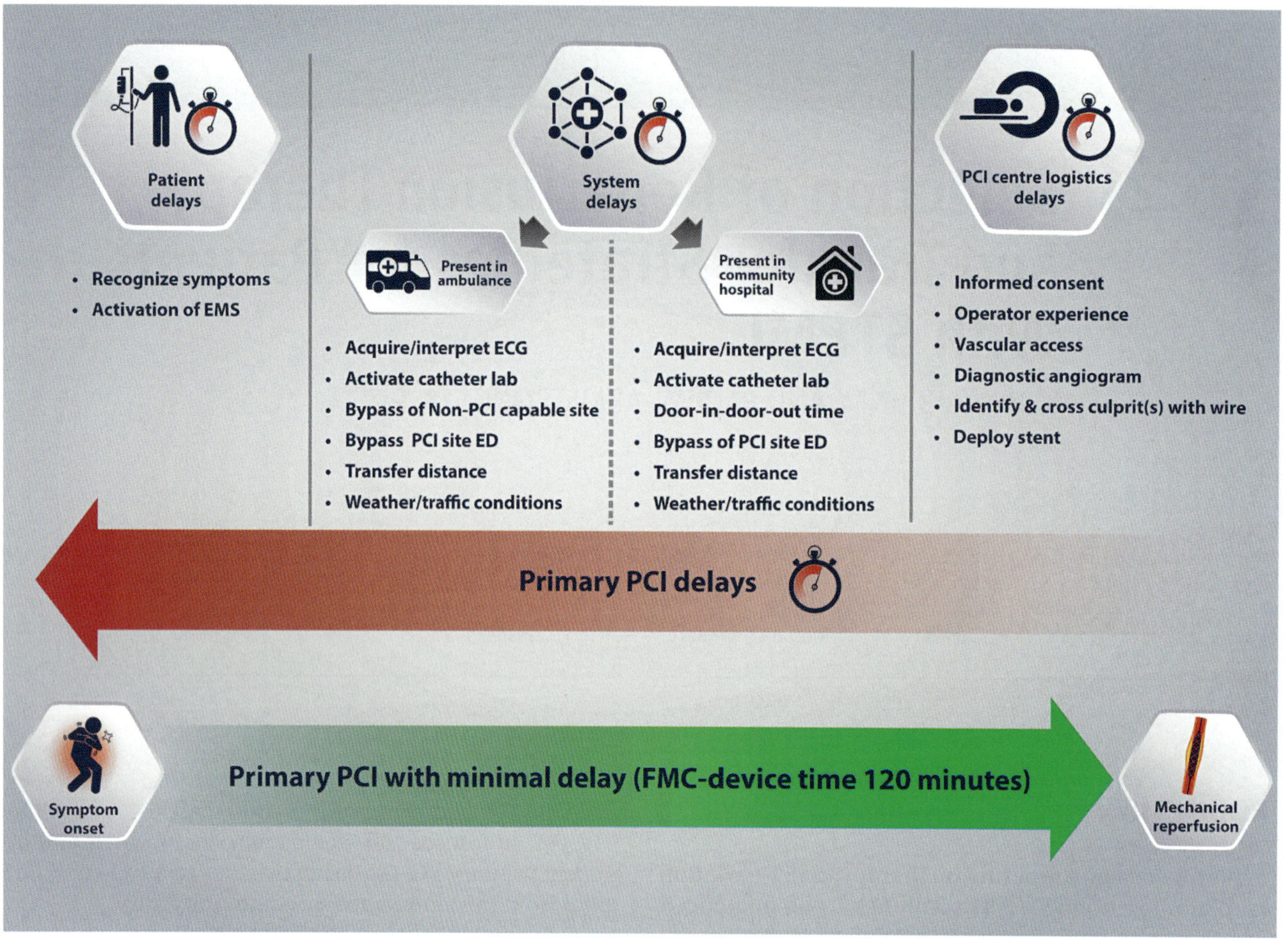

Fig. 8.1 Components of delays in transfer of STEMI for primary PCI. Primary PCI delays (*red arrow*) can occur across three domains. (1) Patient delays can occur in activating the health system. (2) System delays can occur both in the ambulance and in the community hospital delaying the onset of reperfusion. (3) Once transferred to a PCI-capable hospital, cardiac catheterization delays can occur prior to achieving mechanical recanalization. Otherwise, primary PCI with minimal delay should occur with a first medical contact to device time within 120 minutes (*green arrow*).

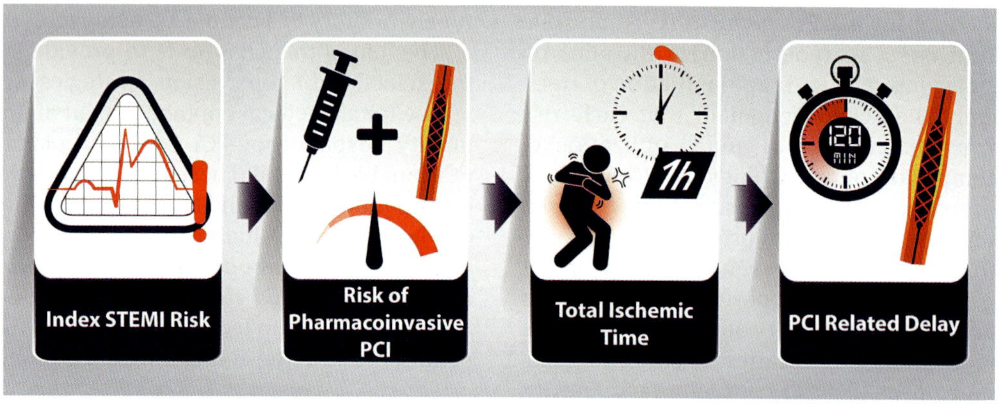

Fig. 8.2 Four principles to consider when choosing a reperfusion strategy in ST-elevation myocardial infarction (STEMI) requiring transfer to a PCI-capable hospital. All four of these foundational principles should be reviewed by the clinician when faced with a STEMI in the pre-hospital (ambulance) setting or in the community hospital.

of any front-line clinician. Evaluating the selection of the best reperfusion strategy in a transfer STEMI patient is highlighted in Fig. 8.2.

Index STEMI Risk

Low-Intermediate Risk STEMI

Since baseline risk strongly intersects with time from symptom onset to reperfusion in modulating reperfusion strategies, an appreciation for the wide spectrum of STEMI risk becomes important. Using the TIMI STEMI risk score, Morrow et al. demonstrated the large majority of patients in the NRMI-3 registry are at low-to-intermediate risk. Similarly, in a cohort of 1791 STEMI patients in the Netherlands with STEMI undergoing primary PCI, the ZWOLLE group found more than two-thirds of STEMI patients were low risk and suitable for early discharge. The CADILLAC PCI risk score (derived from 2082 participants in the CADILLAC STEMI trial and validated in the Stent-PAMI trial) also found more than 80% of STEMI patients were low or intermediate risk. When reperfusion strategies were compared in 5295 STEMI patients from seventy-three Belgian hospitals, mortality was no different with fibrinolysis compared to primary PCI in low risk (0.3% vs. 0.4%, adjusted $P = .60$) or intermediate risk (2.9% vs. 3.1%, adjusted $P = .30$) patients. Importantly, the benefits of primary PCI were *only* seen in patients with high TIMI STEMI risk scores (23.7% vs. 30.6%; adjusted $P = .03$).

Worthy of note is none of the prior studies have addressed the intersection of myocardial territory at risk and ischemic time, as it relates to outcomes. Arguably, the early stable patient with a large territory of ischemic myocardium has the highest potential mortality benefit from reperfusion as compared to patients with smaller territories at risk who present beyond the optimal time period for myocardial salvage. Based on the NRMI registry, a young anterior STEMI patient presenting early with symptoms should be considered for early fibrinolysis rather than waiting for primary PCI (i.e., shorter PCI-related delay). There is now growing acceptance of the need to account for myocardial territory at risk in choosing a reperfusion strategy with a greater imperative for shorter delay from first medical contact to reperfusion in early presenting (<2–3 hours) large territory STEMI patients, with consideration of pharmacoinvasive PCI in those who are at lower risk (Fig. 8.3).

High-Risk STEMI

STEMI presenting in cardiogenic shock portend the worse prognosis with a 40%–50% mortality at 30-days.[1,2] Primary PCI is universally accepted as the choice of reperfusion therapy for this cohort as supported by the SHOCK trial where early coronary angiography and emergent revascularization (PCI or CABG) improved 6-month survival compared to conservative approach (medical stabilization without routine coronary angiography). In a retrospective analysis of 2929 STEMI patients from the Vancouver Heath Authority STEMI registry who received primary PCI, 9.4% presented with cardiogenic shock. When compared to those without cardiogenic shock, median first medical contact to device times was longer (113.5 minutes, IQR 93–145 minutes vs. 103 minute, IQR 85.130 minute), and cardiogenic shock patients were more likely to exceed guideline recommendations for reperfusion. Notably, for every 10-minute increase in first medical contact to device time, absolute mortality increased by 4%–7% reinforcing the need to reduce *total ischemic times* in this high-risk cohort of patients.[3]

In an analysis of sixteen randomized trials of primary angioplasty versus fibrinolysis, baseline STEMI risk was also a major determinant of defining which time delay to primary PCI was acceptable, whereby longer delays with primary PCI offered a survival advantage *only* in the higher-risk patients (acceptable PCI-related delay as much as 200 minutes). Notwithstanding this latitude, when primary PCI is contemplated in high-risk patients, every effort

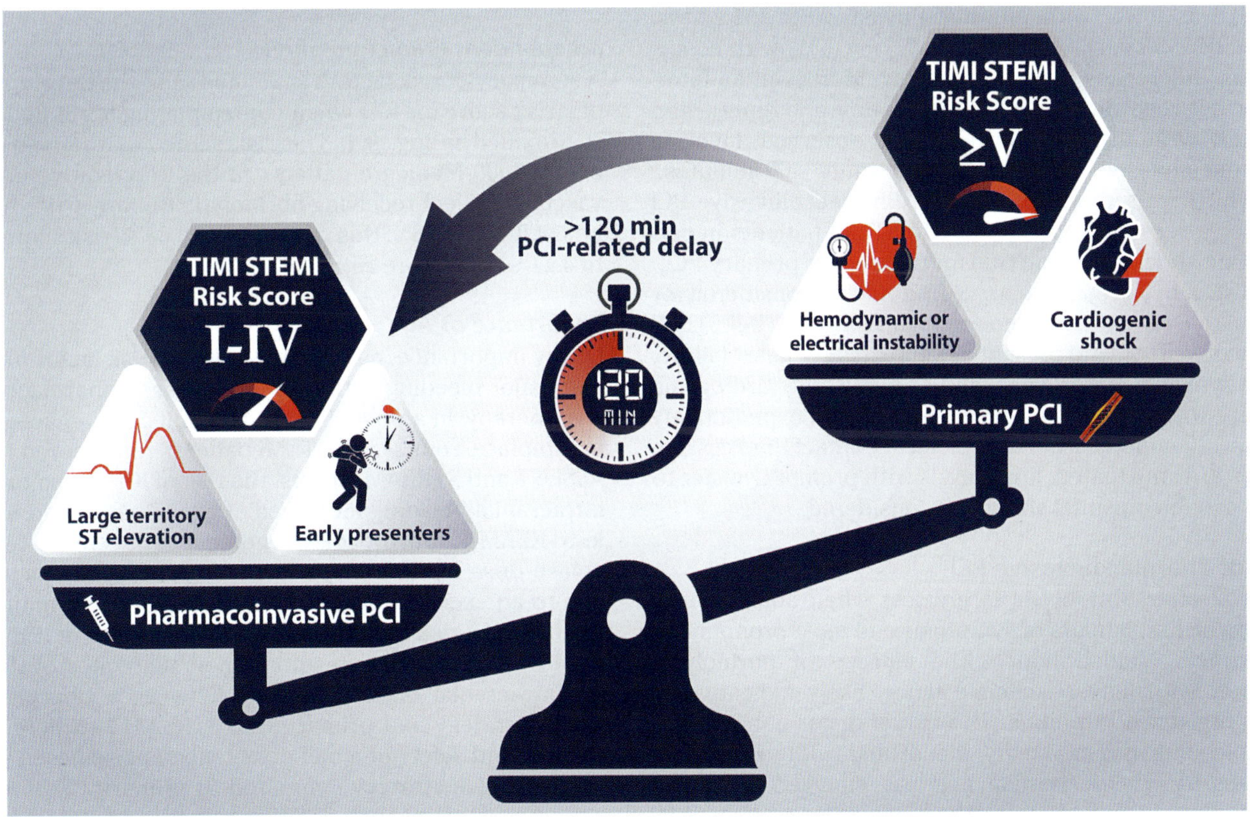

Fig. 8.3 Balancing index (baseline) STEMI risk to inform the best mode of reperfusion. Pharmacoinvasive PCI should be considered in patients who present early, are low-to-intermediate risk (TIMI STEMI risk score <5), especially with large myocardial territory at risk. Primary PCI should be considered in patients who are high risk (TIMI STEMI risk score ≥5) cardiogenic shock or hemodynamic/electrical instability. If primary PCI cannot be achieved in a timely manner (≤120 minutes from first medical contact), pharmacoinvasive PCI should be considered (*arrow*).

TABLE 8.1 Contraindications to Fibrinolysis

ABSOLUTE	RELATIVE
• History of any prior ICH • Prior ischemic stroke within the preceding 3 months, EXCEPT when within 3 h which could be treated with fibrinolysis • Known structural cerebral vascular lesion (e.g., arteriovenous malformation) or known malignant intracranial neoplasm (primary or metastatic) • Suspected aortic dissection • Active bleeding or bleeding diathesis (excluding menses) • Significant closed-head or facial trauma within the preceding 3 months	• History of chronic, severe, poorly controlled hypertension or uncontrolled hypertension on presentation (e.g., SBP >180 mm Hg and/or DBP >110 mm Hg) • History of prior ischemic stroke >3 months • Dementia • Known intracranial pathology not covered in absolute contraindications • Traumatic or prolonged (10 min) CPR • Major surgery within the preceding 3 weeks • Recent (within 2–4 weeks) internal bleeding or active peptic ulcer • Noncompressible vascular punctures • Pregnancy • Current warfarin therapy • For streptokinase or anistreplase, a prior exposure (more than 5 days previously) or allergic reaction to these drugs

should still be made to shorten treatment time given the evidence that survival with primary PCI attenuates for every 10-minute PCI-related delay, particularly in those who present in cardiogenic shock.[4]

We support a primary PCI approach to STEMI with cardiogenic shock (default strategy): however, geographic constraints with excessive transfer times may preclude this as an option. In an observational analysis from the Vital Heart Response STEMI network in Alberta, Canada, 426 patients with cardiogenic shock and STEMI presenting to a non-PCI capable hospital (with excessive transfer times) were studied, 53.8 % receiving pharmacoinvasive PCI and 46.2% receiving primary PCI. Worst lead residual ST-elevation <1 mm was greater with pharmacoinvasive PCI (57.3% vs. 46.3%, $P = .012$) and the primary clinical composite of in-hospital mortality, renal failure requiring dialysis, cardiac arrest, or mechanical circulatory support (MCS) was lower with pharmacoinvasive PCI (35.2% vs. 57.0%; IPW OR 0.44, 95% CI 0.26–0.72, $P = .001$) with no significant differences in major bleeding. Moreover, an interaction between inter-hospital transfer time and reperfusion strategy with all-cause mortality was observed, favoring pharmacoinvasive PCI with transfer times >60 minutes.[5] Until further studies are available, Pharmacoinvasive PCI may be a reasonable alternative to STEMI patients in cardiogenic shock with long transport times for primary PCI.

As seen in Fig. 8.3, primary PCI should be considered for those transfer patients who are high risk (i.e., TIMI STEMI risk score ≥5) or who present in Killip Class IV heart failure, hemodynamic compromise, and/or persistent cardiogenic shock—with the aim to achieve primary PCI expeditiously within 120 minutes from first medical contact. If excessive delays are anticipated, fibrinolysis with prompt transfer to a PCI-capable hospital should be considered.

Risk of Pharmacoinvasive PCI

Survival after fibrinolysis is greatest when administered within the first 3 hours of symptoms and most pronounced within the "golden hour". The efficacy of fibrinolysis declines with longer ischemic times, likely indicative of older organized thrombus. The risk of major nonintracranial bleeding has markedly diminished with transradial catheter-based intervention and has emerged as a preferred strategy including for those requiring rescue intervention when fibrinolysis fails. While the risk of intracranial hemorrhage (ICH) remains real, the perception of its risk is exaggerated by some physicians as recently reported in a survey of French emergency departments where estimates were as high as 5x the actual risk of roughly 1%.[6] In a recent prospective STEMI registry where selection of reperfusion strategy was based on ischemic time and risk of fibrinolysis, ICH rates were 0.6% at one year regardless of reperfusion strategy employed.[7] While these rates of ICH are low, it remains imperative to evaluate the risk of ICH given the associated morbidity and mortality with its occurrence.

Absolute and relative contraindications of fibrinolysis are summarized in Table 8.1. When the risk of ICH with fibrinolysis exceeds 1%, primary PCI should be considered the default strategy. However, the risk of the evolving STEMI needs to be balanced when timely primary PCI is not available. Half-dose tenecteplase may be a reasonable strategy as this regimen appears to have similar efficacy to full-dose tenecteplase and is associated with less major bleeding risk.

Independent Predictors of ICH

A summary of risk factors (modified) and the development of a risk score for ICH when contemplating fibrinolytic use is provided in Fig. 8.4. The risk score was derived from over 30,000 Medicare patients in the Cooperative Cardiovascular Project receiving fibrinolytic therapy with overall risk of ICH of 1.43%; this ranged from 0.69% (risk score 0–1) to 4.11% (risk score ≥5).

Importance of Age

Of key importance, age remains a major risk factor for ICH and major bleeding with fibrinolytic-based pharmacoinvasive therapy. In a pooled analysis of full-dose tenecteplase or alteplase from 24,000 STEMI patients randomized in the ASSENT and STREAM-1 trials, the risk of ICH or major nonintracranial bleeding increased at age 60 years and older.[8] In STREAM-1, a protocol amendment reduced the tenecteplase dose by 50% in patients 75 years of age or older due to an excess of ICH early in the trial which mitigated the bleeding risk and decreased the incidence of ICH from 1.0% to 0.5%, thereby resulting in similar rates of ICH or nonintracranial bleeding events between a pharmacoinvasive strategy and primary PCI. STREAM-2 explored the efficacy and safety of a half-dose tenecteplase-based pharmacoinvasive strategy compared to primary PCI in older patients ≥60 years with STEMI randomized within 3 hours of symptom onset and unable to undergo primary PCI within 1 hour. Despite a remarkably low and similar incidence of major nonintracranial bleeding (1.3% vs. 1.0%),

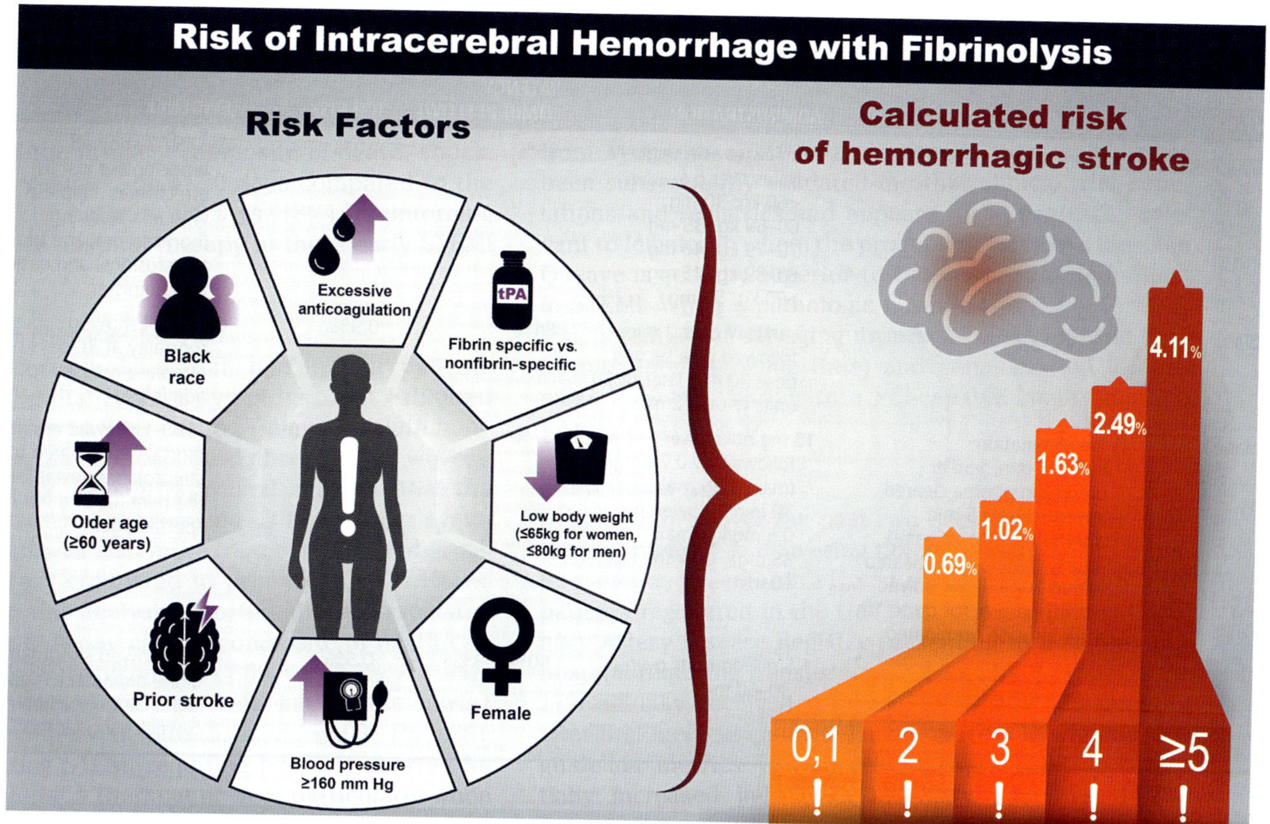

Fig. 8.4 Adapted risk factors for intracranial hemorrhage (left) and calculated risk for hemorrhagic stroke (right). In those with an ICH risk of >1%, careful risk assessment regarding the use of pharmacoinvasive PCI should be considered weighing the risk of delays to primary PCI.

an increased risk of ICH in the pharmacoinvasive strategy versus primary PCI was observed (1.5% vs. 0%)—however attributable to excessive additional anti-thrombotic therapy and protocol deviations.[9] Of note, no ICH cases were observed in those 75 years or older in STREAM-2.[9]

Contemplating Choice of Agent and Contraindications to Fibrinolysis

On balance, we favor tenecteplase as the preferred agent of choice, given the established safety and efficacy facilitated by a simple weight-adjusted single bolus injection which can be administered easily in the pre-hospital and community setting. Other fibrinolytic agents provide a variety of options depending on health economic and other local considerations and their various characteristics along with the risk of ICH as highlighted in Table 8.2.

Influence of Total Ischemic Time

Undoubtably, timely primary PCI reduces infarct size, resulting in reduced mortality and subsequent heart failure. However, when symptom onset to balloon time exceeds 90 minutes, myocardial salvage markedly decreases in tandem with increased microvascular obstruction as demonstrated by cardiac magnetic resonance (CMR) imaging in STEMI. Until recently, shortening *total ischemic times* has largely been ignored, given the preoccupation with abbreviating door-to-balloon times (DBT) for primary PCI. Paradoxically, these efforts in further decreasing DBT have not resulted in parallel reductions in mortality. The key role of total ischemic time on outcomes has been recently validated in a pooled analysis of over 3000 STEMI patients undergoing primary PCI from ten randomized studies. When stratified by both total ischemic time and DBT, CMR imaging showed that infarct size and microvascular obstruction were strongly associated with total ischemic time *but not DBT*.[10] We now know *total ischemic time* is a crucial metric to consider when choosing a reperfusion strategy and can be usefully stratified according to early, delayed, and late presenters with STEMI (Fig. 8.5).

Early Presenters (≤3 Hours of Symptom Onset)

As seen in Fig. 8.5, early presenters have the potential to derive the greatest benefit to minimize myocardial necrosis and preserve LV function (myocardial salvage), thereby avoiding shock and heart failure with the goal of improving overall survival. Early presenters often have "fresh clot" most conducive to fibrinolysis with higher rates of successful reperfusion and are ideal candidates.

In a combined analysis of pharmacoinvasive PCI from the CAPTIM and WEST trials, a temporal interaction was demonstrated in STEMI patients presenting within 2 hours of symptom onset where those receiving early fibrinolysis (with appropriate timely coronary co-intervention) showed improved one-year survival when compared to primary PCI (2.8% vs. 6.9%; HR0.43, 95% CI 0.20–0.91; $P = .021$).

Building on this work, an analysis from the STREAM trial (early presenting patients) evaluated the relationship on ischemic times based on whether the first point of care was a pre-hospital location versus community hospital. Shorter ischemic times with pre-hospital pharmacoinvasive PCI were observed with shorter symptom

TABLE 8.3 Pharmacoinvasive Registry Studies

STUDY	NUMBER OF PATIENTS	AVERAGE AGE	COMPARISON	INTERVENTION	EFFICACY	SAFETY
FAST-MI 2014	1492	60	PI with majority receiving TNK	Primary PCI	5-year survival 88% for PI, 83% for primary PCI, and 59% for no reperfusion. (Adjusted HR for PI vs. primary PCI 0.73, 95% CI 0.50–1.06). (Adjusted HR for prehospital PI vs. primary PCI 0.63, 95% CI 0.34–0.91).	In-hospital major bleeding 1.9% vs. 1.3% vs. 2.2% for no reperfusion, PI and primary PCI ($P = .29$). ICH 0% vs. 0.4% vs. 0.3%, respectively, ($P = .79$).
Korean KAMIR Registry 2016	$N = 9586$	60	PI with TNK, Alteplase, or Urokinase	Primary PCI	Twelve-month rates of death and major adverse cardiac events (composite of death, recurrent myocardial infarction, target-vessel revascularization, and coronary artery bypass graft surgery) were similar between pharmacoinvasive strategy and primary PCI. (4.4% vs. 4.1% and 7.5% vs. 7.8%, respectively).	Incidences of major bleeding and stroke during hospitalization were not different (0.7% vs. 0.3%, $P = .096$; 0.6% vs. 0.5%, $P = .868$, respectively)
Canadian VHR STEMI Registry 2017	$N = 5583$	59	PI with TNK (selected ½ dose in the elderly)	Primary PCI	The primary composite of death CHF, CS, and re-MI was significantly lower with a pharmacoinvasive approach (16.3% vs. 23.1%, IP-weighted hazard ratio, 0.84; 95% CI, 0.72–0.99; $P = .033$) at 1-year	Major bleeding and intracranial hemorrhage were similar between a pharmacoinvasive strategy and primary PCI (7.6% vs. 7.5%, $P = .867$; 0.6% vs. 0.6%; $P = .841$, respectively).
Kuwait REPERFUSE STEMI Registry 2020	$N = 936$	53	PI with either TNK or reteplase	Primary PCI	No significant difference in the composite in in-hospital death, re-MI stroke of CHF (2.4%, vs. 4.2%, $P = .12$; RR = 1.0; 95% CI 0.98–1.02; $P = .96$)	Major bleeding was similar (0.7% vs. 1.5%, $P = .36$)
Mexico City STEMI Registry 2020	$N = 579$	58	PI with TNK (77%), alteplase (21.9%), or streptokinase (1.0%)	Primary PCI	No significant difference in the composite of death, CS, re-MI, or CHF at 30-days (11.3% vs. 14.5%, HR 0.76, 95% CI 0.48–1.21, $P = .24$)	Major bleeding and ICH were similar (5.1% vs. 5.9%, HR 0.92, 95% CI 0.45–1.86, $P = .81$; 0.6% vs. 0.0%, $P = .15$, respectively)
Norway NORMI STEMI Registry 2022	$N = 9787$	64	PI (choice of fibrinolysis unspecified)	Primary PCI	Mortality at median 2.5 years with timely primary PCI ≤120 min was 10.3%, with delayed primary PCI 121–180 min was 14.6%, with late primary PCI >180 min was 15.5%, with PI was 8.9%. Higher mortality with delayed primary PCI and late primary PCI compared to PI (adjusted HR 1.3, 95% CI 1.0–1.5, adjusted HR 1.4, 95% CI 1.1–1.7, respectively)	Major bleeding higher with PI (1.0% for timely primary PCI, 1.4% for delayed primary PCI, 1.2% for late primary PCI, 2.4% for PI)
Australian STEMI Registry 2023	$N = 2091$	59	PI	Primary PCI	Mortality at 3 years was 11.1% after primary PCI (6.7% timely, 20.2% late) and 6.2% after PI (9.4% rescue, 4.8% scheduled); $P < .01$.	BARC 3–5 bleeding 2.2 % vs. 2.3%, $P = .103$; ICH 0.1% vs. 0.2%, $P = .523$

event, and patient health status outcomes) should be collected both in the short and long term. Aggregation of this data should be reviewed by relevant stakeholders at regular intervals to ensure continuous quality improvement. Participation in regional and/or national registries should be encouraged to evaluate how local care compares to other benchmarks. Transfer STEMI networks should be flexible to accommodate evolutions of care guided by new evidence. An example of such a construct is highlighted in Fig. 8.10.

COVID STEMI

The COVID-19 pandemic has had a profound impact on STEMI systems of care. The global threat has overwhelmed emergency medical services, heath care system/infrastructure and health care practitioners worldwide. As COVID-19 infections persist, timely metrics for primary PCI have become even more challenging to achieve,[19] particularly when patient COVID-19 status is unclear and health care workers safety becomes a concern—which

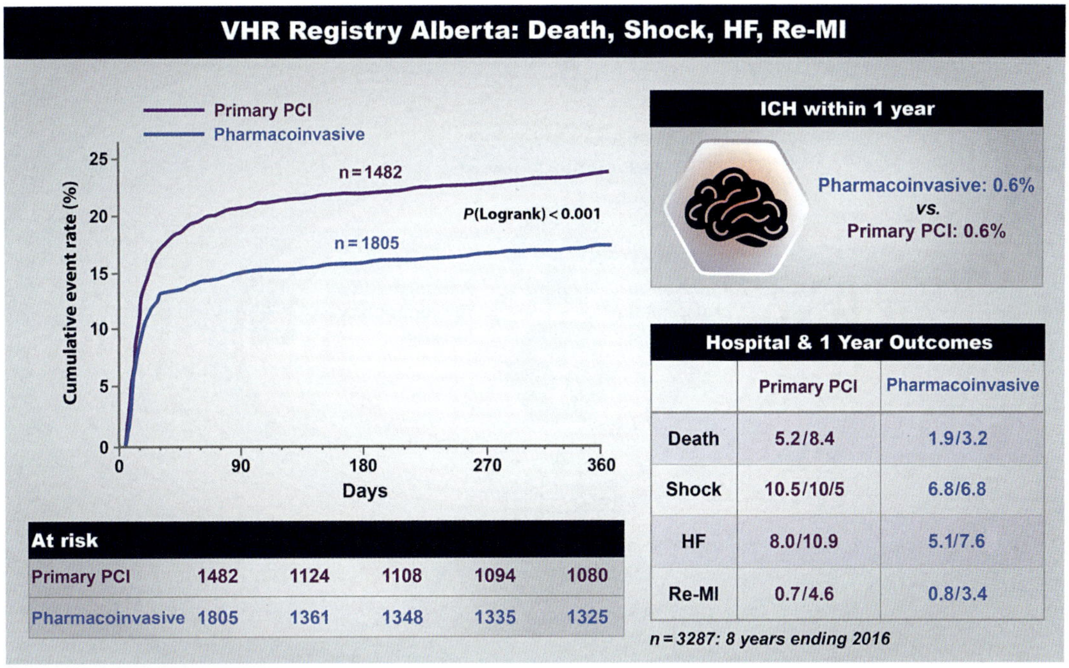

Fig. 8.7 Canadian STEMI registry comparing patients selected for primary PCI versus pharmacoinvasive PCI. Pharmacoinvasive PCI reduced the composite of death, shock, heart failure, and reinfarction compared to primary PCI at one year. Similar reductions were noted for the individual outcomes in-hospital and at one year. Similar rates of intracranial hemorrhage were observed at one year.

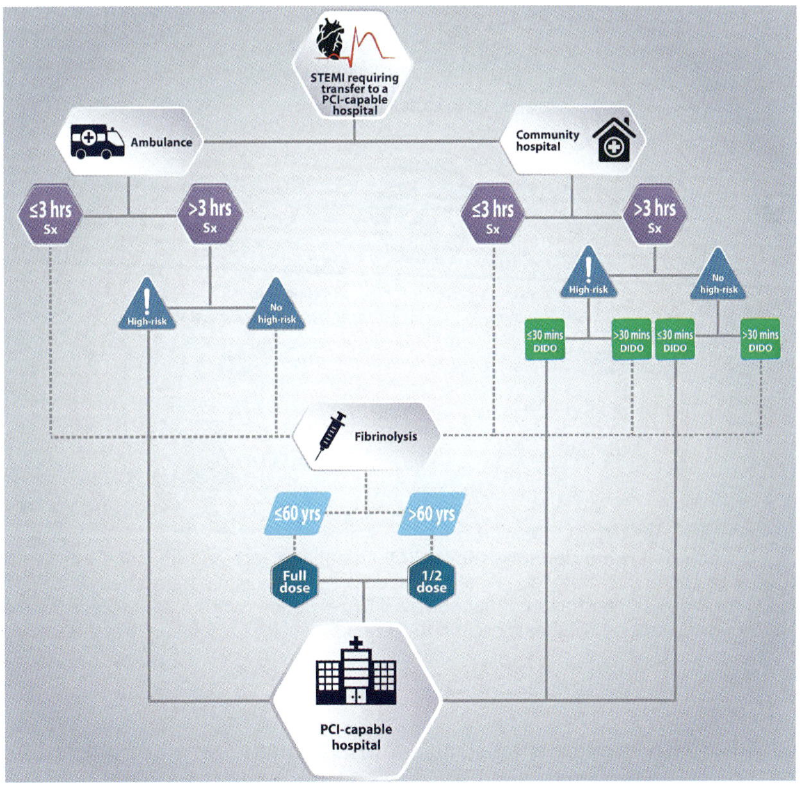

Fig. 8.8 Recommended treatment algorithm for transfer patients with STEMI. If presenting in the ambulance within 3 hours of ischemic symptoms, pre-hospital fibrinolysis should be administered (*dotted line*) with immediate transfer to a PCI-capable hospital. If more than 3 hours of symptoms, patients should be evaluated by considerations of potential benefit and baseline risk. If considered high risk, primary PCI should be considered. If low risk, pre-hospital fibrinolysis should be administered (*dotted line*) with immediate transfer to a PCI-capable hospital. If presenting to a community hospital within 3 hours of ischemic symptoms, pre-hospital fibrinolysis (*dotted line*) should be administered with immediate transfer to a PCI-capable hospital. If more than 3 hours of symptoms, patients should be stratified by baseline risk. If considered high risk, primary PCI should be considered with a door-in-door-out (DIDO) time of <30 minutes. If this cannot be achieved, fibrinolysis should be considered (*dotted line*). If low risk and DIDO time <30 minutes, primary PCI should be considered. Otherwise, fibrinolysis should be administered (*dotted line*) with immediate transfer. If fibrinolysis is considered, a ½ dose tenecteplase strategy should be used in those 60 years of age and older.

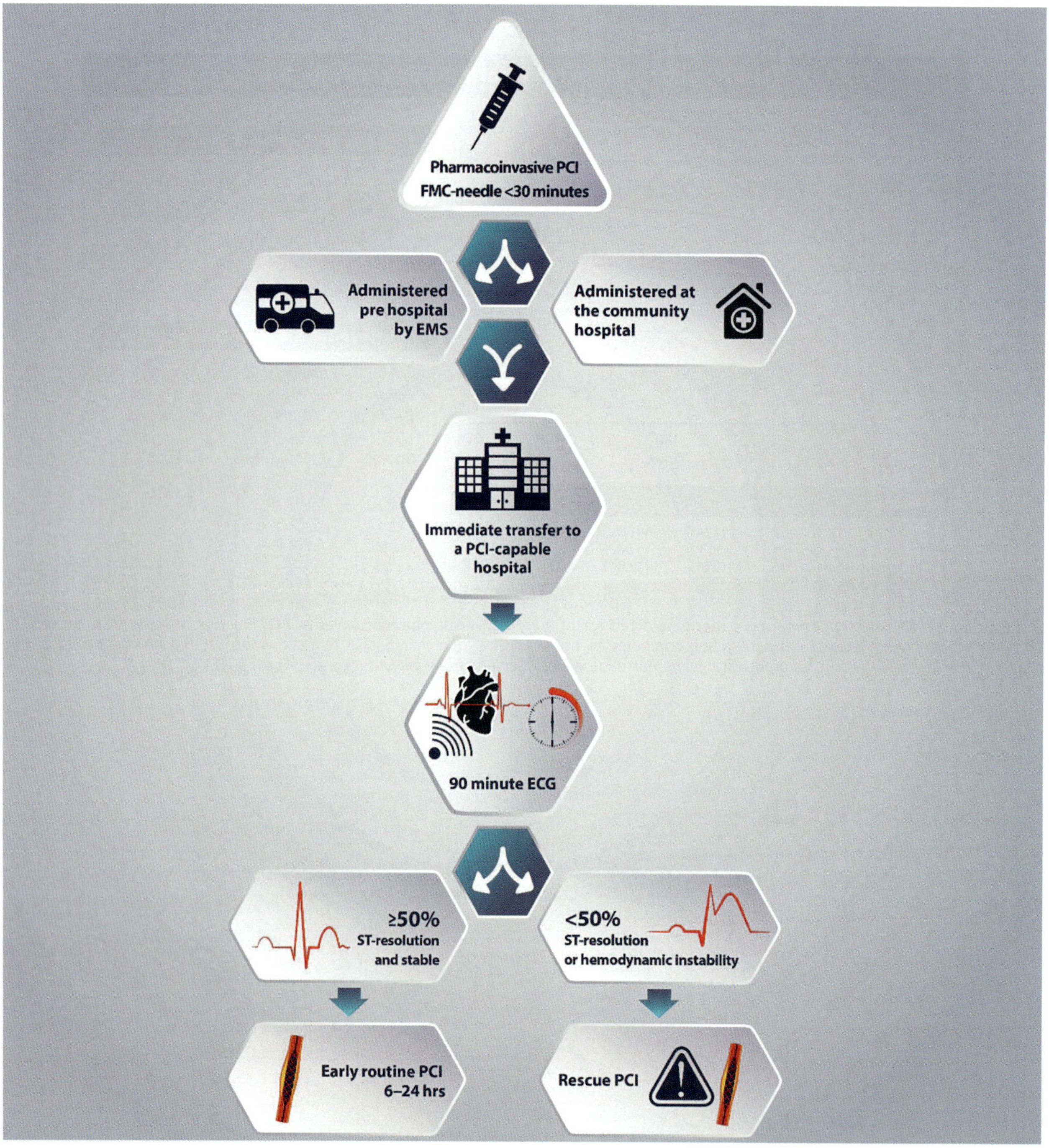

Fig. 8.9 Transfer and evaluation algorithm following fibrinolysis for STEMI. In patients receiving fibrinolysis (first medical contact to needle time of <30 minutes) regardless of ambulance or community hospital, all patients should be immediately transferred to a PCI-capable hospital for reperfusion evaluation with a 60–90-minute ECG following administration of fibrinolysis. If ST resolution (worst lead) exceeds 50% or greater, successful myocardial perfusion has been established, and scheduled routine PCI should occur 6 to 24 hours later. If ST resolution (worst lead) is less than 50%, immediate rescue intervention should ensue.

underscores the need for an alternative reperfusion strategy. Employing a pharmacoinvasive approach facilitates prompt pharmacologic reperfusion, allowing for time for patient transfer and preparation at PCI-capable hospitals for rescue intervention, if needed. Otherwise, scheduled PCI in COVID-19 STEMI allows for a controlled environment prone to less error, ensuring safety to the patient as well as health care workers. Variations in reperfusion strategies differ in North America for COVID-19 STEMI but reassuringly have not altered in-hospital mortality.[20] Fig. 8.11 highlights the need for reappraisal of STEMI care in the peri-COVID-19 era, with consideration of pharmacoinvasive PCI in appropriate patients.[21] Enhancing the state of readiness for alternative reperfusion choices when impediments to achieving timely PCI supervene, such as interventional laboratory engagement, staff shortages, or redeployment due to noncardiovascular emergencies, is a sensible proposition for the future.

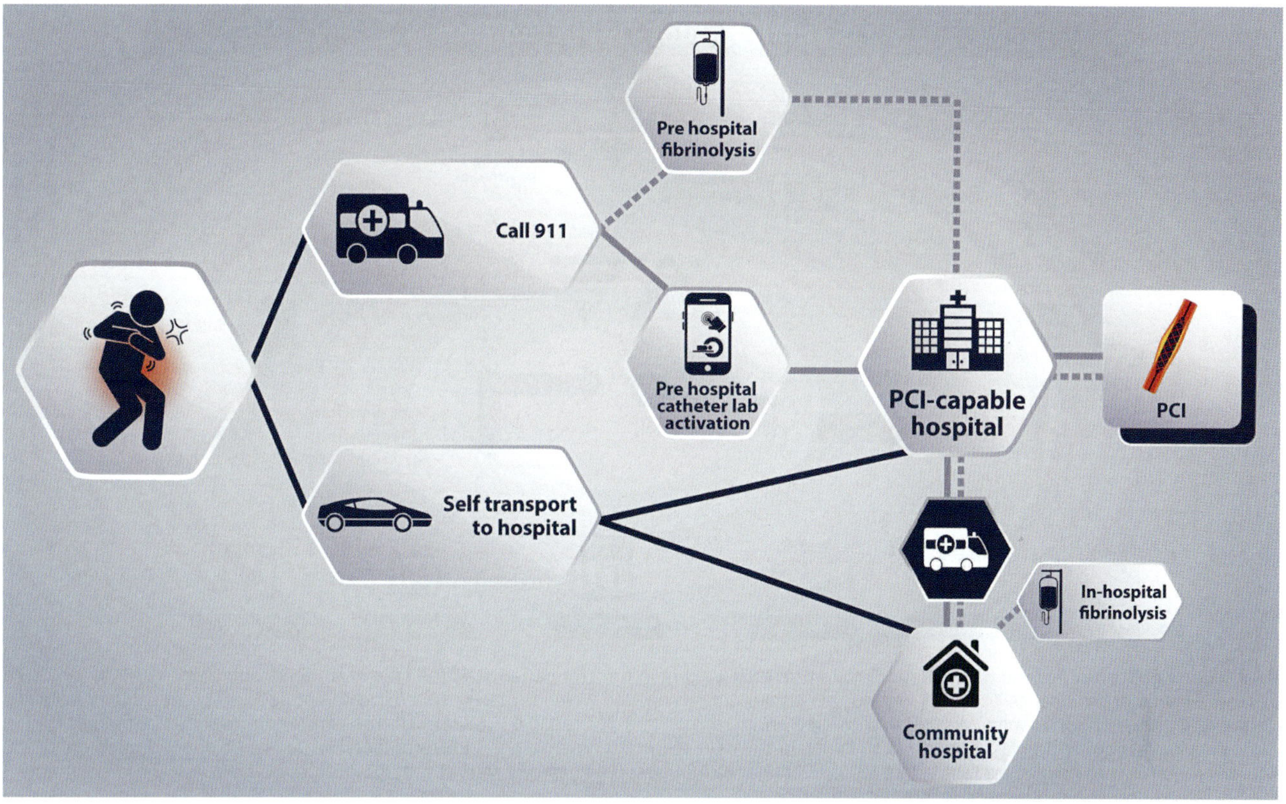

Fig. 8.10 An ideal STEMI network construct governed by the four key factors influencing reperfusion options. If presenting in the ambulance, reperfusion therapy should be decided pre-hospital with administration of fibrinolysis in the ambulance and transfer to a PCI-capable hospital for pharmacoinvasive PCI (*dotted line*) or cardiac catheterization laboratory activation in the ambulance for primary PCI (*solid line*). If self-presenting to a PCI-capable hospital, primary PCI should be the standard reperfusion option (*solid line*). If self-presenting to a community hospital, either activation of the cardiac catheterization laboratory for immediate transfer for primary PCI (*solid line*) or administration of in-hospital fibrinolysis with immediate transfer to a PCI-capable hospital for pharmacoinvasive PCI (*dotted line*) should be considered.

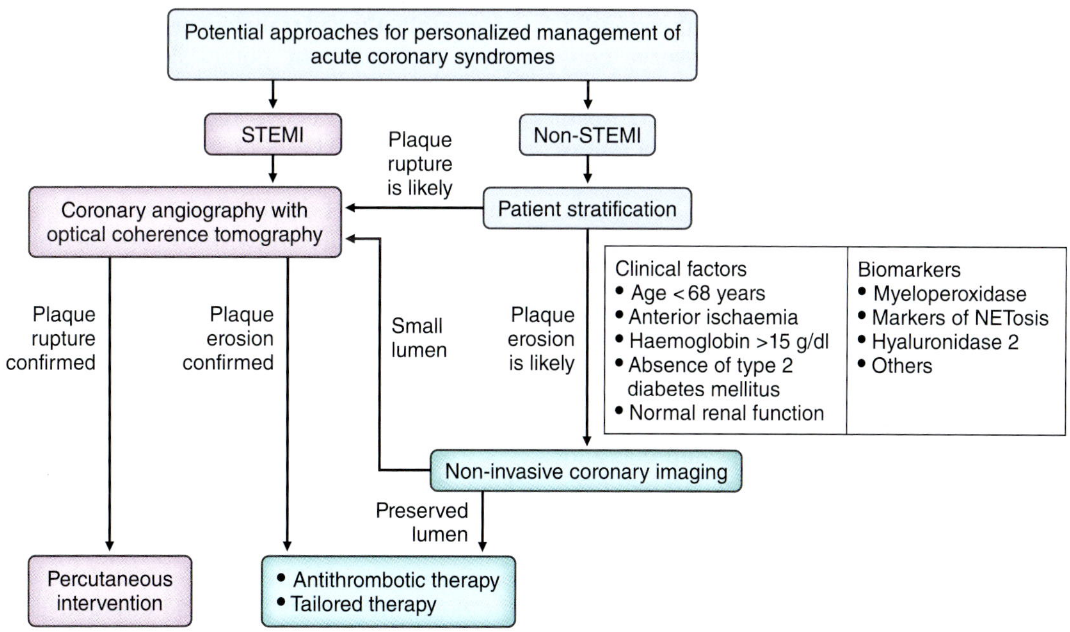

Fig. 8.11 Current situation and proposed redesign for STEMI care during the COIVD-19 pandemic. Assessing the state of STEMI care during a pandemic and suggestions for redesigning systems of STEMI care with a dual reperfusion option with the aim of administering prompt reperfusion and minimizing total ischemic time.

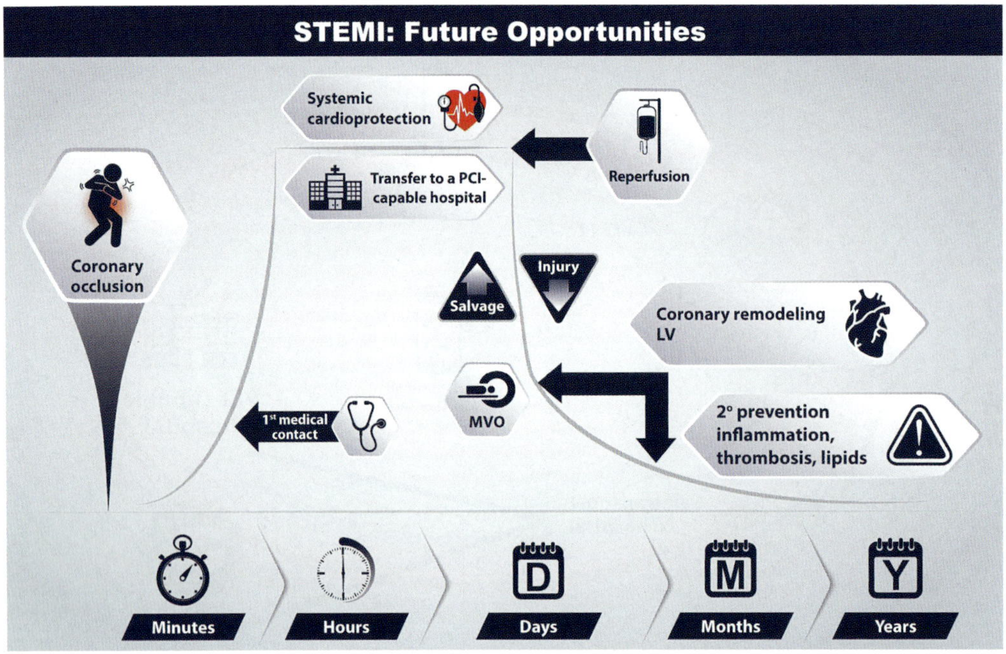

Fig. 8.12 Future opportunities and considerations to improve STEMI care in transfer patients. At the time of coronary occlusion in STEMI, early access to medical care (ambulance or hospital) is critical with further enhancements needed. With diagnosis, systemic cardioprotective agents could be administered (i.e., in the ambulance or community hospital) in those requiring transfer to a PCI-capable hospital with the aim to improve myocardial salvage (reduce microvascular obstruction) and mitigate reperfusion injury. In the days following reperfusion, additional therapies aimed at optimizing coronary and left ventricular remodeling are needed and should be studied. Longer term, investigative efforts should continue to focus on secondary prevention measures targeting inflammation, thrombosis, and lipid optimization.

Future Opportunities for Transfer Patients With STEMI

Prompt reperfusion must continue to be the primary focus for STEMI patients requiring transfer to a PCI-capable facility to mitigate ischemic risk, regardless of ambulance or community presentation. It remains impossible to achieve timely metrics with primary PCI in a large majority of these patients worldwide. While pharmacoinvasive PCI provides a logical evidence-based alternative, future therapeutic strategies aimed at prompt recanalization deserve consideration. Although prior facilitated PCI trials were associated with excessive bleeding risk, given that ½ dose tenecteplase is now an established component of a reperfusion strategy option and radial PCI has become the standard of care for STEMI, re-evaluation of STEMI therapy in transfer patients who are unable to receive timely primary PCI (within 120 minutes of first medical contact) deserves consideration. Ideally, a future trial would involve comparison of a facilitated PCI strategy with ½ dose tenecteplase and mandatory early PCI (regardless of reperfusion status) versus guideline-based primary PCI. Of note is an ongoing multicenter clinical study (OPTIMAL-REPERFUSION) of STEMI patients presenting within 6 hours of symptoms and PCI-related delay of ≥120 minutes, randomized to reduced-dose facilitated PCI (reduced-dose fibrinolysis combined with simultaneous transfer for immediate invasive angiography with intent to PCI <3 hours) versus a standard pharmacoinvasive approach (full-dose fibrinolysis with immediate transfer and rescue intervention or scheduled angiography within 3–24 hours). The primary endpoint is a composite of death, reinfarction, refractory ischemia congestive heart failure, or cardiogenic shock at 30 days.[22]

A further crucial unmet need is to address the contribution of microvascular obstruction (MVO) to myocardial salvage, final infarct size, and clinical outcomes. Therapies given during transfer of STEMI patients to enhance cardioprotection prior to reperfusion therapy (irrespective of pharmacologic or mechanical intervention) are a high priority. One example is the application of novel therapeutics such as IL-6 inhibitors that have been tested for reperfusion injury at the time of STEMI.[23] Earlier initiation of such therapies at the time of transfer (or in the ambulance) may augment its therapeutic potential by "conditioning ischemic myocardium" prior to reperfusion—which should apply to any cardioprotective agent being tested for reperfusion injury. As seen in Fig. 8.12, we contend that the large cohort of transfer patients with STEMI affords a unique opportunity to test novel cardioprotective strategies in the crucial window proximal to reperfusion during which reduction of microvascular obstruction (myocardial edema), enhancement of myocardial salvage, and improved left ventricular remodeling should reduce morbidity and mortality.

CONCLUSION

Remarkable progress has been achieved in the care of STEMI patients over the past two decades. Reflecting on this evolution through a patient-centred lens which focuses on the Institute of Medicine's principles of achieving quality of care seems an appropriate target. This perspective charges us to provide effective and safe therapy in a timely and equitable manner. Provided we incorporate what we have learned and measure how well we apply these learnings in our practice, our patients will be well served. Their future care will be even better if we rise to the challenge of their unmet needs by investigating novel solutions to address them.

ACKNOWLEDGMENT

We would like to thank Lisa Soulard from the Canadian VIGOUR Centre for her editorial assistance and development of our figures.

REFERENCES

1. Thiele H, et al. Management of cardiogenic shock complicating myocardial infarction: an update 2019. *Eur Heart J.* 2019;40:2671–2683.
2. Baran DA, et al. SCAI clinical expert consensus statement on the classification of cardiogenic shock: this document was endorsed by the American College of Cardiology (ACC), the American Heart Association (AHA), the Society of Critical Care Medicine (SCCM), and the society of thoracic surgeons (STS) in April 2019. *Catheter Cardiovasc Interv.* 2019;94:29–37.
3. Kochan A, et al. Reperfusion delays and outcomes among patients with ST-segment-elevation myocardial infarction with and without cardiogenic shock. *Circ Cardiovasc Interv.* 2023;16:e012810.
4. Scholz KH, et al. Impact of treatment delay on mortality in ST-segment elevation myocardial infarction (STEMI) patients presenting with and without haemodynamic instability: results from the German prospective, multicentre FITT-STEMI trial. *Eur Heart J.* 2018;39:1065–1074.
5. Van Diepen S, et al. Reperfusion in ST-segment elevation myocardial infarction patients with cardiogenic shock and prolonged inter-hospital transport times. *Circ Cardiovasc Interv.* 2024;17(2):e013415.
6. Pineda A, et al. Benefit-risk balance of fibrinolytic therapy in ST-elevation myocardial infarction as evaluated by physicians. *Eur J Emerg Med.* 2024;30:216–218.
7. Bainey KR, et al. Pharmacoinvasive strategy versus primary percutaneous coronary intervention in ST-elevation myocardial infarction in clinical practice: insights from the vital heart response registry. *Circ Cardiovasc Interv.* 2019;12:e008059.
8. Armstrong PW, et al. The second strategic reperfusion early after myocardial infarction (STREAM-2) study optimizing pharmacoinvasive reperfusion strategy in older ST-elevation myocardial infarction patients. *Am Heart J.* 2020;226:140–146.
9. Van de Werf F, et al. STREAM-2: half-dose tenecteplase or primary percutaneous coronary intervention in older patients with ST-segment-elevation myocardial infarction: a randomized, open-label trial. *Circulation.* 2023;148(9):753–764.
10. Redfors B, et al. Time delay, infarct size, and microvascular obstruction after primary percutaneous coronary intervention for ST-segment-elevation myocardial infarction. *Circ Cardiovasc Interv.* 2021;14:E009879.
11. Welsh RC, et al. Relationship between community hospital versus pre-hospital location of randomisation and clinical outcomes in ST-elevation myocardial infarction patients: insights from the Stream study. *Eur Hear J Acute Cardiovasc Care.* 2018;7:504–513.
12. Nepper-Christensen L, et al. Benefit from reperfusion with primary percutaneous coronary intervention beyond 12 hours of symptom duration in patients with ST-segment-elevation myocardial infarction. *Circ Cardiovasc Interv.* 2018;11:e006842.
13. Jollis JG, et al. Treatment time and in-hospital mortality among patients with ST-segment elevation myocardial infarction, 2018–2021. *JAMA.* 2022;328:2033–2040.
14. Neumann FJ, et al. 2018 ESC/EACTS guidelines on myocardial revascularization. *Eur Heart J.* 2019;40:87–165.
15. Lawton JS, et al. 2021 ACC/AHA/SCAI guideline for coronary artery revascularization: a report of the American College of Cardiology/American Heart Association joint committee on clinical practice guidelines. *Circulation.* 2022;145:E18–E114.
16. Byrne RA, et al. 2023 ESC guidelines for the management of acute coronary syndromes. *Eur Heart J.* 2023;44(38):3720–3826. https://doi.org/10.1093/eurheartj/ehad191.
17. Vanhaverbeke M, et al. Prevention of cardiogenic shock after acute myocardial infarction. *Circulation.* 2019;139:137–139.
18. Jamal J, et al. Clinical research Interventional cardiology late outcomes of ST-elevation myocardial infarction treated by pharmaco-invasive or primary percutaneous coronary intervention. *Eur Heart J.* 2022;44:516–528.
19. Xiang D, et al. Management and outcomes of patients with STEMI during the COVID-19 pandemic in China. *J Am Coll Cardiol.* 2020;76(11):1318–1324. https://doi.org/10.1016/j.jacc.2020.06.039.
20. Shavadia JS, et al. Comparative analysis of patients with STEMI and COVID-19 between Canada and the United States. *J Soc Cardiovasc Angiogr Interv.* 2023;2:100970. https://doi.org/10.1016/J.JSCAI.2023.100970.
21. Bainey KR, et al. ST-segment-elevation myocardial infarction care and COVID-19: the value proposition of fibrinolytic therapy and the pharmacoinvasive strategy. *Circ Cardiovasc Qual Outcomes.* 2020;13:284–286.
22. Chen Z, et al. Rationale and design of the OPTIMAL-REPERFUSION trial: a prospective randomized multi-center clinical trial comparing different fibrinolysis-transfer percutaneous coronary intervention strategies in acute ST-segment elevation myocardial infarction. *Clin Cardiol.* 2021;44:455–462.
23. Broch K, et al. Randomized trial of interleukin-6 receptor inhibition in patients with acute ST-segment elevation myocardial infarction. *J Am Coll Cardiol.* 2021;77:1845–1855.

9 Fibrinolytic Therapy for Patients With STEMI

PETER R. SINNAEVE AND FRANS J. VAN DE WERF

INTRODUCTION

An ST-segment myocardial infarction (STEMI) is caused by the occlusion of a major epicardial coronary artery and is generally triggered by rupture of a vulnerable plaque, with subsequent formation of an occlusive thrombus.[1] Rapid restoration of coronary blood flow is essential in preventing myocardial necrosis, and early reperfusion of the infarct-related artery limits infarct size and improves outcome. Achieving the shortest possible delay between symptom onset and reperfusion is therefore one of the most critical factors in the management of STEMI. Effective reperfusion of the infarct-related artery can be achieved by mechanical reperfusion, using primary percutaneous coronary intervention (PPCI; see Chapter 8), or by pharmacological reperfusion using fibrinolytic agents. Unfortunately, only a minority of hospitals worldwide have catheterization facility. Moreover, hospitals with a catheterization lab often do not offer PPCI during off-office hours. Fibrinolysis, in contrast, is universally available without the need for advanced logistics (Table 9.1). Thus, despite the impressive benefit and widespread use of PPCI, fibrinolysis remains the only option for reperfusion for many STEMI patients worldwide.[2] In the past decades, remarkable progress has been made in improving fibrinolytic therapies, in identifying patients who benefit from this treatment, and in identifying patients at risk for bleeding. In addition, in the past years, studies have provided the answer to how to fit in fibrinolytic therapy in contemporary hospital networks, especially to when and how to plan an early angiography and PCI in patients who have received fibrinolytic therapy (see Chapter 8).[3]

ROLE OF FIBRINOLYSIS IN CONTEMPORARY CARE

Over the past 2 decades, the proportion of STEMI patients receiving fibrinolytic therapy has gradually declined from 35% to 12% in the most recent European survey.[2] Is fibrinolysis still relevant in the 21st century then, now that guidelines and advocacy groups unequivocally recommend PPCI as the preferred reperfusion strategy?[4] Compared to fibrinolysis, PPCI certainly achieves higher patency rates and is associated with fewer intracranial bleeding complications (Chapter 11). PPCI also immediately deals with the underlying lesion or ruptured plaque and easily gauges the extent of coronary disease (Table 9.1). On aggregate, PPCI is better than lytic therapy in terms of outcome[5] but only if it can be done within 120 minutes after first medical contact by an experienced catheterization team. Achieving such rapid implementation of PPCI is not possible in a considerable proportion of STEMI patients worldwide. Poor weather conditions, long distances to a PCI hospital, traffic jams, and suboptimal local health care organizations are all possible reasons for significant delays. As a consequence, fibrinolysis remains an important option for many patients. For instance, almost half of STEMI patients in Africa or in non-ESC-associated Middle Eastern countries still receive fibrinolytic therapy.[2] It is clear that in remote or sparsely populated areas, fibrinolysis is often the only option for expedited reperfusion.[6,7] Structural and unexpected interhospital transfer delays are often underestimated in urban areas as well.

Once a STEMI patient is committed to be sent to a PPCI-capable center but unanticipated delays occur, an opportunity for early reperfusion is lost. Such patients are likely to have benefited from early fibrinolysis, in the absence of contraindications. Transfer-related delays in PPCI are common, and as door-to-balloon delays increase, the outcome advantage of PPCI over fibrinolysis clearly diminishes (see Chapter 8).[8] In a recent large American registry (n = 114,871), only 17% of patients requiring interhospital transfer for PPCI were treated within the guideline-recommended maximal delay of ≤120 minutes.[9] In-hospital mortality was more than threefold lower in patients treated within this delay: 4.3% versus 14.2%

TABLE 9.1 Comparison of (Dis)advantages of Fibrinolysis versus PPCI

	FIBRINOLYSIS	PRIMARY PCI
Advantage	Universally available	More efficient reperfusion and better outcome
	Independent of physician's experience and can be used by trained paramedics	Less risk of reinfarction or residual ischemia
	Can be administered in prehospital settings or community hospitals	Less risk of systemic and intracranial hemorrhage
Disadvantage	Higher risk of systemic and intracranial bleeding	Dependent on experience of team and on availability of 24/7 facilities
	Reperfusion in 60% of patients	PCI-related time delays can be long
	Not efficient in patients presenting late	

($P < .01$; adjusted OR, 0.44, 95% CI, 0.26–0.71). In essence, although efforts to reduce transfer times and optimize STEMI networks for prompt referral can be successful,[10] a substantial proportion of STEMI might still benefit from lytic therapy.[11] The need for a less resource-dependent alternative to PPCI became pertinent during the 2019 pandemic. Significant delays due to COVID-19 testing and an often inaccessible ambulance system as well as a shortage of staff during the 2019 pandemic led to a renewed interest in fibrinolysis as a more accessible and faster reperfusion option in times of restricted access to overloaded health care systems.[12,13]

In most STEMI networks, fibrinolysis is not isolated from PCI.[14] The optimal combination of fibrinolysis and (rescue or planned) PCI is complex and is the subject of a separate chapter (see Chapter 8).[15] In addition, interest in local intracoronary administration of lytics has attracted renewed interest, especially as an alternative for PPCI patients with a large thrombotic burden. For all these reasons, fibrinolytic therapy is still relevant today in a modern well-established network of STEMI care.

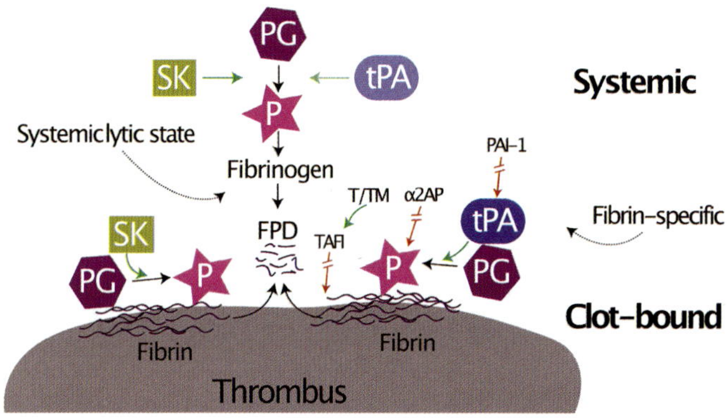

FIG. 9.1 Mechanism of fibrinolysis and fibrinolytic agents: tPA (alteplase) predominantly activates plasminogen bound to the clot's surface (clot-bound), while streptokinase activates clot-bound and fluid-phase plasminogen indiscriminately (systemic). *α2AP*, Alpha-2-antiplasmin; *FPD*, fibrin degradation products; *P*, plasmin; *PG*, plasminogen; *PAI-1*, plasminogen activator inhibitor 1; *SK*, streptokinase; *tPA*, tissue-type plasminogen activator; *TAFI*, thrombin activatable fibrinolysis inhibitor; T/TM, thrombomodulin/-thrombin complex.

TABLE 9.2 Fibrinolytic Agents

Non-fibrin-specific agents	Fibrin-specific agents
Streptokinase	Alteplase and derivates
Saruplase	Reteplase
APSAC (anistreplase)	Tenecteplase Lanoteplase Amediplase Monteplase Pametiplase
	Staphylokinase

HOW DO FIBRINOLYTIC AGENTS WORK?

The goal of administering a fibrinolytic agent is to dissolve the clot that impedes blood flow in a coronary artery. This dissolution of thrombus is achieved pharmacologically by activating the fibrinolytic system. Fibrinolytic agents convert the inactive proenzyme plasminogen to its active state, plasmin (Fig. 9.1).[16] Plasmin then degrades fibrin, a major constituent of thrombi, to soluble fibrin-degradation products, ultimately resulting in clot dissolution.[17] Fibrinolytic agents are traditionally categorized as fibrin-selective versus nonselective agents, depending on whether or not they lyse clots in the absence of systemic plasminogen activation (Table 9.2).

Streptokinase, anistreplase, and urokinase are non-fibrin-selective fibrinolytic agents and indiscriminately activate both circulating and clot-bound plasminogen to plasmin. This activity not only causes local dissolution of a thrombus but also systemic degradation of circulating fibrinogen. In contrast, alteplase and its derivatives, as well as staphylokinase, digest clot-bound fibrinogen relatively selectively and tend not to deplete systemic coagulation factors as much as streptokinase. Fibrin-selective drugs are more efficient in dissolving thrombi. The selective nature of fibrin-specific lytic agents does have some unwanted side effects; however, their lack of systemic fibrinogen depletion might increase the risk of rethrombosis and reocclusion (Chapter 19). Subsequent derivatives of alteplase have been aimed at providing more practical bolus-delivery at the same time as potential improvements in risk-benefit balance due to enhanced fibrin-specificity of some derivatives. New developments in improving the selectivity and safety of fibrinolytic agents include combining them with chemically modified nanoparticles or targeted cell membranes.[18]

Several circulating factors suppress the activation of plasminogen, most notably plasminogen activator inhibitor (PAI)-1 (Fig. 9.1). Resistance or lack of resistance to PAI-1 characterizes, in part, the potency of the different fibrinolytic agents. Consequently, PAI-1 is a major determinant of the resistance of thrombi to lysis by fibrinolytic agents. Other factors can influence the delicate balance of thrombus formation and resolution by endogenous fibrinolysis of intravenous fibrinolytics.[19] Active plasmin for instance is directly inhibited by alpha-2-antiplasmin (α2AP), while thrombin activatable fibrinolysis inhibitor (TAFI) inhibits fibrinolysis by plasmin upon activation through the thrombomodulin/thrombin complex.

SPECIFIC FIBRINOLYTIC AGENTS

Streptokinase

Streptokinase is a non-fibrinogen-specific fibrinolytic agent that indirectly activates plasminogen (Tables 9.3 and 9.4). Streptokinase is a single-chain 414 amino acid long protein, resembling serine proteases but without enzymatic activity on its own. Plasminogen is activated after forming a complex with streptokinase, exposing its active site which catalyzes the conversion to plasmin. This complex is more resistant against inactivation by α_2-antiplasmin than free-circulating plasmin.

TABLE 9.3 Characteristics of Lytic Agents

	FIBRIN SPECIFICITY	HALF-LIFE (MIN)	PAI-1 RESISTANCE
Streptokinase	–	18–23	–
APSAC	–	40–90	–
Alteplase	↑	3–4	–
Reteplase	↓	15–18	–
Tenecteplase	↑↑	20–24	↑
Lanoteplase	↓	30–45	↑
Pametiplase	↑	30–47	–
Monteplase	↑	23	↑
Staphylokinase (PEG)	↑↑↑	13	–

TABLE 9.4 Dosing Regimens of Frequently Used Fibrinolytic Agents ([a]Not Indicated in the Label)

Streptokinase
1.5 million IU/1 h
Alteplase
15 mg bolus
90-min infusion
• 0.75 mg/kg over 30 min (max 50 mg)
• 0.50 mg/kg over next hour (max 35 mg)
• Total dose not to exceed 100 mg
(Alternatively: 8 mg bolus and 42-mg infusion/90 min in a pharmacoinvasive strategy[a])
Reteplase
Initial 10 U bolus, followed by second 10 U bolus 30 min later
Tenecteplase
Weight-adjusted single bolus:
• 30 mg if <60 kg
• 35 mg if 60–69 kg
• 40 mg if 70–79 kg
• 45 mg if 80–89 kg
• 50 mg if ≥90 kg
Half-dose if age >60 years[a] (in a pharmacoinvasive strategy)

In STEMI, 1.5 million units of streptokinase are usually given in a 1-hour infusion. Due to its lack of fibrin-specificity, however, streptokinase generates active plasmin in the circulation and induces a systemic lytic state, when α_2-antiplasmin becomes exhausted. Circulating fibrinogen levels decrease well below 20% of baseline within the first 60 minutes after infusion. As a consequence, additional anticoagulants are not always recommended in combination with streptokinase or other non-fibrin-specific fibrinolytics (Chapter 12).

Because streptokinase is produced by hemolytic streptococci, patients who receive streptokinase invariably develop antistreptococcal antibodies. This immunological reaction often causes fever but would also completely neutralize a new dose of streptokinase in the first 3 months after administration, effectively precluding early readministration. In some patients, high neutralizing antibody titres even persist for years after their treatment. In addition, preexisting antistreptokinase antibodies are relatively common and can impede reperfusion after treatment with streptokinase in patients with STEMI. However, hypotension, a frequent but often transient side effect of streptokinase, is more likely the result of bradykinin release than caused by an acute allergic reaction.

Clinical Trials of Streptokinase

In the open-label GISSI-1 study, 11,806 patients with STEMI presenting within 12 hours of symptom onset were randomized to either intravenous streptokinase or control therapy. In-hospital mortality was 10.7% in patients treated with intravenous streptokinase versus 13.1% in control patients, indicating 23 lives saved per 1000 patients treated. This benefit in mortality was preserved after 1-year and 10-year follow-up (Fig. 9.2). Another landmark trial, the Second International Study of Infarct Survival (ISIS-2) clearly showed the benefit of adding aspirin to streptokinase. 17,187 patients received 1.5 MU streptokinase, 160 mg aspirin daily for 1 month, both treatments, or neither. Treatment with aspirin or streptokinase alone resulted in a significant reduction in 5-week vascular mortality (23% and 24%, respectively). The benefit of aspirin and streptokinase was independent and additive, with a 42% reduction in vascular death when both agents were combined. Aspirin significantly reduced nonfatal reinfarction and was not associated with any significant increase in intracranial hemorrhages (Chapter 13). Reinfarction rate was higher when streptokinase was used alone, an effect that was abolished when aspirin was added.

Tissue-Type Plasminogen Activator

Recombinant tissue-type plasminogen activator (alteplase, rt-PA, tPA) is a single-chain tissue-type plasminogen activator molecule, manufactured by recombinant DNA technology (Tables 9.3 and 9.4).[20] Alteplase is a relatively weak plasminogen activator in the absence of fibrin. The presence of fibrin at the surface of a clot, however, considerably boosts alteplase's activation rate of plasminogen

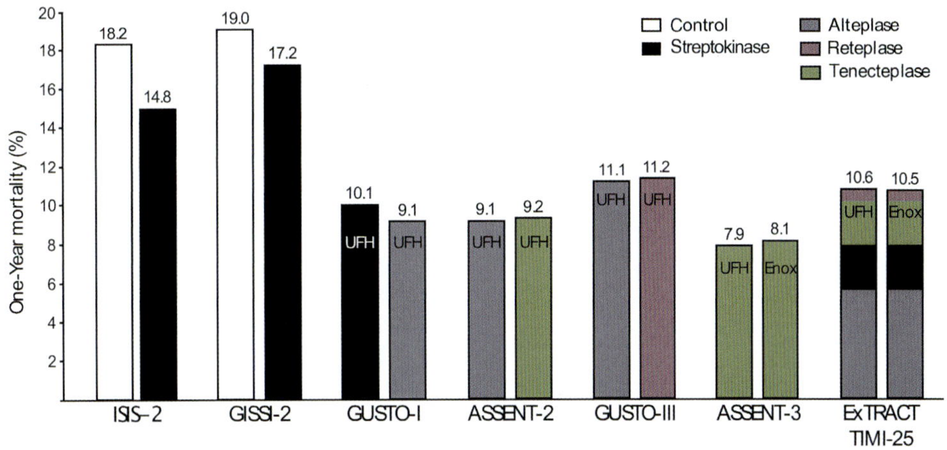

FIG. 9.2 One-year mortality rates in key fibrinolytic trials (*Enox*, Enoxaparin; *UFH*, unfractionated heparin).

by forming a ternary complex. As a consequence, it has considerably greater fibrin-specificity than streptokinase but nevertheless induces mild systemic fibrinogen depletion. Plasmin formed at the surface of fibrin is also more resistant to inactivation by α_2-antiplasmin. The effectiveness of alteplase is also offset to some extent by the PAI-1. Alteplase requires a continuous intravenous infusion due to its short half-life or should be used in front-loaded scheme (Table 9.4). It also needs concomitant anticoagulant therapy as fibrin-specific agents increase the risk of reocclusion by a factor of two in the absence of a generalized systemic lytic state.

Clinical Trials of Alteplase

The question which of the two, streptokinase or alteplase, is the most effective in terms of mortality reduction was finally settled in 1993 in the first Global Utilization of Streptokinase and Tissue Plasminogen Activator for Occluded Coronary Arteries (GUSTO-1) trial. In this trial that included over 40,000 patients, a shorter (front-loaded) 90-minutes dosing regimen of alteplase was used, which had been shown to achieve higher patency rates than the 3-hour scheme. 30-day mortality was 6.3% in patients receiving alteplase and intravenous heparin compared to 7.4% in patients treated with streptokinase and intravenous heparin (*P* = .001), driven by a significantly higher TIMI flow grade 3 at 90 minutes (54% vs. 32% with streptokinase). Early reocclusion was not uncommon in the era before systematic planned angiography and angioplasty after lytic therapy (Chapter 19), in part, because of paradoxical pro-coagulant and platelet-activating side effects of fibrinolytic agents and was associated with a very high 30-day mortality: 12%, compared to just 1.1% in patients with early and persistently patent coronary arteries. In the end, GUSTO-1 together with the TIMI-1 trial from 1988 convincingly showed that early vessel patency following fibrinolysis directly translates into improved outcome, often referred to as the “open artery theory”.

Finally, half-dose alteplase was evaluated in a pharmacoinvasive (PI) strategy in the EARLY-MYO trial.[21] Three hundred and forty-four STEMI patients aged seventy-five or younger presenting within 6 hours after symptom onset and with an expected PPCI delay were randomized to PPCI or pharmacoinvasive management with half-dose alteplase (8 mg bolus followed by 42 mg over 90 minutes). All patients received a loading dose of either clopidogrel (300 or 600 mg) or ticagrelor (180 mg). The PI strategy with half-dose alteplase was superior to PPCI with respect to the primary endpoint of complete epicardial and myocardial tissue reperfusion, assessed angiographically. Importantly, there were no intracranial hemorrhages in both arms. Awaiting a larger outcome trial, it remains unclear whether a PI strategy with half-dose alteplase equals PPCI in reducing cardiovascular events, however.

Reteplase

After the identification of the molecular structure of t-PA, several attempts were made at improving its properties by targeted mutations and deletions. In general, these efforts focused on improving fibrin-specificity and resistance to PAI-1, and especially on prolonging its half-life. Reteplase, a second-generation fibrinolytic agent, was a first attempt to improve on the shortcomings of alteplase (Tables 9.3 and 9.4). It is a mutant of alteplase in which the finger, the kringle-1 domain, and epidermal growth factor domains were removed. This results in a decreased plasma clearance with a longer half-life than alteplase (Table 9.3), allowing administration as (double) bolus injection. The removal of the finger domain diminishes fibrin specificity, however, although inactivation by PAI-1 remains similar as with alteplase.

Clinical Trials of Reteplase

Reteplase was evaluated in two large outcome trials. In the double-blind INJECT trial, 6010 patients with STEMI within 12 hours of symptom onset, were randomized to either double-bolus reteplase (10 U), given 30 minutes apart, or streptokinase. INJECT did not find any difference in 35-day mortality between double-bolus reteplase and streptokinase. The percentage of patients with complete ST-segment resolution was significantly higher with reteplase in a substudy of INJECT, but this did not translate into improved outcomes. In the GUSTO-III trial, which was designed as a superiority trial, 15,059 patients were randomized to double-bolus reteplase, or front-loaded alteplase. Like in INJECT, mortality at 30 days was again similar for both treatment arms (7.47% vs. 7.24%), as was the incidence of hemorrhagic stroke (0.91% vs. 0.93%) or other major bleeding complications. Similar mortality rates were maintained for both treatment groups at one-year follow-up (Fig. 9.2) and were very consistent among various subgroups including the elderly and patients presenting early after symptom onset. Reteplase is still available and in clinical use today.

Tenecteplase

Tenecteplase (TNK-t-PA) is bioengineered from alteplase with mutations at three places (T103, N117, KHRR296-299), which increases its plasma half-life (T103, 20 minutes), improves fibrin binding and fibrin specificity, and increases resistance to PAI-1 (N117 & KHRR296-299).[22] Its slower clearance allows convenient single-bolus administration (Tables 9.3 and 9.4). The higher fibrin specificity of tenecteplase is the result of reduced efficiency of plasminogen activation in the presence of fibrinogen and fibrin degradation products, while efficiency in the presence of fibrin remains equivalent. As a result, tenecteplase leads to faster recanalization compared to alteplase. Tenecteplase also has higher fibrinolytic potency on platelet-rich clots than its parent molecule.

Clinical Trials of Tenecteplase

Efficacy of different doses of tenecteplase with respect to establishing angiographic patency was initially evaluated in the Thrombolysis in Myocardial Infarction (TIMI) 10A and 10B trials. Taken together, patency rates were identical after single-bolus administration of 40 mg tenecteplase compared with alteplase (63%). A 50-mg dose of tenecteplase had to be discontinued early because of an excess of intracranial hemorrhages in the 10B part (Fig. 9.3). Concomitantly, the safety of single-bolus administration of tenecteplase was evaluated in the Assessment of the Safety and Efficacy of a New Thrombolytic (ASSENT) 1 study: 3325 patients received a single bolus of either 30 or 40 mg tenecteplase. Mortality or severe bleeding complications including intracranial hemorrhages occurred in a low proportion of patients, without significant differences among the treatment groups.

In the double-blind ASSENT-2 trial, 16,949 patients were randomized to single-bolus weight-adjusted tenecteplase or weight-adjusted front-loaded alteplase. Specifically designed as an equivalency trial, this study showed that tenecteplase and alteplase were equivalent for 30-day mortality (6.18% vs. 6.15%, 90% CI, 0.917–1.104). The two treatments did not differ significantly in any subgroup analysis, except for a lower 30-day mortality with tenecteplase in patients treated after 4 hours of symptom onset. Although the rates of intracranial hemorrhage were similar for tenecteplase (0.93%) and alteplase (0.94%), female patients, elderly >75 years and patients weighing less than 67 kg tended to have lower rates of intracranial hemorrhage after treatment with tenecteplase. Noncerebral bleeding complications occurred significantly less frequently in the tenecteplase group, a difference that was even more apparent in high-risk females. Thus, increased fibrin specificity of tenecteplase may induce both a better outcome in late-treated patients and fewer noncerebral bleeding complications in high-risk patients.

After the ASSENT trials, different doses of tenecteplase have been used in real-world practice and in clinical trials. In the pharmacoinvasive STREAM study (see Chapter 8), for instance, the dose of tenecteplase was reduced by 50% in patients above 75 years of age, after enrolling about 20% of the ultimate study population because of an excess of bleeding complications including intracranial bleeding in the elderly.[23] After halving the dose (Table 9.4), no more intracranial bleedings were seen in this age category. An analysis of all bleeding complications in almost 24,000 patients from the ASSENT and STREAM-1 trials clearly showed that the risk of intracranial hemorrhage starts to increase around the age of 60 years.[24] Hence, in the STREAM-2 trial, half-bolus tenecteplase was evaluated in a pharmaco-invasively managed population 60 years of age or older (see Chapter 8). Half-dose tenecteplase was found be safe and effective, provided that contraindications to fibrinolysis are observed (e.g., uncontrolled hypertension) and excess anticoagulation is avoided.[25] This study suggests that half-dose tenecteplase may provide a more favorable risk/benefit balance in older patients. Formal professional society guidelines do not yet recommend this regimen.

Staphylokinase

Recombinant staphylokinase has only limited use in some countries and is described briefly here for completeness. Although staphylokinase, a bacterial profibrinolytic agent, was already discovered in 1908, its clinical use in STEMI only regained interest and momentum in the last decade of the 20th century (Tables 9.3 and 9.4). This delay, in contrast with the rapid uptake of streptokinase, was due to the presence of antibody-related neutralizing activity in serum samples of test subjects and massive bleeding in staphylokinase-treated dogs in the 1960s. In retrospect, the choice of this animal model was unfortunate, as staphylokinase lacks fibrin-specificity in dogs, in contrast with other species.[26]

Staphylokinase has a high fibrinolytic potency, is very effective in dissolving platelet-rich thrombi, and possesses high-fibrin specificity in human plasma. In the STAR trial, the effects of staphylokinase versus front-loaded and weight-adjusted alteplase on early coronary artery patency were evaluated in 100 STEMI patients. TIMI-3 flow at 90 minutes was reached in 58% of patients treated with alteplase and in 62% of patients treated with staphylokinase. Staphylokinase proved to be highly fibrin-specific, preserving circulating fibrinogen, plasminogen, and α_2-antiplasmin levels, whereas alteplase caused a significant drop of fibrinogen, plasminogen, and α_2-antiplasmin. Although wild-type staphylokinase induces an antibody response, engineered variants with reduced antigenicity have been shown to decrease the occurrence and magnitude of inactivating antibodies. Staphylokinase has recently regained attention in the treatment of ischemic stroke.[27,28]

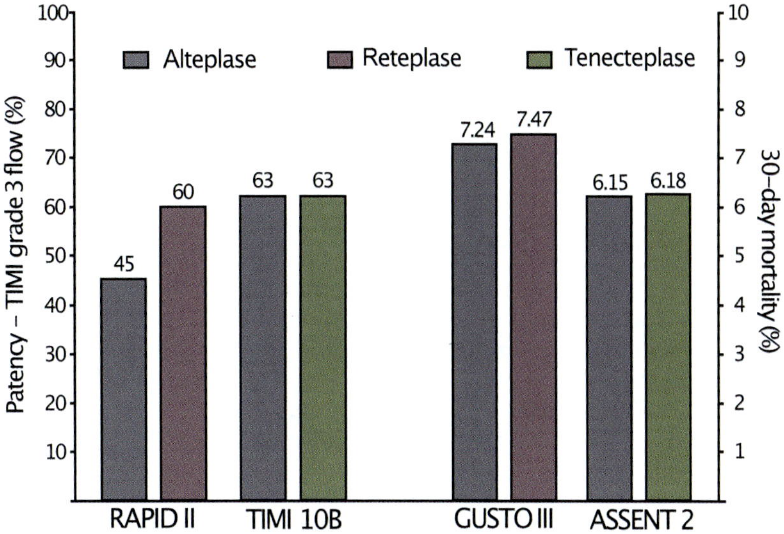

FIG. 9.3 Patency versus outcome in the landmark reteplase and tenecteplase trials.

Prourokinase

Prourokinase, also known as saruplase, is a single-chain recombinant urokinase-type plasminogen activator without immunogenicity. It is not fibrin-specific and has a plasma half-life of 9 minutes. Prourokinase is infrequently used as standard fibrinolytic used in STEMI patients and is not approved in Europe or the United States. It has attracted renewed interest, however, as an intracoronary adjunct in patients undergoing primary PCI, although large trials are lacking.[29,30] Historically, in the Comparison Trial of Saruplase and Streptokinase (COMPASS) trial, 3089 patients were randomized to prourokinase or streptokinase. Thirty-day mortality was numerically lower in the saruplase group (5.7% vs. 6.7% for streptokinase). Intracranial hemorrhage occurred more frequently with prourokinase (0.9% vs. 0.3% for streptokinase), although only a limited number of elderly patients were included in this trial. In another study, the Bolus Administration of Saruplase in Europe (BASE) trial, several dosing regimens were tested. Although the highest dose, a double bolus of 40/40 mg, resulted in the highest patency, it also had the highest complication rate.

CLINICAL USE, INDICATIONS, AND CONTRAINDICATIONS FOR FIBRINOLYTIC THERAPY

Indications for Fibrinolytic Therapy

Traditionally, patients with typical chest pain of up to 12 hours duration presenting with electrocardiographic ST-segment elevations or presumed new bundle-branch block are eligible for fibrinolytic therapy. The clot-lysing efficacy of fibrinolytic therapy is clearly time-dependent; it works best on newly formed clots. In addition, early in the course of STEMI, the thrombus may be smaller and thus faster and easier to lyse. Consequently, treatment delays are associated with less successful ST-segment recovery after fibrinolysis and lead to higher mortality rates.[9] Although administering fibrinolytic agents up to 12 hours after the onset of symptoms may be beneficial in terms of outcome, every minute that reperfusion is postponed will inevitably result in more extensive necrosis and higher mortality rates.

The usual electrocardiographic criterion for administration of fibrinolytic therapy is at least 0.1 mV of ST-segment elevation in two or more contiguous leads. Since mortality is significantly higher in patients with a (new) complete left bundle-branch block, administration of a fibrinolytic agent is also recommended in this population.

Contraindications to Fibrinolysis

Contraindications to fibrinolysis are, in essence, precautionary measures to avoid excessive risk of hemorrhage (Tables 9.5 and 9.6). In these patients, especially those with a previous history of stroke or recent major surgery or bleeding, PPCI should be considered even when this would be associated with a significant treatment delay.

Registries have suggested that there is a greater mortality disadvantage in fibrinolysis-treated patients over 75 years of age, possibly due to an excess of major bleeding complications. This excessive mortality might also be explained, in part, by negative selection, as fitter elderly patients might have been more likely amenable to PPCI.

TABLE 9.5 Contraindications for Fibrinolysis

ABSOLUTE	RELATIVE
- Previous hemorrhagic stroke at any time - Nonhemorrhagic stroke <6 months - CNS malformation, neoplasm, or damage - Recent surgery or significant trauma within 2–4 weeks - Active (uncontrolled) bleeding - Gastrointestinal bleeding within last month - Known bleeding disorder - Suspected aortic dissection	- Transient ischemic attack <6 months - Uncontrolled or refractory hypertension - Traumatic cardiopulmonary resuscitation or prolonged CPR - Current use of anticoagulants - Recent bleeding (2–4 weeks) - Pregnancy

TABLE 9.6 Patients at Increased Risk for Intracranial Hemorrhage

- Prior history of cerebrovascular disease, including CVA and TIA
- Age above 75 years
- Female gender
- Low body weight
- High blood pressure or pulse pressure on admission

Mortality rates in these observational studies, however, contrast with findings from large randomized trials. In the SENIOR PAMI trial, PPCI was not found to be superior to fibrinolytic in 481 elderly patients (≥70 years of age). Furthermore, data from the Fibrinolytic Therapy Trialists (FTT) group in 3300 STEMI patients over the age of 75 showed a significant absolute mortality reduction by fibrinolytic therapy that was even greater than in younger patients (34 vs. 16 patients per 1000 randomized). An ongoing concern is the risk of intracranial bleeding with lytic therapy, especially in the elderly (Fig. 9.4). Results from recent trials including STREAM 1 and 2 as well as registries have suggested that reduced-dose fibrinolysis might be a safe and effective alternative for older patients. Care needs to be taken to avoid inappropriate concomitant antithrombotic therapies or excessive doses, however. In STREAM-2 for instance, six intracranial hemorrhages occurred in the pharmacoinvasive arm (1.5% vs. none in the PPCI arm), three of which were attributed to protocol violations including additional administration of full-dose UFH after full-dose subcutaneous enoxaparin in two patients and uncontrolled hypertension in one.[25]

Intracoronary Fibrinolysis

Intracoronary fibrinolysis has regained attention as an adjunct for PPCI to help prevent microvascular obstruction and reperfusion injury (see Chapter 20) (Fig. 9.5).[31] Several recent small and single-blinded trials evaluated prourokinase as an adjunct to PPCI, with favorable effect on myocardial perfusion and infarct size in a meta-analysis.[29] There are no large randomized trials with adjunct intracoronary prourokinase yet, however. The largest study to date, T-TIME, randomized STEMI patients with a proximal/mid occlusion of a major coronary artery to placebo (n = 151) or low-dose intracoronary alteplase (10 mg [n = 144] or 20 mg [n = 145]) administered after reperfusion but before stent implantation.[32] The primary endpoint, the extent of microvascular obstruction on MRI at day 2 to 7, was not different between the three treatment groups. In a subanalysis, low-dose intracoronary alteplase even appeared to be harmful in patients with a longer ischemic time (more than 4 hours).[33] A meta-analysis of 6 RCT, including T-TIME and representing 890 patients, did not show an improvement in post-PCI epicardial reperfusion, although there was a trend toward improved outcomes (Fig. 9.5).[34] Still, another study reported an increased risk of subacute stent thrombosis and poorer reperfusion after low-dose intracoronary tenecteplase,[35] perhaps in part due to the early procoagulant trait of fibrinolysis. As a result, the systematic use of intracoronary (low-dose) fibrinolysis as an adjunct to primary PCI cannot be recommended.[36] Intracoronary fibrinolysis might still be an option in case of high thrombus burden in selected cases.[37]

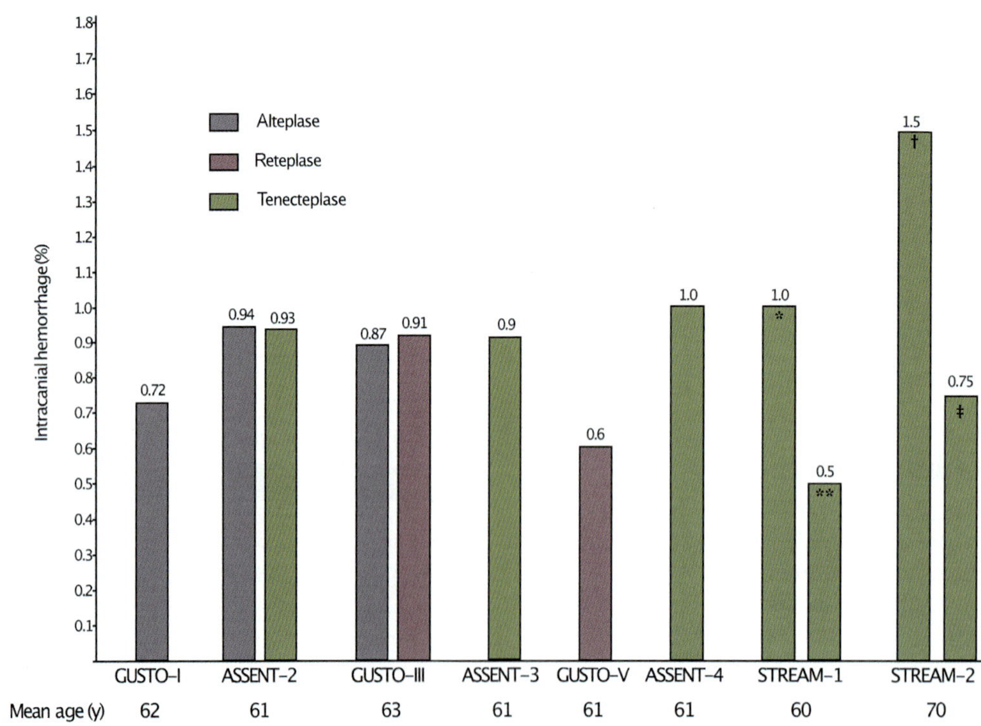

FIG. 9.4 Intracranial hemorrhage rates in randomized fibrinolytic studies. For ASSENT-4 PCI and STREAM 1 & 2, only the rates in the lytic arms are shown (* before and ** after an amendment in STREAM-1 that halved the dose of tenecteplase in patients 75 years of age and older, † all ICH in STREAM-2, ‡ ICH rate excluding protocol violations (excessive anticoagulation and untreated hypertension). Note that only patients older than 60 years were included in STREAM-2.

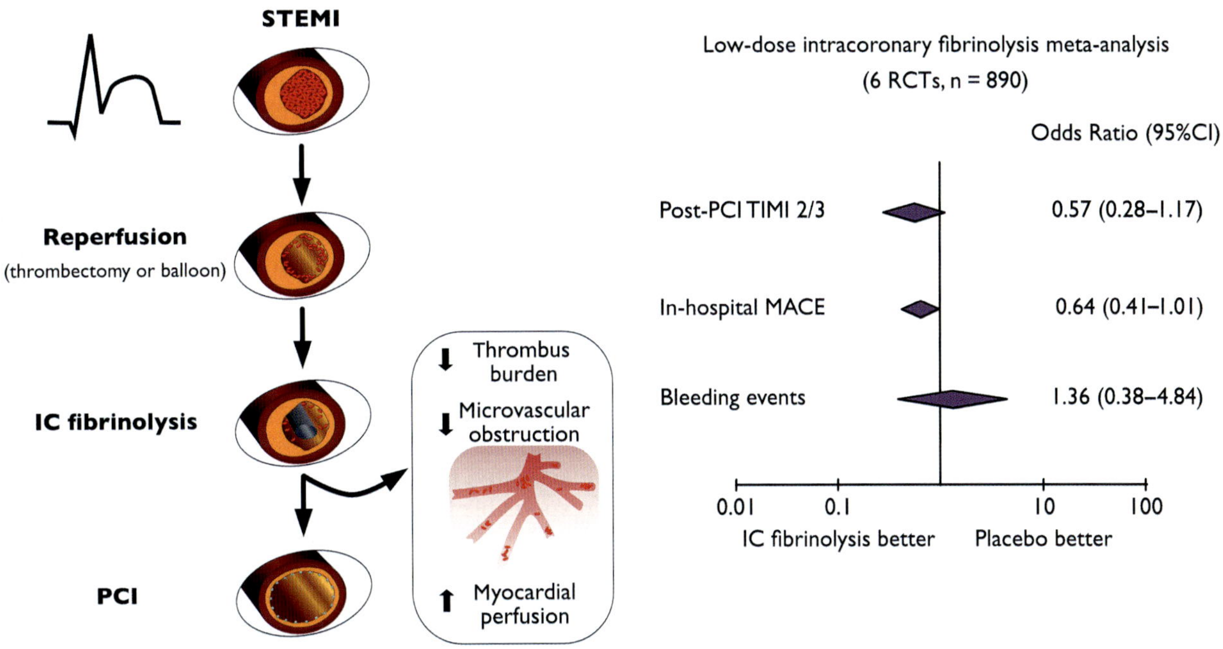

FIG. 9.5 Intracoronary fibrinolysis and its putative advantages. (*IC*, Intracoronary; *MACE*, major adverse cardiac events; *PCI*, percutaneous coronary intervention; *RCT*, randomized clinical trial); odds ratios based on a meta-analysis of 6 RCT representing 890 patients by Alyamani et al.[34]

ASSESSMENT OF REPERFUSION

Early reperfusion in STEMI is associated with smaller infarcts and improved survival.[38] Assessing reperfusion is essential in contemporary pharmacoinvasive strategies, as failed reperfusion early after fibrinolysis leads to worse outcome as well.[39] The early efficacy trials used 60- or 90-minute patency of the infarct-related vessel on angiography as the most important demonstration of successful fibrinolysis. A TIMI flow grade of <3 in the infarct-related artery is associated with poor functional recovery of the left ventricle and increased mortality.[40] Angiography, however, at best represents a snapshot view of a dynamic process of coronary occlusion and recanalization. Myocardial tissue reperfusion as assessed by myocardial blush grade correlates better with outcome than epicardial coronary artery patency, illustrating that restored epicardial blood flow does not necessarily reflect reperfusion at the tissue level.[41] Restoration of reperfusion at the tissue level can be assessed noninvasively with contrast echocardiography (Chapter 15), MRI (Chapter 17), or, more practically, ST-segment monitoring. ST-segment resolution, reflecting myocardial reperfusion, has been shown to be associated with better short-term and long-term mortality. In contemporary practice and clinical trials, ST-segment resolution of 50% or more at 60 to 90 minutes after lytic therapy is also used to assess the early success of reperfusion in the context of a pharmacoinvasive strategy (see Chapter 8).[40] In the presence of evidence of successful fibrinolysis, an angiography and PCI should only be planned between 3 and 24 hours after successful lytic therapy to avoid peri-procedural thrombotic complications while permitting maximal patency of the infarct vessel in a timely fashion.

CONCOMITANT THERAPIES

Because the formation and lysis of a coronary thrombus result from a complex interplay of different pathways involving platelets and the coagulation system, the additional use of agents that target each of these separate components beyond lysis potentially optimizes clot dissolution and prevents reocclusion. Indeed, a major drawback of fibrinolytic therapy is its procoagulant side effect due to increased thrombin generation. Therefore, better as well as safer inhibition of thrombin and platelets improves the efficacy of fibrinolysis. The use of anticoagulants and antiplatelet therapy are described in detail in Chapter 25 and Chapter 26, respectively and are briefly discussed here.

Anticoagulation With Fibrinolysis

Unfractionated Heparin

Intravenous unfractionated heparin (UFH) has been standard adjunctive antithrombotic therapy with fibrin-specific fibrinolytics since the first GUSTO trial. UFH does not necessarily improve early patency rates but improves patency rates at later time points by preventing rethrombosis and reinfarction. It took several large trials and over a decade to settle on the most optimal UFH dosing regimen, balancing bleeding risk versus thrombosis. In three trials (TIMI 9, GUSTO II, and TIMI 10B), heparin doses were reduced during the course of the trial, resulting in lower rates of intracranial bleeding. The current recommended dosing scheme which was first used in the ASSENT-3 trial also includes an early measurement of the activated partial thromboplastin time after 3 hours.

The use of UFH suffers from significant drawbacks. The level of anticoagulation with UFH is highly variable in patients due to low bioavailability and variable clearance, requiring frequent aPTT measurements. UFH is also relatively ineffective in inhibiting clot-associated thrombin and factor X and does not reduce the generation of thrombin associated with fibrinolysis. These properties can result in rebound activation of the coagulation cascade after cessation of an infusion, increasing the risk of reocclusion (Chapter 19). UFH has been largely replaced by low molecular weight heparin as an adjunct to lytic therapy.

Low Molecular Weight Heparins and Pentasaccharides

Low molecular weight heparin (LMWH) has several advantages over conventional UFH, including greater bioavailability, better resistance to inhibition by activated platelets and a lower incidence of heparin-induced thrombocytopenia. Also, a higher anti-Xa:IIa ratio than that of UFH more efficiently promotes the inhibition of thrombin generation. LMWH are much easier to administrate and have a more stable and predictable anticoagulant response that eliminates the need for aPTT monitoring. Subcutaneous administration and a longer half-life significantly facilitate prehospital as well as in-hospital administration when compared to UFH.

Studies have shown a reduction in reinfarction rates and enhanced late patency with the use of LMWH in acute coronary syndromes. Compared to UFH, patency rates after alteplase administration tended to be higher with dalteparin or enoxaparin in the ASSENT (Assessment of the Safety and Efficacy of a New Thrombolytic agent) PLUS and Heparin Aspirin Reperfusion Trial (HART II) trials. In the ENTIRE-TIMI (ENoxaparin and Tenecteplase with or without glycoprotein (GP) IIb/IIIa Inhibitor as Reperfusion strategy in ST elevation MI—Thrombolysis in Myocardial Infarction) 23 trial enoxaparin plus full-dose tenecteplase achieved similar TIMI 3 flow rates compared to UFH plus tenecteplase at 60 minutes.

In the ASSENT-3 study, enoxaparin (30-mg intravenous bolus followed by 1 mg/kg immediately and every 12 hours subcutaneous for 7 days) was compared to UFH in combination with tenecteplase. Enoxaparin significantly reduced the risk of ischemic complications at 30 days. Enoxaparin in combination with tenecteplase was also evaluated in the prehospital setting in the ASSENT-3 PLUS trial. A nonsignificant reduction in ischemic complications with enoxaparin was observed, at the expense of an increase in intracranial bleeding in elderly patients. Using an age-adjusted dose (*no bolus and 75% of the maintenance dose*), however, enoxaparin still increased the risk of major bleeding by 50%, but not the risk of intracranial bleeding after fibrinolytic therapy, while still reducing the risk of ischemic complications in the ExTRACT-TIMI 25 study. Two meta-analyses of trials comparing LMWH to UFH confirm that LMWH reduces the risk of death and reinfarction but is associated with a higher risk of major bleeding complications (OR, 1.45; CI, 1.24–1.91). In the current guidelines, enoxaparin, with an age and weight-adjusted dose as used in the ExTRACT-TIMI 25 trial, is recommended over UFH (class IA recommendation).[4]

Fondaparinux, a synthetic pentasaccharide, is a selective antithrombin-dependent factor Xa inhibitor. As with LMWH, fondaparinux is less biologically variable and does not need monitoring of its anticoagulant effect. In the OASIS-6 trial, fondaparinux was compared with UFH or placebo in 12,092 patients with STEMI. Lytic therapy was used in 45% of patients (n = 5436), most of them receiving a non-fibrin-specific agent. In these patients, fondaparinux was associated with a significant 21% lower risk of death or myocardial infarction when compared to standard heparin or placebo. In addition, the risk of bleeding, including intracranial bleeding, was considerably lower with fondaparinux, irrespective of the type of fibrinolytic agent. Guidelines recommend fondaparinux as adjunctive therapy to streptokinase (ESC, class IIaB).[4]

Intravenous Direct Thrombin Inhibitors

In contrast with UFH, which only inhibits fluid-phase thrombin, direct thrombin inhibitors inhibit both fibrin-bound and circulating thrombin. Because inadequately inactivated thrombin at the site of the thrombus is in part responsible for the procoagulant side effect of fibrinolysis, direct inhibition of thrombin might reduce the occurrence of ischemic complications after reperfusion. Thrombin inhibitors like hirudin or bivalirudin only appear to interact favorably with streptokinase, not with alteplase. In the HERO-2 (Hirulog and Early Reperfusion or Occlusion) trial, 17,073 patients with STEMI were randomized to streptokinase and UFH or streptokinase and bivalirudin. Mortality at 30 days was not different between both regimens, although the reinfarction rate within 96 hours was significantly lower in the bivalirudin group, suggesting that early and more efficient inhibition of thrombin might prevent reocclusion. Mild to moderate bleeding complications were higher in the bivalirudin group, however. Guidelines do not recommend bivalirudin as an adjunct to fibrinolysis except in patients with heparin-induced thrombocytopenia.[4]

Oral Anticoagulants

Chronic use of oral anticoagulants (OAC), including direct OAC (DOAC) or vitamin K antagonists (VKA) is a relative contra-indication for fibrinolytic therapy due to the increased risk of bleeding complications. In a contemporary registry in the United States, STEMI patients with atrial fibrillation on OAC were expectedly less likely to receive fibrinolytic therapy (3% vs. 5% of those not on OAC).[42] The less frequent use of lytics might also have been driven by the typically higher risk profile of patients on OAC, including higher age and a history of cerebrovascular disease. On aggregate, in-hospital major bleeding rates were similar among lytic-treated STEMI patients regardless of chronic OAC use. Still, for VKA, the bleeding risk does depend on the INR level for VKA, with substantially higher risk with an INR above 3. With DOAC, the risk depends on the dose, as well as on the timing of the last dose and the patient's renal function. In STEMI patients who cannot undergo timely primary PCI, the inactivation of the DOAC with the specific reversal agents idarucizumab (for dabigatran) or andexanet (for the FXa inhibitors) can be considered, especially if the last dose was taken recently.

Antiplatelet Agents With Fibrinolysis

In the landmark Second International Study of Infarct Survival (ISIS-2) study, aspirin was clearly beneficial when given to STEMI patients. In addition, the reinfarction rate

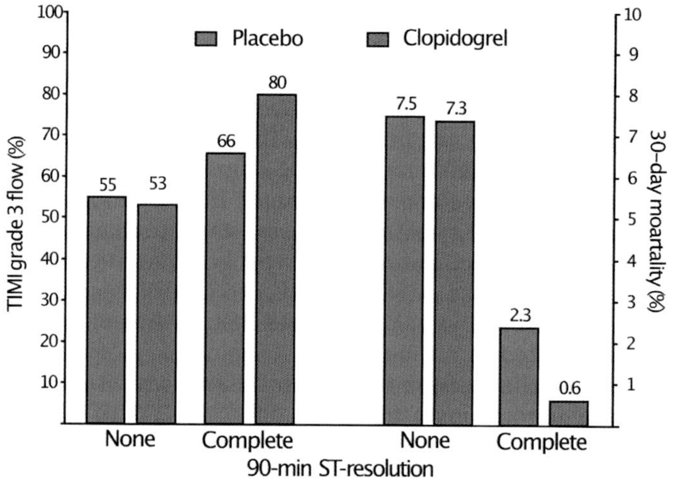

FIG. 9.6 TIMI grade 3 flow rates and outcome versus ST-segment resolution in patients randomized to placebo or clopidogrel in the CLARITY study.

was lower than when streptokinase was used alone. Since then, low-dose aspirin has been standard therapy with fibrinolysis.

Adenosine Diphosphate Receptor ($P2Y_{12}$) Antagonists

Despite the use of aspirin in lytic-treated patients, reocclusion and reinfarction after successful pharmacological reperfusion continues to be a problem, especially when a planned early (3–24 hours) PCI is not possible. The Clopidogrel as Adjunctive Reperfusion Therapy (CLARITY)-TIMI 28 trial examined whether clopidogrel, a $P2Y_{12}$ receptor inhibitor (300 mg bolus followed by 75 mg daily), was associated with higher rates of infarct-related artery patency in patients treated with a fibrinolytic agent and aspirin. Clopidogrel appears to improve patency rates by preventing reocclusion rather than through facilitating early reperfusion (Fig. 9.6). At angiographic follow-up at least 2 days after fibrinolytic therapy, clopidogrel was associated with significantly better patency rates in CLARITY-TIMI 28. No increased risk of bleeding complications including intracranial hemorrhage with clopidogrel was observed. Since no patients over 75 years of age were included in CLARITY-TIMI 28, however, it remains uncertain whether upfront dual antiplatelet therapy is safe in the elderly treated with lytic therapy. In contemporary practice, most lytic-treated patients receive an early coronary angiography (see Chapter 8). When using fibrinolysis in patients who cannot undergo primary PCI but still have access to PCI facilities in a STEMI network, it appears to be sensible to load clopidogrel upfront, at the time of starting lytic therapy, and not wait until the intervention. In the ASSENT-4 PCI study, clopidogrel was only started per protocol when a PCI was deemed necessary; the delay of clopidogrel administration might have been one of the reasons why the patency rate with tenecteplase was lower than expected and the reocclusion rate high. In contrast, in the STREAM-I study, comparing fibrinolysis with rescue or planned PCI versus primary PCI in patients unable to undergo PPCI within 60 minutes, a loading dose of 300 mg clopidogrel was given upfront, followed by a daily dose of 75 mg. In patients above 75 years of age, however, no loading dose was given because of a lack of safety data. In STREAM-2, a loading dose of 300 mg was given to all patients, however.[43]

About two-thirds of pharmacoinvasively managed patients still have unacceptably high residual platelet reactivity when undergoing PCI after the initial loading of clopidogrel. Switching to a more potent and faster-acting $P2Y_{12}$ inhibitor such as prasugrel or ticagrelor might lower the periprocedural thrombotic risk but can also increase the risk of bleeding complications, especially early after fibrinolysis.

Ticagrelor was clearly superior to clopidogrel in STEMI patients in the PLATO trial, but in this study, patients who received fibrinolysis in the previous 24 hours were excluded. An early loading of ticagrelor after fibrinolysis was tested in the TREAT (Ticagrelor in Patients With ST-Elevation Myocardial Infarction Treated With Pharmacological Thrombolysis) trial (Fig. 9.7). In TREAT, 3799 STEMI

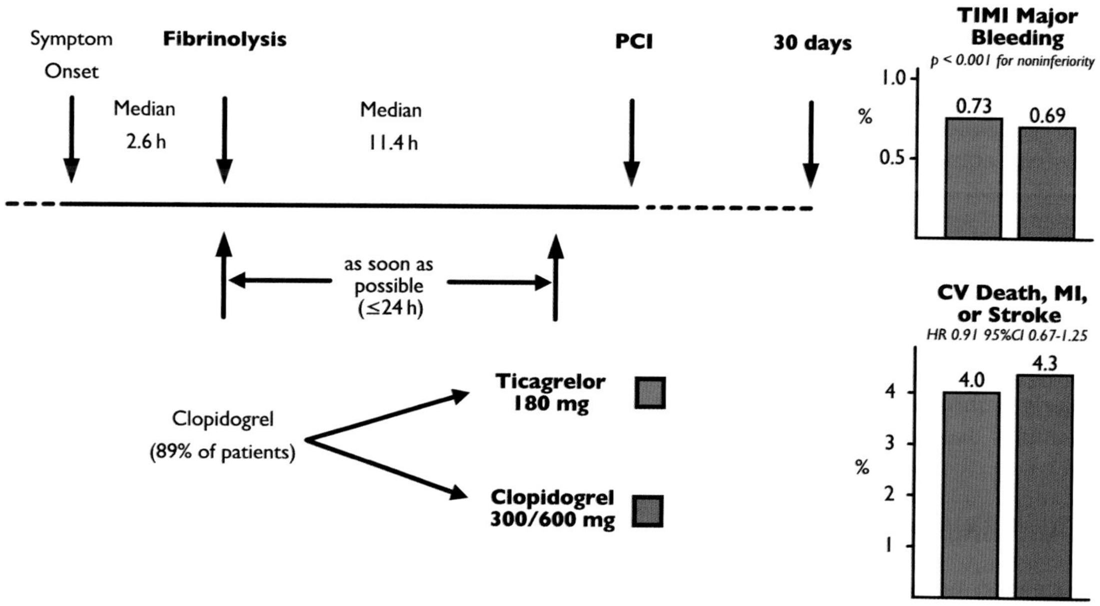

FIG. 9.7 Design and primary (TIMI major bleeding) and secondary (cardiovascular [CV] death, myocardial infarction [MI] or stroke) endpoints at day 30 in the TREAT trial.

22. Berg ES, Tegn NK, Abdelnoor M, et al. Long-term outcomes of invasive vs conservative strategies for older patients with non–ST-segment elevation acute coronary syndromes. *J Am Coll Cardiol*. 2023;82(21):2021–2030. https://doi.org/10.1016/j.jacc.2023.09.809.
23. Lu H, Hatfield LA, Al-Azazi S, et al. Sex-based disparities in acute myocardial infarction treatment patterns and outcomes in older adults hospitalized across 6 high-income countries: an analysis from the International Health Systems Research Collaborative. *Circ Cardiovasc Qual Outcomes*. 2024;17(3):e010144. https://doi.org/10.1161/CIRCOUTCOMES.123.010144.
24. Elgendy IY, Wegermann ZK, Li S, et al. Sex differences in management and outcomes of acute myocardial infarction patients presenting with cardiogenic shock. *JACC Cardiovasc Interv*. 2022;15(6):642–652. https://doi.org/10.1016/j.jcin.2021.12.033.
25. Gaba P, Christiansen EH, Nielsen PH, et al. Percutaneous coronary intervention vs coronary artery bypass graft surgery for left main disease in patients with and without acute coronary syndromes: a pooled analysis of 4 randomized clinical trials. *JAMA Cardiol*. 2023;8(7):631–639. https://doi.org/10.1001/jamacardio.2023.1177.
26. Head SJ, Milojevic M, Daemen J, et al. Mortality after coronary artery bypass grafting versus percutaneous coronary intervention with stenting for coronary artery disease: a pooled analysis of individual patient data. *Lancet*. 2018;391(10124):939–948. https://doi.org/10.1016/S0140-6736(18)30423-9.

11 Approach to Percutaneous Coronary Intervention in Myocardial Infarction

JEREMIAH P. DEPTA AND DEEPAK L. BHATT

INTRODUCTION

Percutaneous coronary intervention (PCI) is the dominant strategy used for coronary revascularization in acute myocardial infarction (MI).[1–6] In the United States, the estimated annual incidence of acute MI is 805,000 (see Chapter 1), which includes a substantial percentage of the primary indications for PCI performed annually.[1] This chapter reviews the evidence and practical considerations for PCI in patients with acute MI, including both ST-elevation MI (STEMI) and non–ST-elevation MI (NSTEMI). Selection among the options for reperfusion therapy for STEMI is addressed in Chapter 8, and selection among strategies for management of NSTEMI is discussed in Chapter 10. Antiplatelet therapy is discussed in Chapters 12, 26, and anticoagulant therapy is discussed in Chapters 12, 25.

TIMING OF PERCUTANEOUS CORONARY INTERVENTION

ST-Elevation Myocardial Infarction Strategies for Reducing Time to Treatment

If performed in a timely fashion by experienced operators, primary PCI is the recommended method for reperfusion in patients presenting with STEMI.[2,4,6] The benefit of reperfusion therapy is greatest in the first 3 hours after symptom onset (see Chapter 8). The development of regional systems for STEMI care and reperfusion therapy to limit the total ischemic time and meet time-to-treatment goals is detailed in Chapter 3. Regardless of the recommended time-to-treatment goals, reperfusion should always be established as rapidly as possible for any individual patient. It is estimated that 90% of STEMI patients presenting to a PCI-capable hospital without a clinical reason for delay achieve the door-to-device time goal of ≤90 minutes. Achieving a door-to-balloon time <90 minutes is associated with a significantly lower risk of in-hospital, 30-day, 6- and 12-month mortality compared with delays >90 minutes.[7] A checklist (Table 11.1) was developed by the American College of Cardiology (ACC)/American Heart Association (AHA) with practical system strategies to minimize door-to-device time.

Non–ST-Elevation Myocardial Infarction: Timing of Angiography

In patients with NSTEMI, routine invasive angiography is associated with improved outcomes and is generally the preferred approach over medical therapy alone.[2] The

TABLE 11.1 Checklist for Reducing Door-to-Device Times in ST-Elevation Myocardial Infarction

Time-to-Treatment Goals
PCI-Capable Hospital
Goal: FMC-to-device time <90 min (ESC: <60 min to wire crossing)
Non–PCI-Capable Hospital
Goal: Transfer to PCI-capable hospital with FMC-to-device time of <120 min (door-in-door-out <30 min; ESC: <90 min to wire crossing after arrival to PCI center) If anticipated FMC-to-device is >120 min, administer fibrinolytic within 30 min of arrival (ESC time to needle <10 min)
Checklist for Reducing Door-to-Device Times
▫ Prehospital ECG to diagnose STEMI and activate PCI team ▫ Emergency room physicians activate the PCI team ▫ A single call to a central paging system activates the PCI team ▫ PCI team arrival to the catheterization laboratory within 20 min ▫ Timely analysis and feedback of time-to-treatment metrics by the STEMI care team

[a]Denotes recommendations in the 2023 ESC ACS Guidelines[6]

ECG, Electrocardiogram; *ESC*, European society of cardiology; *FMC*, first medical contact; *PCI*, percutaneous coronary intervention; *STEMI*, ST-elevation myocardial infarction.

From O'Gara PT, et al. 2013 ACCF/AHA guideline for the management of ST-elevation myocardial infarction: a report of the American College of Cardiology Foundation/American Heart Association task force on practice guidelines. *Circulation*. 2013;127:e362; Lawton, JS, et al. 2021 ACC/AHA/SCAI guideline for coronary artery revascularization: executive summary: a report of the American College of Cardiology/American Heart Association joint committee on clinical practice guidelines. *J Am Coll Cardiol*. 2022;79:197–215; Byrne RA, et al. 2023 ESC Guidelines for the management of acute coronary syndromes. *Eur Heart J*. 2023;44(38):3720–3826.

timing of diagnostic angiography with the intent to perform PCI is driven by risk stratification and clinical stability (see Chapter 10). Immediate invasive evaluation should be performed in NSTEMI patients with cardiogenic shock, refractory symptoms, recurrent dynamic ischemic ECG changes, or electrical instability Chapter 10).[2,6] The timing of angiography in the invasive strategy is stratified based on clinical risk assessment (Fig. 11.1) into immediate (<2 hours), early (<24 hours), or prior to discharge (typically 24–72 hours).[2] If a patient is managed using an ischemia-guided strategy, angiography is recommended after medical treatment has failed with objective evidence of ischemia on noninvasive stress testing or with a high risk for mortality or morbidity.[2]

An early invasive strategy did not improve survival, reduce recurrent MI or heart failure readmissions, or repeat revascularization compared with a delayed invasive strategy in non–ST-elevation acute coronary syndrome (NSTE-ACS).[7,8] In the TIMACS (Timing of Intervention in Patients with Acute Coronary Syndromes) trial, high-risk patients (i.e., GRACE [Global Registry of Acute Coronary Events] risk score >140) who underwent an early invasive strategy had a 38% reduction in death, MI, and stroke at 6 months compared with a delayed invasive strategy.[2] An early invasive strategy is advocated in patients at higher risk for adverse clinical events (Fig. 11.1). Using a validated risk stratification score (e.g., GRACE; https://www.outcomes-umassmed.org/grace/acs_risk2/index.html) can help identify patients at a higher risk of cardiac events and need for early invasive angiography.[2,6]

VASCULAR ACCESS

Vascular access is vitally important for the success of PCI. Historically, femoral access was the most common approach used for PCI in the United States. Adoption of the transradial approach has gained significant popularity and is preferred by many patients and operators. Importantly, bleeding remains the most common PCI-related complication and is associated with higher mortality rates.

Performing Vascular Access

Femoral

Retrograde puncture of the femoral artery (Fig. 11.2) is required for femoral access during diagnostic coronary angiography and PCI. The common femoral artery is used due to its larger size and ability to compress the artery against the femoral head during manual compression. Patients should receive sedation and a local anesthetic before arterial cannulation. Because of variability in patient's body habitus, several landmarks should be noted. A line drawn between the anterior superior iliac spine and pubis demarcates the inguinal ligament. The inguinal crease should not be used to approximate the inguinal ligament, especially in obese patients. Fluoroscopy should be used to mark the femoral head. The common femoral should be entered at a 30- to 45-degree angle approximately 1–2 cm below the inguinal ligament, which is typically at the center of the femoral head. A "low stick" can result in cannulation of the superficial femoral artery, which increases the risk of hematoma, dissection, arterial occlusion, or formation of a pseudoaneurysm or arteriovenous fistula. Conversely, a "high stick" above the inguinal ligament or inferior epigastric artery does not allow for effective manual compression against the femoral head and significantly increases the risk of retroperitoneal hemorrhage. Before administering therapeutic anticoagulation for PCI, limited angiography through the femoral sheath at an oblique ipsilateral angle can be performed to determine the arteriotomy site in relationship to the femoral head, inferior epigastric artery, and femoral bifurcation, which could modify the timing of PCI and/or choice to use a vascular access closure device.

Two commonly used techniques to reduce vascular complications during femoral access include the use of a micropuncture needle and/or ultrasound guidance. Traditionally, an 18-gauge wide open-bore needle has been used for arterial cannulation. A smaller micropuncture 21-gauge needle can be used to access the common femoral artery. After placement of a 0.018-inch wire into the artery, limited angiography can localize the site of cannulation through the needle or inner dilator, and if acceptable, a 4F micropuncture sheath can be advanced over the 0.018 in wire and exchanged for a 5F or 6F sheath over an 0.035 in wire. If the arteriotomy site is too low or high, the needle or inner dilator can be removed with minimal bleeding risks and femoral access at an alternative site can be reattempted. Real-time ultrasound guidance has also been used for femoral access and allows for visualization of needle entrance into the common femoral artery above the bifurcation. Ultrasound guidance is associated with a lower risk of major bleeding and vascular complications. Routine use of ultrasound guidance for femoral access for PCI is recommended.

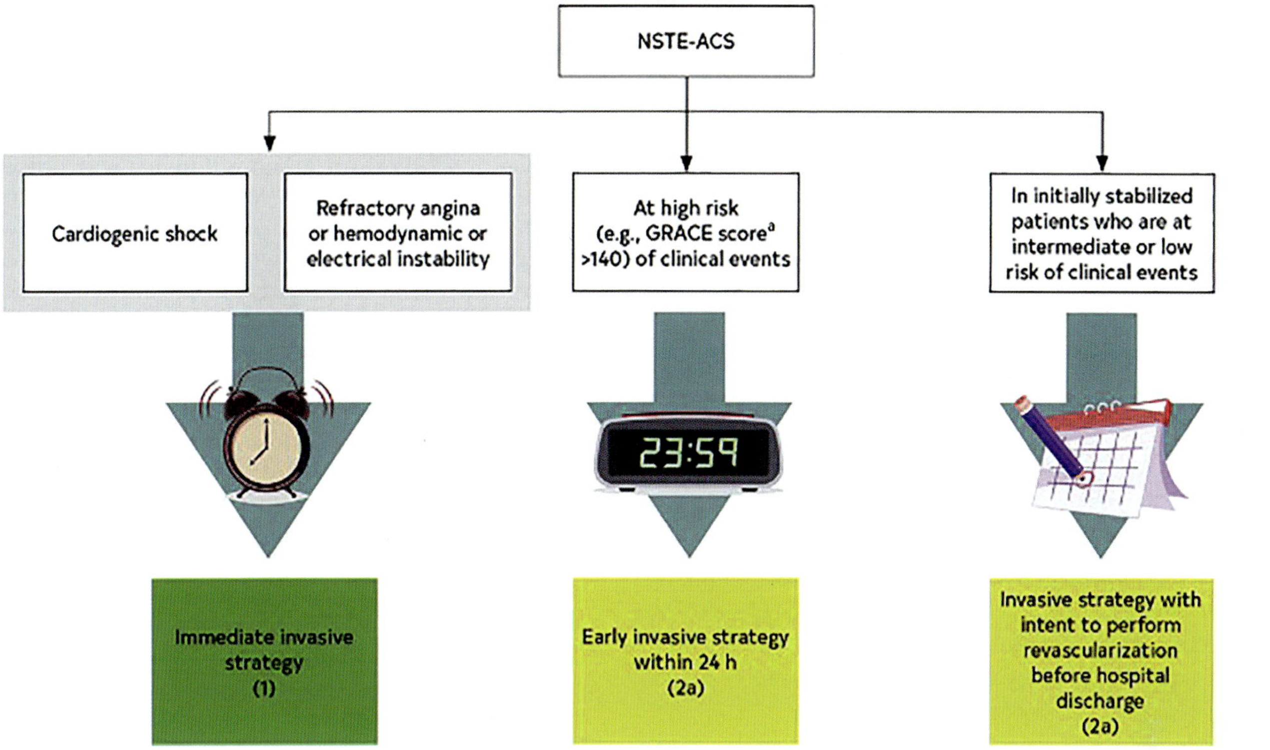

FIG. 11.1 Timing of invasive strategy for Non-ST-segment elevation acute coronary syndrome. The algorithm summarizes the 2021 ACC/AHA.SCAI Coronary Artery Revascularization Guideline recommendations for the timing of coronary angiography with the intent to perform revascularization in patients presenting with NSTE-ACS. *NSTE-ACS*, Non-ST-segment Elevation Acute Coronary Syndrome; *GRACE*, Global Registry of Acute Coronary Events. [a]https://www.mdcalc.com/grace-acs-risk-mortality-calculator. (From Lawton JS, et al. 2021 ACC/AHA/SCAI guideline for coronary artery revascularization: executive summary: a report of the American College of Cardiology/American Heart Association joint committee on clinical practice guidelines. *J Am Coll Cardiol*. 2022;79:197–215.)

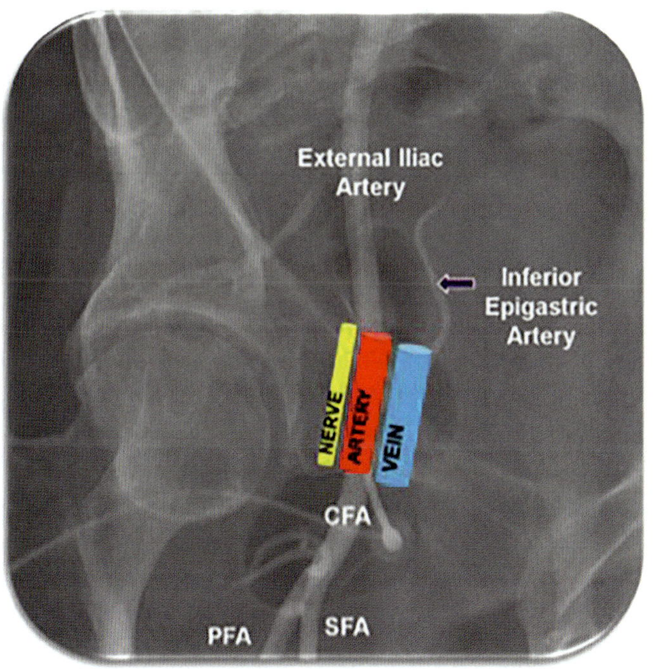

FIG. 11.2 Anatomy of the femoral artery. Femoral angiography of the right femoral artery in a right anterior oblique view. The common femoral artery should be entered below the inguinal ligament in the middle one-third of the femoral head to avoid a low (i.e., at or below the femoral bifurcation) or high stick (i.e., above the inferior epigastric artery). *CFA*, Common femoral artery; *PFA*, profunda femoris artery; *SFA*, superficial femoral artery. (From Bangalore S, Bhatt DL. Femoral arterial access and closure. *Circulation*. 2011;124:e147–156.)

Radial

The learning curve for a radial approach can be longer compared with femoral access. It should not be used in patients with a forearm arteriovenous fistula. Assessment for collateral ulnar circulation via the ulnar-palmar arterial arch is advocated. However, failure to demonstrate dual circulation to the hand (i.e., incomplete palmar arch) is not an absolute contraindication for radial access. Assessment is performed using either the modified Allen's or plethysmo-oxymetric test, the latter of which has a higher specificity. A plethysmo-oxymetric test is an Allen's test with a pulse oximeter placed on the thumb. The examiner assesses the baseline saturation and waveform and then compresses the ulnar and radial arteries until the waveform disappears and the oxygen saturation is zero. The pressure on the ulnar artery is released. If the waveform and oxygen saturation return to baseline, then adequate collateral flow is present. Any abnormal Allen's test should be confirmed by plethysmo-oxymetric testing. When attempting radial access, a smaller amount of lidocaine (1–2 mL) should be administered to minimize the risk of local vasospasm or obscuring the radial pulse. A micropuncture needle is used to access the radial artery and for placement of a hydrophilic radial arterial sheath over a 0.021- to 0.025-inch guidewire. Ultrasound is also useful to minimize the number of attempts needed for successful arterial cannulation.[9]

Vasospasm can be a significant limitation in radial access. Intra-arterial administration of an antispasmolytic drug (e.g., nitroglycerin, diltiazem, verapamil) is mandatory. A number

TABLE 11.2 Comparison of Femoral and Radial Access for Percutaneous Coronary Intervention

	FEMORAL	RADIAL
Anatomic		
Vessel size	6–10 mm	2–3 mm
Vascular course	Less variable	Highly variable
Vessel location	Variable because of body habitus	Superficial
Nearby neurovascular	Yes	No
Procedural		
Procedural success	Marginally higher	Marginally lower
Procedural time	Comparable	Comparable
Contrast load	Comparable	Comparable
Fluoroscopy time	Marginally lower	Marginally higher
Choice of sheath size	Unrestricted	Restricted (typically 6-F)
Learning curve	Shorter	Longer (typically 50 cases)
Patient Care		
Preference	Lower	Higher
Time to ambulation	Typically 2–6 h	Immediate
Length of stay	Longer	Shorter
Complications		
Access site bleeding	Higher	Lower
Vessel occlusion	Rare	0%–10%
Pseudoaneurysm	1%–5%	Rare

From Byrne RA, et al. Vascular access and closure in coronary angiography and percutaneous intervention. *Nat Rev Cardiol*. 2013;10:27–40.

of single agents or "cocktail" regimens have been used to prevent vasospasm. Most operators use verapamil (2.5–5 mg) and/or nitroglycerin (100–200 µg). An intravenous or inter-arterial bolus of unfractionated heparin (e.g., 5000 IU or 50 IU/kg or higher a dose) is recommended after radial artery cannulation and the use of ipsilateral ulnar artery compression is recommended to reduce the risk for radial artery occlusion.[9] Patent hemostasis is essential following any transradial approach. Access via the left radial may be advantageous over the right radial because of the higher prevalence of right-handed individuals; the aortic path approximates a transfemoral approach, which allows for easier coronary cannulation with standard Judkins guide catheters and easier access to the left internal mammary artery in coronary artery bypass graft (CABG) patients. If radial access fails, femoral access should be considered. Ipsilateral ulnar access is a reasonable alternative when radial or femoral access is not feasible.[9]

Advantages and Disadvantages of Radial Versus Femoral Access

When considering vascular access, operators should consider important differences between femoral and radial access (Table 11.2). In the United States, rates of radial access for PCI in 2004–2007 were less than 2% because of unfamiliarity with the radial approach and concern for increased procedure length and radiation exposure. However, rates in the United States have increased exponentially, with utilization rates above 50% and as high as 70% to 80% in one study.[10]

Current Evidence: Radial Versus Femoral

Radial access is associated with a lower rate of vascular complications, major bleeding, and a lower rate of adverse cardiac events in patients with ACS compared with femoral access. In the radial vs. femoral access for coronary intervention (RIVAL) trial, no difference was observed in the composite rate of death, MI, stroke, or non-CABG major bleeding in patients who presented with ACS without ST-segment elevation and who were randomized to femoral versus radial access. However, mortality at 30 days and vascular complications were significantly lower with radial access.[9] Patients who presented with STEMI in the radial vs. femoral randomized investigation in ST-elevation acute coronary syndrome (RIFLE-STEACS) and ST "elevation myocardial infarction treated by radial or femoral approach (STEMI-RADIAL) trials also demonstrated a significant reduction in bleeding and vascular complications,[9] which translated into shorter hospital stays and lower mortality compared with the femoral approach.[11] The lower mortality in STEMI with radial catheterization was confirmed in observational data from the National Cardiovascular Data Registry. The minimizing adverse haemorrhagic events by transradial access site and systemic implementation of AngioX (MATRIX) trial demonstrated a lower rate of net adverse clinical events (mortality, nonfatal MI and stroke, and non-CABG major bleeding) with a radial versus a femoral approach in ACS patients with or without STEMI, predominantly driven by fewer major bleeding complications and lower mortality.[9]

Considerations for Radial Approach in ST-Elevation Myocardial Infarction

Despite evidence that the radial approach reduces vascular complications, major bleeding, and mortality in STEMI patients, its use is paradoxically lower in this population than in patients with NSTEMI. One concern is that the increased time required for the radial approach may prolong the time-to-treatment goal in STEMI. However, the potential door-to-device delay for radial access is often minimal and the time difference would not offset the mortality benefit of radial PCI over femoral PCI in STEMI. Because of the higher risk for cardiogenic shock in STEMI, the groin should always be prepped for immediate venous access or additional arterial access for hemodynamic support.

Vascular Closure Devices: When to Consider Use

Vascular closure devices were designed to improve the safety of PCI by reducing access site bleeding and vascular complications. Clinical trials have not demonstrated that vascular closure devices lower bleeding and/or vascular complications compared with manual compression. Current guidelines do not recommend routine use of vascular closure.

When manual compression (e.g., 3 minutes per sheath French size [e.g., 6F = 18 minutes]) is used, femoral arterial sheaths can typically be pulled when the activated clotting time (ACT) is less than 160 to 180 seconds with heparin use or 2 hours after bivalirudin is stopped without measuring the ACT. Manual compression can be performed digitally or using a manual compression assist device (e.g., FemoStop, Abbott, Plymouth, Minnesota). Vascular closure devices achieve faster hemostasis, which allows for earlier ambulation, improved patient satisfaction, and shorter hospital length of stay. In the absence of a radial approach, obese patients, whose body habitus may limit effective manual compression, or individuals who cannot tolerate prolonged periods in a supine position, a vascular closure device should be considered. Arteriotomy sites at the femoral bifurcation, in the superficial femoral artery, or in a smaller femoral artery (<5 mm) are associated with a higher risk for device failure and possible arterial occlusion. For these anatomical situations, manual compression is typically favored over a vascular closure device. A number of femoral vascular closure devices are currently approved (https://evtoday.com/device-guide/us/closure-devices) and available with different mechanisms used for closure. No sizeable randomized trial comparing the safety and efficacy of femoral vascular closure devices in PCI has been conducted.

With a transradial approach, a hemostatic band is necessary to achieve hemostasis but also to achieve patent hemostasis.[9] Radial artery occlusion occurs in approximately 2% to 10% of patients.[9] A bolus of intravenous or intra-arterial unfractionated heparin (5000 U or 50 U/kg or higher) should be administered after sheath placement. The optimal duration for hemostatic banding following PCI is 120 to 180 minutes.[12] A recent network meta-analysis demonstrated that 2 hours of hemostatic compression was the best time duration to prevent bleeding and artery occlusion.[12] During hemostatic compression, ipsilateral ulnar artery compression is recommended to maximize patent hemostasis.[9] Using a plethysmography, the ipsilateral ulnar artery is compressed while the hemostatic band is in place. If the waveform or reading suggests the radial artery is occluded, then the band can be deflated (and inflated) as needed to re-establish antegrade flow and minimize bleeding.

Management of Vascular Complications

Vascular complications are one of the most common adverse events following PCI and are associated with an increase in cost, length of stay, morbidity, and mortality. The two most common complications are hematoma and pseudoaneurysm; whereas, less common complications include: dissection, arteriovenous fistula, arterial occlusion, retroperitoneal hemorrhage (RPH), femoral nerve damage, and infection. A hematoma is typically managed conservatively with local compression and rarely requires blood transfusion. The presence of a palpable bruit or pulsatile mass should prompt evaluation with an ultrasound. Small pseudoaneurysms (<3 cm) can be followed with serial ultrasounds. Pseudoaneurysms larger than 3 cm are often treated with ultrasound-guided thrombin injection. Surgical repair may be required for large pseudoaneurysms that are not anatomically suitable for thrombin injection. RPH should be suspected in any patient with a sudden onset of hypotension and flank pain ipsilateral to the vascular access site. Prompt recognition with concomitant volume and blood support is essential for the management of a suspected RPH. Anticoagulation reversal or platelet infusion may also be necessary, despite the theoretical risks for stent thrombosis. Early computed tomography may be useful to diagnose RPH, but should not delay aggressive supportive measures. Most RPHs can be managed conservatively, and endovascular or open-surgical treatment may be necessary in patients who cannot be stabilized hemodynamically. Arterial occlusion should be suspected in any patient with sudden onset of leg pain, paresthesia, decreased or absent pulses, or a cool and/or cyanotic limb. Suspected arterial occlusion is a vascular emergency and should be treated with intravenous (IV) anticoagulation and emergent endovascular or surgical repair.

INTERVENTIONAL PHARMACOTHERAPY

Procedural Sedation

PCI is typically performed using minimal to moderate sedation. The goal is for patients to be comfortable with depressed consciousness while maintaining the ability to follow verbal commands. Patients should receive supplemental oxygen during PCI as needed. Due to the potential risk for respiratory depression leading to hypoxia and/or hypercarbia, all patients should be assessed for a history of or clinical predictors for difficult intubation (e.g., obesity). If present, anesthesiology should be consulted to consider the need for monitored anesthesia care. Typically, an IV sedative and/or analgesic are administered in small incremental dosages during PCI. The two most common agents used are midazolam (0.5–1 mg IV boluses) as a sedative and fentanyl (25–50 µg IV bolus) as an analgesic. Both have a rapid onset of action (2–5 minutes), are rapidly metabolized within 30–60 minutes after administration, and their effects are reversible with flumazenil and naloxone, respectively.

Oral Antiplatelet Therapy

Antiplatelet therapy is essential for PCI in acute MI (see Chapters 13 and 26). In this section, we focus on the practical aspects of oral antiplatelet therapy for operators performing PCI. All patients should receive an oral loading dose of aspirin (US: 325 mg oral; EU: 150–300 mg) or a 600-mg rectal suppository (US)/75 to 250 mg IV (EU) if unable to swallow or vomiting.[2,6] Most patients with STEMI and NSTEMI should receive a loading dose of an adenosine diphosphate (ADP) $P2Y_{12}$ inhibitor. Pretreatment (i.e., prior to coronary angiography) with a loading dose of an oral ADP $P2Y_{12}$ inhibitor in patients with acute MI was previously recommended. However, conflicting data on the benefits of pretreatment with an oral ADP $P2Y_{12}$ before establishing the coronary anatomy do not support routine pretreatment in ACS.[2,3,6]

Anticoagulation Strategies

To prevent the risk of intra- and early postprocedural catheter- and device-related thrombosis, anticoagulant therapy must be administered to all patients undergoing PCI.[2,6] Selecting an initial agent will be discussed in detail

restenosis eliminating the need for a polymer for drug elution. Bioresorbable stents have also been developed to be fully biodegradable, where the stent platform or scaffold is completely reabsorbed after a given period following implantation. Both technologies were designed to reduce the need to reduce the risk of late restenosis/stent thrombosis and shorten the duration of DAPT. Despite the theoretical benefit of these stent platforms, the current evidence has not demonstrated a clinical benefit compared with the currently available DESs.

Drug-coated balloons (DCB) have also been studied for coronary revascularization with the goal of delivering a single dose of drug to a coronary lesion to reduce the risk of restenosis without leaving a stent scaffold behind (i.e., risk of stent thrombosis). In the United States, DCBs are not currently commercially available for coronary PCI. In Europe, DCBs are approved and recommended for treatment for in-stent restenosis of BMS and DES.[23] Newer-generation DCBs have been developed and compared against currently available second-generation DESs for certain *de novo* coronary lesions.[24,25] Patients with small vessel disease are one potential *de* novo coronary lesion subset where DCBs have encouraging clinical evidence compared with DESs.[25,26] DCBs are also being evaluated for other clinical indications, including patients with a high bleeding risk, diffuse coronary disease, and bifurcation lesions.[24]

ADJUNCTIVE DIAGNOSTIC AND THERAPEUTIC DEVICES

Practical Use of Intravascular Imaging

Coronary angiography is a two-dimensional image that has certain limitations, namely, that it is a "luminogram" that accurately describes the vessel lumen, but it provides limited information about plaque composition, size, and distribution. Intravascular imaging allows for real-time assessment of coronary stenoses, which can be used at various times during PCI. Two devices, intravascular ultrasound (IVUS) and optical coherence tomography (OCT), are the most commonly used intravascular imaging devices in clinical practice. Near-infrared spectroscopy may be useful for detecting the lipid composition and potential vulnerability of a plaque, but it is not commonly used to support PCI. Each of these devices is discussed in Chapter 18.

IVUS and OCT are used at various stages of PCI. Before PCI, intravascular imaging can be used to determine plaque morphology, vessel size, location, and distribution. Lesion composition can change interventional strategies for revascularization. For example, if a lesion is heavily calcified (e.g., circumferential calcium), devices that can modify the calcium (e.g., rotational atherectomy) may be used to prepare the lesion before balloon angioplasty. In addition, plaque location and distribution can significantly alter the stenting strategy of bifurcation lesions, especially in left main lesions. Another important use of intravascular imaging is to determine the cause of stent failure in stent thrombosis or in-stent restenosis (Fig. 11.e1). OCT may have some advantages over IVUS for this purpose because it can accurately assess endothelial coverage of the stent struts (i.e., a potential cause of late and very late stent thrombosis) or detect neoatherosclerosis, a potential cause of late stent failure.

Recent evidence demonstrated the benefit of IVUS during PCI. The multicenter randomized ULTIMATE (Intravascular Ultrasound Guided Drug Eluting Stents Implantation in "All-Comers" Coronary Lesions) trial revealed that IVUS-guided PCI with DES significantly reduces target vessel failure and stent thrombosis among all comers compared with angiographic guidance alone.[27] A pooled patient-level analysis of the ULTIMATE and IVUS-XPL (Impact of Intravascular Ultrasound Guidance on the Outcomes of Xience Prime Stents in Long Lesions) trials demonstrated that IVUS guidance reduced cardiac death compared with angiography alone in long lesions requiring stent lengths >28 mm.[28] Observational data suggest that IVUS use for left main PCI is associated with lower rates of coronary complications and major adverse cardiac events at 30 days and 12-month mortality.[29] Current guidelines recommend the use of IVUS during PCI to reduce ischemic events,[2,6] especially for left main or complex lesions.

When to Use Fractional Flow Reserve in Acute Myocardial Infarction?

Coronary angiography does not always accurately predict the hemodynamic significance of a coronary lesion. Only angiographic stenoses of more than 80% to 90% can accurately predict a hemodynamically significant lesion by fractional flow reserve (FFR).[30] Invasive physiologic assessment of a lesion's severity is recommended for intermediate stenoses (i.e., 50%–70%) to determine if PCI should be performed.[2] The two most common methods used to measure a lesion's physiological significance are FFR and instantaneous wave-free ratio (iFR). FFR measures the hemodynamic significance of a coronary lesion by measuring the distal mean coronary and aortic pressures during maximal hyperemia, typically IV adenosine. iFr measures the distal mean coronary and aortic pressures during a wave-free period of diastole and does not require administration of adenosine (i.e., maximal hyperemia). Both measurement tools have a wealth of data supporting its use and clinical benefit compared with PCI-guided by angiography alone.[31]

Despite its utility in stable ischemic heart disease, its use in the setting of acute myocardial infarction remains undefined. In AMI (especially STEMI), culprit lesions should not undergo physiologic assessment by FFR or iFR, namely, due to the abnormal coronary flow in acutely injured myocardium that can cause a false negative result. In NSTEMI, it may be particularly difficult to determine the culprit lesion in patients with multivessel CAD, and physiologic assessment can be used to assess which lesion(s) should be revascularized.[30,31] In STEMI, physiologic assessment of nonculprit lesions may be helpful. In DANAMI-3—PRIMULTI, FFR-guided complete revascularization during the index admission reduced the risk of future revascularization at 12 months compared with culprit-vessel only PCI.[2,3,6,31] The Compare-Acute trial also demonstrated a reduction in cardiovascular events at 12 months with FFR-guided complete revascularization at 12 months compared with culprit-lesion only PCI in STEMI patients.[2,6,31]

Aspiration Thrombectomy

Thrombectomy can be performed by manual aspiration catheters or use of a mechanical thrombectomy catheter system (e.g., Indigo System CAT RX, Penumbra, Inc, Alameda, California). Manual aspiration catheters are simple to use, have a lower profile, and are preferred by many operators. A meta-analysis of 11,321 patients from 20 randomized controlled trials demonstrated that major adverse cardiac events, including stent thrombosis, were significantly reduced in STEMI patients using aspiration thrombectomy before primary PCI compared with primary PCI alone.[2,6,32] However, randomized evidence from adequately sized trials of cardiovascular outcomes does not support its routine use.[2,6,32] The TASTE (Thrombus Aspiration in ST-Elevation Myocardial Infarction in Scandinavia) trial did not show any reduction in death, MI, and stent thrombosis in STEMI patients (n = 7244) randomized to manual aspiration compared with primary PCI alone.[2,6,32] The TOTAL (Trial of Routine Aspiration Thrombectomy with PCI versus PCI Alone in Patients with STEMI) trial of 10,732 STEMI patients who underwent primary PCI randomized to bailout or upfront routine manual aspiration thrombectomy did not find any clinical benefit at 180 days with routine aspiration thrombectomy; moreover, a higher rate of stroke at 180 days was observed with routine aspiration thrombectomy compared with primary PCI alone.[2,6,32] A patient-level meta-analysis of TASTE, TOTAL, and TAPAS (Thrombus Aspiration during Percutaneous coronary intervention in Acute myocardial infarction Study) did not show any clinical benefit for routine aspiration thrombectomy, but a subgroup analysis of patients with a high thrombus burden did have fewer cardiovascular deaths but also a higher risk of stroke predominantly driven by the TOTAL trial.[2,6,32] In STEMI, current guidelines do not recommend routine aspiration thrombectomy,[2,3,6] and it is reserved for selected patients with a large thrombus burden or as bailout following primary PCI.[2]

Distal Embolic Protection

Embolic protection devices have the potential to capture any atherosclerotic debris or thrombus that may be embolized during PCI. A number of embolic protection devices have been developed that use either proximal occlusion or a distal filter to catch embolic debris. The proximal occlusion device is no longer available in the United States. Thus, the filter-based devices (Fig. 11.4) can be used for PCI and can capture debris that is more than 120 µm. One advantage to this device is that anterograde flow is maintained throughout PCI. Currently, embolic protection devices should be used for PCI of saphenous vein grafts (SVGs), which typically contain more friable atherosclerotic debris.[2] In the absence of an SVG, embolic protection is not indicated in PCI for MI, including STEMI. Distal embolic protection has not been shown to improve clinical outcomes or infarct size compared with primary PCI alone.[2]

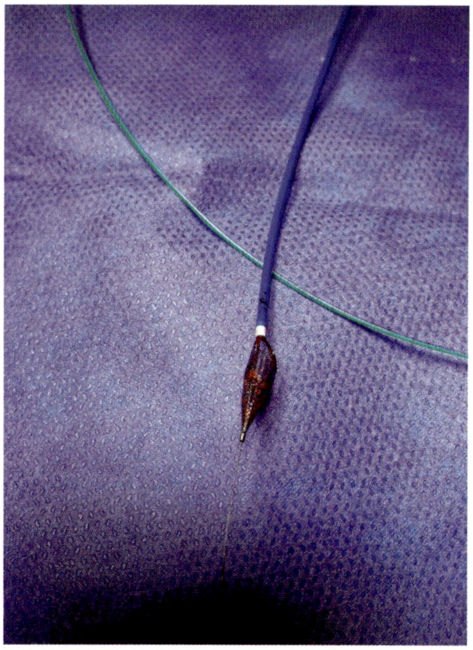

FIG. 11.4 **Filter embolic protection device.** Atherosclerotic debris that was captured using a filter-based embolic protection device following percutaneous coronary intervention of a saphenous vein graft.

LESION-SPECIFIC PERCUTANEOUS CORONARY INTERVENTION STRATEGIES

Bifurcation Lesions

Coronary bifurcation lesions occur at or near a division of a major coronary artery and are found in up to 20% of PCIs. In STEMI, bifurcation lesions comprise approximately 10% of target lesions in primary PCI. Procedural and clinical outcomes associated with PCI of bifurcation lesions remain suboptimal because of the complexity of anatomy and the dynamic changes that occur to the lesion during revascularization. Selection of the optimal PCI strategy to manage bifurcation lesions is challenging. When considering bifurcation PCI, it is important to carefully assess the distribution and morphology (e.g., calcium distribution) of atherosclerotic disease, the relative size of the proximal and distal main branch and side branch, and the bifurcation angle of the main and side branches. During main branch stenting, side branch compromise that requires stenting may be required. Dynamic changes can occur during stenting of the main branch that can compromise coronary blood flow to a side branch, including plaque or a carina shift, bifurcation angle change, vessel spasm, dissection, stent strut protrusion, and conformational changes to the side branch ostium.

The Medina classification remains the most widely accepted scheme used to classify bifurcation lesions (Fig. 11.5). IVUS can be used to assess the distribution and morphology of plaque in a bifurcation lesion and will frequently reclassify lesions compared with angiographic classification. During bifurcation PCI, it is important to determine if a bifurcation lesion will be managed using a one-stent (i.e., provisional) or two-stent approach. In the provisional strategy, the main branch is stented and the side branch may require further treatment including provisional stenting if clinical symptoms and/or angiographic

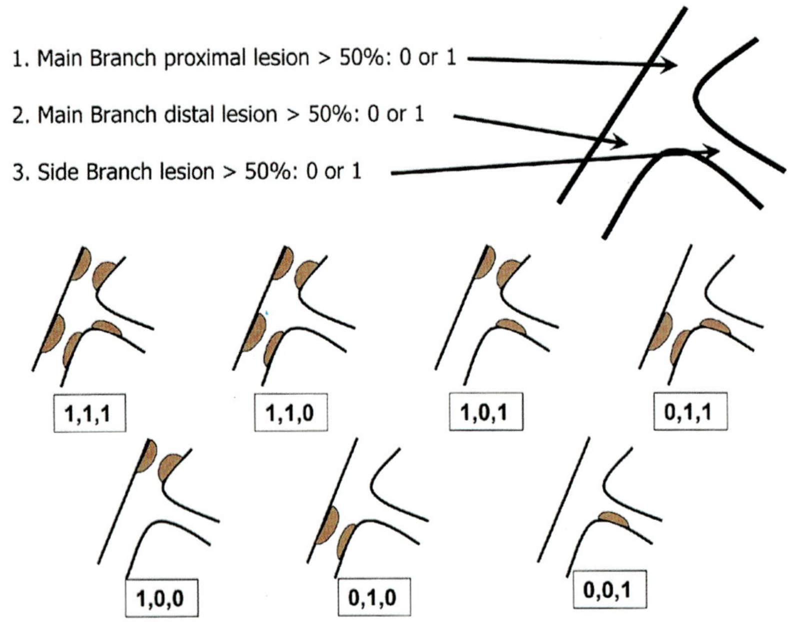

FIG. 11.5 Medina classification of bifurcation lesions. (Redrawn From Latib A, Colombo A. Bifurcation disease: what do we know, what should we do? *JACC Cardiovasc Interv.* 2008;1:218–26.)

(e.g., thrombolysis in myocardial infarction [TIMI] <3 flow) or adjunctive measurements (e.g., FFR ≤0.80 or iFR ≤0.89) warrant intervention. A second stent is required in approximately 5%–25% of provisional stenting cases.[33] A two-stent strategy involves stenting both the main and side branches. Randomized and observational data suggest that provisional side branch stenting compared with planned side branch stenting (i.e., two-stent approach) have similar clinical outcomes, except procedural time and contrast volume are reduced with a provisional approach.[33] Thus, most bifurcation lesions can be treated using a provisional strategy.[33]

Historically, a "true" bifurcation lesion was categorized as a complex bifurcation lesion with significant (>50%) stenosis in both the main and side branches.[33] However, the side branch length, bifurcation angle, and lesion characteristics are also important considerations that help determine the interventional approach for revascularization. The DEFINITION registry used additional major and minor criteria to further define a complex bifurcation lesion (Table 11.4).[33] This study demonstrated that for lesions classified as complex, a two-stent strategy was associated with a lower risk of in-hospital major adverse cardiac events and cardiac death at 1-year compared with provisional stenting. True bifurcation lesions do not always mandate a two-stent approach. Lesions with a side branch lesion <10 mm can often be treated with a provisional approach.[34]

TABLE 11.4 Definition Criteria for Coronary Bifurcation Lesions

MAJOR CRITERIA	MINOR CRITERIA
Distal left main: Side branch lesion length ≥10 mm AND Side branch diameter stenosis ≥70% *Non left main:* Side branch lesion length ≥10 mm AND Side branch diameter stenosis ≥90%	Moderate to severe calcification Multiple lesions Bifurcation angle <45° or >70° Main vessel reference diameter <2.5 mm Thrombus-containing lesions Main vessel lesion length ≥25 mm
Complex Bifurcation Lesion = 1 major and ≥2 minor	

From Chen SL, et al. Impact of the complexity of bifurcation lesions treated with drug-eluting stents: the DEFINITION study (Definitions and impact of complEx biFurcation leslons on clinical outcomes after percutaNeous coronary IntervenTIOn using drug-eluting steNts). *JACC Cardiovasc Interv.* 2014;7:1266–1276.

Left Main Coronary Artery

Strategies used for left main coronary artery (LMCA) PCI will depend on the plaque distribution (i.e., ostium, body, distal), LMCA length and size, and the bifurcation angle. Focal LMCA stenoses at the ostium or body that do not involve the distal left main artery can often be treated with a short single stent. However, the same strategies used to perform bifurcation PCI also apply to LMCA disease that involves the distal left main and/or ostium of the left anterior descending or left circumflex arteries. Because of the limitations of angiography, IVUS use should be used when technically feasible to accurately assess the distribution of plaque in the LMCA and its branches.[2] In STEMI, if the LMCA is the culprit vessel, then PCI should be considered in patients with TIMI grade <3 flow.[2] In NSTEMI, the decision to treat LMCA disease with PCI or CABG should undergo a prompt evaluation using a heart team approach to assess the complexity of coronary disease (i.e., SYNTAX [Synergy Between Percutaneous Coronary Intervention with TAXUS and Cardiac Surgery] score), surgical risk (i.e., STS [Society of Thoracic Surgery] score), and other co-morbidities to determine the best revascularization strategy using local expertise and patient preferences.[2] In patients with a high SYNTAX score (>33), diabetes mellitus, or multivessel CAD, CABG is typically preferred over PCI, and PCI is favored in patients with a low SYNTAX score (<22) or a high surgical risk (STS >5%).

Aorto-Ostial Lesions

Aorto-ostial lesions are typically defined as lesions within 3 mm of the vessel origin (i.e., left main, right coronary artery, or anomalous coronary vessel). Aorto-ostial disease may be difficult to diagnose with angiography alone, and a high suspicion for its presence should be considered with dampening of the pressure waveform with coronary catheter engagement. IVUS and FFR or iFR are useful for determining the degree of stenosis or hemodynamic significance, respectively, in lesions that are intermediate or indeterminate on angiography. IVUS can also be used to assess plaque distribution and vessel size and mark the ostium during stent deployment. It is important to rule out catheter-induced spasm from engagement of the coronary ostium; where spasm will typically resolve with intracoronary administration of nitroglycerin (100–200 µg). Aorto-ostial disease can be resistant to angioplasty and stenting because of recoil from the muscular and elastic layers of the aorta.

Saphenous Vein Graft

PCI of SVGs is associated with a significantly higher rate of periprocedural MI and acute complications because of atheroembolization and release of vasoactive substances to the downstream microcirculation, which can lead to no-reflow. SVGs are more friable than native coronary disease and prone to distal embolization with manipulation during PCI. In STEMI, approximately 2% to 3% of patients have a history of CABG and approximately half of previous CABG patients will have an SVG that is the culprit vessel. Primary PCI of patients with a history of CABG has a significant delay in door-to-device times (i.e., reperfusion), worse angiographic outcomes, and higher rates of adverse clinical outcomes, including death. As mentioned previously, embolic protection devices should be considered during SVG PCI to improve clinical outcomes.

Arterial Bypass Grafts

PCI of arterial bypass grafts (in situ or free) is rarely performed but can be performed with a high procedural success and short- and long-term efficacy with a low risk of complications. Unlike PCI of SVGs, distal embolic protection is typically not necessary for arterial bypass grafts.

Calcified Lesions

Calcified lesions are less likely to cause ACS with or without ST-segment elevation compared with plaque rupture or erosion. However, a subset of patients with a heavily calcified culprit lesion will present with an MI. During PCI, extensive calcification can be technically challenging and affect delivery of guidewires, balloons, or stents in calcified, rigid arteries. Calcification can also be incredibly resistant to high-pressure balloon dilation, which can lead to stent under expansion (i.e., a predictor of acute stent thrombosis). IVUS should be used to further evaluate the distribution of calcium. In lesions with thick, calcified segments, calcified nodules, or calcium distribution involving >270° of the vessel circumference, lesion modification can be considered.[2] Devices used to modify calcium include rotational and orbital atherectomy, cutting balloons, laser atherectomy, and intravascular lithotripsy (IVL). Routine use of these devices does not improve clinical outcomes, but it does enhance the likelihood of procedural success in selected calcified lesions.[2] These devices can be considered for calcified arteries when balloon dilation is inadequate or there is an inability to cross a lesion with a balloon or stent.[2] The most commonly used rotational atherectomy device is the Rotablator rotational atherectomy device (Boston Scientific, Marlborough, Massachusetts), which removes plaque using a rapidly rotating (150,000–160,000 rpm) atherectomy burr with diamond chips embedded on the surface. Most operators will use a single smaller (1.5 or 1.75 mm) burr for plaque modification to allow for effective balloon dilation and complete stent expansion. IVL using a Shockwave balloon (Shockwave Medical, Santa Clara, California) is an emerging device that significantly improves procedural success in severely calcified vessels.[35]

NONCULPRIT REVASCULARIZATION

An important area in PCI in acute MI, primarily in patients with STEMI, is the management of nonculprit lesions. A heart team approach is essential to determine the optimal revascularization strategy in patients presenting with STEMI and multivessel CAD.[2,6] In acute MI, patients with multivessel CAD have a significantly higher rate of adverse cardiac events, including death and reinfarction compared with patients with single-vessel CAD. During an acute MI, it has been suggested that the pathophysiologic derangements leading to plaque rupture of the culprit vessel may be generalized throughout the entire coronary vasculature, leading to plaque destabilization and vulnerability in nonculprit territories.

Historically, observational and prospective studies were inconclusive on the efficacy and safety of multivessel revascularization in STEMI.[2,6] Recent randomized clinical trials now support revascularization of the nonculprit lesions in STEMI.[2,6,36] Based on this evidence, the 2021 ACC/AHA/SCAI Coronary Revascularization guidelines proposed an algorithm for PCI of nonculprit vessels in STEMI (Fig. 11.6).[2] Staged PCI (i.e., prior to or after discharge) is the preferred strategy due to a reduction in the risk of major adverse cardiac events compared with culprit vessel-only PCI.[2,6] Staged-PCI is ideal for patients with nonculprit lesions that supply a large area of myocardium and do not have comorbidities that increase the risk of PCI (e.g., chronic kidney disease).[2] Nonculprit PCI at the time of primary PCI can be performed on carefully selected patients with nonculprit lesions that are not complex and have normal renal function and volume status. If a patient has complex nonculprit vessel CAD (e.g., left main, chronic total occlusion, severe calcification), elective CABG should also be considered as a potential option for revascularization following primary PCI of the culprit vessel. In patients with cardiogenic shock and STEMI or NSTEMI, culprit vessel-only PCI is recommended due to a significantly lower risk of death and need for hemodialysis at 30 days compared

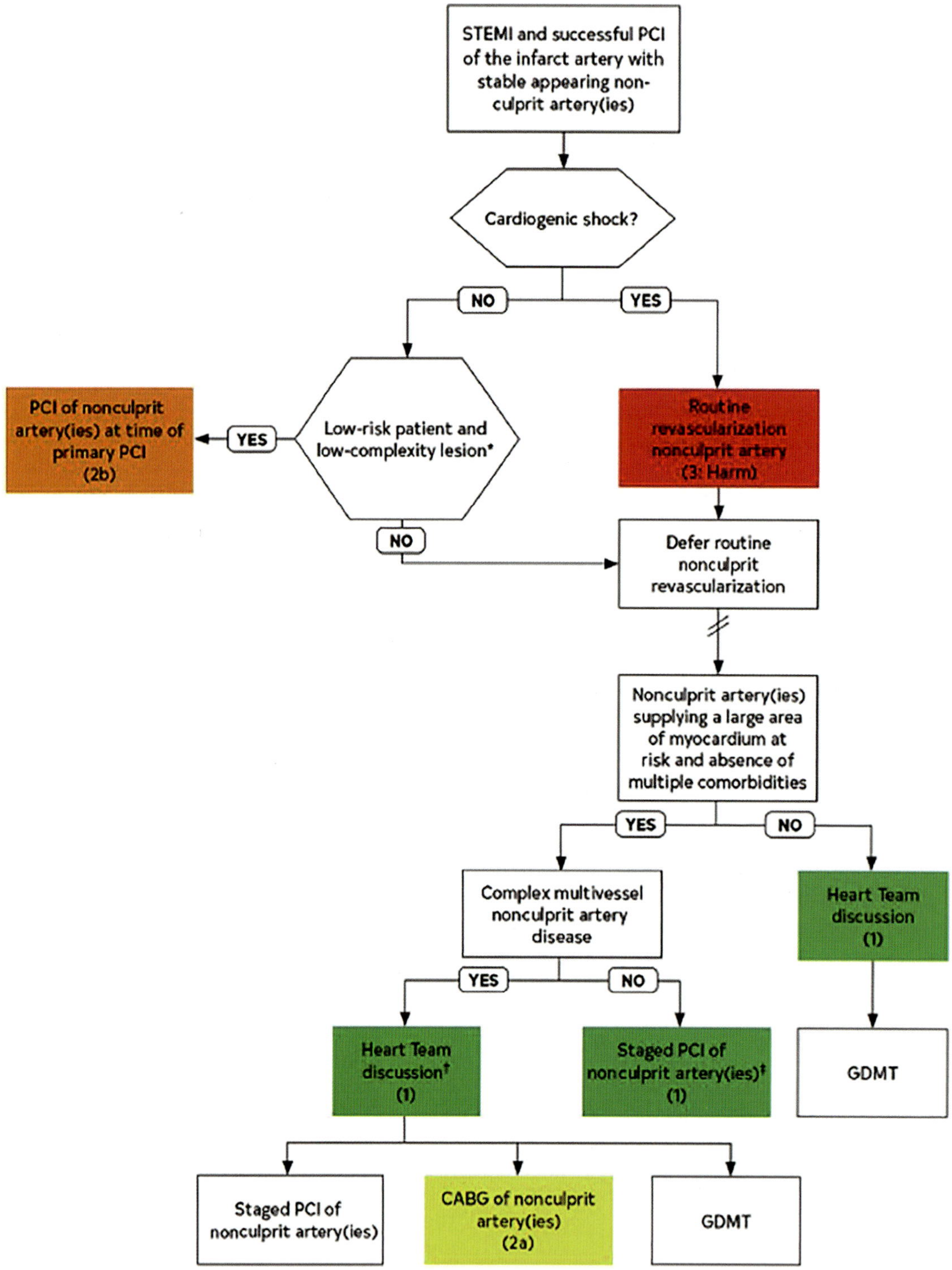

FIG. 11.6 2021 ACC/AHA/SCAI coronary revascularization guidelines algorithm for revascularization of nonculprit vessels in STEMI. [a]Normal blood pressure and heart rate left ventricular end-diastolic pressure <20 mm Hg, no chronic renal insufficiency or acute kidney injury, and expected total contrast volume <3 glomerular filtration rate, simple lesion anatomy. [b]In making the decision about the need for and mode of revascularization the Heart Team should consider the suitability of the nonculprit artery for PCI, the coronary complexity and the risk of revascularization, the extent of myocardium at risk, and patient comorbidities, including life expectancy or other significant patient comorbidities, such as chronic renal insufficiency or acute kidney injury. [c]Staged PCI can be performed in hospital or after discharge, up to 45 days post MI. *CABG*, coronary artery bypass graft; *GDMT*, guideline-directed medical therapy; *PCI*, percutaneous coronary intervention; *STEMI*, ST-segment–elevation myocardial infarction. (From Lawton, JS, et al. 2021 ACC/AHA/SCAI guideline for coronary artery revascularization: executive summary: a report of the American College of Cardiology/American Heart Association joint committee on clinical practice guidelines. *J Am Coll Cardiol.* 2022;79:197–215.)

with multivessel PCI.[2,6,37] In observational studies, complete revascularization may be beneficial in patients who present with NSTEMI. No randomized trials have studied complete versus incomplete revascularization in an NSTEMI-only patient population, but only in subgroups. Thus, the benefits and risks of nonculprit PCI in NSTEMI should be discussed using a heart team approach.[2] Functional hemodynamic assessment of lesions in nonculprit vessels can be considered to determine which lesions should be revascularized.[2,6,30,31]

ST-ELEVATION MYOCARDIAL INFARCTION: WHEN IS CORONARY ARTERY BYPASS GRAFTING NEEDED?

Emergent or urgent CABG (<1%) is rarely needed in patients who present with STEMI. CABG should be considered in patients with suitable anatomy for CABG if: (1) PCI cannot be performed or is unsuccessful, and there is persistent ischemia and/or hemodynamic instability; (2) for surgical repair of a postinfarction mechanical complication; or (3) for a life-threatening ventricular arrhythmia caused by ischemia and left main stenosis (>50%) or three-vessel CAD.[2] CABG should not be performed for persistent angina and a small area of viable myocardium in hemodynamically stable patients or PCI complicated by no-reflow.[2] In stable patients with coronary anatomy that is unsuitable for PCI and a patent infarct-related artery (i.e., TIMI 3 flow), CABG may also be considered if a large area of myocardium is at risk and the nonculprit lesions are complex.[2,6]

PERCUTANEOUS HEMODYNAMIC SUPPORT

Percutaneous hemodynamic assist devices provide superior circulatory support compared with pharmacotherapy.[38] Benefits include (1) maintenance of organ perfusion, (2) prevention of systemic shock, (3) reduction of intracardiac filling pressures to relieve pulmonary congestion, and (4) reduced left ventricular end-diastolic volumes and improved myocardial perfusion. Despite these hemodynamic advantages, a reduction in cardiovascular events has not been demonstrated with these devices.[2] The available devices, their indications, and complications are discussed in Chapter 21. In STEMI with cardiogenic shock refractory to medical therapy, mechanical circulatory support should be initiated before PCI, despite the delay in door-to-device time. Mechanical circulatory support may also be considered in selected patients undergoing higher-risk PCI to prevent hemodynamic compromise during PCI, including LMCA disease, severe multivessel CAD, or a last remaining conduit with an ejection fraction of less than 35% undergoing challenging or prolonged PCI.[2]

CORONARY COMPLICATIONS AND MANAGEMENT

No-Reflow

No-reflow is a known complication of PCI and is defined as reduced coronary blood flow or perfusion despite reestablishing epicardial patency. In acute MI, the incidence of no-reflow is 2% to 3% and occurs more frequently in older patients, STEMI, delayed presentation from symptom onset, cardiogenic shock, longer lesion length, complex lesions (type C), bifurcation lesions, or TIMI less than grade 3 flow before revascularization. No-reflow is associated with ongoing chest discomfort, lack of ST-segment resolution, and a significantly higher risk of in-hospital mortality. It can also occur during PCI of SVG lesions or the use of rotational or orbital atherectomy. The mechanisms responsible for no-reflow are multifactorial and include ischemia-reperfusion injury, microcirculatory injury and dysfunction, and distal embolization (see Chapter 20). Despite inconclusive results on the clinical efficacy of thrombus aspiration during primary PCI, aspiration thrombectomy reduces the risk of no-reflow and may be useful in selected STEMI patients with a large thrombus burden. A number of pharmacologic agents have been studied for the prevention or treatment of no-reflow, including adenosine, calcium channel blockers (e.g., verapamil), epinephrine, GPIs, nitroglycerin, nitroprusside, and thrombolytics. Evidence favoring a definitive pharmacologic agent or regimen for the prevention or treatment of no-reflow is lacking. When no-reflow occurs, a reasonable approach would be to use adenosine, nitroprusside, or verapamil. GPIs and manual aspiration thrombectomy can be used if no-reflow occurs in the setting of a large residual thrombus burden.[2,6]

Coronary Perforation

During PCI, coronary perforation occurs in 0.2% to 0.6% of patients and is higher in patients with complex lesions or with the use of rotational or orbital atherectomy. Most coronary perforations are self-limited, can be classified according to the Ellis criteria (Table 11.5) and are managed based on severity. Immediate recognition of any coronary perforation and prompt balloon occlusion proximal to the area of contrast extravasation in the perforated vessel is essential. Prolonged balloon inflations are typically required (>10 minutes), which should stop blood flow into the pericardium. During this time, patients can be stabilized hemodynamically. Transthoracic echocardiography should be performed to assess if pericardial effusion is present, its size, and for evidence of echocardiographic features of cardiac tamponade. The decision to perform emergent pericardiocentesis should be dictated by the patient's hemodynamics. If available, a perfusion balloon catheter can be used to provide distal blood flow beyond the site of balloon occlusion to perfuse the myocardium during prolonged balloon inflations. Subsequent management will depend on its severity, location, and response to balloon occlusion. Small perforations may be completely sealed with balloon inflation alone. Distal coronary perforation from coronary guidewires can be managed with balloon occlusion or microcatheter aspiration to collapse the distal vessel. If bleeding persists, then embolization can be considered with the use of coils, vascular plugs, thrombus, subcutaneous fat, or fibrin glue. One caveat to distal embolization is that it typically results in an occluded vessel at the site of embolization. If bleeding persists despite prolonged balloon occlusion, a covered stent (e.g., PK Papyrus, Biotronik Inc, Lake Oswego, Oregon) can be placed. Type III coronary perforations usually result in cardiac tamponade, and a covered stent should be implanted for this type of perforation. Reversal of intraprocedural anticoagulation should be avoided in patients undergoing covered stenting due to the risk of stent thrombosis when anticoagulation is fully reversed. In certain patients (e.g., previous CABG surgery), a hemorrhagic effusion may be focal and can self-tamponade the perforation. Emergency cardiac surgery should be

TABLE 11.5 Ellis Classification of Coronary Perforations

PERFORATION TYPE (%)	DESCRIPTION	DEATH	MI	TAMPONADE	EMERGENCY CARDIAC SURGERY
Type I (21%)	Extraluminal crater without myocardial blush, extravasation, or evidence of dissection	0%	0%	8%	15%
Type II (50%)	Myocardial or pericardial blush without extravasation	0%	14%	13%	10%
Type III (29%)	Extravasation through a >1-mm perforation or cavity spilling	19%	50%	63%	66%

MI, Myocardial infarction.
From Ellis SG, et al. Increased coronary perforation in the new device era. Incidence, classification, management, and outcome. *Circulation*. 1994;90:2725.

considered for persistent bleeding and/or hemodynamic compromise despite pericardiocentesis.

Stent Thrombosis: Intraprocedural and Acute

The Academic Research Consortium-2 reclassified the definition of stent thrombosis into definite, probable, or silent.[39] Timing of stent thrombosis is defined as intraprocedural (before completion of PCI), acute (<24 hours), subacute (24 hours to 30 days), late (>30 days to 1 year), or very late (>1 year). The incidence of stent thrombosis in the first year is approximately 1%, with most occurring within the first 30 days. In acute MI, the risk for stent thrombosis increases incrementally in patients undergoing PCI in the setting of NSTEMI and STEMI. Clinical predictors associated with stent thrombosis include clinical, anatomic, and procedural factors (Table 11.6), with discontinuation of DAPT being a major contributing factor for stent thrombosis.

Development of intraprocedural stent thrombosis (i.e., new or increasing thrombus in or near a recently deployed stent before the end of PCI) is a major concern and risk for serious adverse clinical events. Acute MI, large thrombus burden, no-reflow, and bifurcation lesions increase the risk for intraprocedural stent thrombosis. Most cases of intraprocedural stent thrombosis occur in patients undergoing PCI for acute MI. If intraprocedural or acute stent thrombosis occurs, acute occlusion of the stented vessel occurs and should be managed accordingly. If intraprocedural stent thrombosis occurs, it is important to measure the ACT to determine if subtherapeutic anticoagulation may have contributed to the event. Aspiration thrombectomy is usually required with acute stent thrombosis. Intravascular imaging (IVUS or OCT) is key to determining if a mechanical issue led to stent thrombosis (e.g., flow-limiting edge dissection), which will determine the best treatment strategy. Additional pharmacotherapy including GPIs may be useful. If stent thrombosis occurs on clopidogrel, and compliance has been verified, switching to a more potent ADP $P2Y_{12}$ inhibitor is recommended. One important consideration in preventing stent thrombosis in patients who present with MI complicated by cardiogenic shock is the potential for poor gastrointestinal absorption of oral medications. In these cases, it may be necessary to give a prolonged infusion of a GPI or cangrelor to ensure adequate platelet inhibition until oral intake of medications is adequate.

TABLE 11.6 Predictors Associated with Stent Thrombosis

Clinical Variables
• Acute MI (STEMI >> NSTEMI) • Clopidogrel noncompliance or discontinuation • Decreased clopidogrel bioavailability • Diabetes mellitus • Kidney failure • Heart failure, especially left ventricular dysfunction • Previous brachytherapy • Malignancy • Cocaine use
Anatomic Variables
• Long lesions • Smaller vessels • Multivessel disease • Bifurcation lesions
Procedural Factors
• Side branch stenting • Stent under expansion • Incomplete wall apposition (for late or very late stent thrombosis) • Residual inflow and outflow disease • Persistent dissection • Crush technique • Overlapping stent • Residual thrombus • Subtherapeutic anticoagulation during PCI • Post-PCI TIMI flow <3 • No aspirin before PCI

MI, Myocardial infarction; *NSTEMI*, non–ST-elevation myocardial infarction; *PCI*, percutaneous coronary intervention; *STEMI*, ST-elevation myocardial infarction; *TIMI*, Thrombolysis in Myocardial Infarction.
From Mauri L, Bhatt DL. Percutaneous coronary intervention. In: Mann DL, Zipes DP, Libby P, Bonow RO, eds. *Braunwald's Heart Disease: A Textbook of Cardiovascular Medicine*. 10th ed. Philadelphia, PA: Saunders; 2015: 1258.

Optimal Duration of Dual Antiplatelet Therapy After Percutaneous Coronary Intervention: Prevention of Stent Thrombosis

Current guidelines recommend that DAPT should be continued for 12 months following PCI in the setting of acute MI.[2,3,6] A shorter duration of DAPT (1–3 months) with continuation of an ADP $P2Y_{12}$ inhibitor monotherapy may be considered for selected patients, especially in patients with a higher risk of bleeding.[2,6] Second-generation DESs have lower rates of stent thrombosis than first-generation DESs.[40] Considerations that guide the duration of DAPT in patients with acute MI, including those treated with PCI, are detailed in Chapter 26. A careful discussion of the risks, benefits, and alternative therapies when considering DAPT duration in candidates for PCI is essential.

PRACTICAL HOSPITAL FOLLOW-UP AFTER PRIMARY PERCUTANEOUS CORONARY INTERVENTION

Assessment the Day After Percutaneous Coronary Intervention

Following PCI after MI, the site(s) of vascular access should be closely examined for complications. Patients should be encouraged to ambulate early in the hospital to assess for symptom recurrence and for any femoral vascular access complications that can be exacerbated with ambulation. For radial access, the presence of finger discomfort, discoloration, reduced temperature, weakness, or sensory deficit should prompt immediate evaluation with a vascular ultrasound to assess for radial artery occlusion.[41] Patients undergoing radial PCI can resume full activities of daily living the following day and activities with aggressive wrist use in several days.[41] Assessment of the patient's vitals, ECG, rhythm monitoring, and clinical signs/symptoms of heart failure is essential. In STEMI, it is also important to screen (exam and echocardiography) for post-MI complications (e.g., left ventricular thrombus in a large anterior wall MI or ischemic mitral regurgitation). Cardiac magnetic resonance imaging may be considered if echocardiography images are suboptimal.[6] Importantly, a review of the current medications is vital, especially a discussion of use and adverse effects of the antiplatelet medications used for prevention of stent thrombosis. In addition, it is important to have a discussion on what to expect after discharge, with plans for an initial follow-up visit (see Chapter 29).

Biomarker Assessment

Routine assessment of cardiac biomarkers following revascularization is not recommended after PCI. Most patients will have elevated cardiac biomarkers at the time of PCI in acute MI. The clinical utility of routinely measuring cardiac biomarkers following successful revascularization in PCI is minimal and should only be used for patients with recurrent symptoms before discharge. It is difficult to assess for reinfarction using cardiac biomarkers in the acute infarct period after PCI, especially with cardiac troponins, which can remain elevated for 14 days after an acute MI (see Chapter 19).

Management of Recurrent Chest Discomfort

Chest discomfort following PCI is not uncommon (up to 40% of patients). The cause can range from noncardiac to life-threatening (e.g., stent thrombosis). Initial assessment should include an electrocardiogram (ECG) and cardiac biomarkers, and evaluation of use of anti-ischemic medications, predominantly nitroglycerin. The ECG should be assessed carefully for any new or worsening ischemic changes or other causes of chest discomfort in MI (e.g., postinfarction pericarditis). It can be difficult to assess for reinfarction on an ECG in patients with MI, especially STEMI (see Chapter 19). All patients should get an ECG immediately post-PCI, regardless of clinical presentation, which can be useful for comparison in patients with recurrent chest discomfort. If ST-segment elevations are worse or new following PCI, coronary angiography should be performed immediately to rule out stent thrombosis. Despite the frequency of recurrent chest discomfort, most patients will not have any new ECG changes. If chest discomfort is severe and refractory to medical treatment, repeat coronary angiography is also warranted. In patients with recurrent chest discomfort, it is important to review the PCI films, which may reveal a missed coronary complication or potential unrevascularized territories that could account for ischemic symptoms. Patients may also develop discomfort from local vascular injury to the stented vessel (i.e., stretch pain), which is typically benign.

Monitoring for Renal Dysfunction

Acute kidney injury (or contrast-induced nephropathy) occurs in approximately 7% of patients following PCI, and 0.3% of these patients will require hemodialysis.[2,6] Importantly, the risk for in-hospital mortality is significantly higher in patients with acute kidney injury.[2,6] STEMI, cardiogenic shock, and severe baseline chronic kidney disease (glomerular filtration rate [GFR] <30 mL/min per 1.73 m^2) are strong independent predictors of acute kidney injury. Renal function does not have to be monitored routinely following PCI but should be followed closely in patients with chronic kidney disease (GFR <60 mL/min per 1.73 m^2) or those who received a large contrast volume (milliliter of contrast/GFR >2). Intravenous hydration with normal saline (1–1.5 mL/kg/hour) for 12 to 24 hours following PCI can be used in patients without an elevated LVEDP and/or with clinical signs/symptoms of heart failure. Use of N-acetylcysteine, sodium bicarbonate infusion, and diuretics do not reduce the risk of contrast-induced nephropathy. The use of intravascular ultrasound can reduce the volume of contrast needed for PCI and should be considered in patients with renal dysfunction undergoing PCI.

When Is It Safe to Discharge Following ST-Elevation Myocardial Infarction Treated with Primary Percutaneous Coronary Intervention?

Historically, the median length of stay in the era of primary PCI as the dominant approach to reperfusion therapy is approximately 3 days for STEMI patients in the United States, which is significantly shorter compared with other countries.[42] The 30-day clinical outcomes following primary PCI in STEMI patients aged older than 65 years discharged 48 hours following primary PCI have similar rates of mortality and major adverse cardiac events compared with hospital lengths of stay of 4 to 5 days.[2] A prospective observational study evaluated the safety and feasibility of early hospital discharge (<48 hours) in low-risk STEMI patients following successful primary PCI.[43] The study revealed that patients who met the eligibility criteria for early discharge (i.e., successful PCI with TIMI 3 flow, LVEF >40%, absence of CAD requiring revascularization, ambulatory, adequate social support, and the absence of symptoms, heart failure, or ventricular arrhythmias) could be safely discharged <48 hours (median length of stay was 24.6 hours) with a structured virtual follow-up schedule. Early discharge with structured follow-up visits can be considered for selected low-risk STEMI patients following primary PCI.

SUMMARY

PCI is the principal treatment strategy for STEMI and most type 1 NSTEMI patients. The innovations in vascular access, equipment, stent design, adjunctive diagnostic and therapeutic devices, and intravascular imaging have improved the safety and efficacy of PCI in MI. The pharmacotherapy used during and after PCI continues to evolve to reduce ischemic events and minimize bleeding. As new technologies emerge, PCI will continue to evolve as the treatment of choice for acute MI.

REFERENCES

1. Martin SS, Aday AW, Allen NB, et al. Heart disease and stroke statistics-2025 update: a report from the American Heart Association, *Circulation*. 2025;151:e1–e620.
2. Lawton JS, Tamis-Holland JE, Bangalore S, et al. 2021 ACC/AHA/SCAI guideline for coronary artery revascularization: executive summary: a report of the American College of Cardiology/American Heart Association joint committee on clinical practice guidelines. *J Am Coll Cardiol*. 2022;79:197–215.
3. Bhatt DL, Sandhu A, Parikh MA. Diagnosis and treatment of acute coronary syndromes: a review. *JAMA*. 2022;327:662–675.
4. Collet JP, Thiele H, Barbato E, et al. 2020 ESC guidelines for the management of acute coronary syndromes in patients presenting without persistent ST-segment elevation. *Eur Heart J*. 2021;42:1289–1367.
5. Gulati M, Levy PD, Mukherjee D, et al. 2021 AHA/ACC/ASE/CHEST/SAEM/SCCT/SCMR guideline for the evaluation and diagnosis of chest pain: a report of the American College of Cardiology/American Heart Association joint committee on clinical practice guidelines. *J Am Coll Cardiol*. 2021;78:e187–e285.
6. Byrne RA, Rossello X, Coughlan JJ, et al. 2023 ESC guidelines for the management of acute coronary syndromes. *Eur Heart J*. 2023;44(38):3720–3826.
7. Foo CY, Bonsu KO, Nallamothu BK, et al. Coronary intervention door-to-balloon time and outcomes in ST-elevation myocardial infarction: a meta-analysis. *Heart*. 2018;104:1362–1369.
8. Kite TA, Kurmani SA, Bountziouka V, et al. Timing of invasive strategy in non-ST-elevation acute coronary syndrome: a meta-analysis of randomized controlled trials. *Eur Heart J*. 2022;43:3148–3161.
9. Shroff AR, Gulati R, Drachman DE, et al. SCAI expert consensus statement update on best practices for transradial angiography and intervention. *Catheter Cardiovasc Interv*. 2020;95:245–252.
10. Doll JA, Rao SV, Cohen MG, et al. Trends in arterial access site selection and bleeding outcomes following coronary procedures, 2011–2018. *Circ Cardiovasc Qual Outcomes*. 2022;15:e008359.
11. Watanabe H, Domei T, Morimoto T, et al. Effect of 1-month dual antiplatelet therapy followed by clopidogrel vs 12-month dual antiplatelet therapy on cardiovascular and bleeding events in patients receiving PCI: the STOPDAPT-2 randomized clinical trial. *JAMA*. 2019;321:2414–2427.
12. Maqsood MH, Ahmad F, Awad H, et al. Optimal hemostatic band duration after transradial angiography or intervention: insights from a mixed treatment comparison meta-analysis of randomized trials. *Circ Cardiovasc Interv*. 2023;16:e012781.
13. De Luca L, Pavasini R, Biscaglia S, et al. Cangrelor: clinical data, contemporary use, and future perspectives. *J Am Heart Assoc*. 2021;10:e022125.
14. Angiolillo DJ, Bhatt DL, Cannon CP, et al. Antithrombotic therapy in patients with atrial fibrillation treated with oral anticoagulation undergoing percutaneous coronary intervention: a North American perspective: 2021 update. *Circulation*. 2021;143:583–596.
15. Lopes RD, Heizer G, Aronson R, et al. AUGUSTUS investigators Antithrombotic therapy after acute coronary syndrome or PCI in atrial fibrillation. *N Engl J Med*. 2019;380:1509–1524.
16. Vranckx P, Valgimigli M, Eckardt L, et al. Edoxaban-based versus vitamin K antagonist-based antithrombotic regimen after successful coronary stenting in patients with atrial fibrillation (ENTRUST-AF PCI): a randomised, open-label, phase 3b trial. *Lancet*. 2019;394:1335–1343.
17. Mehran R, Baber U, Sharma SK, et al. Ticagrelor with or without aspirin in high-risk patients after PCI. *N Engl J Med*. 2019;381:2032–2042.
18. Hahn JY, Song YB, Oh JH, et al. Effect of P2Y12 inhibitor monotherapy vs dual antiplatelet therapy on cardiovascular events in patients undergoing percutaneous coronary intervention: the SMART CHOICE randomized clinical trial. *JAMA*. 2019;321:2428–2437.
19. Kim BK, Hong SJ, Cho YH, et al. Effect of ticagrelor monotherapy vs ticagrelor with aspirin on major bleeding and cardiovascular events in patients with acute coronary syndrome: the TICO randomized clinical trial. *JAMA*. 2020;323:2407–2416.
20. Vranckx P, Valgimigli M, Jüni P, et al. Ticagrelor plus aspirin for 1 month, followed by ticagrelor monotherapy for 23 months vs aspirin plus clopidogrel or ticagrelor for 12 months, followed by aspirin monotherapy for 12 months after implantation of a drug eluting stent: a multicentre, open-label, randomized superiority trial. *Lancet*. 2018;392:940m–949m.
21. Lee YJ, Han YL, Kim HS, et al. Impact of one-month DAPT followed by aspirin monotherapy in patients undergoing percutaneous coronary intervention according to clinical presentation: a post hoc analysis of the randomised one-month DAPT trial. *EuroIntervention*. 2022;18:471–481.
22. Ploumen EH, von Birgelen C, Kok MM, et al. Final 5-year report of the randomized BIO-RESORT trial comparing 3 contemporary drug-eluting stents in all-comers. *J Am Heart Assoc*. 2022;11:e026041.
23. Neumann FJ, Sousa-Uva M, Ahlsson A, et al. 2018 ESC/EACTS guidelines on myocardial revascularization. *Eur Heart J*. 2019;40:87–165.
24. Jeger RV, Eccleshall S, Wan Ahmad WA, et al. Drug-coated balloons for coronary artery disease: third report of the international DCB consensus group. *JACC Cardiovasc Interv*. 2020;13:1391–1402.
25. Sánchez JS, Nozari Y, Abdollahi P, et al. Drug-coated balloons vs drug-eluting stents for the treatment of small coronary artery disease: a meta-analysis of randomized trials. *Catheter Cardiovasc Interv*. 2021;98:66–75.
26. Abbott JD, Benedetto D, Bhatt DL. Drug-coated balloons in small vessels: preferred strategy to drug-eluting stents? *J Am Coll Cardiol Intv*. 2023;16(9):1062–1064..
27. Gao XF, Zhang YJ, Tian NL, et al. 3-year outcomes of the ULTIMATE trial comparing intravascular ultrasound versus angiography-guided drug-eluting stent implantation. *JACC Cardiovasc Interv*. 2021;14:247–257.
28. Hong SJ, Mintz GS, Ahn CM, et al. Improved 3-year cardiac survival after IVUS-guided long DES implantation: a patient-level analysis from 2 randomized trials. *JACC Cardiovasc Interv*. 2022;15:208–216.
29. Kinnaird T, Johnson T, Anderson R, et al. Intravascular imaging and 12-month mortality after unprotected left main stem PCI: an analysis from the British cardiovascular intervention society database. *JACC Cardiovasc Interv*. 2020;13:346–357.
30. Bhatt DL. Fractional flow reserve measurement for the physiological assessment of coronary artery stenosis severity. *JAMA*. 2018;320:1275–1276.
31. Lotfi A, Davies JE, Fearon WF, Grines CL, Kern MJ, Klein LW. Focused update of expert consensus statement: use of invasive assessments of coronary physiology and structure: a position statement of the society of cardiac angiography and interventions. *Catheter Cardiovasc Interv*. 2018;92:336–347.
32. Pruthi S, Bangalore S. The state of coronary thrombus aspiration. *J Am Heart Assoc*. 2022;11:e026849.
33. Albiero R, Burzotta F, Caiazzo G, et al. Treatment of coronary bifurcation lesions, part I: implanting the first stent in the provisional pathway. The 16th expert consensus document of the European bifurcation Club. *EuroIntervention*. 2022;18:e362–e376.
34. Hildick-Smith D, Egred M, Banning A, et al. The European bifurcation club left main coronary stent study: a randomized comparison of stepwise provisional vs. systematic dual stenting strategies (EBC MAIN). *Eur Heart J*. 2021;42:3829–3839.
35. Kereiakes DJ, Hill JM, Ben-Yehuda O, et al. Intravascular lithotripsy for treatment of calcified coronary lesions: patient-level pooled analysis of the disrupt CAD studies. *JACC Cardiovasc Interv*. 2021;14:1337–1348.
36. Mehta SR, Wood DA, Storey RF, et al. Complete revascularization with multivessel PCI for myocardial infarction. *N Engl J Med*. 2019;381:1411–1421.
37. Thiele H, Akin I, Sandri M, et al. One-year outcomes after PCI strategies in cardiogenic shock. *N Engl J Med*. 2018;379:1699–1710.
38. Jentzer JC, Rao SV, Baran DA, et al. Mechanical circulatory devices in acute myocardial infarction-cardiogenic shock: current studies and future directions. *J Soc Cardiovasc Angiogr Interv*. 2023;2:100586.
39. Garcia-Garcia HM, McFadden EP, Farb A, et al. Standardized end point definitions for coronary intervention trials: the academic research consortium-2 consensus document. *Circulation*. 2018;137:2635–2650.
40. Kuramitsu S, Sonoda S, Ando K, et al. Risk factors and long-term clinical outcomes of second-generation drug-eluting stent thrombosis. *Circ Cardiovasc Interv*. 2019;12:e007822.
41. Mason PJ, Shah B, Tamis-Holland JE, et al. An update on radial artery access and best practices for transradial coronary angiography and intervention in acute coronary syndrome: a scientific statement from the American Heart Association. *Circ Cardiovasc Interv*. 2018;11:e000035.
42. Rashidi A, Whitehead L, Newson R, et al. Factors affecting hospital readmission rates following an acute coronary syndrome: a systematic review. *J Clin Nurs*. 2021;31:2377–2397.
43. Rathod KS, Koganti S, Jain AK, et al. Early hospital discharge following PCI for patients with STEMI. *J Am Coll Cardiol*. 2021;78:2550–2560.

12 Acute Coronary Syndrome: Selection of Initial Anticoagulant Therapy

JOHANNE SILVAIN, MICHEL ZEITOUNI, AND GILLES MONTALESCOT

INTRODUCTION

Acute coronary syndrome (ACS) includes patients presenting with ST-segment elevation myocardial infarction (STEMI) and those without ST-segment elevation (NSTEMI) and although they share a common physiopathology and principles of treatment (Chapter 13), the approaches to management of anticoagulant therapy for these conditions differ by myocardial infarction (MI) type and overall management strategy (invasive vs. conservative).

Rationale for Anticoagulant Therapy in Acute Coronary Syndrome

The rationale for administering anticoagulant therapy acutely in STEMI patients is strong and includes the following treatment goals:[1,2]

- Establishing and maintaining patency of the infarct-related artery whatever the reperfusion strategy used (fibrinolysis, primary angioplasty, or no reperfusion therapy)
- Prevention of ventricular thrombus formation and embolization (stroke and noncerebral circulation)
- Prevention of complications related to PCI, such as catheter thrombosis, distal embolization of fragmented thrombus, slow or no flow post-PCI, abrupt vessel closure, acute stent thrombosis, and ischemic stroke.

Other objectives are common to acute medical conditions and bed rest such as prevention of deep venous thrombosis and possible subsequent pulmonary embolism.

In NSTEMI, the objectives are similar, although the artery is rarely fully occluded[1]:

1. Maintaining patency of the infarct-related artery whatever strategy is decided by the treating physician (invasive strategy or medical therapy)
2. Prevention of PCI-related complications
3. Prevention of complications of bed rest

Containing Thrombus Formation and Propagation

During the acute phase of MI, most myocytes loss in the infarct zone occurs via coagulation necrosis and proceeds to inflammation, phagocytosis of necrotic myocytes, and repair eventuating in scar formation (Chapter 30). Successful and durable myocardial reperfusion is therefore the final goal of the initial antithrombotic therapy, including anticoagulation and antiplatelet therapy (Chapter 19). After the initial disruption or rupture of vulnerable plaque (Chapter 3), the common pathophysiological substrate of ACS, the damaged endothelium, and the exposition of the lipid core leads to platelet adhesion and aggregation followed almost instantly by activation of the coagulation cascade and formation of an initial platelet-rich thrombus (Fig. 12.1A).

A key step in this process is the activation of prothrombin to thrombin (Factor IIa), which will transform the circulating fibrinogen into fibrin fibers, forming the scaffold of the coronary thrombus and leading to its stabilization (Figs. 12.1B and 12.1C). The evolution of the thrombus may culminate in resolution with asymptomatic healing, a subtotal coronary artery occlusion leading to an NSTEMI, or to fully occlusive thrombus presenting as a STEMI. As a result, an initial anticoagulation therapy is indicated in all patients with MI, in the absence of contraindications. The class of anticoagulant and dose regimen will depend on the type of MI and whether the anticoagulant is to be used as adjunct to PCI, or fibrinolysis.

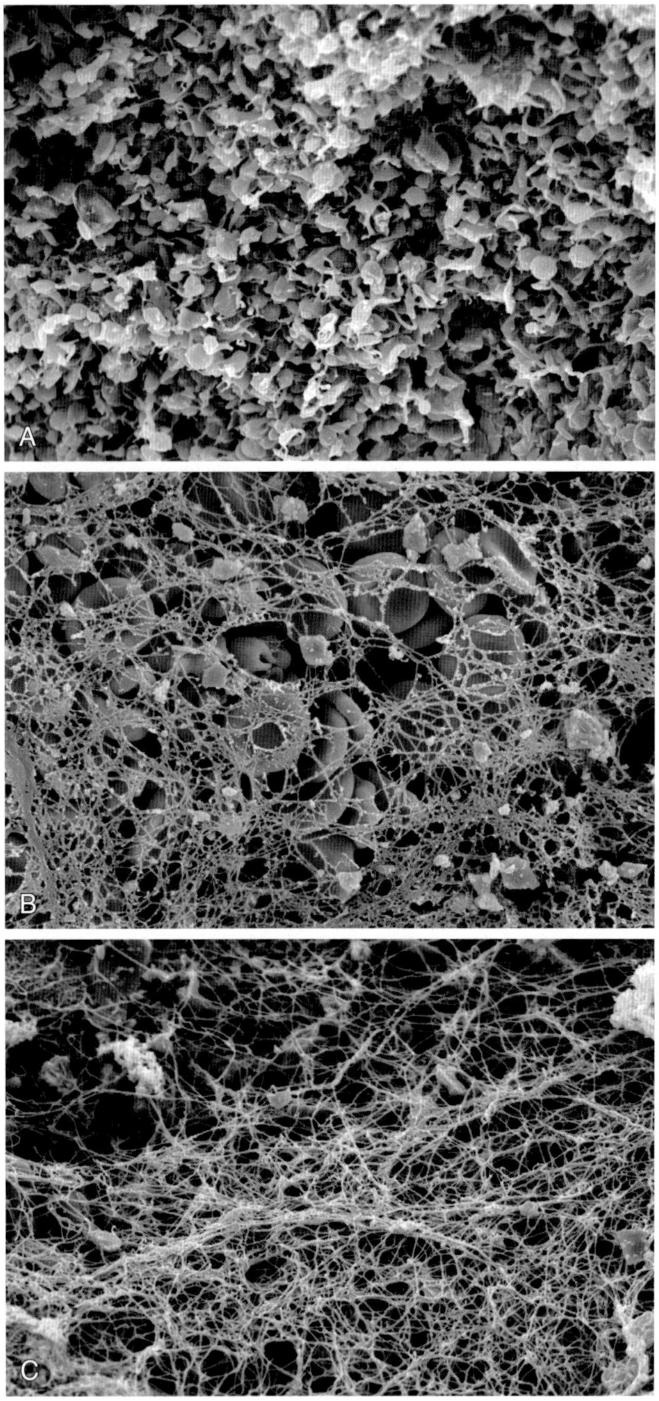

FIG. 12.1 (A) Platelet-rich thrombus. (B) Stabilization of thrombus with fibrin fibers. (C) Fibrin-rich thrombus. *(From Silvain J et al, classic references.)*

Although treatment with unfractionated heparin (UFH), as the prototypical parenteral anticoagulant, has a strong pathobiological rationale and has become entrenched in the clinical management of MI, the evidence from clinical studies directly demonstrating the efficacy of UFH in MI is modest. However, the rationale for the use of anticoagulants in MI has been bolstered by subsequent trials of newer anticoagulants, such as the low-molecular weight heparins (LMWHs), for example, enoxaparin, and the synthetics drugs such as the indirect Factor Xa inhibitor fondaparinux and bivalirudin, a direct thrombin inhibitor.

OVERVIEW OF AVAILABLE ANTICOAGULANT DRUGS

While adjuvant anticoagulant therapy may result in a small improvement in the initial restoration of flow in the thrombotic coronary artery, its main roles are maintaining patency after successful reperfusion, preventing reocclusion, and reducing the risk of thrombotic complications of PCI. The options for initial anticoagulant therapy include four main drugs: UFH and LMWHs, such as enoxaparin, fondaparinux, and bivalirudin. UFH and enoxaparin are the most frequently used anticoagulants worldwide. They are both biological products, derived from mucosal tissues, such as porcine bovine intestines. Inherent drawbacks led to the development of synthetic anticoagulants such as fondaparinux and bivalirudin. The mechanism of action of each of these four agents is illustrated in Fig. 12.2 and compared in Table 12.1.

Unfractionated Heparin

UFH was the first anticoagulant used in the treatment of MI. UFH is a heterogeneous mixture of mucopolysaccharides, with a molecular weight ranging from 2000 to 30,000 (mostly 15,000–18,000) Da that bind and activate the antithrombin, greatly increasing the inhibitory effects of antithrombin on thrombin. Activated antithrombin inhibits several coagulation factors, including factor Xa, resulting in an anticoagulant effect. Because its actions are via binding to antithrombin, UFH is classified as an indirect thrombin inhibitor (Fig. 12.2). Because UFH is poorly absorbed when injected via the SC route, IV administration is the preferred route of administration.

A major drawback of UFH is the significant variability of its therapeutic response. The heterogeneous composition and variable elimination of UFH through the endoplasmic reticulum result in a marked interpatient variability of therapeutic response and necessitate close monitoring of anticoagulant intensity with the activated clotting time (ACT) or with the activated partial thromboplastin time (aPTT). UFH can also cause immunologically mediated thrombocytopenia also known as heparin-induced thrombocytopenia (HIT) which is rare (2%–3% of patients) but potentially life threatening. Other drawbacks of UFH include an increase in platelet activation and aggregation, a dependency on binding antithrombin-III for inhibition of thrombin activity, a sensitivity to platelet factor 4 (PF4), an inability to inhibit clot-bound thrombin, and the need for frequent monitoring.

Even with standardized weight-based dosing nomograms, less than a third of initial aPTT measurements are within the therapeutic range. The anticoagulant effect of UFH is lost rapidly, within a few hours after interruption. During the first 24 hours after UFH cessation, there is a risk of reactivation of the coagulation process and thereby a transiently increased risk of recurrent ischemic events despite adjunctive aspirin treatment. A desire to overcome the disadvantages of UFH has stimulated interest in the development of alternative anticoagulants within the past decades.

Historically high doses of UFH were used in fibrinolysis or PCI to overcome thrombotic complications, however, studies have shown that these higher doses were only

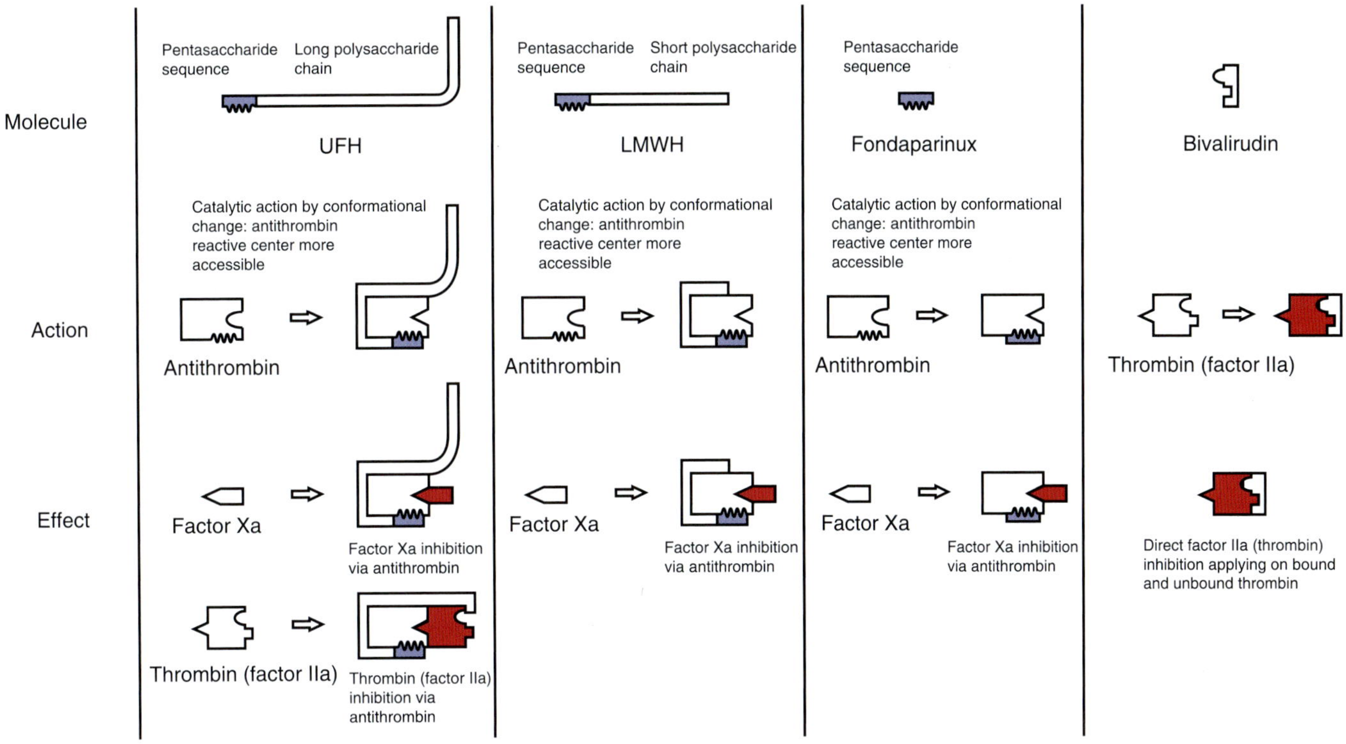

FIG. 12.2 Action of available anticoagulant.

TABLE 12.1 Pharmacologic Properties of Parenteral Anticoagulants

MEDICATION	UNFRACTIONATED HEPARIN	ENOXAPARIN	FONDAPARINUX	BIVALIRUDIN
Mechanism	AT-III mediated factor Xa and thrombin inhibitor	AT-III mediated factor Xa and thrombin inhibitor	Indirect factor Xa inhibitor	Direct thrombin inhibitor, reversible
Route of administration	IV– SC	IV – SC	IV – SC	IV
Half-life	1–2 h	5–7 h	17–21 h	25 min
Molecular weight	3– 0 kDa	2–8 kDa	1.7 kDa	2.2 kDa
Metabolism	Hepatic	Hepatic	Excreted largely as unchanged drug	Plasma proteases
Elimination	Extra-renal	Renal	Renal	Renal
Onset	Immediate (IV)	- Immediate (IV) - 3–5 h (SC)	2–3 h (SC)	Immediate
Notes	Inactive on clot associated thrombin	- Inactive on clot associated thrombin - More factor Xa selectivity	Inactive on clot associated thrombin	Inhibits clot-associated thrombin
Incidence of HIT (heparin-induced thrombocytopenia)	0.5 %	<0.1%	negligible	negligible
Antidote	protamine	Andexanet Alfa (full) protamine (partial)	None[a]	None[a]

[a]The options of 4-factor prothrombin concentrates and recombinant factor VIIa to manage bleeding may be used in the case of life-threatening bleeding, taking into account that there is an increased risk of thrombosis with the latter option.

associated with higher rate of bleeding (including intracranial hemorrhage) without impact on ischemic endpoints and that efficacy was preserved at the lower doses. The initial doses of UFH used in PCI (up to 175 UI/kg were gradually lowered to 140 UI/kg, 100 UI/kg, 85 UI/kg, 70 UI/kg, 60 UI/kg, and even 50 UI/kg in the latest trials when glycoprotein (GP) IIb/IIIa receptor inhibitor is used. A similar pattern was shown with the target ACT for the optimal ranging of UFH efficacy suggesting that the therapeutic window for UFH is relatively narrow.

Enoxaparin

LMWHs are a class of heparin-derived compounds with molecular weights ranging from 2000 to 8000 Da (Table 12.2). By virtue of enhanced binding of LMWH-antithrombin to factor Xa, LMWHs have balanced anti-Xa and anti-IIa activity, with the relative activity against factor Xa versus. IIa depending on the molecular weight of the molecule; the heavier the LMWH is, the greater relative anti-IIa activity it has (Fig. 12.2). Enoxaparin is the most studied and widely used LMWH for the treatment of

TABLE 12.2 Comparison of Low-Molecular Weight Heparin Preparations[a]

GENERIC NAME (TRADE NAME OR SYNONYM)	MEAN MOLECULAR WEIGHT	ANTI-XA: ANTI-IIA RATIO	FDA INDICATION FOR ACS
Enoxaparin (Lovenox, Clexane)	4200	3.8	Yes
Nadroparin (Fraxiparine, Sleparina)	4500	3.6	Yes
Reviparin (Clivaparine)	4000	3.5	No
Dalteparin (Fragmin)	6000	2.7	Yes
Parnaparin (Fluxum, Minidalton)	4500–5000	2.4	No
Ardeparin (Normiflo)	6000	1.9	No
Tinzaparin (Innohep, Logiparin)	4500	1.9	No
Certoparin (Alphaparin, Sandoparin, Embolex)	4200–6200		n/a

[a]In descending order of relative anti-Xa:anti-IIa activity.
FDA, Food and drug administration.

ACS. LMWHs are approximately one-third of the molecular weight of UFH, conferring greater bioavailability that enables administration via the subcutaneous (SC) route. Other advantages of enoxaparin include a stable and reliable anticoagulant effect without any need for monitoring, provided that weight-based dosing is used, and renal failure is absent.

Once bound to antithrombin, enoxaparin provides a greater specificity for factor Xa when compared with UFH, producing enhanced blockade of the coagulation cascade upstream of thrombin generation. The ratio of inhibition of factor Xa/IIa varies between agents and is 3 to 1 for enoxaparin. HIT is 20 times less common with enoxaparin than with UFH but can still occur. On top of these anticoagulant actions, enoxaparin may have some anti-inflammatory properties and does not activate platelets.

The main drawback of enoxaparin is its renal elimination, which, in the presence of renal dysfunction, can result in accumulation over time with repeated injections (>3 injections). Furthermore, in case of active bleeding, protamine enables only a partial reversibility of enoxaparin. Similarly, to UFH, enoxaparin was used at high doses in the first phase 2 trials such as *The Thrombolysis in Myocardial Infarction* 11A trial, which demonstrated that doses higher than 1.0 mg/kg should not be used due to excess bleeding.

Fondaparinux

Fondaparinux is a synthetic pentasaccharide that was developed to have a chemical structure similar to the antithrombin binding active site domain of UFH (Fig. 12.2). This highly selective drug induces a conformational change leading to a potent inhibition of factor Xa reducing thrombin generation. Unlike UFH and LMWH, fondaparinux has no inhibitory effect on thrombin (Factor IIa) itself. Fondaparinux inhibits factor Xa indirectly, by binding reversibly, noncovalently, and with high affinity to antithrombin. Like LMWH, but in a more selective manner, it targets this upstream step in the coagulation cascade of thrombin generation (Fig. 12.3).

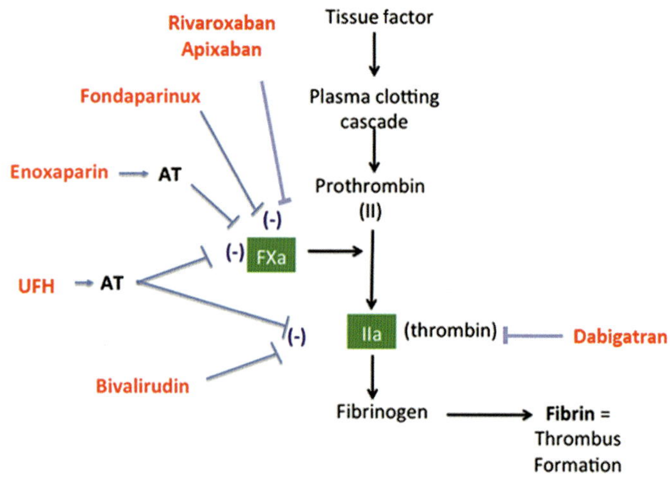

FIG. 12.3 Anticoagulation targets.

Advantages of fondaparinux include 100% bioavailability after SC injection and a long half-life of 15–17 hours, allowing for once daily administration. Fondaparinux is eliminated mainly by the kidneys and is contraindicated if CrCl is <30 mL/min. It has a predictable anticoagulant effect with no requirement for monitoring, and no cross-reactivity with antibodies associated with HIT. Fondaparinux is insensitive to inactivation by platelet-released heparin neutralization proteins. Therefore, monitoring the platelet count is unnecessary, as is monitoring of anti-Xa activity. Phase 2 trials evaluated different doses of intravenous fondaparinux (2.5 and 5.0 mg) as compared to UFH, and the lower dose of 2.5 mg was selected because of its more favorable safety profile.

Bivalirudin

Bivalirudin and hirudin are synthetic drugs with the ability of being direct thrombin (IIa) inhibitors (DTI). Several DTIs have been tested over time, but only bivalirudin reached clinical use in PCI and ACS settings. Unlike UFH, bivalirudin inactivates both fluid-phase thrombin and clot-bound thrombin, with less activation of platelets. As it does not bind to plasma proteins, the anticoagulant effect of bivalirudin is more predictable. Bivalirudin is eliminated by the kidney. The effect of bivalirudin can be followed with routine coagulation tests (aPTT and ACT).

Initial phase 2 studies tested different regimens of the drug starting with low bolus doses of 0.5 mg/kg and 0.75 mg/kg that were considered not sufficient for PCI and the first large trial used a higher dose (bolus dose of 1.0 mg/kg followed by a 4-hour infusion of 2.5 mg/kg/h and a 14- to 20-hour infusion of 0.2 mg/kg/h) as compared to high doses of UFH (175 UI/kg) in PCI. Subsequently, both the bolus and the infusion doses were lowered (0.75-mg/kg bolus plus 1.75 mg/kg/h for the duration of PCI) with uncertainty about the optimal duration of infusion after the PCI.

Future Parenteral Anticoagulants

Factor XI inhibitors are the next potential generation of anticoagulant, and several agents have been developed to inhibit factor XI at different stages including antisense oligonucleotides, monoclonal antibodies, small synthetic molecules, natural peptides, and aptamers, with promising preliminary data bringing new evidence that the intrinsic pathway is essential in the process of thrombus formation. Several agents are undergoing phase 3 clinical trials with the hope that they may be as efficient and safer than actual parenteral anticoagulants in ACS.

Monitoring of Available Anticoagulant Therapy

Biological bedside monitoring of the anticoagulation effect of the various available drugs is not mandatory for all and depends essentially on the stability of the anticoagulant hence, their therapeutic window.

Biological monitoring of the anticoagulant effect of the various available drugs is not mandatory for all agents. For UFH, the therapeutic window is narrow thus requiring frequent monitoring of its anticoagulant activity. Two different biomarkers exist: aPTT, which can be obtained in <1 hour, has an optimal target of 50–75 seconds, corresponding to 1.5–2.5 times the upper limit of normal (ULN). Above these values, the risk of bleeding complications is increased, without further antithrombotic benefits; below them, the antithrombotic effect is insufficient. The second biomarker available is ACT which can be used for monitoring of UFH during PCI but has a very narrow therapeutic window and difficulties in reaching its target values (<40% in PCI).

Enoxaparin can reliably be monitored by assessing the anti-Xa activity level in a standard chromogenic laboratory assay. Although data showed that with a standard protocol adjusted for weight and renal function, more than 95% patients are in the therapeutic window; insufficient levels of anti-Xa during PCI of patients with ACS have been linked to an increased risk of death and ischemic events in the peri-procedural period. There is no easy bedside approach to monitoring of enoxaparin. ACT is not discriminant enough for monitoring LMWH therapy. Tests such as the Hemonox bedside test were developed and validated in a cohort of patients[3] but have not been adopted into routine use in practice because the enoxaparin level is within the therapeutic window in 95% of patients.

Fondaparinux has no significant influence on the usual variables that monitor anticoagulant activity, such as aPTT, ACT, prothrombin, and thrombin times and requires an adapted anti-Xa assay that uses an appropriate standard curve.

Bivalirudin plasma concentration correlates well with coagulation tests (aPTT and ACT), which can be used to monitor the anticoagulant activity of bivalirudin in the same manner as UFH. In the *Randomized Evaluation in PCI Linking Angiomax to Reduced Clinical Events (REPLACE)-2 trial*, it was mandated to measure the ACT after the initial bivalirudin bolus with an additional bolus in case of low ACT. However, the pharmacokinetics and pharmacodynamics of bivalirudin are such that low ACTs were only found in 2%–3% of the patients, and it is considered that there is no need to routinely monitor the degree of anticoagulation for short-term use as an adjunct to PCI. In summary, the only anticoagulant which may need to be monitored is UFH. However, meta-analyses have shown that the available bedside test ACT poorly correlates with ischemic or bleeding complications.

Reversal of Anticoagulant Therapy

Protamine sulfate can be used in an equimolar concentration to inhibit UFH and to a lesser degree inhibits the anticoagulant effect of enoxaparin. Protamine has no effect on fondaparinux or bivalirudin. Due to the very short half-life of bivalirudin, waiting until the end of its effect after drug cessation is a potential strategy to reduce bleeding complications. In the case of fondaparinux, presently, there is no available specific antidote. Recombinant factor VIIa has been recommended but is associated with an increased risk of thrombotic complications. Four-factor prothrombin complex concentrates, which are effective for urgent reversal of vitamin K antagonist therapy in major bleeding events, can be used in patients with severe bleeding under enoxaparin, fondaparinux, or bivalirudin, although data on their efficacy is limited.

One important advancement in the past decade has been the development and validation of andexanet alfa for reversing anticoagulation associated with FXa inhibitors, whether oral or parenteral. The phase 3 ANNEXA-4 trial[4] using a bolus of andexanet, followed by a 2-hour infusion efficiently reversed 75% of anti-factor Xa inhibition after 30 in patients treated by enoxaparin with acute major bleeding. All antagonists require close monitoring for signs and symptoms of thromboembolic events and need to have their anticoagulation regimen resume shortly after the resolution of the bleeding event.

INITIAL ANTICOAGULATION THERAPY

STEMI Patients Treated With Primary Percutaneous Intervention

Although extensively studied, anticoagulation during primary PCI remains controversial (see also Chapter 17). Patients undergoing primary PCI should receive a combination of dual antiplatelet therapy (Chapter 19) with a combination of a parenteral anticoagulant. Fondaparinux carries a possible hazard related to catheter thrombosis, is not recommended as an anticoagulant in this setting, and will not be discussed in this section. Three options are used to support primary PCI: UFH, bivalirudin, or enoxaparin, all administered intravenously. Professional society guidelines for anticoagulant therapy in STEMI treated with primary PCI are summarized in Table 12.3.

Unfractionated Heparin During Primary PCI

An intravenous UFH bolus adapted to the concomitant use of a GPIIb/IIIa inhibitor (GPI) and titrated to an appropriate ACT time is a familiar and well-tested strategy for initial anticoagulant therapy at the time of primary PCI for STEMI. UFH has a class I recommendation in both the American College of Cardiology Foundation (ACCF)/American Heart Association (AHA) and European Society of Cardiology (ESC) guidelines but with a level of evidence C due to the absence of placebo-controlled trials evaluating UFH in primary PCI. Dosing should follow standard recommendations for PCI [Initial treatment: i.v. bolus 70–100 U/kg followed by

TABLE 12.3 Initial Anticoagulation Therapy Recommended to Support Primary PCI in STEMI

ANTICOAGULATION THERAPY	ESC[b] COR	ESC[b] LOE	ACC/AHA/SCAI[a]
UFH Initial treatment: i.v. bolus 70–100 U/kg followed by i.v. infusion titrated to achieve an aPTT of 60–80 sec During PCI: 70–100 U/kg i.v. bolus or according to ACT in case of UFH pretreatment	I	C	No specific recommendations
Enoxaparin: 0.5 mg/kg i.v. bolus with or without GP IIb/IIIa inhibitor	IIa	A	
Bivalirudin: During PPCI: 0.75 mg/kg i.v. bolus followed by i.v. infusion of 1.75 mg/kg/h for 4 h after the procedure. In patients whose CrCl is below 30 mL/min, maintenance infusion should be reduced to 1 mg/kg/h.	IIa	A	
Fondaparinux: not recommended as sole anticoagulant for primary PCI	III	B	

[a]Adapted from Lawton JS, Tamis-Holland JE, Bangalore S, et al. 2021. ACC/AHA/SCAI guideline for coronary artery revascularization: executive summary: a report of the American College of Cardiology/American Heart Association joint committee on clinical practice guidelines. *Circulation*. 2022;145(3):e4–e17.
[b]Adapted from Ibanez B, James S, Agewall S, et al. 2017 ESC Guidelines for the management of acute myocardial infarction in patients presenting with ST-segment elevation: The Task Force for the management of acute myocardial infarction in patients presenting with ST-segment elevation of the European Society of Cardiology (ESC) guideline. *Eur Heart J.* 2018;39:119–177. doi:10.1093/eurheartj/ehx393 and Byrne RA, Rossello X, Coughlan JJ, et al. 2023 ESC Guidelines for the management of acute coronary syndromes: Developed by the task force on the management of acute coronary syndromes of the European Society of Cardiology (ESC) guideline. *Eur Heart J.* 2023;44:3720–3826. doi:10.1093/eurheartj/ehad191.

i.v. infusion titrated to achieve an aPTT of 60–80 seconds. During PCI: 70–100 U/kg i.v. bolus or according to ACT in case of UFH pretreatment].[5]

Enoxaparin Versus UFH for Primary PCI

Enoxaparin is not used widely in the US as adjunctive therapy for primary PCI, in contrast with Europe. Nevertheless, intravenous enoxaparin (0.5 mg/kg followed by prophylactic 40 mg SC) has been suggested by several nonrandomized studies and an international, open-label, randomized trial to be more predictable and reliable than UFH in primary PCI: the Acute myocardial infarction Treated with primary angioplasty and intravenous enoxaparin or UFH to Lower ischemic and bleeding events at short- and Long-term follow-up (ATOLL) trial. The primary composite endpoint of 30-day death, complication of MI, procedural failure, and major bleeding was not significantly reduced (relative risk reduction 17%, $P = .063$), but there were reductions in the main secondary endpoint of death, recurrent MI, or ACS or urgent revascularization, and in other secondary composite endpoints such as death or resuscitated cardiac arrest and death or complication of MI. Importantly, bleeding was not increased with enoxaparin versus UFH. In the per-protocol analysis of the ATOLL trial—pertinent to more than 87% of the study population—IV enoxaparin was superior to UFH in reducing the primary endpoint (RR, 0.76; 95% CI, 0.62–0.94; $P = .012$) as well as ischemic endpoints, mortality (RR, 0.36; 95% CI, 0.18–0.74; $P = .003$) and major bleeding (RR, 0.46; 95% CI 0.21–1.01; $P = .050$), contributing to the improvement of the net clinical benefit (RR 0.46; 95% CI, 0.3–0.74; $P = .0002$) in patients undergoing primary PCI.

In a systematic review and meta-analysis of enoxaparin versus UFH in PCI, including nonrandomized studies, post-hoc analysis of randomized trial, and the ATOLL randomized trial, 10,243 patients underwent primary PCI for STEMI with either enoxaparin or UFH (Fig. 12.4).

Study	No. needed to treat	No. of events/No. in group: Enoxaparin	No. of events/No. in group: Unfractionated heparin	Relative risk (95% CI) random	P value	Cochran Q for heterogeneity
All PCIs						
Death	60	278/13,943	622/17,023	0.66 (0.57 to 0.76)	<.001	0.46
Death or MI	50	836/11,924	1351/14,968	0.68 (0.57 to 0.81)	<.001	0.42
Complications of MI	66	765/13,943	1135/17,023	0.75 (0.66 to 0.85)	<.001	0.55
Major bleeding	83	295/13,852	564/16,923	0.80 (0.68 to 0.95)	.009	0.58
Minor bleeding	-	718/13,150	793/13,669	0.92 (0.74 to 1.14)	.45	0.21
Primary PCI for STEMI						
Death	34	112/3590	401/6653	0.52 (0.42 to 0.64)	<.001	0.53
Death or MI	28	139/3590	499/6653	0.56 (0.42 to 0.76)	<.001	0.50
Complications of MI	68	96/3590	275/6653	0.76 (0.60 to 0.96)	.022	0.80
Major bleeding	53	92/3499	298/6553	0.72 (0.56 to 0.93)	.01	0.69
Minor bleeding	-	138/3216	177/4372	0.94 (0.60 to 1.47)	.78	0.56

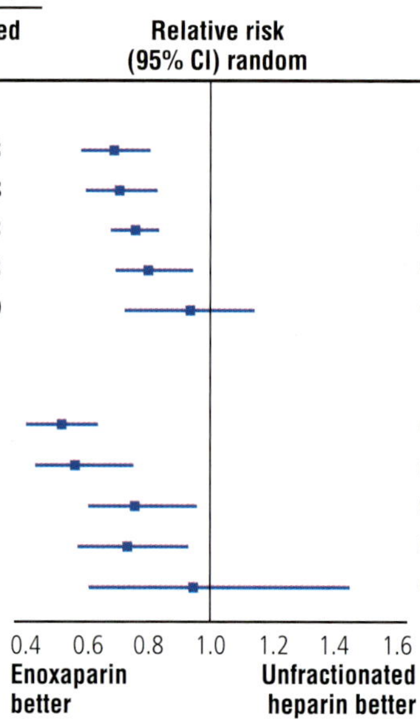

FIG. 12.4 Metanalysis of enoxaparin vs. UFH in PCI in all settings and in STEMI. *(From Silvain J et al, classic references)*

Anticoagulant	2013 ACC-AHA guidelines	2014 ESC guidelines	Ranking for efficacy or safety		Considerations for current practice
			MACE	Major bleeding	
Unfractionated heparin + GPI	COR I	COR I	2nd	4th	Likely worse bleeding with newer $P2Y_{12}$ inhibitors Bleeding risk somewhat mitigated with transradial procedure
LMWH + GPI	None	COR IIa	1st	3rd	Likely worse bleeding with newer $P2Y_{12}$ inhibitors Bleeding risk somewhat mitigated with transradial procedure
Unfractionated heparin	COR I	COR I	4th	2nd	Likely improved MACE with newer $P2Y_{12}$ inhibitors but may negate bleeding advantage
Bivalirudin	COR I Preferred over unfractionated heparin + GPI in those at high risk of bleeding (COR IIa)	COR IIa	3rd	1st	Likely improved MACE with newer $P2Y_{12}$ inhibitors but may negate bleeding advantage
Fondaparinux	COR III	COR III	5th	5th	Should not be recommended based on current data

ACC-AHA, American College of Cardiology Foundation and American Heart Association; *ESC*, European Society of Cardiology; *MACE*, major adverse cardiovascular event; *COR*, class of recommendation; *GPI*, glycoprotein IIb/IIIa inhibitor; *LMWH*, low molecular weight heparin.

FIG. 12.5 Ranking for efficacy and safety of different anticoagulation regimens. *(From Bangalore S, Toklu B, Kotwal A, et al. Anticoagulant therapy during primary percutaneous coronary intervention for acute myocardial infarction: a meta-analysis of randomized trials in the era of stents and P2Y12 inhibitors. BMJ. 2014;349:g6419. https://doi.org/10.1136/bmj.g6419. classic references)*

In this meta-analysis enoxaparin was associated with a significant 48% relative risk reduction of mortality with enoxaparin relative reduction (RR, 0.52; 95% CI, 0.42–0.64; $P < .001$, a reduction of death or MI (RR, 0.61; 95% CI, 0.47–0.79; $P < .001$), complications of MI (RR, 0.70; 95% CI, 0.62–0.80; $P < .001$) and also a reduction in the incidence of major bleeding (RR, 0.72; 95% CI, 0.56–0.93; $P = .01$). Such results were corroborated by others such as the *Trial of Routine Angioplasty and Stenting After Fibrinolysis to Enhance Reperfusion in Acute Myocardial Infarction - TRANSFER-AMI trial.* In another meta-analysis, the combination of LMWH with a GPI was considered the first choice for efficacy and the third choice for safety after bivalirudin and UFH (Fig. 12.5). The authors also concluded that bleeding can also be reduced by using radial arterial access as in ATOLL, which subsequently became the preferred arterial access site in clinical practice in Europe and North America and is endorsed by recent guidelines (see also Chapter 17). The combination of radial access and LMWH combination was considered the best approach to reach efficacy with preserved safety.

Based on these considerations and on the clinical experience with enoxaparin in other PCI settings, enoxaparin has been upgraded in the ESC guidelines (Class IIa) and may be preferred over UFH (Table 12.3). In the latest 2021 ACC/AHA guidelines, no prioritization is given between UFH, enoxaparin, and bivalirudin, regarding anticoagulation in STEMI and primary PCI, although it is noted that "*Enoxaparin is considered a safe alternative to UFH following the results of SYNERGY and ATOLL trials.*"6 In the latest 2023 ESC guidelines, UFH is a Class IC recommendation as the standard of care and enoxaparin is an alternative given a class IIa recommendation for STEMI and NSTE-ACS managed invasivly, while bivalirudin is an option for STEMI with a class IIa recommendation.[5]

Bivalirudin versus UFH for Primary PCI

Multiple randomized trials have evaluated bivalirudin in the primary PCI setting (Fig. 12.6). After the initial findings of the *Harmonizing Outcomes with Revascularization and Stents in Acute Myocardial Infarction* (HORIZONS-AMI) trial (see Chapter 17 to be adapted), bivalirudin was given a Class I recommendation in international guidelines. Notably, bivalirudin was observed to have similar results in terms of ischemic events, an increase in early stent thrombosis, and a reduction of the primary endpoint due to the reduction of major bleeding compared with UFH along with routine use of a GPI in this open-label randomized trial (Fig. 12.7). Subsequent trials have included control groups with contemporary P2Y12 antagonists and without routine use of a GPI.

The open-label *European Ambulance Acute Coronary Syndrome Angiography* (EUROMAX) trial compared a strategy of prehospital bivalirudin with heparin (mostly UFH) with a lower use (69%) of GPI in the heparin group. Bivalirudin was associated with a 40% reduction of the primary composite endpoint of death and non-CABG major bleeding at 30 days, but the mortality benefit observed in the HORIZONS-AMI trial was not confirmed by EUROMAX, and an excess of stent thrombosis was confirmed despite prolonged infusion of bivalirudin and despite the use of novel $P2Y_{12}$ inhibitors in more than half of the patients. The increase in acute stent thrombosis was paralleled by a trend toward a higher rate of reinfarction (1.7% vs. 0.9%, respectively; RR, 1.93; 95% CI, 0.90–4.14; $P = .08$).

A third randomized trial, the *How Effective are Antithrombotic Therapies in PPCI* (HEAT-PPCI) randomized all comers with STEMI planned to undergo primary PCI in a single center to either bivalirudin or UFH in an open-label fashion. The study was representative of contemporary practice with symmetrical and low use of GPI in both arms (15%), the frequent use of novel P2Y12 inhibitors (89%), and a high rate of

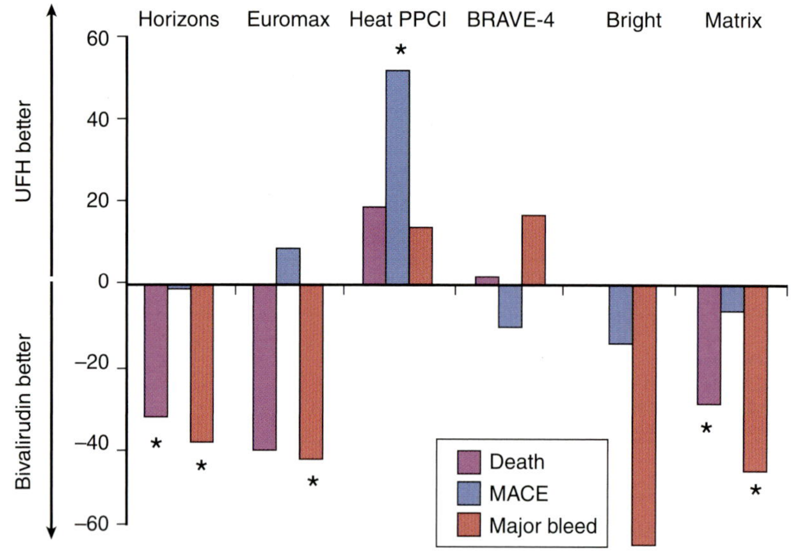

FIG. 12.6 **Summary of clinical trials of bivalirudin.** *Indicates a significant result. Bars indicates relative differences. For the BRIGHT trial only the comparison between UFH and bivalirudin alone was used.

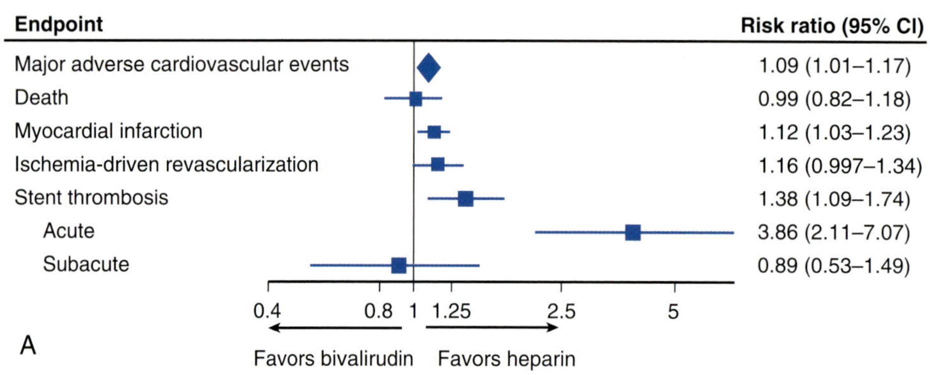

FIG. 12.7 Metanalysis of bivalirudin vs. UFH on MACE. *(From Cavender MA, Sabatine MS. Bivalirudin vs. heparin in patients planned for percutaneous coronary intervention: a meta-analysis of randomised controlled trials. Lancet. 2014;384(9943):599–606. https://doi.org/10.1016/S0140-6736(14)61216-2. classic references)*

radial approach to lower procedure-related major bleeding events. In this trial, UFH was superior to bivalirudin with respect to the primary composite of all-cause mortality, stroke, recurrent infarction, and unplanned target lesion revascularization, with more ischemic events in the bivalirudin group as compared with the UFH group (8.7% vs. 5.7%, respectively; HR: 1.52; 95% CI, 1.09–2.13; $P = .01$), including an increase in stent thrombosis (3.4% vs. 0.9%, RR, 3.91; 95% CI, 1.61–9.52; $P = .001$). Major bleeding was not reduced by bivalirudin (3.5% vs. 3.1%; $P = .59$).

The *Bavarian Reperfusion Alternatives Evaluation* (BRAVE) 4 open-label randomized trial examined whether a strategy of prasugrel plus bivalirudin was superior to a strategy with clopidogrel plus UFH in primary PCI patients. No differences were found in the primary endpoint in a trial that was interrupted due to slow patient recruitment. In the Chinese *Bivalirudin in Acute Myocardial Infarction versus Heparin and GPI Plus Heparin Trial* (BRIGHT) open-label trial ($n = 2194$ patients), three arms were compared, bivalirudin with a post-PCI infusion of 1.75 mg/kg/h for a median duration of 3 hours ($n = 735$), UFH alone ($n = 729$), or UFH plus tirofiban with a post-PCI infusion ($n = 730$). At 30 days, bivalirudin resulted in a decrease in net adverse clinical events (all-cause death, reinfarction, ischemia-driven target vessel revascularization, stroke, or any bleeding) compared with both UFH alone and UFH plus tirofiban (8.8% vs. 13.2% vs. 17%, respectively), primarily due to a reduction in bleeding events including minor bleedings with bivalirudin (4.1% vs. 7.5% vs. 12.3%, respectively) without significant differences in major adverse cardiac, cerebral events, or stent thrombosis.

The *Minimizing Adverse Haemorrhagic Events by TRansradial Access Site and Systemic Implementation of angioX* (MATRIX trial) ($n = 7213$ patients) open-label trial found that bivalirudin was not statistically superior to UFH at 30 days for both coprimary endpoints of death, MI, or stroke (MACE) and net adverse clinical events (death, MI, or stroke and non-CABG bleeding). Several secondary endpoints, including major bleeding (1.4% vs. 2.5%, $P = .001$) and all-cause death (1.7% vs. 2.3%, $P = .042$) favored bivalirudin. Ultimately GPI was administrated in 4.6% of the bivalirudin group and 25.8% of the UFH group. However, definite stent thrombosis was more common in the bivalirudin-treated patients (1.0% vs. 0.6%, $P = .048$). In MATRIX, bivalirudin was dosed according to drug labeling (a bolus of 0.75 mg/kg followed by an infusion of 1.75 mg/kg/h until the end of PCI), which included a prolonged infusion according to the randomized group (full dose for up to 4 h).

In the *Bivalirudin versus Heparin in NSTEMI and STEMI in Patients on Modern Antiplatelet Therapy in SWEDEHEART* (VALIDATE) multicenter, randomized, registry-based, open-label clinical trial among 6066 patients with ACS undergoing coronary revascularization, bivalirudin was not effective at preventing death, MI, or major bleeding with UFH. Individual outcomes, including major bleeding and stent thrombosis, were also similar between treatment arms. Similarly to HEAT-PPCI, this large, open-label trial included patients with a high rate of radial artery access (>90%), potent P2Y12 inhibitors, and no GP IIb/IIIa inhibitors.

Lastly, the *Bivalirudin with prolonged full-dose Infusion during primary PCI versus Heparin Trial* - BRIGHT-4 open-label, randomized controlled trial including 6016 patients, demonstrated that bivalirudin is superior to UFH monotherapy in reducing bleeding and ischemic events at 30 days among patients with STEMI undergoing primary PCI.[7] A major difference compared with prior trials is the routine continuation of full dose bivalirudin infusion for 2–4 hours (mean 3 hours) post-PCI. Most of these patients received ticagrelor and were treated via radial access.

Thus, when putting in perspective all the trials and various meta-analyses bivalirudin, the reduction of bleeding events with bivalirudin was mostly found in open-label trials with an imbalanced use of GP IIb/IIIa inhibitors in conjunction with UFH and is mitigated by the use of radial access. In a pragmatic contemporary setting, a signal of increased stent thrombosis and subsequent myocardial infarction in patients treated with bivalirudin led to a cautious use, although this signal was inconsistent and may be reduced with a post-PCI infusion as demonstrated in BRIGHT-4 (but not in the MATRIX trial). Hence, the ESC and European Association for Cardio-Thoracic Surgery downgraded the recommendation for bivalirudin from class I to IIa in patients with STEMI undergoing PCI in its 2014 guidelines on myocardial revascularization, the 2017 and the 2023 ESC guidelines. Latest 2021 ACC/AHA/SCAI Guideline for Coronary Artery Revascularization provided a similar IIa recommendation in STEMI.

Continuing Anticoagulation After Primary PCI

Previous studies suggested that acute thrombotic complications of primary PCI occur mostly within the first 48 hours after the procedure, probably because of the delayed effect of oral P2Y12 inhibitors and residual thrombosis. In the MATRIX trial, prolonging bivalirudin infusion after PCI did not improve the outcomes compared with bivalirudin infusion confined to the duration of PCI. In the BRIGHT-4 trial, anticoagulation with bivalirudin plus a post-PCI high-dose infusion for 2–4 hours significantly reduced the 30-day composite rate of all-cause mortality or BARC types 3–5 major bleeding compared with UFH monotherapy. The RIGHT trial (NCT03664180) which compared a strategy of continued anticoagulant post PCI (with enoxaparin, ACT-guided unfractionated UFH or bivalirudin) versus only periprocedural anticoagulation in 2989 patients admitted for STEMI undergoing primary PCI[8] showed that overall anticoagulation after primary PCI for STEMI is safe but does not appear to reduce ischemic events in the low-to-intermediate risk population of the trial with a significant interaction suggesting that enoxaparin anticoagulation may be beneficial as compared to the other drugs.

STEMI Patients Treated With Fibrinolysis

The potential benefits of acute therapy with anticoagulants in STEMI treated with fibrinolysis are multiple, including facilitating more rapid and durable patency of the infarct-related artery, and prevention of venous thromboembolism. Nevertheless, the data from clinical trials have engendered debate over the clinical benefit of anticoagulants as part of acute therapy. In particular, as reperfusion therapy has evolved, the relevance of data from previous clinical trials has become less certain. However, placebo-controlled data with LMWHs used as an adjunct to contemporary reperfusion regimens have provided additional support for the acute administration of anticoagulants in patients with STEMI treated with fibrinolytic. As such, current professional society guidelines recommend that adequate anticoagulation therapies need to be administered during and after fibrinolysis to optimize patency and should preferably be given until revascularization (if performed) (Tables 12.4 and 12.5).

TABLE 12.4 Initial Anticoagulation Therapy to Support Reperfusion with Fibrinolytic Therapy STEMI guideline

	ACCF/AHA[a]		ESC[b]	
ANTICOAGULATION THERAPY	COR	LOE	COR	LOE
Enoxaparin i.v. followed by s.c. is recommended as the preferred anticoagulant - if age <75 y, 30 mg i.v. bolus followed in 15 min by 1 mg/kg subcutaneously every 12 h (max 100 mg for the first 2 doses) - if age >75 y, no bolus, 0.75 mg/kg subcutaneously every 12 h (max 75 mg for the first 2 doses) - regardless of age, if CrCl< 30 mL/min, 1 mg/kg subcutaneously every 24 h - Duration : for the index hospitalization, up to 8 d or until revascularization	I	A	I	A
UFH: When enoxaparin is not available, UFH is recommended as a weight-adjusted i.v. bolus, followed by infusion - i.v. bolus of 60 U/kg (max 4000 U) followed by infusion of 12 U/kg/h (max 1000 U) initially, adjusted to maintain aPTT at 1.5–2.0 times control for 48 h or until revascularization	I	C	I	B
Fondaparinux: - initial dose 2.5 mg IV, then 2.5 mg subcutaneously daily starting the following day, for the index hospitalization, up to 8 d or until revascularization - Contraindicated if CrCl <30 mL/min	I	B	II[a]	B

[a]Adapted from Silvain J, Beygui F, Barthélémy O, et al. Efficacy and safety of enoxaparin versus unfractionated heparin during percutaneous coronary intervention: systematic review and meta-analysis. *BMJ*. 2012;344:e553. doi:10.1136/bmj.e553.
[b]Adapted from Byrne RA, Rossello X, Coughlan JJ, et al. 2023 ESC Guidelines for the management of acute coronary syndromes: Developed by the task force on the management of acute coronary syndromes of the European Society of Cardiology (ESC) guideline. *Eur Heart J*. 2023;44:3720–3826. doi:10.1093/eurheartj/ehad191.

TABLE 12.5 Adjunctive Antithrombotic Therapy to Support Rescue PCI After Fibrinolytic Therapy

ANTICOAGULATION THERAPY	AHA COR	AHA LOE
Enoxaparin: continue through PCI - no additional drug if last dose was within previous 8 h - 0.3 mg/kg i.v. bolus if last dose was 8–12 h earlier	I	B
UFH continue through PCI, administering i.v. boluses as needed to maintain therapeutic ACT depending on use of GP IIb/IIIa receptor antagonist	I	C
Fondaparinux: As sole anticoagulant for PCI	III	C

UFH as an Adjunct to Fibrinolysis

In trials performed before the introduction of fibrinolytic therapy or the widespread and routine use of ASA, early administration of intravenous UFH reduced venous thromboembolic events, stroke, and reinfarction. Subsequent trials in the reperfusion era are challenging to interpret considering important differences regarding the use of aspirin, the type of fibrinolytic used, and the dose of UFH administered. Meta-analysis of randomized trials in which patients received fibrinolysis have failed to show a clear benefit of UFH compared to placebo for the reduction of reinfarction or death. Nonetheless, overall, data from clinical trials at least raise the possibility that adjunctive therapy with UFH may enhance late patency after the administration of fibrin-specific fibrinolytics. In the absence of randomized clinical trials designed to detect differences in clinical events, expert guidelines have concluded (Class IIa) that it is judicious to use UFH for ≥48 hours with fibrin-specific fibrinolytics.

If used, the recommended dose of UFH is an i.v. bolus of 60 U/kg (maximum of 4000 IU) followed by an IV infusion of 12 U/kg (maximum of 1000 U/h for 24–48 hours). If administrated during fibrinolysis, careful dosing and close monitoring are mandatory (at 3, 6, 12, and 24 hours); with target aPTT of 50–70 seconds as a high value of aPTT values (>70 seconds) need to be avoided as they are associated with a higher likelihood of bleeding, reinfarction, and death.

Enoxaparin as an Adjunct to Fibrinolysis

In contrast to the uncertain evidence with UFH, trials of LMWHs have demonstrated a clear benefit compared with placebo as well as UFH and supported LMWHs as the treatment of choice for adjunctive anticoagulant therapy with fibrinolytics. Specifically, placebo-controlled studies with LMWH have confirmed the importance of an adjuvant anticoagulant strategy in fibrinolysis therapy with improvement of patency, ST-segment resolution, and composite endpoints of death, reinfarction and recurrent angina or stroke weighed against an increase of major bleeding.

In the *Assessment of the Safety and Efficacy of a New Thrombolytic3* (ASSENT 3) trial, enoxaparin compared with UFH resulted in a similar rate of reperfusion of the infarct artery but reduced rates of reocclusion, reinfarction, or recurrent ischemic events. In the ExTRACT-TIMI 25 trial (n = 20,475 patients), enoxaparin significantly reduced death or re-MI balanced against an increase in major bleeding events. The benefits of enoxaparin over UFH are evident regardless of the type of fibrinolytic administered (streptokinase or fibrin-specific) and across a wide range of patient subgroups. In patients who were not treated with post-lytic PCI, the recommended dose is 30 mg i.v. bolus followed 15 minutes later by 1 mg/kg SC BID (with a maximum of 100 mg for the first two doses) until hospital discharge for a maximum of 8 days. However, a lower dose of enoxaparin should be used in patients >75 years of age (no bolus and 0.75 mg/kg SC BID, with a maximum of 75 mg for the first two doses) and in those with impaired renal function (estimated creatinine clearance <30 mL/min) with SC doses given only once every 24 hours.

Fondaparinux as an Adjunct to Fibrinolysis

Fondaparinux reduces the rate of reocclusion of the infarct-related artery. Moreover, in the large *Sixth Organization to Assess Strategies in Ischemic Syndromes* (OASIS-6) trial (n = 12,092 patients), fondaparinux was superior to placebo with respect to the rate of death or reinfarction (HR: 0.79 [95% CI 0.68–0.92]) and not superior to UFH in fibrinolytic-treated patients (HR: 0.96 [95% CI 0.81–1.13]). Nevertheless, the trial established the efficacy of an antithrombin and compared with UFH, fondaparinux offered an attractive alternative with the convenience of a once-daily SC injections (2.5 mg once daily for up to 8 days). However, its use is complicated by the need for coadministration of an additional antithrombin with anti-IIa activity if PCI is to be performed. Fondaparinux should not be given as the sole anticoagulant to patients referred for PCI and is contraindicated for patients with a creatinine clearance <30 mL/min. In patients treated with streptokinase, the latest ESC guidelines recommend an intravenous bolus of fondaparinux followed by a subcutaneous dose at 24 hours.

Bivalirudin as an Adjunct to Fibrinolysis

The direct thrombin inhibitors hirudin and bivalirudin were compared to UFH in several randomized trials of patients with STEMI undergoing fibrinolysis – *Global Utilization of Streptokinase and Tissue Plasminogen Activator for Occluded Coronary Arteries trial* (GUSTO IIb) (n = 2274), *Hirudin for the Improvement of Thrombolysis* (HIT-4) (n = 1208), and *Hirulog Early Reperfusion/Occlusion Study* (HERO-2) (n = 17,073), showing a reduction in the incidence of recurrent MI by 25%–30% compared with UFH without improving mortality. In GUSTO IIb, hirudin, lowered 30-day death/reinfarction (8.6% vs. 14.4%; P = 0.004) in conjunction with streptokinase but did not confer a benefit in patients treated with tissue-type plasminogen activator. Additionally, at the studied doses, both hirudin and bivalirudin are associated with higher rates of major bleeding, including intracranial hemorrhage, compared to UFH when used alongside fibrinolytic agents. Notably, bivalirudin has not been evaluated in combination with fibrin-specific agents.

In patients with a known history of HIT, it is recommended to substitute bivalirudin as an alternative to UFH or LMWH in conjunction with streptokinase (Class IIa recommendation). Dosing according to the HERO 2 regimen (a bolus of 0.25 mg/kg followed by an IV infusion of 0.5 mg/kg/h for the first 12 hours, and 0.25 mg/kg/h for the subsequent 36 hours) is recommended but with a reduction in the infusion rate if the aPTT is longer than 75 seconds within the first 12 hours.

Anticoagulant Therapy NSTEMI Patients Managed Invasively

In addition to antiplatelet therapy, an anticoagulant should be added in patients with NSTEMI as soon as possible after presentation. Anticoagulation is effective in addition to platelet inhibition and the combination of the two is more effective than either treatment alone.[1] Several options are available for the treatment of NSTEMI (UFH, enoxaparin, fondaparinux, and bivalirudin). Selection of the optimal regimen is based on considerations of the strategy used (invasive or medical conservative), the ease of use, renal function, and the cost. Importantly, pretreatment with an anticoagulant should not delay angiography and revascularization. A general rule is to avoid crossover between antithrombins (except for adding UFH to fondaparinux), especially between UFH and LMWH, and to discontinue anticoagulation after PCI in most cases. An overview of anticoagulation therapy in NSTEMI is summarized in Fig. 12.8. Discrepancies appeared between the latest 2018 and 2020 ESC guidelines and 2021 ACC/AHA/SCAI guidelines. The ESC downgraded the use of bivalirudin from class I to IIb, putting UFH and fondaparinux first (Class I) and enoxaparin as the first alternative (Class IIa). In the latest 2023 ESC guidelines, bivalirudin is not an option for NSTE-ACS anymore.[5] In contrast, the latest 2021 ACC/AHA/SCAI guidelines maintained bivalirudin as a first alternative to UFH (class IIb) in front of enoxaparin (Class IIb, level of evidence B based on randomized data) and only mentioned fondaparinux for specific situations. Professional society recommendations for anticoagulation in NSTEMI are summarized in Table 12.6

UFH in Treatment of NSTEMI

Anticoagulation, traditionally with UFH, has been a cornerstone of therapy for patients with NSTEMI. A meta-analysis regrouping six trials comparing UFH versus placebo or untreated controls showed a 33% risk reduction in death and MI (OR, 0.67; 95% CI, 0.45–0.99; $P = .04$), with a reduction in MI accounting for practically all the beneficial effects. The benefit was observed at the cost of an increased risk of bleeding. In initial therapy, a recommended weight-adjusted bolus of UFH (60 U/kg) followed by continued infusion of 12 units/kg/h recommended with frequent monitoring (every 6 h until the target range is reached and every 12–24 hours thereafter) and adjustment of dose if necessary.

In the PCI setting, UFH is given as an i.v. bolus either under ACT guidance (ACT in the range of 250–350 seconds) or in a weight-adjusted manner (usually 70–100 IU/kg). Doses need to be lower if GPI is used. Because of marked variability in UFH bioavailability, ACT-guided dosing is

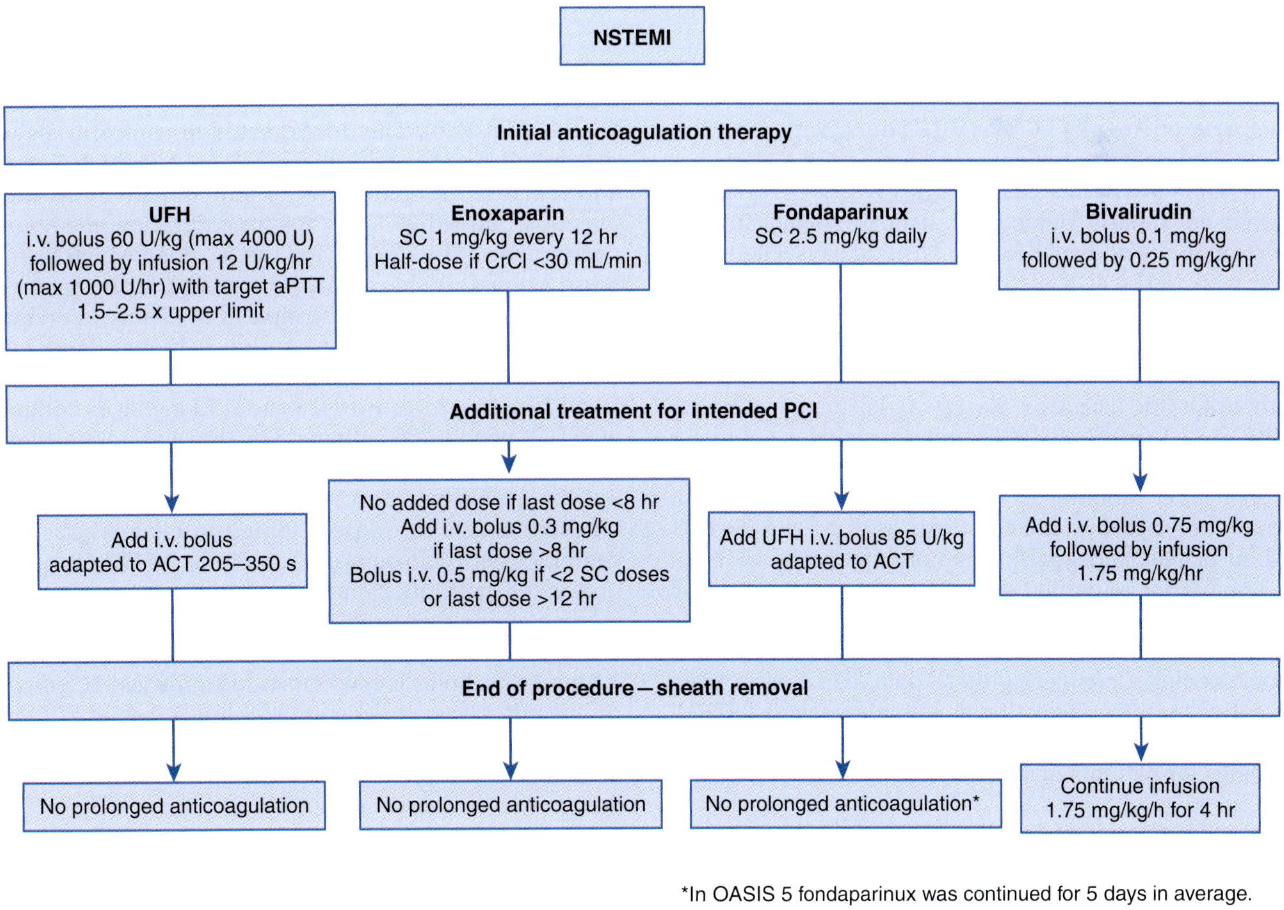

FIG. 12.8 Summary of dose of anticoagulation therapy in NSTEMI.

TABLE 12.6 **Recommended Anticoagulation Therapy in NSTEMI/NSTE-ACS Treated by PCI**

ANTICOAGULATION THERAPY IN PATIENTS WITH NSTE-ACS UNDERGOING PCI	ACC/AHA/SCAI[a] COE	ACC/AHA/SCAI[a] LOE	ESC[b] COE	ESC[b] LOE
UFH (weight-adjusted i.v. bolus during PCI of 70–100 IU/kg or 50–70 IU/kg in combination with a GP IIb/IIIa inhibitor; activated clotting time target range of 250–350 sec or 200–250 sec if a GP IIb/IIIa inhibitor is given) is recommended in patients undergoing PCI.	I	B	I	C
For patients with NSTE-ACS in whom early invasive angiography (i.e., within 24 h) is anticipated (or patients treated previously by SC enoxaparin), **enoxaparin** should be considered as an alternative to UFH.	IIb	B-R	IIa	B
For patients with NSTE-ACS in whom early invasive angiography (i.e., within 24 h) is not anticipated, **fondaparinux** is recommended.	Not recommended		I	B
Bivalirudin may be considered as an alternative to UFH	IIb	A	Not recommended	
Crossover of UFH and LMWH is not recommended			III	B

[a]Adapted from Lawton JS, Tamis-Holland JE, Bangalore S, et al. 2021. ACC/AHA/SCAI guideline for coronary artery revascularization: executive summary: a report of the American College of Cardiology/American Heart Association joint committee on clinical practice guidelines. *Circulation*. 2022;145(3):e4–e17.
[b]Adapted from Byrne RA, Rossello X, Coughlan JJ, et al. 2023 ESC Guidelines for the management of acute coronary syndromes: Developed by the task force on the management of acute coronary syndromes of the European Society of Cardiology (ESC) guideline. *Eur Heart J*. 2023;44:3720–3826. doi:10.1093/eurheartj/ehad191.

necessary and recommended, especially for prolonged procedures when additional dosing may be required. Monitoring of the anticoagulant response by aPTT can also be made according to a standardized nomogram, aiming for an APTT of 50–70 seconds or 1.5–2.5 times control. If the patient is already treated with an ongoing IV infusion of UFH, an additional i.v. bolus of UFH should be adapted according to the ACT values. HIT occurs in approximately 0.5% of patients with the use of UFH and is more common with longer durations of treatment. Both monitoring and safety (bleeding and HIT) are the major drawbacks of this traditional anticoagulant therapy.

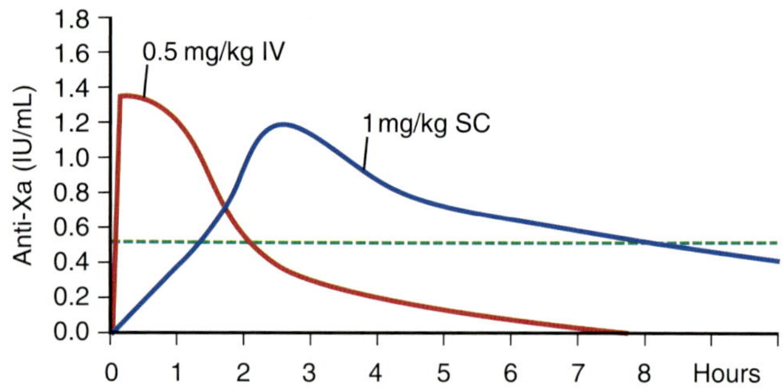

FIG. 12.9 Pharmacodynamics of IV enoxaparin vs. SC enoxaparin.

Enoxaparin in Treatment of NSTEMI

LMWHs, including enoxaparin, have proven effective in the medical management of NSTEMI. The standard dose of enoxaparin is 1 mg/kg SC every 12 hours, with modification to once daily for patients with a creatinine clearance <30 mL/min LMWH. In a meta-analysis of 21,945 NSTE-ACS patients, enoxaparin yielded a statistically significant 10% reduction in the odds of death or MI at 30 days when compared with UFH, OR 0.90, 95% CI 0.81–0.99, P = .043. In a meta-analysis of patients with NSTEMI and STEMI managed invasively (n = 30,966), enoxaparin significantly reduced death (RR, 0.66; 95% CI, 0.57–0.76; P <.001), the composite of death, or MI (RR, 0.68, 0.57–0.81; P <.001), complications of MI (RR, 0.75, 0.6–0.85; P <.001), and the incidence of major bleeding (RR, 0.80; 0.68–0.95; P = .009). However, in the largest open-label randomized trial (N = 9978, SYNERGY) to evaluate enoxaparin among patients with NSTEACS managed invasively, enoxaparin was not superior to UFH but was noninferior regarding death or myocardial infarction at 30 days (0.96; 95% CI, 0.86–1.06). Enoxaparin was a safe and effective alternative to UFH with a modest excess of major bleeding. Considering these data, enoxaparin is an alternative for anticoagulation in all patients with NSTEMI treated with PCI (Table 12.6) and favored in the ACCF/AHA guidelines for patients managed noninvasively.

Pharmacodynamics of Enoxaparin and the Invasive Strategy

Enoxaparin pharmacology was well studied and is quite predictable due to its pharmacological proprieties and its renal elimination. The IV use of enoxaparin has a different pharmacokinetic or pharmacodynamic profile from the SC use (Fig. 12.9). The doses tested in clinical trials were generally lower than SC doses (0.5 mg/kg and 0.75 mg/kg) and reached the same peak of anti-Xa activity as the SC injection but within 3 minutes for a duration of 2 hours in comparison with 2 hours for the SC dose which lasts for 8 to 12 hours. IV enoxaparin was tested in the Safety and Efficacy of Intravenous Enoxaparin in Elective Percutaneous Coronary Intervention: An International Randomized Evaluation (STEEPLE) study (n = 3528 patients) showing lower bleeding rates with 0.5 and 0.75 mg/kg as compared with UFH in non-ACS patients. The trial was not powered to detect a difference in efficacy between enoxaparin groups but the lower dose of 0.5 mg/kg exhibited a lower rate of bleeding and is the dose adopted in clinical practice in centers where enoxaparin is used. In NSTEACS patients pretreated with enoxaparin, no additional enoxaparin is recommended during PCI if the last SC enoxaparin injection was administered <8 hours before PCI. An additional 0.3 mg/kg i.v. bolus is recommended if the last SC enoxaparin injection was administered >8 hours before PCI. A full dose of enoxaparin 0.5 mg/kg IV is recommended if the last dose was >12 hours or if the patients did not receive 2 SC doses or if the delays are unknown.

Fondaparinux in NSTEMI

In ACS, a 2.5-mg fixed daily dose of fondaparinux is an alternative (Class I) as the initial anticoagulation therapy.

In the *Fifth Organization to Assess Strategies in Ischemic Syndromes (*OASIS-5) trial (*n* = 20,078) of NSTEACS patients, fondaparinux was compared with SC enoxaparin 1 mg/kg twice daily for 8 days maximum (average 5.2 vs. 5.4 days, respectively) which is unusually long. The primary efficacy outcome (death, MI, or refractory ischemia at 9 days) was similar in both groups, 5.7% for enoxaparin versus 5.8% for fondaparinux (HR: 1.01; 95% CI 0.90–1.13), fulfilling the criteria for noninferiority. Compared with enoxaparin, fondaparinux reduced major bleeding by 48% (2.2% vs. 4.1%; HR: 0.52; 95% CI, 0.44–0.61; *P* <.001). A reduction in mortality with fondaparinux at 30 days (2.9% vs. 3.5%; HR: 0.83; 95% CI, 0.71– 0.97; *P* = .02) and at 6 months (5.8% vs. 6.5%; HR: 0.89; 95% CI, 0.80–1.00; *P* = .05) has been ascribed to the reduction in major bleeding. Of note with respect to the design of the comparator (enoxaparin) in the trial, it is possible that excessive dosing of enoxaparin occurred because no dose adjustment was made in the elderly, or in patients with renal failure. Moreover, a full dose of UFH was administered in the cath lab for PCI; a strategy associated with more bleeding in the *Superior Yield of the New strategy of Enoxaparin, Revascularization, and GlYcoprotein IIb/IIIa inhibitors* (SYNERGY) trial.

Despite the demonstrated efficacy for medical therapy, fondaparinux is associated with a higher rate of abrupt vessel closure and unexpected thrombus formation during coronary angiography/PCI than UFH or enoxaparin. In the PCI population in OASIS-5, catheter thrombus occurred more frequently with fondaparinux (0.9%) than with enoxaparin (0.4%). This excess appears to be avoided by a bolus of UFH at the time of PCI. Therefore, professional guidelines recommend that fondaparinux should not be used as a sole anticoagulant for patients undergoing PCI. The optimal dose of UFH to be administered during PCI in patients initially treated with fondaparinux was investigated in the *Fondaparinux Trial With Unfractionated Heparin During Revascularization in Acute Coronary Syndromes* (FUTURA/OASIS-8, *n* = 2026 patients) and found to be the standard dose of 85 IU/kg adjusted by ACT.

Direct Thrombin Inhibitors

Overall, bivalirudin offers similar efficacy, while significantly lowering the risk of major bleeding, compared with UFH plus systematic GPI for patients with NSTEACS undergoing PCI. In NSTEACS patients, bivalirudin is recommended at a very low dose of 0.1 mg/kg i.v. bolus followed by an infusion of 0.25 mg/kg/h until PCI, and the dose must be changed for urgent or elective PCI to a 0.75 mg/kg i.v. bolus followed by 1.75 mg/kg/h infusion. *The Acute Catheterization and Urgent Intervention Triage Strategy trial* (ACUITY) was an open-label trial testing bivalirudin specifically in the setting of NSTEACS (*n* = 13,819) planned for an invasive strategy. There was no significant difference between standard UFH/enoxaparin plus systematic GPI, and the combination of bivalirudin plus systematic GPI, for the composite ischemia endpoint at 30 days (7.3% vs. 7.7%, respectively; RR, 1.07; 95% CI, 0.92–1.23; *P* = .39) or for major bleeding (5.7% vs. 5.3%; RR, 0.93; 95% CI, 0.78–1.10; *P* = .38). An arm of the trial with bivalirudin alone was noninferior to UFH/enoxaparin plus systematic GPI with respect to the composite ischemia endpoint (7.8% vs. 7.3%; RR, 1.08; 95% CI, 0.93–1.24; *P* = .32) but was associated with a significantly lower rate of major bleeding (3.0% vs. 5.7%; RR, 0.53; 95% CI, 0.43–0.65; *P* < .001) translating into better 30-day net clinical outcome (combining efficacy and bleeding endpoints).

However, in patients not pretreated with clopidogrel prior to PCI, a significant excess of ischemic endpoints was observed (9.1% vs. 7.1%; RR, 1.29, 95% CI, 1.03–1.63) with bivalirudin alone compared with UFH/enoxaparin and GPI. The *Intracoronary Stenting and Antithrombotic Regimen: Rapid Early Action for Coronary Treatment* 3 (ISAR–REACT 3) trial (*n* = 4750 stable and unstable patients) compared double-blinded UFH versus bivalirudin in patients who had received 600 mg of clopidogrel. A reduced rate of major bleeding with bivalirudin was offset by an increase in ischemic events. However, patients in the heparin group received a bolus of 140 U of heparin per kilogram, which is twice the current recommended dose. For NSTEMI patients undergoing PCI, the *Intracoronary Stenting and Antithrombotic Regimen: Rapid Early Action for Coronary Treatment* 4 (ISAR-REACT 4) trial provided additional evidence in favor of the safety of bivalirudin in terms of bleeding when compared with a combination of UFH and GPI (abciximab) in a double-blind manner. It should be noted that most of the evidence in support of bivalirudin is derived from trials in which the comparator was either very high doses of UFH or UFH plus systematic use of GPI, a combination that is no longer routinely used. In the VALIDATE open-label randomized trial, the rate of the composite of death from any cause, myocardial infarction, or major bleeding was not lower among those who received bivalirudin than among those who received heparin monotherapy. Of importance, GPI was only used as a rescue therapy and in only <3% of patients in both arms.

Myocardial Infarction Patients Treated Without Reperfusion Therapy

The OASIS-6 double-blinded trial included 12,092 patients with STEMI who were stratified according to whether they received reperfusion therapy and thus did not need UFH (stratum 1, *n* = 5658) or did require UFH therapy because of fibrinolytics, scheduled PCI, or medical conservative treatment (stratum 2, *n* = 6494). In patients with STEMI not receiving reperfusion treatment, fondaparinux reduced the composite of death or myocardial reinfarction without an increase in severe bleedings or strokes as compared to placebo or UF heparin.

In the *Treatment of Enoxaparin and Tirofiban in Acute Myocardial Infarction* (TETAMI) trial, patients with STEMI and no reperfusion therapy were randomized in a 2 × 2 factorial fashion to enoxaparin versus UFH and to tirofiban versus placebo (*n* = 1224). Treatment with enoxaparin did not provide benefits over UFH, and there were no differences in bleeding events. Additionally, treatment with the GP IIb/IIIa inhibitor tirofiban did not provide additional benefit to aspirin.

Anticoagulation with fondaparinux and enoxaparin in patients with nonreperfused MI (STEMI or NSTEMI) is a reasonable option. If PCI is needed in a patient receiving

13 Overview of Antiplatelet Therapy for Acute Coronary Syndrome

LUIS ORTEGA-PAZ, FRANCESCO FRANCHI, AND DOMINICK J. ANGIOLILLO

INTRODUCTION

Atherosclerotic plaque rupture followed by arterial thrombosis is the major determinant leading to an acute coronary syndrome (ACS).[1–3] Platelet adhesion, activation, and aggregation have a pivotal role in the cascade of events leading to arterial thrombosis, and therefore, antiplatelet therapy is essential in the treatment of patients with ACS.[1–3] Multiple platelet signaling pathways are involved in thrombus formation, which represents potential targets for antiplatelet agents. Currently, several classes of antiplatelet therapies are clinically available for both oral and intravenous administration for the treatment of patients with ACS, including unstable angina, non-ST-segment elevation (NSTE) ACS (MI), and ST-segment elevation MI (STEMI).[1–3] This chapter provides an overview of these antiplatelet therapies used in the setting of acute MI, including describing the rationale for use, pharmacological principles, pivotal clinical trial data, and guidance for selecting the initial antiplatelet regimen in the early phase of management.

RATIONALE FOR USE OF ANTIPLATELET THERAPY

The pathobiology of atherothrombosis is discussed in Chapter 1 and the fundamental principles underlying the rationale for antiplatelet therapy are described in Chapter 13. Injury to the arterial vessel wall, such as plaque rupture, fissure, or erosion, exposes the subendothelial layer and leads to recruitment and activation of platelets, as well as generation of excessive levels of thrombin. These events ultimately result in the formation of a fibrin-rich thrombus.[3]

Platelet-mediated thrombosis follows three principal steps: (1) platelet adhesion, (2) activation and additional recruitment, and (3) aggregation (Fig. 13.1).[1,3,4] Adhesion of platelets to the subendothelium during the rolling phase is mediated by the interaction between the glycoprotein (GP) Ib/V/IX receptor complex located on the platelet surface and the von Willebrand factor (vWf), and between collagen exposed at the site of vascular injury and platelets collagen receptors.[1,3,4] After adhesion, binding of collagen to these receptor triggers intracellular mechanisms that shift platelet integrins to a high-affinity state and induce the release of activating factors, which enhance the interactions among adherent platelets and promote further recruitment and activation of circulating platelets.[1,3,4] Activating factors include thromboxane A_2 (TXA_2), adenosine diphosphate (ADP), serotonin, epinephrine, and thrombin.[1,3,4] Platelet activation by these mediators leads to a change in platelet shape, expression of pro-inflammatory molecules (e.g., soluble CD40 ligand and P-selectin), and expression of platelet procoagulant activity. The final pathway for all agonists is the conversion of the platelet GP IIb/IIIa receptor, the main receptor mediating platelet aggregation, into its active form.[1,3,4] Activated GP IIb/IIIa receptors bind to soluble adhesive substrates, including fibrinogen and vWf, leading to platelet aggregation and thrombus formation mediated by platelet-platelet interactions.[1,3,4]

Vascular injury also exposes subendothelial tissue factor, which activates the clotting cascade leading to thrombin generation.[1–4] However, only a modest amount of thrombin is produced as a result of the coagulation cascade.[1–4] In fact, thrombin is one of the most potent platelet activators and the surface of activated platelets is the main source of circulating thrombin.[1–4] During arterial thrombosis, thrombin converts fibrinogen to fibrin, generating a fibrin-rich clot, and further activates platelets by binding to protease-activated receptors (PARs) on the platelet membrane.[1–4] Therefore, pathogenic thrombosis is a complex interplay between cellular (i.e., platelets) and plasma (i.e., coagulation factors) components, which interact in an auto-amplified process (Fig. 13.1).

Multiple receptors and signaling pathways are involved in arterial thrombosis. Therefore, several antiplatelet

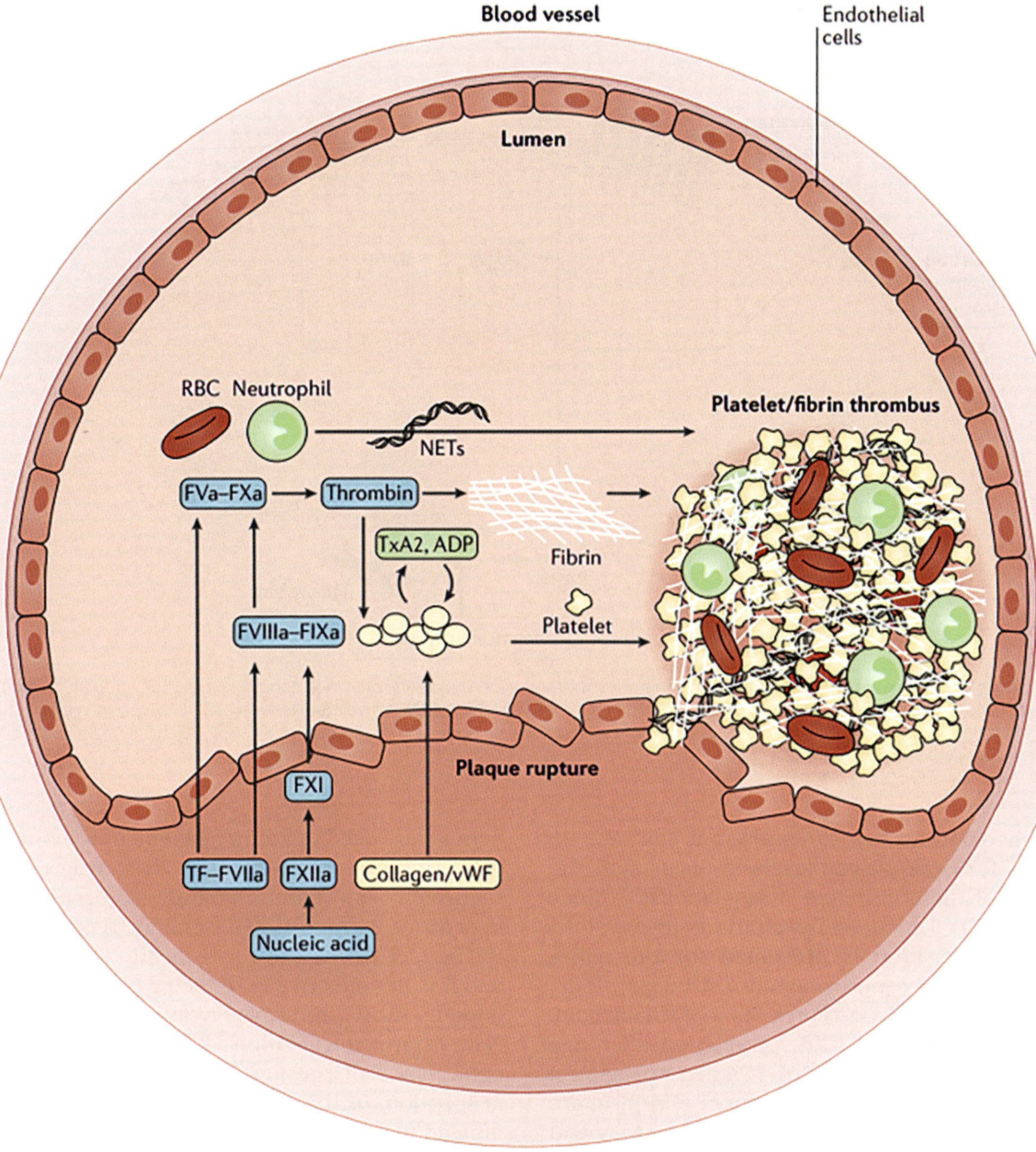

FIG. 13.1 Formation of an occlusive arterial thrombosis. Rupture of an atherosclerotic plaque exposes collagen and von Willebrand factor (vWF), which bind and activate platelets. Released second messengers, such as ADP and thromboxane A2 (TxA2), further activate platelets. Tissue factor (TF) within the plaque binds factor VIIa (FVIIa), and this complex activates the clotting cascade, resulting in fibrin formation. In addition, FXII is activated by nucleic acid and other negatively charged surfaces and contributes to thrombin generation. Neutrophils are incorporated into the thrombus and extrude neutrophil extracellular traps (NETs). Red blood cells (RBCs) are also incorporated into thrombi. (Adapted with permission from Mackman N, Bergmeier W, Stouffer GA, Weitz JI. Therapeutic strategies for thrombosis: new targets and approaches. *Nat Rev Drug Discov.* 2020;19:333–352.)

agents have been developed to target different components of this complex process as described below (Fig. 13.2).

ANTIPLATELET THERAPIES IN MYOCARDIAL INFARCTION

Several classes of antiplatelet agents, available for both oral and intravenous administration, are currently approved for clinical use in the management of patients with ACS. These include: (1) COX-1 inhibitors (aspirin); (2) ADP $P2Y_{12}$ receptor antagonists (ticlopidine, clopidogrel, prasugrel, ticagrelor, cangrelor); (3) GP IIb/IIIa receptor inhibitors (abciximab, eptifibatide, tirofiban); (4) PAR-1 receptor inhibitors (vorapaxar).[5–7] Details on the pharmacology and clinical trial development of these classes of antiplatelet agents are provided below.

Aspirin

Aspirin exerts its antiplatelet effects by irreversibly blocking, by means of acetylation, the COX-1 enzyme, which is responsible for the generation of TXA_2 from arachidonic acid; in turn, it decreases platelet activation mediated by the G-coupled thromboxane and prostaglandin endoperoxide (TP) receptors (Fig. 13.2).[8,9] Aspirin is rapidly absorbed in the upper gastrointestinal tract and is associated with measurable platelet inhibition within 60 minutes. The plasma half-life of aspirin is approximately 20 minutes, and peak plasma levels are achieved 30 to 40 minutes after

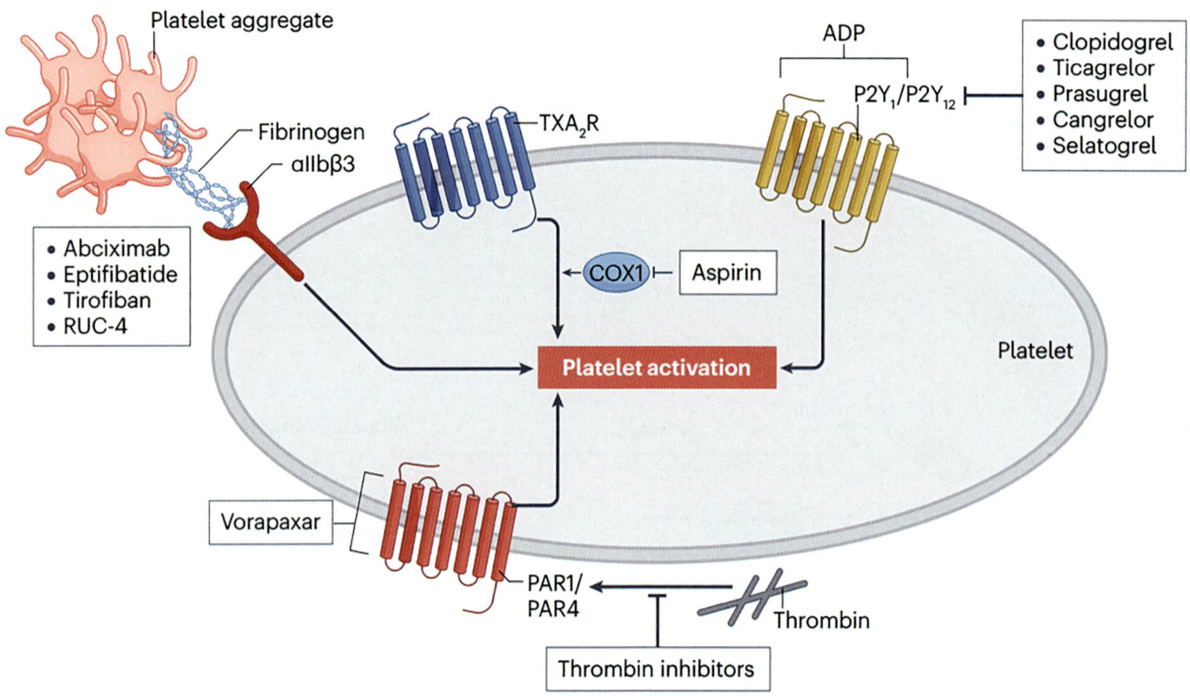

FIG. 13.2 Pharmacological targets for contemporary antiplatelet therapy. Contemporary pharmacological targets for antiplatelet therapy are shown and include receptors on the surface of platelets that are involved in platelet activation. *COX1*, Cyclooxygenase 1; *GDF15*, growth differentiation factor 15; *PAR*, protease-activated receptor; *TXA2R*, thromboxane A2 receptor. (Adapted with permission from Gawaz M, Geisler T, Borst O. Current concepts and novel targets for antiplatelet therapy. *Nat Rev Cardiol*. 2023;20:583–599.)

ingestion of uncoated aspirin. In contrast, it can take up to 3 to 4 hours for peak plasma levels to occur after the administration of enteric-coated formulations.[8,9] Since the blockade of COX-1 induced by aspirin is irreversible, TXA_2-mediated aggregation is prevented for the entire life span of the platelet (approximately 7–10 days). Daily administration of 30 mg of aspirin results in virtually complete suppression of platelet TXA_2 production after one week. In clinical practice, standard regimens of aspirin range from 75 to 325 mg daily. Higher doses of aspirin are required to block COX-2, which has antiinflammatory and analgesic effects through inhibition of the vascular PGI2 (prostacyclin), a platelet inhibitor, and a vasodilator.[8,9]

In the ISIS-2 (International Study of Infarct Survival-2) trial, aspirin therapy was associated with a significant reduction in vascular mortality in patients with suspected acute MI randomized to receive either aspirin, streptokinase, both agents, or placebo. Several other trials have consistently demonstrated an important 40%–50% reduction in cardiovascular events with aspirin treatment in MI patients. The clinical benefit of aspirin is achieved at low doses (75–100 mg daily), with no additional benefit provided by higher doses. In contrast, a dose-dependent increase in the risk of bleeding has been shown, in particular for upper gastrointestinal bleeding.[10] Despite the therapeutic benefit of aspirin, some patients receiving long-term therapy are at risk of thrombotic events due to insufficient inhibition of platelets, giving rise to the term "aspirin resistance."[10] However, the association between variability in response to aspirin and cardiovascular events has led to inconsistent findings.[2] This is likely attributable to the type of tests being utilized for pharmacodynamic (PD) evaluation of aspirin effects. In fact, when tests specific for COX-1 activity are used, "aspirin resistance" is extremely rare and is likely due to noncompliance; drug-drug interactions (i.e., ibuprofen), and enteric coating also represent contributing causes.[11] The residual ischemic risk is thus mainly due to the fact that aspirin specifically targets TXA_2 pathway and it is not effective in reducing platelet activation stimulated by other pathways involved in arterial thrombosis.[11] New aspirin formulations have been developed to overcome some of the limitations, in particular the delayed absorption, in the setting of ACS. To this extent, a novel inhaled nanoparticle aspirin formulation has shown to be associated with earlier and greater drug exposure, resulting in faster and stronger platelet inhibition compared to oral aspirin.[12] Moreover, a novel formulation of the phospholipid-aspirin complex has been designed to overcome common limitations of aspirin by improving erratic gastrointestinal absorption, unpredictable antiplatelet efficacy, and gastrointestinal toxicity. Thus potentially leading to less dyspeptic symptoms, bleeding, and improved adherence.[8,9]

$P2Y_{12}$ Receptor Antagonists

The agonist ADP exerts its effects on platelets through the purinergic G-protein-coupled $P2Y_1$ and $P2Y_{12}$ receptors (Fig. 13.2).[2] Although both receptors are involved in aggregation, ADP-stimulated effects on platelets are mediated mainly by G_i-coupled $P2Y_{12}$ receptor activation, which leads to sustained platelet aggregation and stabilization of platelet aggregates, while $P2Y_1$ is responsible for an initial weak and transient phase of aggregation and change in platelet shape.[2] The addition of a $P2Y_{12}$ receptor inhibitor to aspirin reduces platelet aggregation more than what

TABLE 13.1 Pharmacological Properties of $P2Y_{12}$ Receptor Inhibitors

	CLOPIDOGREL	PRASUGREL	TICAGRELOR	CANGRELOR
Pharmacological class	Thienopyridine	Thienopyridine	CPTP	ATP analogue
Receptor blockade	Irreversible	Irreversible	Reversible	Reversible
Administration route	Oral	Oral	Oral	IV
Frequency	Once daily	Once daily	Twice daily	Bolus plus infusion
Pro-drug	Yes	Yes	No[a]	No
Onset of action	2–8 h	30 min–4 h[b]	30 min–4 h[b]	2 min
Offset of action	7–10 days	7–10 days	3–5 days	30–60 min
CYP drug interaction	CYP2C19	No	CYP3A	No
Approved settings	ACS and stable CAD PCI	ACS undergoing PCI	ACS (full spectrum)	$P2Y_{12}$ receptor inhibitors naïve patients and are not being given a GPI undergoing PCI

[a]Although, most of ticagrelor-mediated antiplatelet effects are direct, approximately 30%–40% are attributed to an active metabolite (AR-C124910XX).
[b]Depending on clinical setting.
ACS, Acute coronary syndrome; *CAD*, Coronary artery disease; *CYP*, cytochrome P450; *CPTP*, cyclopentyltriazolopyrimidine; *GPI*, a glycoprotein IIb/IIIa inhibitor; *IV*, intravenous; *PCI*, percutaneous coronary intervention.

each single drug can achieve and this synergism has been shown to be beneficial in the multitude of clinical trials assessing the optimal antithrombotic regimen in patients undergoing coronary stent implantation.[5–7]

Several oral $P2Y_{12}$ receptor inhibitors (ticlopidine, clopidogrel, prasugrel, and ticagrelor) have been developed to be used in addition to aspirin for the prevention of ischemic events during the acute management and secondary prevention after an MI (Table 13.1). The first available $P2Y_{12}$ receptor inhibitor was the first-generation thienopyridine ticlopidine.[5–7] Although ticlopidine in combination with aspirin showed to be superior compared with either aspirin alone or anticoagulation in combination with aspirin for prevention of thrombotic events in patients undergoing PCI, its use has been largely abandoned due to its frequent side effects, including life-threatening hematologic disorders.[5–7] The following sections will provide an overview on pharmacology and clinical trial development of $P2Y_{12}$ receptor inhibitors currently approved for clinical use, focusing on studies performed in the acute phase of ACS.

Clopidogrel

Clopidogrel (Fig. 13.2) is a second-generation thienopyridine with a more favorable safety profile compared with ticlopidine.[5–7] Further, clopidogrel has a pharmacological advantage over ticlopidine, as it achieves a faster onset on action through administration of a loading dose (LD).[5–7] Clopidogrel is orally administrated and is a pro-drug that requires metabolic transformation in order to exert its antiplatelet effect (Table 13.1).[5–7] After intestinal absorption, approximately 85% of clopidogrel is hydrolyzed by carboxylase to an *inactive* metabolite. The remaining approximately 15% is rapidly metabolized by hepatic cytochrome P450 (CYP) isoenzymes, in particular CYP2C19, in a 2-step oxidation process with the generation of a highly unstable active metabolite which irreversibly binds to the $P2Y_{12}$ receptor (Fig. 13.3).[5–7]

Several clinical trials have shown the benefit of dual antiplatelet therapy (DAPT) with a combination of aspirin and clopidogrel in patients with ACS or undergoing PCI (Table 13.2).[5–7] In the CURE (Clopidogrel in Unstable Angina to Prevent Recurrent Events) trial, the administration of clopidogrel (300 mg LD followed by 75 mg once daily) in addition to aspirin significantly reduced by 20% a composite of death from cardiovascular causes, nonfatal MI or stroke, compared with aspirin alone in patients with NSTE-ACS (n = 12,562), who were medically managed or underwent revascularization (PCI or CABG). However, this occurred at the expense of an increased risk of major bleeding complications. A posthoc analysis of aspirin dose showed that bleeding events were less likely to occur with lower doses of aspirin (≤100 mg) without any trade-off in efficacy. The clinical benefit of DAPT with aspirin and clopidogrel was also shown in a lower-risk population of patients undergoing elective PCI (including patients with ACS) in the CREDO (Clopidogrel for the Reduction of Events During Observation) trial as well as in patients with STEMI in the COMMIT (Clopidogrel and Metoprolol in Myocardial Infarction) and CLARITY (Clopidogrel as Adjunctive Reperfusion Therapy) trials.

Although clopidogrel is still the most widely used $P2Y_{12}$ receptor antagonist, a considerable number of patients still continue to experience recurrent thrombotic events while receiving clopidogrel.[5–7] This risk has been in part attributed to the high interindividual variability which characterizes the response to clopidogrel.[13] Several factors have been associated with clopidogrel response variability, including clinical [i.e., poor absorption, drug-drug interactions, ACS, diabetes mellitus (DM), obesity, chronic kidney disease], genetic (i.e., CYP polymorphisms) and cellular (i.e., accelerated platelet turnover, reduced CYP3A4 metabolic activity, or upregulation of $P2Y_{12}$ pathway) factors.[14] Pharmacodynamic studies have shown that approximately 30% to 40% of patients have high platelet reactivity (HPR) while on-clopidogrel treatment, which translates into worse outcomes.[13] Overall, these observations underscore the need for more potent antiplatelet agents for the treatment of MI patients.

Prasugrel

Prasugrel is an irreversible orally administered third-generation thienopyridine. It is a pro-drug which, after intestinal absorption, requires a single-step oxidation process through hepatic CYP in order to generate its active metabolite (Table 13.1 and Fig. 13.3).[5–7,13] Even though prasugrel's active metabolite has the same *in vitro* affinity for the $P2Y_{12}$

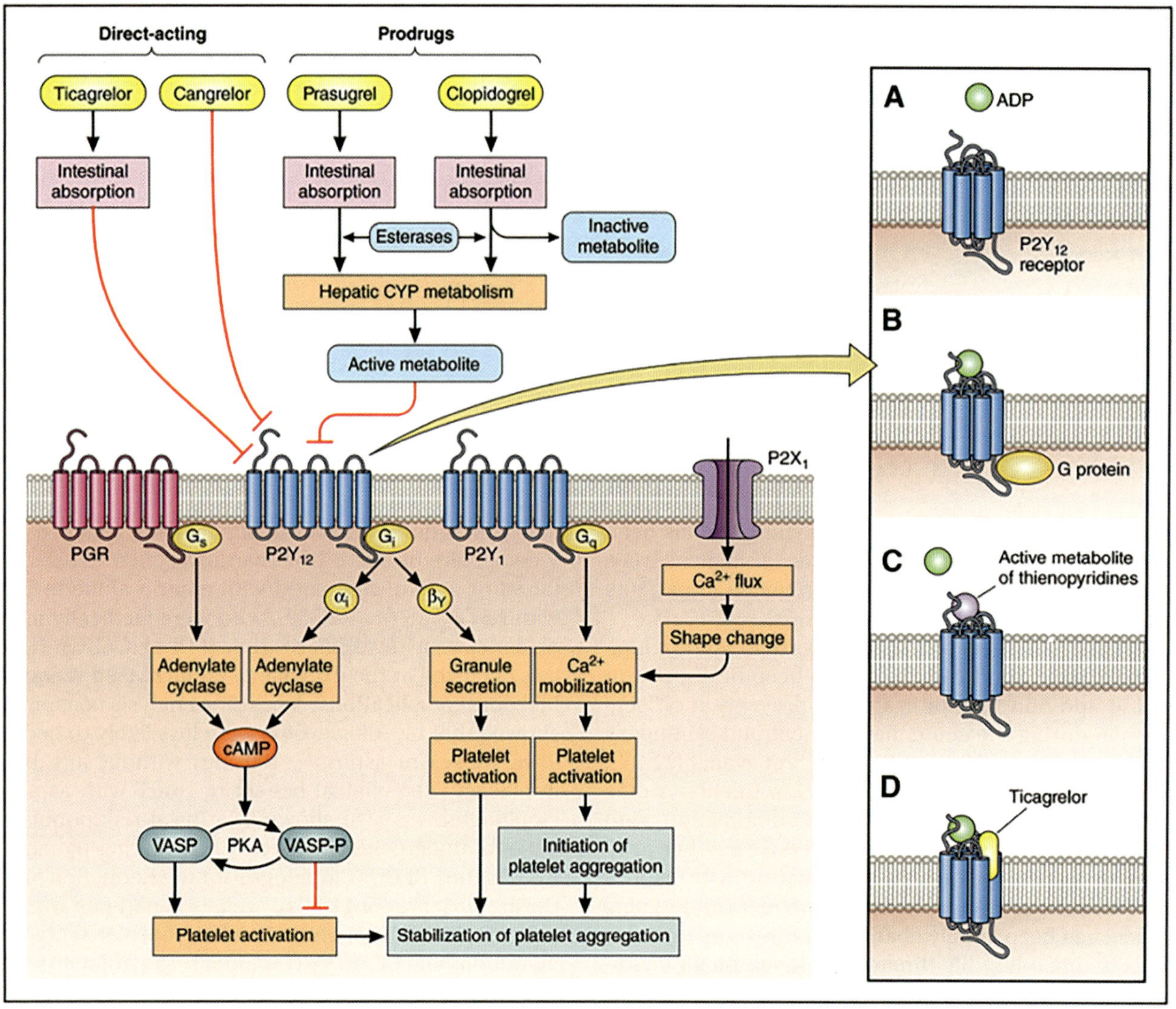

FIG. 13.3 **Mechanisms of action and binding properties of $P2Y_{12}$ inhibitors.** Left, Mechanism of action. Activation of the $P2Y_{12}$ receptor inhibits adenylyl cyclase, causing a decrease in cAMP and phosphorylated (P) vasodilator-stimulated phosphoprotein (VASP) levels, and activation of $P2Y_{12}$ causes an increase in intracellular Ca^{2+} levels. These changes promote platelet aggregation by altering the ligand-binding properties of the glycoprotein IIb/IIIa receptor. Inhibition of the $P2Y_{12}$ receptor therefore suppresses platelet activation. Clopidogrel and prasugrel are oral prodrugs requiring hepatic metabolism to generate an active metabolite that irreversibly inhibits the $P2Y_{12}$ receptor. Ticagrelor is a direct-acting (no metabolism required) oral agent that reversibly inhibits the $P2Y_{12}$ receptor. Cangrelor is a direct-acting intravenous agent that reversibly inhibits the $P2Y_{12}$ receptor. Right, Binding properties. (A) ADP binds to the $P2Y_{12}$ receptor, which (B) leads to a conformational change of the receptor and to G-protein activation. (C) The active metabolite of thienopyridines occupies the ADP-binding site on the $P2Y_{12}$ receptor. Binding is irreversible, which renders the receptor nonfunctional for the life of the platelet. (D) Ticagrelor binds reversibly to the $P2Y_{12}$ receptor at a site that is distinct from the ADP-binding site. *CYP*, Cytochrome P450; *PGR*, prostaglandin receptor; *PKA*, protein kinase A. (Adapted with permission from Angiolillo DJ, Rollini F, Storey RF, et al. International expert consensus on switching platelet $P2Y_{12}$ receptor-inhibiting therapies. *Circulation*. 2017;136(20):1955–1975.)

receptor as clopidogrel's active metabolite, the metabolic conversion of prasugrel is more efficient, leading to higher *in vivo* availability.[5–7,13] These pharmacological properties translate into a more prompt (faster onset of action), potent (enhanced platelet inhibition) and predictable (lower inter-individual variability in effects) antiplatelet effect compared with clopidogrel.[5–7,13] In particular, a 60 mg LD of prasugrel achieves 50% platelet inhibition by 30 minutes and 80% to 90% inhibition by 2 hours.[5–7,13]

In the TRITON-TIMI 38 (Trial to Assess Improvement in Therapeutic Outcomes by Optimizing Platelet Inhibition with Prasugrel-Thrombolysis in Myocardial Infarction 38) trial, patients (n = 13,608) with moderate-to-high-risk ACS scheduled for PCI were randomized to receive either prasugrel 60 mg LD followed by 10 mg daily maintenance dose (MD) or clopidogrel 300 mg LD and 75 mg daily MD, in addition to aspirin (Tables 13.3 and 13.e1). Prasugrel significantly reduced the primary efficacy end point (a composite of cardiovascular death, nonfatal MI, or nonfatal stroke) as compared with clopidogrel over a median follow-up of 14.5 months (9.9% vs. 12.1%; hazard ratio [HR], 0.81; 95% confidence interval [CI], 0.73–0.90; $P < .001$), mainly driven by a reduction in nonfatal MI. A significant 52% reduction in the rate of stent thrombosis, irrespective of stent type, and 34% in need for urgent target vessel revascularization was also achieved by prasugrel.

This effect was hampered by significantly increased rates of noncoronary artery bypass graft (CABG)-related thrombolysis in myocardial infarction (TIMI) major

TABLE 13.2 Major Clinical Trials on Clopidogrel in Patients with Acute Coronary Syndrome

TRIAL	PATIENTS (N)	SETTING	TREATMENT ARMS	PRIMARY ENDPOINT	RESULTS
CURE	12,562	NSTE-ACS	Aspirin + clopidogrel vs. aspirin	CV death, nonfatal MI, or stroke at 1 year	9.3% vs. 11.4% HR, 0.80 [0.72–0.90] *P* < .001
PCI-CURE	2658	NSTE-ACS treated with PCI	Aspirin + clopidogrel vs. aspirin	CV death, MI, or revascularization within 30 days	4.5% vs. 6.4% RR, 0.70 [0.50–0.97] *P* = .03
CREDO	2116	Patients undergoing PCI (including ACS)	Aspirin + clopidogrel vs. aspirin	CV death, MI, or stroke at 1 year	8.5% vs. 11.5% RRR, 26.9% [3.9–44.4%] *P* = .02
COMMIT	45,852	STEMI	Aspirin + clopidogrel vs. aspirin	Death, reinfarction, or stroke at 28 days	9.2% vs. 10.1% OR, 0.91 [0.86–0.97] *P* = .002
CLARITY-TIMI 28	3491	STEMI	Aspirin + clopidogrel + FA vs. Aspirin + FA	Occluded infarct-related artery, death, or recurrent MI before angiography	15.0% vs. 21.7% OR, 0.64 [0.53–0.76] *P* < .001
CURRENT-OASIS 7	25,087	ACS referred for an early invasive strategy	Aspirin + double-dose clopidogrel vs. aspirin + standard-dose clopidogrel	CV death, MI, or stroke at 30 days	4.2% vs. 4.4% HR, 0.94 [0.83–1.06] *P* = .30
POPular AGE[45]	1002	Patients ≥70 years with NSTE-ACS	Aspirin + clopidogrel vs. aspirin + ticagrelor	NACE and PLATO major and minor bleeding at 1 year	NACE: ARD −4%, 95% CI, −10.0–1.4; $P_{noninferiority}$ = 0.03 Bleeding: 18% vs. 24%, HR, 0.71 [0.54–0.94] *P* = .02
STOPDAPT 2 ACS[40]	4169	ACS who underwent successful PCI with EES	Aspirin + clopidogrel for 1–2 months followed by clopidogrel monotherapy vs. aspirin + clopidogrel for 12 months	CV death, MI, any stroke, definite stent thrombosis, or bleeding at 12 months	3.2% vs. 2.8%, ARD −0.37%, 95% CI, −0.68–1.42; $P_{noninferiority}$ = 0.06

Clopidogrel was given as a 300-mg loading dose and then 75 mg daily in CURE, PCI-CURE, CREDO, COMMIT, and CLARITY-TIMI 28. In CURRENT-OASIS 7, double-dose clopidogrel was defined as a 600-mg loading dose and 150 mg once daily for 7 days, followed by 75 mg once daily; standard-dose clopidogrel was defined as a 300-mg loading dose, followed by 75 mg once daily. Patients were also randomized to receive low-dose (75–100 mg/day) or high-dose (300–325 mg/day) aspirin.
ACS, Acute coronary syndrome; ARD, absolute risk difference; *CV*, cardiovascular; *EES*, everolimus-eluting stents; *FA*, fibrinolytic agent; *HR*, hazard ratio; *MI*, myocardial infarction; *NSTE-ACS*, non-ST-segment elevation acute coronary syndrome; *NACE*, net clinical benefit; *OR*, odds ratio; *PLATO*, PLATelet inhibition and patient Outcomes; *PCI*, percutaneous coronary intervention; *RR*, relative risk; *RRR*, relative risk reduction; *STEMI*, ST-segment elevation myocardial infarction.

bleeding; CABG-related TIMI major bleeding, life-threatening bleeding, and fatal bleeding were also increased. However, the net clinical benefit was still in favor of prasugrel-treated patients. The benefit achieved by prasugrel over clopidogrel was consistent in patients with STEMI and was particularly notable in patients with DM and in those experiencing recurrent events.[5–7] Clinical outcomes with prasugrel treatment were not affected by CYP polymorphisms or drug interfering with CYP2C19 enzymes.[13] Also, results were consistent irrespective of aspirin dose.[5–7] In contrast, a neutral effect was found in low body weight patients (<60 kg) and elderly (≥75 years), and a net harm was shown in patients with a history of stroke or transient ischemic attack.[5–7] Among patients (*n* = 346) undergoing isolated CABG and receiving the study drug before the procedure, although there was a higher 12-hours chest tube blood loss, a reduction in all-cause and cardiovascular mortality with prasugrel compared with clopidogrel was shown.[5–7]

The efficacy of prasugrel compared to clopidogrel in medically managed ACS was tested in the TRILOGY-ACS (TaRgeted platelet Inhibition to cLarify the Optimal strateGy to medicallY manage Acute Coronary Syndromes) trial (Table 13.2). Aspirin-treated patients (*n* = 9326) with a NSTE ACS in whom medical management was chosen were randomized to receive either prasugrel (30 mg LD followed by 10 mg MD) or clopidogrel (300 mg LD and 75 mg MD). Prasugrel MD was adjusted to 5 mg for patients with age ≥75 years or who weighed less than 60 kg. Clopidogrel pretreatment prior to randomization occurred in approximately 96% of patients. The primary endpoint was a composite of cardiac death, MI, or stroke among patients with age <75 years (*n* = 7243). After a median follow-up of 17 months, there were no differences between prasugrel and clopidogrel in the primary ischemic endpoint (13.9% vs. 16%; HR, 0.91; 95% CI, 0.79–1.05; *P* = .21). Importantly, the rates of non-CABG-related severe or life-threatening bleeding according to Global Use of Strategies to Open Occluded Coronary Arteries (GUSTO) criteria, TIMI major bleeding, and intracranial bleeding were overall low and similar between groups. Moreover, in the secondary analysis on patients (*n* = 2083) aged 75 years or older, prasugrel 5 mg was not associated with an ischemic benefit compared to standard clopidogrel, although there was no increase in bleeding. Importantly, in the prespecified

TABLE 13.3 Major Completed Phase III Clinical Trials on Novel Antiplatelet Agents in ACS

TRIAL	PATIENTS (N)	SETTING	TREATMENT ARMS	PRIMARY ENDPOINT	RESULTS
TRITON-TIMI 38	13,608	ACS patients undergoing PCI	Aspirin + prasugrel vs. aspirin + clopidogrel	CV death, nonfatal, MI, or nonfatal stroke at 14.5 months	9.9% vs. 12.1% HR, 0.81 [0.73–0.90] *P* < .001
TRILOGY-ACS	9326	Medically managed NSTE-ACS	Aspirin + prasugrel vs. aspirin + clopidogrel	CV death, MI, or stroke at 17 months in patients with age <75 years	13.9% vs. 16.0% HR, 0.91 [0.79–1.05] *P* = .21
ACCOAST	4033	NSTE-ACS scheduled for angiography	pretreatment with prasugrel 30 mg vs. placebo	CV death, MI, stroke, GPI bailout, or urgent revascularization at 7 days	10.0% vs. 9.8% HR, 1.02 [0.84–1.25] *P* = .81
PLATO	18,624	ACS	Aspirin + ticagrelor vs. aspirin + clopidogrel	Death from vascular causes, MI, or stroke at 12 months	9.8% vs. 11.7% HR, 0.84 [0.77–0.92] *P* < .001
TICAKOREA[52]	800	ACS	Aspirin + ticagrelor vs. aspirin + clopidogrel	PLATO major and minor bleeding at 1 year	11.7% vs. 5.3% HR, 2.26 [1.34–3.79] *P* = .002
ISAR-REACT 5[27]	4018	ACS	Aspirin + ticagrelor vs. aspirin + prasugrel	Death, MI, or stroke at 12 months	9.3% vs. 6.9% HR, 1.36 [1.09–1.70] *P* = .006
DUBIUS[28]	1449	NSTE-ACS	Pretreatment with ticagrelor vs. No pretreatment with ticagrelor or prasugrel	Vascular death, MI, stroke, and BARC type 3, 4, and 5 bleeding	2.9% vs. 3.3%, ARD −0.46; [−2.90–1.90]
CHAMPION PHOENIX	11,145	Patients undergoing PCI	Aspirin + clopidogrel + cangrelor vs. aspirin + clopidogrel	Death from any cause, MI, IDR, and stent thrombosis at 48 h	4.7% vs. 5.9% OR, 0.78 [0.66–0.93] *P* = .005
TRACER	12,944	NSTE-ACS	standard APT + vorapaxar vs. standard APT + placebo	CV death, MI, stroke, recurrent ischemia with rehospitalization, or urgent coronary revascularization at 2 years	18.5% vs. 19.9% HR, 0.92 [0.85–1.01] *P* = .07
TRA 2P-TIMI 50	26,449	Patients with history of MI, ischemic stroke, or PAD	standard APT + vorapaxar vs. standard APT + placebo	CV death, MI, or stroke at 36 months	9.3% vs. 10.5% HR, 0.87 [0.80–0.94] *P* < .001

ACS, Acute coronary syndrome; *APT*, antiplatelet therapy; *ARD*, absolute risk reduction; *BARC*, bleeding academic research consortium; *CV*, cardiovascular; *GPI*, glycoprotein IIb/IIIa inhibitor; *HR*, hazard ratio; *IDR*, ischemia-driven revascularization; *MI*, myocardial infarction; *NSTE*, non-ST-elevation; *OR*, odds ratio; *PAD*, peripheral artery disease; *PLATO*, PLATelet inhibition and patient Outcomes; *PCI*, percutaneous coronary intervention.

sub-study on patients <75 years who underwent angiography before randomization (n = 3085), prasugrel led to a significant reduction in the risks of the composite primary endpoint compared with clopidogrel, with a trend toward increased risk of major bleeding. These data suggest that when angiography is performed for ACS and anatomic coronary disease is confirmed, the benefits and risks of a more intense antiplatelet therapy exist whether the patient is treated with drugs or PCI.[5–7]

Ticagrelor

Ticagrelor is an orally administered cyclopentyltriazolopyrimidine (CPTP), which directly and reversibly inhibits the platelet $P2Y_{12}$ receptor (Table 13.1 and Fig. 13.3).[5–7] Ticagrelor is not a pro-drug and does not require metabolic activation, although approximately 30%–40% of its antiplatelet effects are attributed to an active metabolite (AR-C124910XX) generated through the hepatic CYP3A system (CYP3A4 and CYP3A5).[5–7] Ticagrelor does not bind directly to the platelet ADP binding site on the $P2Y_{12}$ receptor but reversibly binds to a distinct site on the receptor and prevents ADP from causing activation of the $P2Y_{12}$ pathway in a noncompetitive fashion through allosteric modulation.[5–7] Ticagrelor is rapidly absorbed after oral administration and has a half-life of 7 to 12 hours, thus requiring twice daily dosing. Compared to clopidogrel, ticagrelor achieves a faster, more potent, and more predictable antiplatelet effect, with a faster offset of action.[5–7]

The efficacy and safety of ticagrelor in patients with ACS were evaluated in the phase III PLATO (Platelet Inhibition and Patient Outcomes) trial (Table 13.3). There are key differences between the PLATO and TRITON-TIMI 38 trial designs, as summarized in Table 13.e1. In the PLATO trial, ACS patients (n = 18,624) were randomized to receive either ticagrelor (180 mg LD followed by 90 mg b.i.d. MD) or clopidogrel (300–600 mg LD followed by 75 mg daily MD) in addition to aspirin for 12 months. The trial embraced the whole spectrum of patients with ACS, including both those intended to undergo invasive and noninvasive management. Patients pretreated with clopidogrel were eligible for study entry and study drug LD administration occurred before or after angiography, but before PCI. Compared with clopidogrel, ticagrelor significantly reduced the primary endpoint (a composite of death from vascular causes, MI, or stroke) at 12 months (9.8% vs. 11.7%; HR, 0.84; 95% CI, 0.77–0.92; $P < .001$), including a significant 21% reduction in cardiovascular death and a 16% reduction of MI. Ticagrelor treatment also significantly reduced the rates of definite or probable stent thrombosis.

Even though protocol-defined major bleeding was similar between groups (11.6% vs. 11.2%; $P = .43$), ticagrelor led to a significantly increased hazard of non-CABG-related PLATO and TIMI major bleeding, as well as fatal intracranial hemorrhage. Importantly, the benefit of ticagrelor over clopidogrel was consistent across multiple prespecified subgroups, including patients treated initially with a noninvasive or invasive (followed by PCI or CABG) strategy.[5–7] Accordingly, patients with STEMI, DM, >75 years of age, <60 kg, with prior stroke or transient ischemic attack, with recurrent cardiovascular events, chronic kidney disease, and with or without CYP2C19 loss-of-function polymorphisms were also favored by ticagrelor therapy. Bleeding outcomes were also consistent across subgroups, with no groups experiencing harm with ticagrelor.[5–7]

Importantly, a geographic interaction was found in the trial, with patients enrolled in North America not receiving a reduction in the primary endpoint by ticagrelor treatment. While these findings can be attributed to play of chance, a posthoc assessment found this to be possibly attributed to the use of high-dose (≥300 mg/daily) aspirin, which was more common in North America.[15] Although subsequent studies failed to demonstrate any effect of aspirin dosing on the pharmacokinetic and pharmacodynamic profile of ticagrelor, the use of low-dose aspirin (≤100 mg) is currently recommended in ticagrelor-treated patients.[16,17]

Non-$P2Y_{12}$-mediated effects of ticagrelor related to increased plasma levels of adenosine have been described.[15] Under normal conditions, adenosine has a very short half-life and is rapidly up-taken by red blood cells and metabolized.[15] Ticagrelor has been shown to significantly inhibit cellular uptake of adenosine by blocking the sodium-dependent equilabrative nucleoside transporters (ENT 1) and thus increasing adenosine plasma concentrations.[15] Adenosine has multiple cardiac and extra-cardiac properties, which include inhibition of platelet aggregation (mainly through the activation of A_{2A} G-coupled receptors), arterial vasodilation, reduction in inflammatory response, negative chronotropic and dromotropic effect, stimulation of pulmonary vagal C fibers mediating the sensation of dyspnea, and a role in the regulation of kidney glomerular filtration.[15] Although ticagrelor does not directly act on adenosine receptors, it enhances biological effects of adenosine, which may contribute to the overall benefits of ticagrelor, including reduction in cardiovascular mortality, as well as to the non bleeding side effects of ticagrelor, such as higher incidence of dyspnea (15%–22% of ticagrelor treated patients) and ventricular pauses and increased levels of creatinine and uric acid during treatment compared with clopidogrel (Fig. 13.4).[15] These side effects are usually self-limiting and have no impact on clinical outcomes but were responsible for the higher discontinuation rate of ticagrelor compared with clopidogrel in the PLATO trial. However, some studies have challenged the relationship between increased

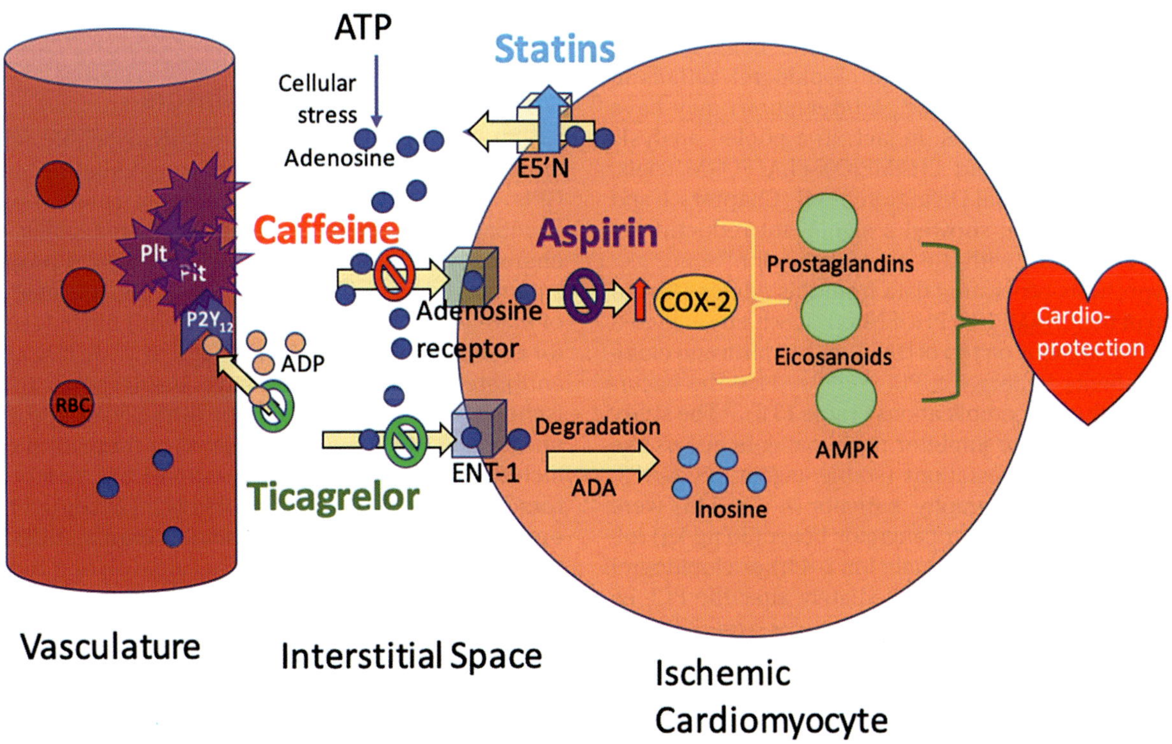

FIG. 13.4 The adenosine-mediated pleiotropic effects of ticagrelor and its interactions with statins, aspirin, and caffeine. *AMPK,* adenosine monophosphate-activated protein kinase. *ATP*, Adenosine triphosphate; *ADP*, adenosine diphosphate; *ADA*, adenosine deaminase; *COX-2*, cyclooxygenase 2; *ENT-1*, equilibrate nucleoside transporter-1; *E5′N*, ecto5′-nucleotidase; *Plt*, platelet; *RBC*, red blood cell; (Adapted with permission from From Triska J, Maitra N, Deshotels MR, et al. A comprehensive review of the pleiotropic effects of ticagrelor. *Cardiovasc Drugs Ther*. 2024;38(4):775–797.)

circulating adenosine levels and the development of ticagrelor-induced dyspnea.[18] Importantly, no effect of ticagrelor on specific pulmonary function parameters, such as spirometry, lung volumes, diffusion capacity, and pulse oximetry, has been shown.[15]

Cangrelor

Although prasugrel and ticagrelor are characterized by more prompt, potent, and predictable antiplatelet effects leading to greater clinical efficacy over clopidogrel, these drugs still present limitations inherent to orally administered antiplatelet agents, including delayed pharmacodynamic effect in patients with STEMI, slow offset of action, and inability to exert reliable and predictable platelet inhibition in patients hemodynamically unstable or sedated, intubated, in shock, under therapeutic hypothermia or with nausea or vomiting.[5–7] Cangrelor is an analog of adenosine triphosphate (ATP) and is the first reversible intravenous $P2Y_{12}$ inhibitor. It directly binds to the $P2Y_{12}$ receptor in a predominantly competitive manner without the need for being metabolized (Table 13.1 and Fig. 13.3).[19] Cangrelor achieves very potent (>80%) antiplatelet effects reaching steady-state concentrations within few minutes and is characterized by a linear dose-dependent pharmacokinetic profile which leads to very stable pharmacodynamic effects. Owing to its very short half-life (3–5 min), cangrelor has a fast offset of action, with platelet aggregation returning to baseline levels within 30–60 minutes.[19]

The role of cangrelor as adjunctive antiplatelet therapy in patients requiring PCI has been tested in three large-scale phase III clinical trials. Although the first two trials, namely the CHAMPION (Cangrelor vs. Standard Therapy to Achieve Optimal Management of Platelet Inhibition)-PCI and the CHAMPION-PLATFORM trials, were interrupted for futility and failed to document any ischemic benefit of cangrelor over DAPT with aspirin and clopidogrel, pitfalls in study end point definitions (i.e., MI definition) may have contributed to these results. In fact, in a pooled analysis of the CHAMPION-PCI and CHAMPION-PLATFORM trials, which used the Universal Definition of MI (Chapters 1 and 2) to define MI events, showed a significant reduction in the primary endpoint with the use of cangrelor.[19]

The hypothesis-generating data from this analysis led to the design of the CHAMPION PHOENIX trial, which evaluated if addition of cangrelor on top of DAPT with aspirin and clopidogrel in patients undergoing PCI could reduce the occurrence acute ischemic complications (Table 13.3).[19] The study included $P2Y_{12}$ receptor inhibitor naïve patients across the spectrum of CAD manifestations (stable angina, NSTE-ACS, and STEMI). After angiography, patients (n = 11,145) were randomized to receive either cangrelor bolus (30 µg/kg) followed by infusion (4 µg/kg per min for 2–4 h) or clopidogrel LD (300 or 600 mg before or immediately after the PCI, as per institutional standard). In the cangrelor arm, patients received 600 mg of clopidogrel at the end of infusion. The primary efficacy endpoint was a composite of death from any cause, MI, ischemia-drive revascularization, and stent thrombosis at 48 hours. Adjunctive cangrelor therapy significantly reduced the primary efficacy end point (a composite of death from any cause, MI, ischemia-driven revascularization, and stent thrombosis) at 48 hours (4.7% vs. 5.9%; adjusted odds ratio [OR] with cangrelor, 0.78; 95% CI, 0.66–0.93; P = .005), primarily driven by a reduction in the hazard of MI (3.8% vs. 4.7%; P = .02). The use of cangrelor led to a significant reduction in the rate of stent thrombosis at 48 hours (0.8% vs. 1.4%; OR, 0.62; 95% CI, 0.43–0.90; P = .01). Intra-procedural stent thrombosis, which was shown to be associated with an increase in adverse outcomes at 48 hours and 30 days, was also significantly reduced.

The rate of severe bleeding at 48 hours was not significantly increased by cangrelor with GUSTO criteria, as well as with other definitions of bleeding. However, the rate of major bleeding according to the more sensitive ACUITY criteria was significantly higher in patients treated with cangrelor, primarily driven by a higher incidence of hematoma at the site of vascular access. Overall, the net rate of adverse clinical events (ischemic plus bleeding events) was significantly reduced by the use of cangrelor. The clinical benefit of adjunctive cangrelor therapy was consistent at 30 days and across multiple prespecified subgroups, such as different clinical presentation (stable angina, NSTE-ACS, or STEMI), dose and timing of clopidogrel loading, stent type, and duration of study drug infusion.

These results were further confirmed by a pooled analysis of approximately 25,000 patients enrolled in the three CHAMPION trials, which showed consistent results using the PHOENIX definition of MI.[19] Cangrelor has also been tested as a bridging strategy in patients (n = 210) on thienopyridine treatment (including patients with a recent MI) and requiring CABG, showing high and stable levels of platelet inhibition up to 7 days of infusion, with a rapid offset after discontinuation prior to surgery. This strategy was not associated with an increased risk of major bleeding or side effects before or during CABG, although these findings need to be interpreted with caution as the study was not powered for clinical outcomes.[2,19]

Glycoprotein IIb/IIIa Inhibitors

GP IIb/IIIa inhibitors (GPIs) are only available for intravenous use and include abciximab, eptifibatide, tirofiban.[20] GPIs are classified into two groups: small (eptifibatide, tirofiban) and nonsmall (abciximab) molecules. GPIs are characterized by different pharmacological properties as summarized in Table 13.4. They target the final pathway of platelet aggregation, competing with fibrinogen and vWf for GP IIb/IIIa receptor binding, and provide fast and potent antiplatelet effects.[20] GPIs have been shown to improve ischemic outcomes in patients with STEMI and NSTE-ACS undergoing PCI, even though most of these studies did not include the use of novel generation $P2Y_{12}$ receptor inhibitors.[20] The administration of GPIs is an accepted treatment option in high-risk ACS patients undergoing PCI. However, their role is currently reduced because of their high rates of bleeding complications, as well as the development of alternative treatment strategies with a more favorable safety profile. Indeed, available data support a selective (i.e., bail-out in case of large residual thrombus) rather than a routine use of GPIs for patients with ACS treated with PCI.[20] Intracoronary administration of GPIs has been tested in several small studies and associated with some benefits, as compared with intravenous administration, but these have not been confirmed in large-scale clinical trials.[20]

TABLE 13.4 Pharmacology of Glycoprotein IIb/IIIa Inhibitors

	ABCIXIMAB[a]	EPTIFIBATIDE	TIROFIBAN
Trade name	ReoPro	Integrilin	Aggrastat
Molecule	Fragment antigen binding (Fab)[7E3]	Synthetic peptide	Nonpeptide mimetic
Molecular weight	approximately 50,000	approximately 800	approximately 500
Stoichiometry (drug to GP IIb/IIIa)	approximately 1.5:1	>>100:1	>>100:1
Binding	Noncompetitive	Competitive	Competitive
Half-life	Plasma: 10–15 h Biologic: 12–24 h	Plasma: 2–2.5 h Biologic = plasma	Plasma: 2–2.5 h Biologic = plasma
PCI dosing	Bolus: 0.25 mg/kg (10–60 min) Infusion: 0.125 µg/kg/min (12 h)	Bolus: 180 µg/kg[b] + 180 µg/kg (after 10 min) Infusion: 2 µg/kg/min (24–48 h)[c]	Bolus: 25 µg/kg (30 min) Infusion: 0.10 µg/kg/min (48 h)
Renal adjustment	No	Bolus: 180 µg/kg Infusion: 1 µg/kg/min (24–48 h)	Bolus: 12.5 µg/kg (30 min) Infusion: 0.10 µg/kg/min (48 h)

[a]Since 2018, the original drug maker is no longer supplying abciximab, but generic formulations are available in some countries.
[b]Started immediately before PCI.
[c]Started immediately after the first bolus.
GP, Glycoprotein; *PCI*, percutaneous coronary intervention.
From Muñiz-Lozano A, Rollini F, Franchi F, Angiolillo DJ. Update on platelet glycoprotein IIb/IIIa inhibitors: recommendations for clinical practice. Ther Adv Cardiovasc Dis. 2013;7(4):197–213. doi:10.1177/1753944713487781.

PAR-1 Antagonists

The serine protease thrombin is one of the most potent platelet activators and the surface of activated platelets is the main source of circulating thrombin Fig. 13.2.[1,2] PARs are a family of G-protein-coupled receptors and, in humans, four types of PARs have been described; PAR-1 and PAR-4 are expressed on human platelets, but PAR-1 has the principal role of mediating platelet activation at low concentrations of thrombin, while PAR-4 reacts only at high concentrations.[1,2] Several PAR1 antagonists have been developed so far,[21,22] of which only vorapaxar has completed phase III clinical investigations and is available for clinical use. Vorapaxar was tested in two large-scale phase III clinical trials: TRACER (Thrombin Receptor Antagonist for Clinical Event Reduction in Acute Coronary Syndrome) and TRA 2°P-TIMI 50 (Thrombin Receptor Antagonist in Secondary Prevention of Atherothrombotic Ischemic Events - TIMI 50) trial (Table 13.3).[23] Although vorapaxar did not have a favorable balance of efficacy and bleeding in the acute management of ACS in the TRACER trial, this PAR-1 antagonist was effective for long-term secondary prevention after MI in TRA 2°P-TIMI 50. In a substudy of the TRA 2°P-TIMI 50, vorapaxar significantly reduced acute limb ischemia and peripheral revascularization but was accompanied by an increased risk of bleeding. Currently, vorapaxar use in clinical practice is predominantly limited to peripheral artery disease.[23,24]

PRACTICAL RECOMMENDATIONS AND GUIDELINES

Guidelines recommendation from the American College of Cardiology (ACC)/American Heart Association (AHA)[16] and the European Society of Cardiology (ESC)[17] for the use of antiplatelet therapy in patients with MI are summarized in Tables 13.5 and 13.6. The following sections will provide practical considerations for the initial management of antiplatelet strategies in patients with NSTE-ACS and STEMI.

Indications and Dosing of Antiplatelet Therapies

Oral Antiplatelet Therapies

Aspirin: Aspirin is the established first-line therapy in patients with ACS. Non-enteric-coated aspirin (150–325 mg) should be administered promptly after presentation in patients with both NSTE-ACS and STEMI and then continued indefinitely irrespective of the treatment strategy. Aspirin LD should preferably be given orally including chewing to ensure complete inhibition of TXA_2-dependent platelet aggregation. However, an intravenous formulation is available in certain countries and can be used as a 300–500 mg dose in patients who are unable to swallow. Even if the optimal dosing regimen for the prevention of cardiovascular events has been the subject of controversy, current evidence suggests the use of low-dose aspirin (≤100 mg) following the initial LD of administration of aspirin. In aspirin-treated patients, the use of nonsteroidal anti-inflammatory drugs should be avoided because of their competition for the COX-1 active site.[16,17]

Clopidogrel: Clopidogrel (300–600 mg LD and 75 mg daily maintenance dose) is currently approved for the treatment of patients with ACS, irrespective of the clinical presentation or the treatment strategy, and in patients undergoing PCI. Although the LD regimen varies according to different guidelines, available data suggest that a 600 mg LD should be preferred in ACS patients undergoing PCI.[16,17] In patients with STEMI treated with fibrinolytics, clopidogrel is also

INITIAL TREATMENT

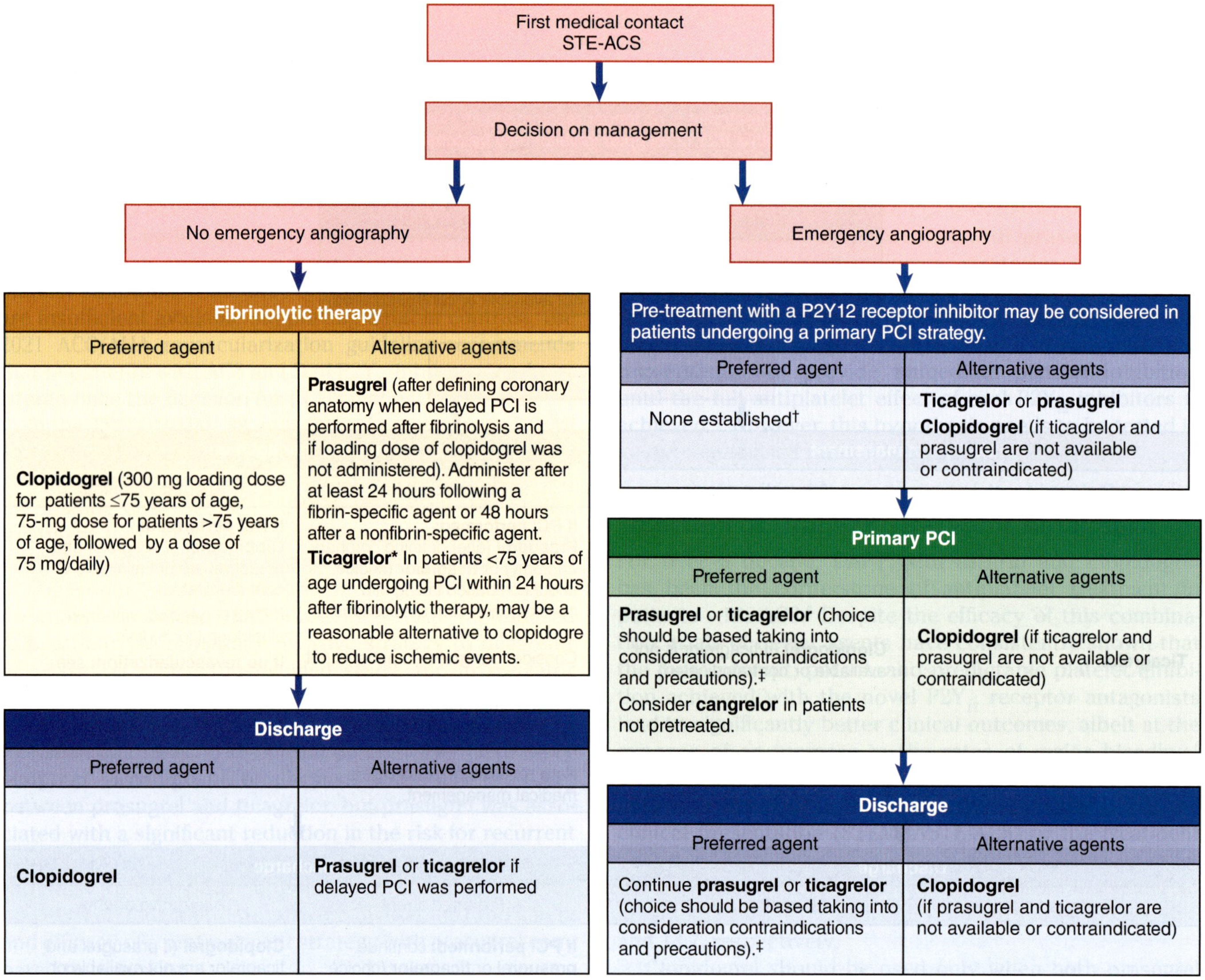

FIG. 13.7 Algorithm for choice of $P2Y_{12}$ receptor antagonists in patients with STE-ACS. *Tested only in few small nonrandomized studies of patients undergoing delayed PCI. †The choice to pretreat with a $P2Y_{12}$ receptor antagonist should be based on the risk/benefit ratio of such approach, taking into consideration the thrombotic and bleeding risk. Early administration of antiplatelet therapy may protect the patient from thrombotic events in the vulnerable period before and immediately after PCI. However, pretreatment may result in an unnecessary excess of platelet inhibition and related bleeding risk when patients do not undergo PCI, such as patients found not to have coronary artery disease or patients requiring CABG. ‡If patient was previously treated with clopidogrel, switching to prasugrel or ticagrelor should be considered. *STE-ACS*, ST-segment elevation acute coronary syndrome *PCI*, percutaneous coronary intervention.

in a smaller randomized trial (n = 1230), there was no difference between ticagrelor and prasugrel in the primary efficacy endpoint (a composite of death, reinfarction, urgent target vessel revascularization, stroke, or serious bleeding requiring transfusion or prolonging hospitalization) at 7 days (4.0% vs. 4.1%; OR, 0.98; 95% CI; 0.55–1.73; P = .939).[42]

Based on these data, the 2020 ESC guidelines for the management of ACS in patients presenting without persistent ST-segment recommended that prasugrel should be considered in preference to ticagrelor for NSTE-ACS patients who proceed to PCI.[32] The 2021 ACC/AHA revascularization guideline recommend ticagrelor or prasugrel over clopidogrel but give the same level of recommendation to ticagrelor and prasugrel.[16] Of note, the ACC/AHA guideline provides a specific recommendation in patients undergoing PCI who have a history of stroke or transient ischemic attack, stating that prasugrel should not be administered. In clinical practice, the selection of one drug should also take into account the specific contraindications of each drug and patient characteristics. Although platelet function and genetic testing have been proposed to help identify patients who may benefit from treatment with the novel $P2Y_{12}$ receptor inhibitors, these agents should be used based on clinical grounds. In acute settings, platelet function testing (PFT) and genotyping provide valuable prognostic data for patients receiving $P2Y_{12}$ inhibitor treatment after PCI for ACS, predicting cardiovascular risks such as bleeding and ischemic events. Specifically, PFTs can guide both escalation and de-escalation of $P2Y_{12}$ inhibitor treatment, while genotyping is recommended only for de-escalation.[43,44]

Given its reversible binding to the $P2Y_{12}$ receptor and its plasma half-life of 8 to 12 hours, ticagrelor requires twice/daily administration.[5–7] Therefore, patients with poor compliance may not be optimal candidates for ticagrelor, and the use of an irreversible inhibitor, which requires only a once daily administration with $P2Y_{12}$ receptors blocked for the lifetime of a platelet (7–10 days), could be the preferred choice. However, the reversible binding property of ticagrelor also translates into a faster offset of action, leading to a shorter wash-out period before surgery and potentially to reduced peri-procedural-related bleeding.[5–7] It may also be hypothesized that reversible agents with twice daily dosing such as ticagrelor, which provides stable plasma concentrations, may enable more effective antiplatelet effects in patients with high platelet turnover rates, such as those with MI or diabetes mellitus, characterized by higher levels of reticulated platelets, which are hyperreactive and associated with worse outcomes.[5–7]

The type of management strategy should also be considered in the choice of the $P2Y_{12}$ receptor inhibitor. In patients with MI who are treated with PCI all three agents, clopidogrel, prasugrel, and ticagrelor, can be used.[5–7] While in patients with STEMI the probability of performing PCI is usually high, thus allowing to choose among all drugs, in patients with NSTE-ACS, either the choice to pretreat or uncertainties about the following management strategy can limit the choice between clopidogrel and ticagrelor. These agents, but not prasugrel, are approved for pretreatment and for treatment of NSTE-ACS patients who are medically managed.[5–7] In this latter scenario, ticagrelor represents the first-line treatment due to the benefit showed over clopidogrel in the medically managed subgroup of the PLATO trial.[5–7]

Elderly patients with ACS represent a population of interest as their bleeding risk is substantially higher than young patients, yielding a different risk/benefit balance when selecting antiplatelet agents. The Optimization of Antiplatelet Treatment in High-risk Elderly (POPular AGE) trial randomized patients ≥70 years old with NSTE-ACS (n = 1002) to clopidogrel-based DAPT or a potent-$P2Y_{12}$-based DAPT (ticagrelor or prasugrel) strategy.[45] At 1 year, compared to potent-$P2Y_{12}$-based DAPT, clopidogrel-based DAPT significantly reduced the rate of bleeding without an increase in the composite of all-cause death, MI, and stroke. Moreover, in the Swedish Web-System for Enhancement and Development of Evidence-Based Care in Heart Disease Evaluated According to Recommended Therapies (SWEDEHEART) registry, in patients ≥80 years, ticagrelor use among elderly patients with MI was associated with a higher risk of bleeding and death compared with clopidogrel, but with a lower risk of MI.[46]

When to Use an Intravenous Antiplatelet Agent

The ACC/AHA revascularization and ESC guidelines provide a similar recommendation, stating that in patients with ACS undergoing PCI with large thrombus burden, no-reflow, or slow flow, intravenous GPI agents are reasonable to improve procedural success.[16,32,47] The ESC guidelines emphasize that GPI should not be used if the coronary anatomy is unknown.

Most recent guidelines have added cangrelor among their recommended antiplatelet agents. The ACC/AHA revascularization and ESC guidelines provide similar recommendations, stating that in patients undergoing PCI who are $P2Y_{12}$ inhibitor naïve, intravenous cangrelor may be reasonable to reduce periprocedural ischemic events.

In clinical practice, intravenous antiplatelet agents could be a reasonable option in patients with high-risk NSTE-ACS or STEMI. In particular, because of its pharmacological properties and favorable safety profile, cangrelor could be the agent of choice, especially in combination with ticagrelor, given the practicality of switching between these two agents. Nevertheless, GPIs (preferably bolus with or without short duration of infusion) can be considered in patients with high-thrombotic burden, including patients with stent thrombosis and recurrent MI while on DAPT, as well as for bail-out.

A PD study randomized $P2Y_{12}$ naïve, troponin-negative patients with ACS (n = 100) to crushed ticagrelor (180 mg) or eptifibatide bolus plus clopidogrel (600 mg) at the time of PCI.[48] Eptifibatide plus clopidogrel was associated with lower rates of high platelet reactivity and periprocedural MI than crusher ticagrelor, without differences in hemoglobin between groups. The clinical implications of these findings are unknown as these strategies have not been compared in outcome-based studies.

Switching $P2Y_{12}$ Receptor Antagonists

Switching $P2Y_{12}$ inhibiting therapies occurs very commonly in clinical practice, particularly in the acute setting of patients presenting with an MI.[5–7] Several circumstances may lead clinicians to switch antiplatelet agents in the acute phase of an MI. Switching from clopidogrel to a newer agent usually occurs in patients who are pretreated with clopidogrel due to the better clinical profile of prasugrel and ticagrelor.[5–7] Switching from clopidogrel to ticagrelor occurred in nearly half of the patients enrolled in the PLATO trial, which showed consistent safety and efficacy results irrespective of prior exposure to clopidogrel. In the trial, patients randomized to ticagrelor therapy were treated with a 180 mg LD irrespective of the timing of the last dose of clopidogrel. Accordingly, a similar approach should be applied in clinical practice whenever switching from clopidogrel to ticagrelor in the acute phase of MI (Fig. 13.8).

Switching from clopidogrel to prasugrel was not explored in the TRITON TIMI 38 trial. Data from registries have not shown any major safety concerns (i.e., bleeding) related to switching.[5–7] Surrogate data from dedicated pharmacodynamic studies showed that patients pretreated with clopidogrel can switch to prasugrel, which leads to enhanced levels of platelet inhibition. These are achieved more promptly when switching using a 60-mg LD rather than a 10-mg MD, and without any drug interactions, irrespective of whether a patient was on maintenance 75 mg/d therapy or recently exposed to a 600-mg LD of clopidogrel. Therefore, administering a 60-mg LD should be the strategy to use when switching from clopidogrel to prasugrel in patients with acute MI.[5–7]

Switching from a novel $P2Y_{12}$ receptor inhibitor to clopidogrel occurs very commonly in clinical practice but with limited data to support this approach.[5–7] Reduced costs associated with a generic formulation of clopidogrel as well as concerns about bleeding with prasugrel and ticagrelor remain key reasons for switching to clopidogrel. In the absence of clinical studies investigating the effects of such strategy based on pharmacodynamic

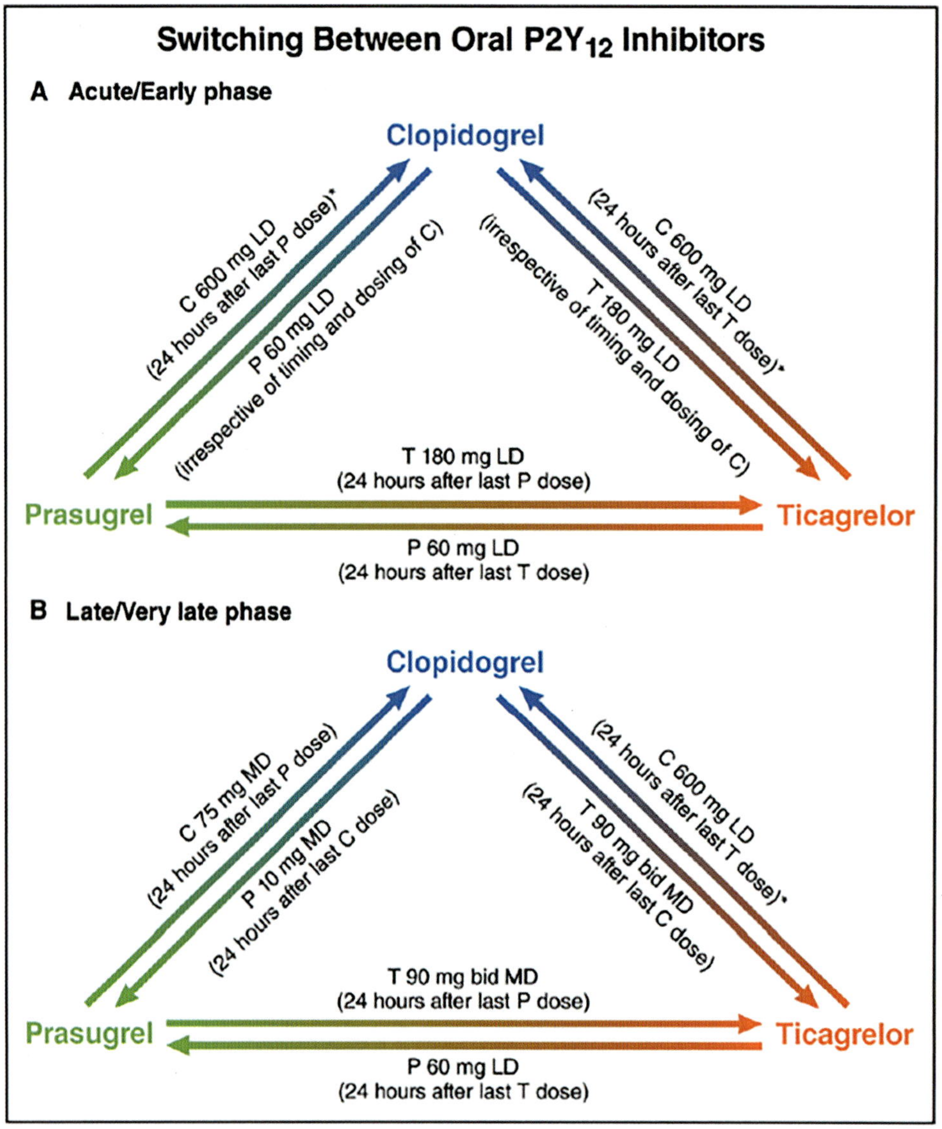

FIG. 13.8 Consensus recommendations on switching between oral P2Y12 inhibitors. (**A**), Switching between oral agents in the acute/early phase. In the acute/early phase (≤30 days from the index event), switching should occur with the administration of a loading dose (LD) in most cases, with the exception of patients who are deescalating therapy because of bleeding or bleeding concerns, in whom a maintenance dose (MD) of clopidogrel (C) should be considered. Timing of switching should be 24 hours after the last dose of a given drug, with the exception of when escalating to prasugrel (P) or ticagrelor (T), when the LD can be given regardless of the timing and dosing of the previous clopidogrel regimen. *Consider de-escalation with clopidogrel 75-mg. (**B**), Switching between oral agents in the late/very late phase. In the late/very late phase (>30 days from the index event), switching should occur with the administration of an MD 24 hours after the last dose of a given drug, with the exception of patients changing from ticagrelor to prasugrel therapy, for whom an LD should be considered. De-escalation from ticagrelor to clopidogrel should occur with administration of an LD 24 hours after the last dose of ticagrelor (but in patients in whom de-escalation occurs because of bleeding or bleeding concerns, an MD of clopidogrel should be considered). *Consider de-escalation with clopidogrel 75-mg MD (24 hours after last prasugrel or ticagrelor dose) in patients with bleeding or bleeding concerns. (*With permission from: Angiolillo DJ, Rollini F, Storey RF, Bhatt DL, James S, Schneider DJ, Sibbing D, So DYF, Trenk D, Alexopoulos D, Gurbel PA, Hochholzer W, De Luca L, Bonello L, Aradi D, Cuisset T, Tantry US, Wang TY, Valgimigli M, Waksman R, Mehran R, Montalescot G, Franchi F, Price MJ. International Expert Consensus on Switching Platelet P2Y12 Receptor-Inhibiting Therapies. Circulation. 2017;136(20):1955–1975.* doi: 10.1161/CIRCULATIONAHA.117.031164.)

considerations, whenever switching from prasugrel or ticagrelor is required, clopidogrel should be administered with a 600-mg LD, given its unpredictable platelet inhibitory profile.[5–7]

Registry data indicate that switches between novel $P2Y_{12}$ receptor inhibitors occur rarely, ranging from 2% to 4% of patients[5–7] In this setting, clinical data are lacking and also pharmacodynamic studies are limited. However, switching from ticagrelor to prasugrel has shown to be associated with an acute (24–48 hours) increase in platelet reactivity, potentially due to a drug interaction, which is reduced with the administration of a 60-mg LD. Conversely, small PD investigations showed that platelet inhibition is enhanced when switching from prasugrel to ticagrelor. Based on the best available evidence, the administration of an LD is preferred when switching between new $P2Y_{12}$ receptor inhibitors.[5–7]

Switching from the intravenous cangrelor to clopidogrel has been tested in large-scale clinical trials, while data on switching to the new agents derive from small pharmacodynamic studies. Overall, available data suggest that clopidogrel and prasugrel should be administered immediately after discontinuation of cangrelor infusion to avoid a pharmacodynamic interaction given that these agents compete

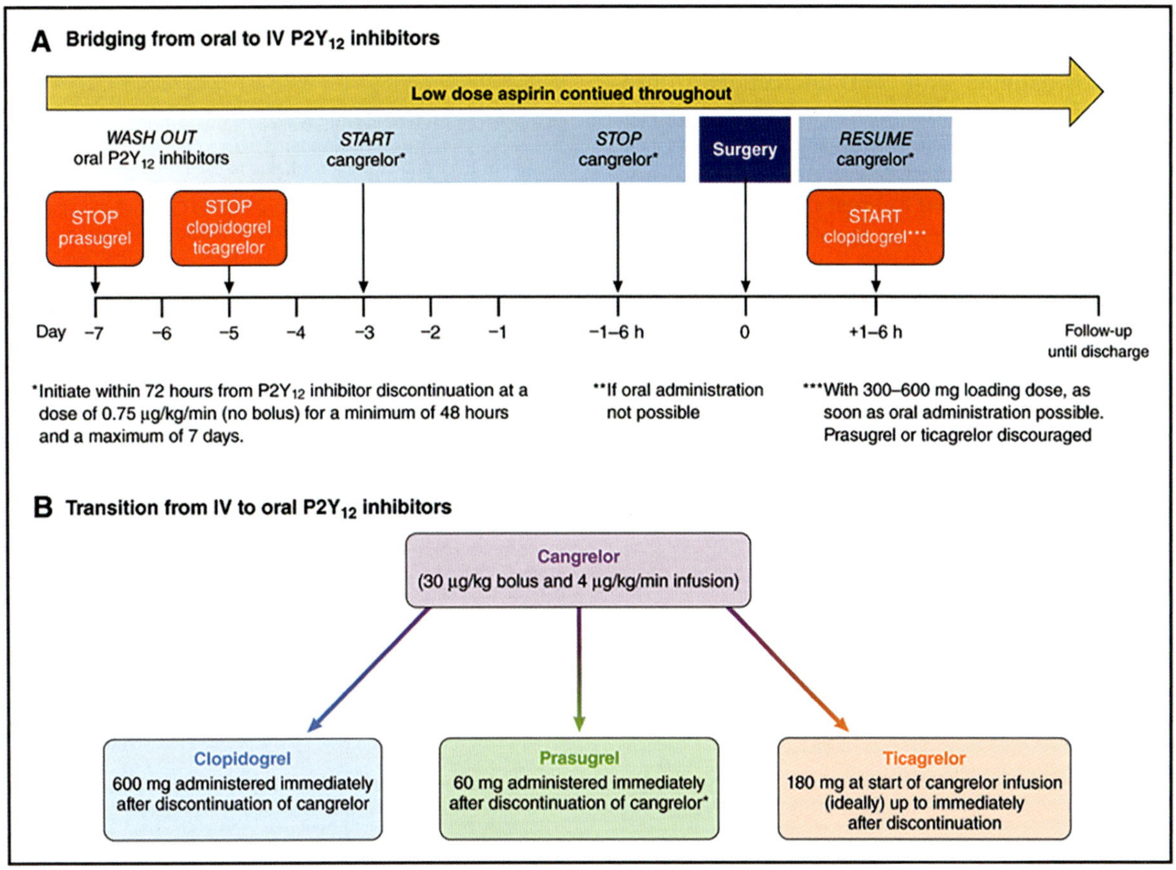

FIG. 13.9 Consensus recommendations on switching between oral and intravenous P2Y12 inhibitors. (**A**) Bridging from oral to intravenous agents. For both cardiac and noncardiac surgery, if withdrawal of P2Y12-inhibiting therapy is needed, clopidogrel and ticagrelor should be discontinued for 5 days and prasugrel for 7 days. It is reasonable to start cangrelor bridging up to 3 to 4 days after prasugrel discontinuation and 2 to 3 days of clopidogrel and ticagrelor discontinuation. Platelet function testing may be considered to help guide timing of starting cangrelor infusion. After surgery, regardless of bridging strategy, clopidogrel should be resumed with a loading dose (LD) as soon as oral administration is possible and the risk of severe bleeding is acceptable (prasugrel and ticagrelor administration should be discouraged). If the use of oral P2Y12-inhibiting therapy is not possible, postsurgery bridging with an intravenous agent should be considered. (**B**) Transition from intravenous to oral agents. An LD should always be used when transitioning from cangrelor to an oral agent. In the case of thienopyridines (clopidogrel or prasugrel), this should be administered immediately after discontinuation of cangrelor infusion. Ticagrelor can be administered before, during, or immediately after cangrelor infusion, although earlier administration (eg, at the time of percutaneous coronary intervention) should be considered. *According to the package insert of the European Medical Agency, but not that of the US Food and Drug Administration, prasugrel may also be administered 30 minutes before infusion is stopped. Preliminary studies have shown that prasugrel given at the start of a 2-hour infusion of cangrelor results in sufficient platelet inhibition, but this strategy cannot be routinely recommended until more data are available. (With *permission from: Angiolillo DJ, Rollini F, Storey RF, Bhatt DL, James S, Schneider DJ, Sibbing D, So DYF, Trenk D, Alexopoulos D, Gurbel PA, Hochholzer W, De Luca L, Bonello L, Aradi D, Cuisset T, Tantry US, Wang TY, Valgimigli M, Waksman R, Mehran R, Montalescot G, Franchi F, Price MJ. International Expert Consensus on Switching Platelet P2Y12 Receptor-Inhibiting Therapies. Circulation. 2017;136(20):1955-1975.* doi: 10.1161/CIRCULATIONAHA.117.031164.)

for the same ADP binding site[5–7] (Fig. 13.9). Indeed, in a PD study that enrolled patients with ACS undergoing PCI, concomitant administration of prasugrel with cangrelor leads to a marked increase in platelet reactivity after stopping cangrelor infusion, supporting the presence of a drug-drug interaction (DDI).[49]

In contrast, ticagrelor is a noncompetitive ADP antagonist and thus can be administered before, during, or after cangrelor infusion. Although cangrelor is approved for $P2Y_{12}$-naïve patients, its use in patients treated with ticagrelor is not infrequent in clinical practice.[50] Two translational studies have assessed these clinical questions. First, a pharmacodynamic study reported that ticagrelor could be administered as a crushed formulation concomitantly (i.e., administered simultaneously) with cangrelor without apparent DDI in patients undergoing primary PCI.[38] Furthermore, a second pharmacodynamic study suggested that cangrelor can be used without apparent DDI in patients with stable CAD pretreated with ticagrelor.[51] In both studies, cangrelor was an effective strategy to bridge the platelet inhibition gap associated with oral $P2Y_{12}$ inhibition induced by ticagrelor.

Ultimately, no drug interaction has been described when transitioning from any oral $P2Y_{12}$ receptor inhibitor to cangrelor, which can thus be started at any time.[5–7]

SUMMARY

Antiplatelet therapy has a pivotal role in the treatment of patients with MI. Currently, DAPT with a combination of aspirin and either prasugrel or ticagrelor should be considered the treatment of choice in the setting of acute MI as these agents achieve a faster and more potent platelet inhibition compared with clopidogrel and improve outcomes with an overall satisfactory safety profile. Clopidogrel should be considered for patients with contraindications to prasugrel and ticagrelor and for those who require adjunctive oral anticoagulant therapy. The findings that patients still continue to experience ischemic events despite COX-1 and $P2Y_{12}$ receptor blockade, raised interest toward alternative antithrombotic strategies, such as agents targeting different pathways involved in thrombosis or intravenous drugs, particularly attractive to achieve an immediate antiplatelet effect in the early phase of an ACS. Results from ongoing clinical trials are warranted to provide more insights on the optimal antithrombotic regimen to maximize ischemic benefit and minimize hemorrhagic risk.

CLASSIC REFERENCES

Bhatt DL, Lincoff AM, Gibson CM, et al. Intravenous platelet blockade with cangrelor during PCI. *N Engl J Med*. 2009;361(24):2330–2341.

Chen ZM, Jiang LX, Chen YP, et al. Addition of clopidogrel to aspirin in 45,852 patients with acute myocardial infarction: randomised placebo-controlled trial. *Lancet*. 2005;366:1607.

Harrington RA, Stone GW, McNulty S, et al. Platelet inhibition with cangrelor in patients undergoing PCI. *N Engl J Med*. 2009;361:2318.

ISIS-2 (Second International Study of Infarct Survival) Collaborative Group. Randomised trial of intravenous streptokinase, oral aspirin, both, or neither among 17,187 cases of suspected acute myocardial infarction: ISIS-2. ISIS-2 (second international study of infarct survival) collaborative group. *Lancet*. 1988;2:349.

Roe MT, Armstrong PW, Fox KA, et al. Prasugrel versus clopidogrel for acute coronary syndromes without revascularization. *N Engl J Med*. 2012;367(14):1297–1309.

Sabatine MS, Cannon CP, Gibson CM, et al. Addition of clopidogrel to aspirin and fibrinolytic therapy for myocardial infarction with ST-segment elevation. *N Engl J Med*. 2005;352:1179.

Steinhubl SR, Berger PB, Mann JT 3rd, et al. Early and sustained dual oral antiplatelet therapy following percutaneous coronary intervention: a randomized controlled trial. *JAMA*. 2002;288:2411.

Wiviott SD, Braunwald E, McCabe CH, et al. Prasugrel versus clopidogrel in patients with acute coronary syndromes. *N Engl J Med*. 2007;357:2001.

Wallentin L, Becker RC, Budaj A, et al. Ticagrelor versus clopidogrel in patients with acute coronary syndromes. *N Engl J Med*. 2009;361(11):1045–1057.

Yusuf S, Zhao F, Mehta SR, et al. Effects of clopidogrel in addition to aspirin in patients with acute coronary syndromes without ST-segment elevation. *N Engl J Med*. 2001;345:494.

REFERENCES

1. Libby P, Pasterkamp G, Crea F, Jang IK. Reassessing the mechanisms of acute coronary syndromes. *Circ Res*. 2019;124:150–160.
2. Gawaz M, Geisler T, Borst O. Current concepts and novel targets for antiplatelet therapy. *Nat Rev Cardiol*. 2023;20:583–599.
3. Huynh K. Inflammation in plaque erosion and rupture. *Nat Rev Cardiol*. 2022;19:80.
4. Mackman N, Bergmeier W, Stouffer GA, Weitz JI. Therapeutic strategies for thrombosis: new targets and approaches. *Nat Rev Drug Discov*. 2020;19:333–352.
5. Kamran H, Jneid H, Kayani WT, et al. Oral antiplatelet therapy after acute coronary syndrome: a review. *JAMA*. 2021;325:1545–1555.
6. Angiolillo DJ, Galli M, Collet JP, et al. Antiplatelet therapy after percutaneous coronary intervention. *EuroIntervention*. 2022;17:e1371–e1396.
7. Rodriguez F, Harrington RA. Management of antithrombotic therapy after acute coronary syndromes. *N Engl J Med*. 2021;384:452–460.
8. Angiolillo DJ, Bhatt DL, Lanza F, et al. Pharmacokinetic/pharmacodynamic assessment of a novel, pharmaceutical lipid-aspirin complex: results of a randomized, crossover, bioequivalence study. *J Thromb Thrombolysis*. 2019;48:554–562.
9. Franchi F, Schneider DJ, Prats J, et al. Pharmacokinetic and pharmacodynamic profiles of a novel phospholipid-aspirin complex liquid formulation and low dose enteric-coated aspirin: results from a prospective, randomized, crossover study. *J Thromb Thrombolysis*. 2022;54:373–381.
10. Capodanno D, Angiolillo DJ. Personalised antiplatelet therapies for coronary artery disease: what the future holds. *Eur Heart J*. 2023;44:3059–3072.
11. Patti G, Cavallari I, Andreotti F, et al. Prevention of atherothrombotic events in patients with diabetes mellitus: from antithrombotic therapies to new-generation glucose-lowering drugs. *Nat Rev Cardiol*. 2019;16:113–130.
12. Gurbel PA, Bliden KP, Chaudhary R, Tantry US. First in-human experience with inhaled acetylsalicylic acid for immediate platelet inhibition: comparison with chewed and swallowed acetylsalicylic acid. *Circulation*. 2020;142:1305–1307.
13. Galli M, Ortega-Paz L, Franchi F, et al. Precision medicine in interventional cardiology: implications for antiplatelet therapy in patients undergoing percutaneous coronary intervention. *Pharmacogenomics*. 2022;23:723–737.
14. Angiolillo DJ, Capodanno D, Danchin N, et al. Derivation, validation, and prognostic utility of a prediction rule for nonresponse to clopidogrel: the ABCD-GENE score. *JACC Cardiovasc Interv*. 2020;13:606–617.
15. Triska J, Maitra N, Deshotels MR, et al. A comprehensive review of the pleiotropic effects of ticagrelor. *Cardiovasc Drugs Ther*. 2024;38(4):775–797.
16. Lawton JS, Tamis-Holland JE, Bangalore S, et al. 2021 ACC/AHA/SCAI guideline for coronary artery revascularization: a report of the American College of Cardiology/American Heart Association joint committee on clinical practice guidelines. *Circulation*. 2022;145:e18–e114.
17. Byrne RA, Rossello X, Coughlan JJ, et al. 2023 ESC guidelines for the management of acute coronary syndromes. *Eur Heart J*. 2023;44:3720–3826.
18. Ortega-Paz L, Brugaletta S, Ariotti S, et al. Adenosine and ticagrelor plasma levels in patients with and without ticagrelor-related dyspnea. *Circulation*. 2018;138:646–648.
19. De Luca L, Steg PG, Bhatt DL, et al. Cangrelor: clinical data, contemporary use, and future perspectives. *J Am Heart Assoc*. 2021;10:e022125.
20. Capodanno D, Milluzzo RP, Angiolillo DJ. Intravenous antiplatelet therapies (glycoprotein IIb/IIIa receptor inhibitors and cangrelor) in percutaneous coronary intervention: from pharmacology to indications for clinical use. *Ther Adv Cardiovasc Dis*. 2019;13:1753944719893274.
21. Franchi F, Rollini F, Faz G, et al. Pharmacodynamic effects of vorapaxar in prior myocardial infarction patients treated with potent oral P2Y(12) receptor inhibitors with and without aspirin: results of the VORA-PRATIC study. *J Am Heart Assoc*. 2020;9:e015865.
22. Franchi F, Rollini F, Kairouz V, et al. Pharmacodynamic effects of vorapaxar in patients with and without diabetes mellitus: results of the OPTIMUS-5 study. *JACC Basic Transl Sci*. 2019;4:763–775.
23. Canonico ME, Piccolo R, Avvedimento M, et al. Antithrombotic therapy in peripheral artery disease: current evidence and future directions. *J Cardiovasc Dev Dis*. 2023;10:164.
24. Morrison JT, Govsyeyev N, Hess CN, Bonaca MP. Vorapaxar for prevention of major adverse cardiovascular and limb events in peripheral artery disease. *J Cardiovasc Pharmacol Ther*. 2022;27:10742484211056115.
25. Halvorsen S, Mehilli J, Cassese S, et al. 2022 ESC guidelines on cardiovascular assessment and management of patients undergoing non-cardiac surgery. *Eur Heart J*. 2022;43:3826–3924.
26. Cao D, Chandiramani R, Capodanno D, et al. Non-cardiac surgery in patients with coronary artery disease: risk evaluation and periprocedural management. *Nat Rev Cardiol*. 2021;18:37–57.
27. Schupke S, Neumann FJ, Menichelli M, et al. Ticagrelor or prasugrel in patients with acute coronary syndromes. *N Engl J Med*. 2019;381:1524–1534.
28. Tarantini G, Mojoli M, Varbella F, et al. Timing of oral P2Y(12) inhibitor administration in patients with non-ST-segment elevation acute coronary syndrome. *J Am Coll Cardiol*. 2020;76:2450–2459.
29. Capodanno D, Angiolillo DJ. Timing, selection, modulation, and duration of P2Y(12) inhibitors for patients with acute coronary syndromes undergoing PCI. *JACC Cardiovasc Interv*. 2023;16:1–18.
30. Ahrens I, Averkov O, Zuniga EC, et al. Invasive and antiplatelet treatment of patients with non-ST-segment elevation myocardial infarction: Understanding and addressing the global risk-treatment paradox. *Clin Cardiol*. 2019;42:1028–1040.
31. Angiolillo DJ, Erlinge D, Ferreiro JL, et al. European practice patterns for antiplatelet management in NSTE-ACS patients: results from the REal-world ADoption survey focus on acute antiPlatelet treatment (READAPT) survey. *Int J Cardiol*. 2023;386:8–16.
32. Collet JP, Thiele H, Barbato E, et al. 2020 ESC guidelines for the management of acute coronary syndromes in patients presenting without persistent ST-segment elevation. *Eur Heart J*. 2021;42:1289–1367.
33. Pollack CV Jr, Peacock WF, Bhandary DD, et al. Oral antiplatelet therapy administered upstream to patients with NSTEMI. *Crit Pathw Cardiol*. 2020;19:166–172.
34. Capodanno D, Bhatt DL, Gibson CM, et al. Bleeding avoidance strategies in percutaneous coronary intervention. *Nat Rev Cardiol*. 2022;19:117–132.
35. Dawson LP, Chen D, Dagan M, et al. Assessment of pretreatment with oral P2Y12 inhibitors and cardiovascular and bleeding outcomes in patients with non-ST elevation acute coronary syndromes: a systematic review and meta-analysis. *JAMA Netw Open*. 2021;4:e2134322.
36. Dworeck C, Redfors B, Angeras O, et al. Association of pretreatment with P2Y12 receptor antagonists preceding percutaneous coronary intervention in non-ST-segment elevation acute coronary syndromes with outcomes. *JAMA Netw Open*. 2020;3:e2018735.
37. Capodanno D, Alfonso F, Levine GN, et al. ACC/AHA versus ESC guidelines on dual antiplatelet therapy: JACC guideline comparison. *J Am Coll Cardiol*. 2018;72:2915–2931.
38. Franchi F, Rollini F, Rivas A, et al. Platelet inhibition with cangrelor and crushed ticagrelor in patients with ST-segment-elevation myocardial infarction undergoing primary percutaneous coronary intervention. *Circulation*. 2019;139:1661–1670.
39. Capodanno D, Baber U, Bhatt DL, et al. P2Y(12) inhibitor monotherapy in patients undergoing percutaneous coronary intervention. *Nat Rev Cardiol*. 2022;19:829–844.
40. Watanabe H, Morimoto T, Natsuaki M, et al. Comparison of clopidogrel monotherapy after 1 to 2 months of dual antiplatelet therapy with 12 months of dual antiplatelet therapy in patients with acute coronary syndrome: the STOPDAPT-2 ACS randomized clinical trial. *JAMA Cardiol*. 2022;7:407–417.
41. Zhou X, Angiolillo DJ, Ortega-Paz L. P2Y(12) inhibitor monotherapy after percutaneous coronary intervention. *J Cardiovasc Dev Dis*. 2022;9:340. doi:10.3390/jcdd9100340.
42. Motovska Z, Hlinomaz O, Kala P, et al. 1-year outcomes of patients undergoing primary angioplasty for myocardial infarction treated with prasugrel versus ticagrelor. *J Am Coll Cardiol*. 2018;71:371–381.

43. Sibbing D, Aradi D, Alexopoulos D, et al. Updated expert consensus statement on platelet function and genetic testing for guiding P2Y(12) receptor inhibitor treatment in percutaneous coronary intervention. *JACC Cardiovasc Interv*. 2019;12:1521–1537.
44. Capodanno D, Mehran R, Krucoff MW, et al. Defining strategies of modulation of antiplatelet therapy in patients with coronary artery disease: a consensus document from the academic research consortium. *Circulation*. 2023;147:1933–1944.
45. Gimbel M, Qaderdan K, Willemsen L, et al. Clopidogrel versus ticagrelor or prasugrel in patients aged 70 years or older with non-ST-elevation acute coronary syndrome (POPular AGE): the randomised, open-label, non-inferiority trial. *Lancet*. 2020;395:1374–1381.
46. Szummer K, Montez-Rath ME, Alfredsson J, et al. Comparison between ticagrelor and clopidogrel in elderly patients with an acute coronary syndrome: insights from the SWEDEHEART registry. *Circulation*. 2020;142:1700–1708.
47. Ibanez B, James S, Agewall S, et al. 2017 ESC guidelines for the management of acute myocardial infarction in patients presenting with ST-segment elevation: the task force for the management of acute myocardial infarction in patients presenting with ST-segment elevation of the European society of cardiology (ESC). *Eur Heart J*. 2018;39:119–177.
48. Marian MJ, Abu Daya H, Chatterjee A, et al. Effects of crushed ticagrelor versus eptifibatide bolus plus clopidogrel in troponin-negative acute coronary syndrome patients undergoing percutaneous coronary intervention: a randomized clinical trial. *J Am Heart Assoc*. 2019;8:e012844.
49. Franchi F, Rollini F, Ortega-Paz L, et al. Switching from cangrelor to prasugrel in patients undergoing percutaneous coronary intervention: the switching antiplatelet-6 (SWAP-6) study. *JACC Cardiovasc Interv*. 2023;16(20):2528–2539.
50. Rymer JA, Bhatt DL, Angiolillo DJ, et al. Cangrelor use patterns and transition to oral P2Y(12) inhibitors among patients with myocardial infarction: initial results from the CAMEO registry. *J Am Heart Assoc*. 2022;11:e024513.
51. Franchi F, Ortega-Paz L, Rollini F, et al. Cangrelor in patients with coronary artery disease pretreated with ticagrelor: the switching antiplatelet (SWAP)-5 study. *JACC Cardiovasc Interv*. 2023;16:36–46.
52. Park DW, Kwon O, Jang JS, et al. Clinically significant bleeding with ticagrelor versus clopidogrel in korean patients with acute coronary syndromes intended for invasive management: a randomized clinical trial. *Circulation*. 2019;140:1865–1877.

14 Approach to Noninvasive Testing After Presentation with Acute Coronary Syndrome

HAYAN JOUNI AND NANDAN S. ANAVEKAR

INTRODUCTION

Commonly utilized noninvasive tests after presentation with ACS include resting echocardiography, exercise stress testing with electrocardiogram (ECG) monitoring alone, stress imaging with nuclear myocardial perfusion imaging (MPI) or echocardiography, and increasingly rest and stress cardiac magnetic resonance imaging (CMR). Selection among these options depend on the temporal evolution of the presenting ACS and the goals of testing. Resting echocardiography is commonly used for early imaging within the first 72 hours. Exercise ECG or stress imaging is often used for intermediate testing between day 3 and week 6. Late imaging, beyond 6 weeks, uses any of the techniques for selected patient subsets to measure LVEF for implantable cardiac defibrillator (ICD) consideration and viability assessment.

In this chapter, we discuss the role of noninvasive testing after MI, patient selection, and considerations for selection among the alternatives for noninvasive testing. Detailed discussions on each modality, such as echocardiography, MPI, and CMR, can be found in Chapters 15, 16, and 17 respectively. While computed tomography angiography has gained importance in evaluating patients with acute chest pain in the emergency department, it is not widely used in pateients with confirmed ACS and is therefore not included in this chapter (see Chapter 5).

PATHOPHYSIOLOGY OF MYOCARDIAL INFARCTION AS THE BASIS FOR NONINVASIVE TESTING

The pathophysiology of ACS is discussed in detail in Chapter 32. The underlying pathophysiology establishes the foundation of the rationale for noninvasive testing in patients with ACS. The amount of myocardium that is jeopardized by insufficient flow in a coronary artery is referred to as myocardium at risk (Chapter 19). This territory is the amount of myocardium that is expected to scar in the absence of spontaneous reperfusion or treatment with reperfusion therapy. The amount of myocardium that ultimately turns into a scar is referred to as the final infarct size. The difference between myocardium at risk and final infarct size represents that myocardial mass that survives and is accordingly labeled myocardial salvage. Both final infarct size and myocardial salvage reflect in part the efficacy of reperfusion therapy (Chapter 8). These measurements can be quantitated by nuclear MPI or CMR techniques. These imaging modalities are used as an endpoint in research studies comparing reperfusion strategies or examining the efficacy of new MI therapies. Myocardial salvage measurement is not commonly performed in clinical practice due to its logistical demands and lack of direct impact on patient management. MI results in worsening wall motion in the infarct zone and compensatory hyperkinesia in noninfarct zones. Partial or complete recovery in the motion of these stunned segments after reperfusion can take several days up to 6 weeks, with similar durations for resolution of compensatory hyperkinesia in noninfarct zones.

Two of the most important prognostic variables in patients with ACS are global LV function and the extent of coronary artery disease (CAD). Measurement of these variables is a primary objective of noninvasive testing in this setting. Global LV function is most commonly expressed as LV ejection fraction (LVEF). Current professional society practice guidelines recommend measurement of LVEF in all patients with ST-elevation MI (STEMI) and recognize the relationship with prognosis among patients with non-ST-elevation ACS. LVEF and regional wall motion can be measured in the catheterization laboratory by contrast ventriculography or by noninvasive methods. In contemporary practice, LVEF is predominantly performed noninvasively, due to depth and breadth in expertise, and wide and expedited availability of these modalities. Other indices of global LV structure and/or function, including end-diastolic and end-systolic volumes, wall motion score index, and diastolic function can also be measured to compliment the assessment; however, it is important to be cognizant that LVEF has remained the most powerful predictor of outcomes in this clinical setting. Selected patients being considered for ICD may require repeated LVEF measurement beyond 40 days due to the effects of stunning on early LVEF. Remodeling, which is associated with higher mortality and risk of heart failure, occurs in some patients with reduced LVEF (Chapter 30). ACE-inhibitors, angiotensin receptor blockers, and aldosterone antagonists can favorably impact remodeling, making it important to measure LVEF early after MI to identify eligible patients for these medications. As the panoply of medical therapeutics continue to evolve in the management of LV dysfunction and heart failure, early imaging has become more mainstream, especially within the inpatient setting.

RATIONAL USE OF NONINVASIVE TESTING

Noninvasive testing is an important adjunct to clinical assessment for risk stratification and aids in management decisions. Patient care is initiated upstream with appropriate clinical risk assessment, which can be aided by calculating a clinical risk score (see Chapter 6). Occasionally, clinical estimates are sufficient for risk assessment in some patients without additional evaluation. This knowledge can improve the efficiency of noninvasive testing. Testing is least useful for managing patients at very low or very high risk, based on available prognostic information. Although measurement of LVEF is categorized as a class I indication in STEMI guidelines, the measurement reasonably could be avoided in very low risk scenarios, given the very high likelihood of normal LVEF on the basis of clinical assessment. At the other end of the risk spectrum, there are an increasing number of patients with end-stage CAD who are living longer and present with multiple MIs during their lifetime. If prior evaluation has demonstrated that coronary anatomy is not amenable to further revascularization, or if LVEF is severely reduced and the patient is already taking an ACE-inhibitor and has an ICD, there is little to be gained from further noninvasive testing. Universally, testing should therefore, be performed only when the results are likely to impact clinical management. Noninvasive testing should also be performed in a cost-effective manner. Furthermore, redundant testing should be avoided to emphasize the importance of economy of care. For example, if a patient undergoes left ventriculography as part of the early catheterization procedure, performance of echocardiography generally does not add incremental value in the clinical assessment and therefore may not be necessary.

NONINVASIVE TESTING ACCORDING TO TEMPORAL SEQUENCE OF MYOCARDIAL INFARCTION EVOLUTION

The time course of recovery after ACS can be separated into three general phases: early (within 72 hours); intermediate (day 3 to week 6); late (beyond 6 weeks). These phases provide a useful framework in which to consider the goals and alternatives for noninvasive testing (Table 14.1). Resting echocardiography (Chapter 15) is commonly used to evaluate LVEF and regional wall motion in the early phase after MI. It can also help identify mechanical complications of MI (Chapter 22) and conditions that mimic MI (Chapter 4). Although this practice has become less common with routine early invasive management of ACS, early submaximal stress testing (between days 3 and 5 and before hospital discharge), with or without imaging, has typically been performed in lower-risk patients who did not undergo early coronary angiography. Delayed symptom-limited stress testing may be helpful for guiding revascularization decisions in patients with significant CAD in vessels other than the infarct-related artery, typically performed between 3 and 6 weeks after MI. Delayed imaging (beyond 40 days)

TABLE 14.1 Time Course and Noninvasive Testing Strategies after Myocardial Infarction

TIME	MAIN MODALITY[a]	GOAL	IMPACT ON MANAGEMENT
Early (≤72 h)	Rest echo (radionuclide angiogram or MRI)	Measure global and regional LV Identify AMI complications Identify conditions mimicking AMI	Use of ACE-inhibitor Selection of revascularization strategy Select specific treatment Select appropriate treatment
Intermediate (days 3–5) (weeks 3–6)	Submaximal stress test[b] Symptom limited stress test[b]	Assess residual ischemic burden Same as submax test (if not performed) Assess ischemia noninfarct artery[c]	Identify pts for cor angio Identify pts for cor angio Select pts for additional PCI/CABG
Late (≥40 days)	Echo (nuclear or MRI) Nuclear PET or MRI (echo)	Measure LVEF (after stunning resolves) Assess myocardial viability	Eligibility for ICD Revascularization (usually CABG)

[a]The generally preferred and most commonly applied modality is shown first. Modalities listed in parentheses indicate secondary choices.
[b]Selection between a standard stress test and stress imaging is based primarily upon the ability to exercise and the interpretability of the ECG.
[c]If testing is performed to assess ischemia in the noninfarct vessel, stress imaging is recommended over standard stress testing.

with any of the imaging techniques can be performed in selected patients primarily to assess (1) LVEF to determine eligibility for an ICD; (2) evaluate for ischemia as an etiology for interval symptom development.

Early Imaging (Within 72 Hours) After Presentation

Resting Echocardiography

The mainstay of early imaging is resting echocardiography (see Fig. 14.1). Echocardiography (see also Chapter 15) possesses certain advantages over other imaging modalities, including its more widespread availability and portability, the latter facilitates bringing the machine to the bedside. Transthoracic echocardiography provides a comprehensive cardiac assessment that encompasses global and regional left ventricular systolic function, global right ventricular function, chamber sizes, wall thickness, left ventricular diastolic function, valve status, estimated right ventricular systolic pressure, and pericardial fluid. Myocardial contrast can be administered to enhance image quality in patients with technically poor images. Transesophageal echocardiography provides an alternative to transthoracic echocardiography in critically ill patients who may have limited acoustic windows. The performance of transesophageal echocardiography solely to assess cardiac function is an uncommon indication. Transesophageal echocardiography has particular utility in assessment of the thoracic aorta and main pulmonary arteries to diagnose conditions which can mimic ACS. Myocardial strain imaging represents a compliment in the assessment of systolic function and may provide incremental prognostication, especially in patients with normal or mildly reduced LV ejection fraction. In MI patients with ejection fraction >40%, those with global LV strain >-14% have a three-fold higher rate of all-cause mortality or heart failure hospitalization compared to patients with LV strain <-14%.[1] Myocardial contrast echocardiography with microbubbles has been used to assess myocardial perfusion and anecdotally has been used to distinguish stress cardiomyopathy from coronary occlusive disease,[2] but this technique is not commonly performed clinically.

The major reason for performing resting echocardiography early in the course of ACS is measurement of global left ventricular function. Knowledge of LVEF can influence medical decision-making. Treatment with ACE inhibitors and aldosterone antagonists are Class I guideline recommendations in patients with reduced LVEF (Chapter 21 and Chapter 30). Knowledge of LVEF may also influence selection of a specific revascularization procedure, particularly in patients with non-ST-elevation ACS (Chapter 10). In patients with multivessel CAD and reduced LVEF, CABG is preferred over multivessel PCI for non-ST-elevation ACS or stabilized patients after STEMI. Regional wall motion assessment can estimate infarct size, while global LV function can be measured using the wall motion score index, which is a more accurate predictor of outcome than LVEF according to some studies.

A second reason to perform early echocardiography is to aid in the identification of conditions that can mimic ACS, including pulmonary embolism, aortic dissection,

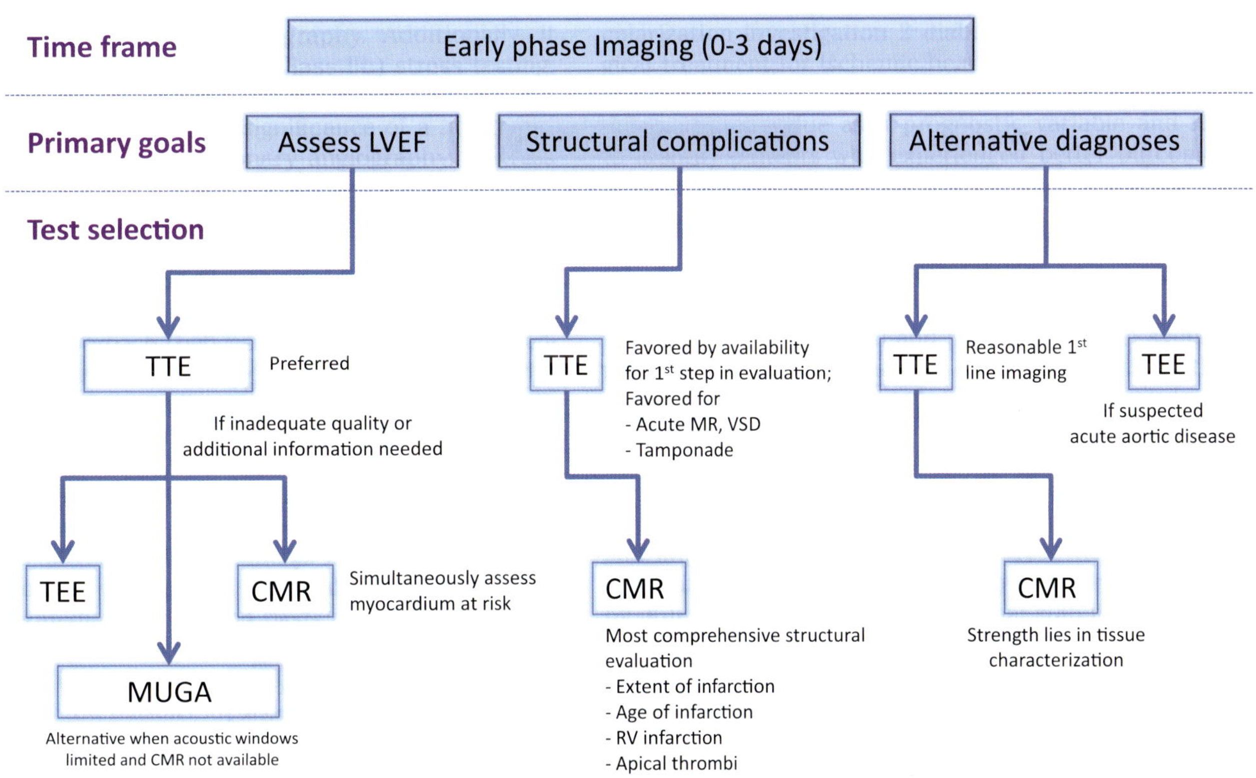

FIG. 14.1 Imaging options in the acute phase of treatment in the setting of acute coronary syndrome. Echocardiography remains the mainstay. Cardiac MRI is an evolving technology that is developing applications in this setting but remains limited by availability. MUGA is applied in selected patients.

In addition, as ischemia may lead to inhomogeneous ventricular electrical conduction and contraction, the strain may be able to detect subtle changes in the timing of contraction.

Mechanical dispersion has been proposed as a marker of this inhomogenous ventricular contraction, which is a presumed reflection of the electromechanical changes in a scarred myocardium. It can be measured as the standard deviation of the time from the peak R-wave to peak negative strain and seems to predict arrhythmic events late after MI (>40 days) independently of LVEF.[8]

Three-Dimensional (3D) Echocardiography

Unlike conventional 2D echocardiography, 3D imaging provides volumetric images of the heart, allowing for more precise and reproducible measurements of critical parameters after ACS, such as left ventricular volumes, mass, and EF. It can better identify and quantify wall motion abnormalities and be especially useful for RV assessment.[9] It may also be a useful adjunct in the evaluation of potential mechanical complications and for guiding interventions during percutaneous procedures.[10]

Contrast Echocardiography

In situations where standard images are suboptimal, such as obesity or lung disease, which account for up to 20% of cases, contrast echocardiography may be helpful. Contrast agents are lipid-shelled, gas-filled encapsulated microbubbles that reflect ultrasound waves and consequently improve visualization of endocardial borders and increase the number of interpretable segments. They can be useful for quantification of LVEF, diagnosis of thrombus, (Fig. 15.10; Video 15.8) LV aneurysm or tissue perfusion. Indeed, by highlighting areas of impaired myocardial perfusion, it can detect ischemic regions and provide evidence on myocardial viability, with the persistence of a perfusion defect after 4-weeks being linked with worse LV remodeling.

Overall, these advanced echocardiographic techniques provide a more comprehensive assessment of myocardial structure and function in ACS. They enhance our diagnostic capabilities, offer better risk stratification, and guide personalized therapeutic strategies. However, as with any technology, it is crucial to recognize their strengths and limitations.

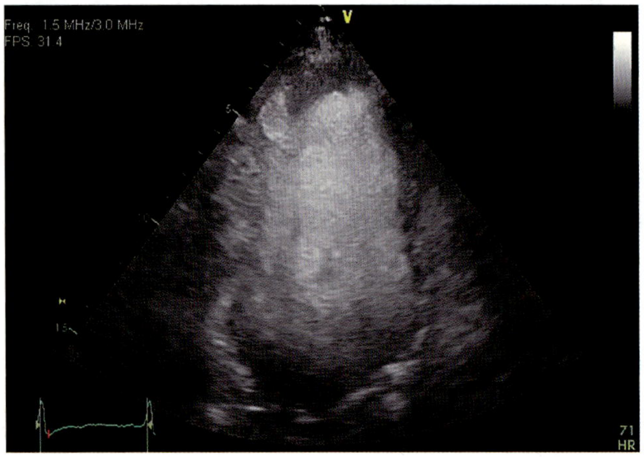

FIG. 15.10 LV opacification using contrast ultrasound agent. An apical thrombus is well visualized after injection of lipid-shelled, gas-filled encapsulated microbubbles (echocardiographic contrast agent, Definity).

ECHOCARDIOGRAPHY IN THE POST-ACUTE CORONARY SYNDROME EVALUATION

Following an acute coronary event, echocardiography is also useful for evaluating myocardial recovery. Repeat exams can monitor improvements or worsening in function, guide ongoing treatment strategies, and provide prognostic information.

Risk Stratification

In addition to detecting the mechanical complications described, echocardiography provides essential information for risk stratification. Reduced LVEF, increased LV volume, and the presence of RWMAs are all associated with poorer prognosis.

Assessment of Left Ventricular Function

A reduced LVEF after ACS is a strong predictor of poor outcome, but LV systolic function can also improve over time and reevaluation of the LVEF 40 days later may be useful.[1] Echocardiography is the favored method to measure LVEF since it can identify other abnormalities that are associated with a poorer prognosis such as RWMAs, diastolic dysfunction, concomitant RV involvement, left atrial volume, and MR.[11,12]

Qualitative and Semi-Quantitative Evaluation of Left Ventricular Systolic Function

The correlation between the visual LVEF estimation and its radionuclide determination is good, but this ***eyeball method*** requires experience, and clinicians should validate their own performance with quantitative methods. Another semi-quantitative assessment of regional LV contraction is the ***wall motion score index*** (WMSI). A 16-segment model (Fig. 15.11) is recommended since the apical cap does not contract.[13] A good correlation exists between the WMSI and the LVEF measured by radionuclide ventriculography. Because CAD causes segmental dysfunction, which can be accompanied by compensatory hyperkinesis of nonischemic segments, regional assessment of systolic function is more sensitive than global approaches.

Quantitative Evaluation of Global Left Ventricular Systolic Function

Quantitative evaluation of global LV systolic function is based on endocardial border tracing at end-diastole and end-systole in two orthogonal views. Evaluation of regional wall thickening is not influenced by cardiac translation or rotation, as opposed to wall motion, but requires excellent definition of the borders. Volume estimations are based on geometric assumptions about ventricular shape, which range from a simple ellipsoid to a complex hemi-cylindrical, hemi-ellipsoid shape. The American Society

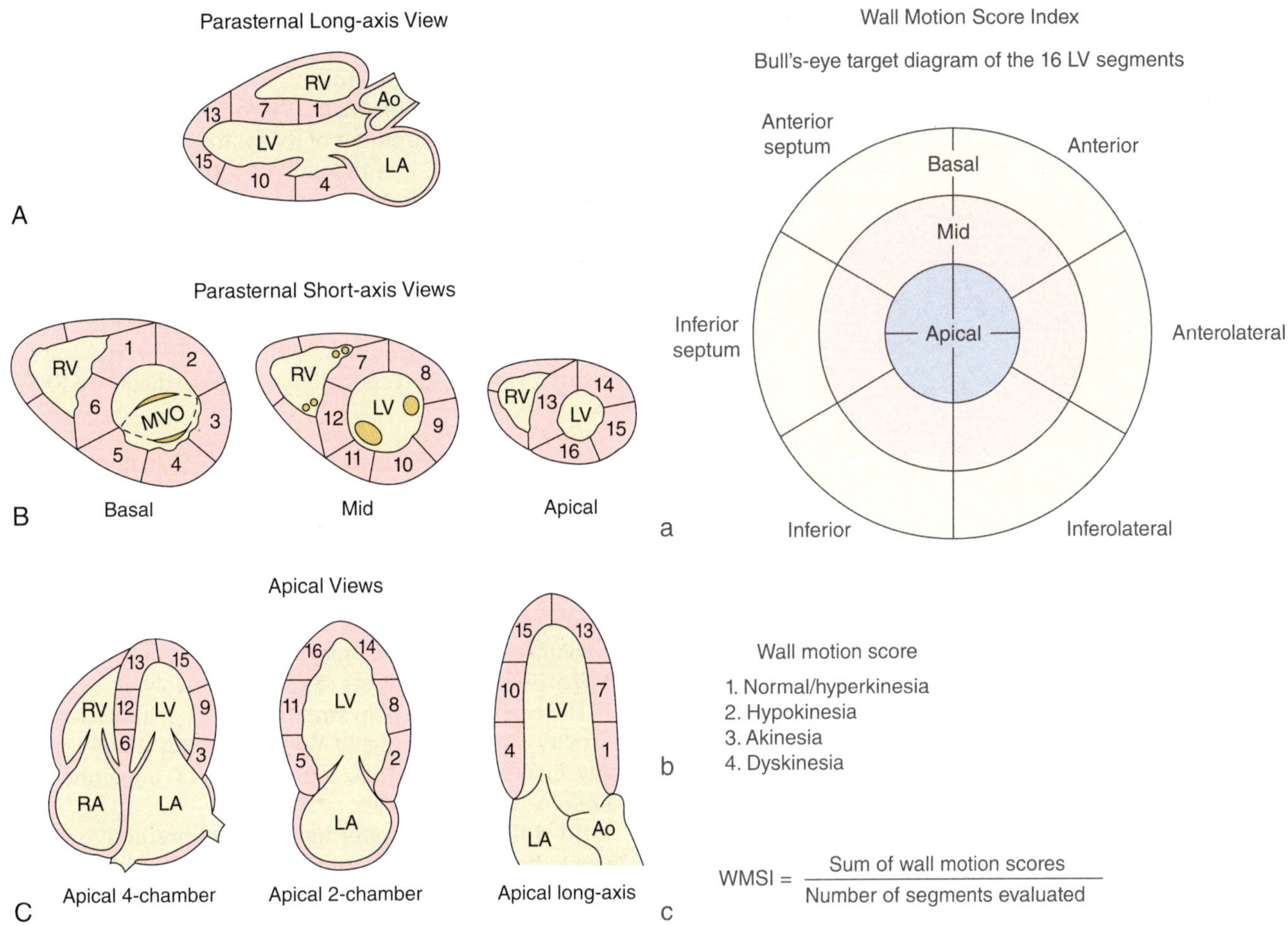

FIG. 15.11 (A) Schematic of the 16 segments of the LV as described by the American Society of Echocardiography. a, Parasternal long-axis view. b, Parasternal short-axis views. c, Apical views. The numbers in the diagram correspond to the following segments: 1, basal anteroseptum; 2, basal anterior wall; 3, basal anterolateral wall; 4, basal inferolateral wall; 5, basal inferior wall; 6, basal inferior septum; 7, mid anterior septum; 8, mid anterior wall; 9, mid anterolateral wall; 10, mid inferolateral wall; 11, mid inferior wall; l2, mid inferior septum; 13, septal apex; 14, anterior apex; 15, lateral apex; 16, inferior apex. *Ao*, Aorta; *LA*, left atrium; *LV*, left ventricle, *MVO*, mitral valve orifice; *RA*, right atrium; *RV*, right ventricle. (B) a, The 16 segments of the LV displayed as a bull's eye. b, The wall motion score: A score is assigned to each segment, according to its contractility: 1) normal or hyperkinetic, 2) hypokinetic, 3) akinetic (absent or negligible thickening) and 4) dyskinetic (systolic thinning or stretching, e.g. aneurysm). c, The WMSI is calculated by dividing the sum of the regional scores by the number of evaluable segments and can vary between 1 (for normal ventricular contraction) and 3.9 (for severe systolic dysfunction).

of Echocardiography (ASE) recommends the ***modified Simpson's biplane*** method for LV volumes and ejection fraction.[13] (Fig. 15.12; Video 15.10). In patients with good image quality, ***three-dimensional echocardiography*** (3D)-based measurements are accurate and reproducible and should be used when available (Fig. 15.13; Video 15.11) as it is superior to 2D echocardiography for LV volumes and mass and showed excellent correlations with cardiac magnetic resonance imaging (r = 0.98 for EDV, 0.99 for ESV, and 0.97 for LVEF, $P < .0001$) in patients with LVEF < 40%.

Echocardiographic Assessment of Right Ventricular Function

Echocardiography is an excellent tool to identify RV infarction, including RV regional or global dysfunction occurring with LV inferior wall MI. Because RV infarction may be revealed only by dysfunction of its inferior wall, attention should be paid to this region in optimized parasternal short-axis views. Indirect signs such as RV dilatation, tricuspid regurgitation, reduced excursion of the tricuspid annulus, and dilatation of the inferior vena cavae can also

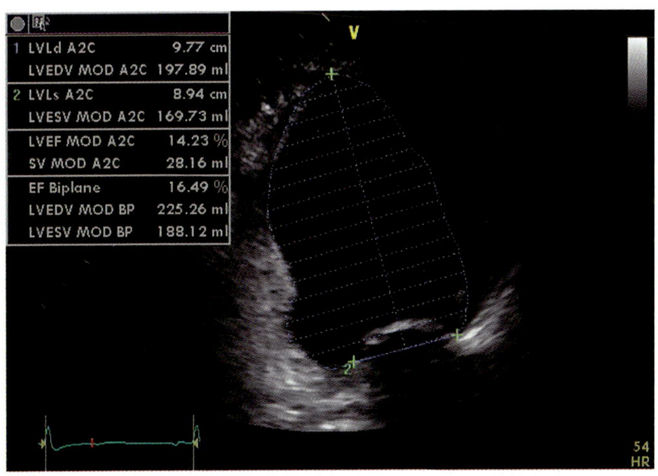

FIG. 15.12 Evaluation of LV volumes and systolic function using the Simpson's method of disks. The LV endocardial borders are traced at end-systole and end-diastole in two orthogonal views, the apical 4- and 2-chamber views (shown), and the LVEF is derived. Determination of the LV end-diastolic (EDV) and end-systolic volumes (ESV) allows calculation of the stroke volume (EDV-ESV = SV), cardiac output (SV × heart rate), and ejection fraction ([SV/EDV] × 100).

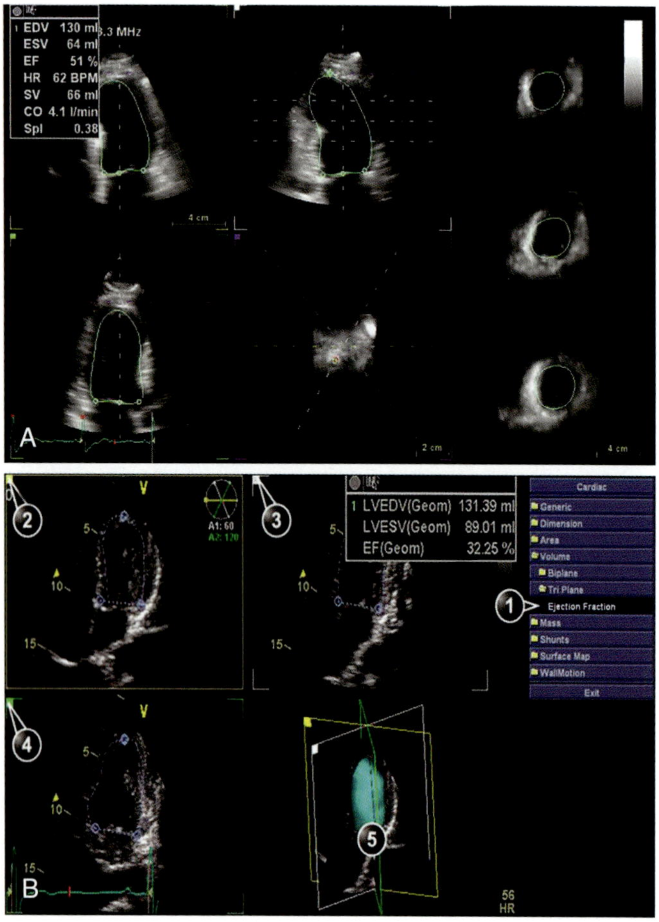

FIG. 15.13 Three-dimensional (3D) assessment of LV function. (A) Automated determination of LVEF using volumetric assessment and multislice (5–12) short axis volumes. (B) 3D full-volume of the LV can be processed from apical 4-chamber, 2-chamber, and long-axis views with special analytical software to create a dynamic 3D cast.

TABLE 15.1 Normal Values and Threshold for Echocardiographic Parameters of RV Function

PARAMETER	MEAN ± SD	ABNORMALITY THRESHOLD
TAPSE (mm)	24 ± 3.5	<17
Pulsed Doppler S wave (cm/sec)	14.1 ± 2.3	<9.5
Color Doppler S wave (cm/sec)	9.7 ± 1.85	<6.0
RV fractional area change (%)	49 ± 7	<35
RV free wall 2D strain[a] (%)	−29 ± 4.5	
RV 3D EF (%)	58 ± 6.5	<45
Pulsed Doppler MP	0.26 ± 0.085	>0.43
Tissue Doppler MPI	0.38 ± 0.08	>0.54
E-wave deceleration time (m/sec)	180 ± 31	<119 or >242
E/A	1.4 ± 0.3	<0.8 or >2.0
e/a′	1.18 ± 0.33	<0.52
e′	14.0 ± 3.1	<7.8
E/e′	4.0 ± 1.0	>6.0

MPI, Myocardial performance index.
[a]Limited data; values may vary depending on vendor and software version.
Reproduced with permission from Liga R, Colli A, Taggart DP, Boden WE, De Caterina R. Myocardial Revascularization in patients with ischemic cardiomyopathy: for whom and how. *J Am Heart Assoc*. 2023;12:e026943.

often be found. Many methods are available to quantify RV systolic function, with good correlation with MRI and radionuclide ventriculography (Table 15.1, Fig. 15.14, and Video 15.12).[13]

Fractional area change from the apical 4-chamber view expresses the percentage of RV area change between end-systole and end-diastole.

Tricuspid Annular Plane Systolic Excursion (TAPSE) is an indirect measurement of RV systolic function achieved by M-Mode or TDI. It is the shift of the RV base during systole and diastole measured in apical 4-C; an excursion of <1.5 cm (M-Mode) or <10 cm/s (TDI) is very specific for the detection of a RVEF < 50%.

To overcome the RV's complex geometry, ***3D echocardiography*** showed good correlations with MRI despite measuring smaller volumes, with 3D RVEF < 51% having a sensitivity of 91% and specificity of 80% to diagnose RV-MI.[14]

Prognosis After Acute Coronary Syndrome

The prognosis after ACS is determined in part by LV size, severity of systolic dysfunction, and the presence and extent of ischemic myocardium. Patients with LVEF <40% and end-systolic volume (ESV) >130 cc have a 5-year-survival rate of 65% and 52%, respectively; in general, the lower the LVEF and the larger the volumes, the worse the mortality and morbidity. Likewise, a WMSI ≥ 1.7 usually suggests dysfunction involving >20% of the LV.[12] Hence, WMSI can help stratify patients at increased risk of mortality after ACS, a higher WMSI reflecting a larger number of dysfunctional segments, more severe LV impairment, and therefore, worse prognosis.

Mid-wall GLS may offer incremental predictive value of myocardial injury as it correlates better with infarct size than LVEF and is independently predictive of arrhythmic events and mortality.

Furthermore, echocardiography may help to distinguish infarct extension from recurrent ischemia and to quantify the amount of myocardium at risk. Indeed, during MI, the nonaffected ventricular segments are usually hyperdynamic as a compensatory mechanism. The absence of such compensation suggests multivessel coronary disease and is associated with worse outcomes. Left atrial enlargement is also associated with inferior prognosis.

Left Ventricular Diastolic Dysfunction and Hemodynamic Assessment

After coronary occlusion, changes in the transmitral flow profile by pulsed-wave Doppler parallel the worsening of diastolic function measured invasively (peak-dP/dt, LVEDP, and tau) and may be present even when systolic function remains normal. A *restrictive filling pattern*, defined by an elevated E to A ratio and a short deceleration time, is indicative of stage 3 or 4 diastolic dysfunction (Fig. 15.15) and is an independent predictor of mortality after ACS (hazard ratio 2.7; 95% CI 2.2–3.2), even after multivariate analysis including age, sex, and LVEF.[15] TDI is a useful adjunct to pulsed-wave Doppler, with a ratio of *transmitral flow velocity to early mitral annulus velocity (E/E′)* >15 being predictive of LV remodeling and all-cause mortality.

Echocardiography can determine the *hemodynamic profile* of a patient, with measurement of the cardiac output and estimation of capillary wedge pressure (PCWP). A mitral deceleration time <120 milliseconds is highly predictive of a PCWP greater than 20 mmHg. Likewise, the deceleration

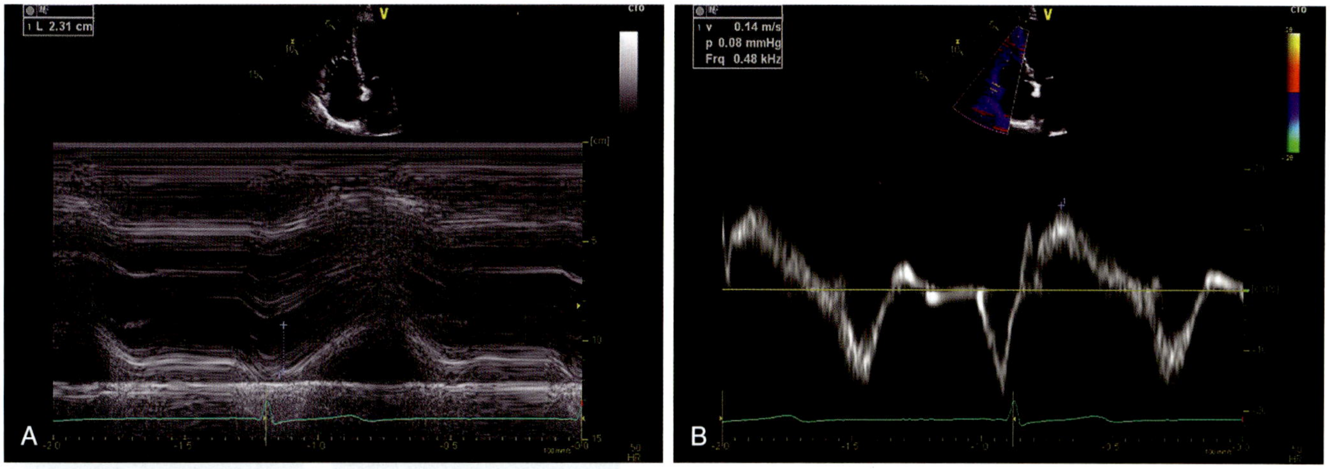

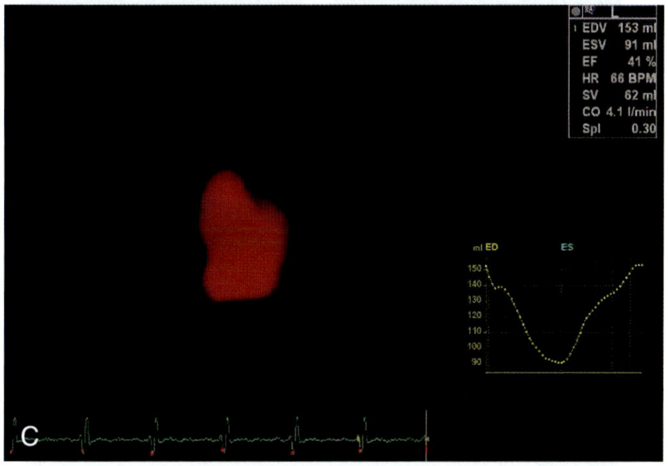

FIG. 15.14 Methods to quantify RV systolic function. (A) In this example, RV systolic function estimated by the tricuspid annular systolic plane excursion (TAPSE) by M-Mode is normal; (B) TDI of the RV lateral anulus (RV-TDI) showing a systolic velocity of the RV of 14 cm/s; to overcome the limitations of the complex geometry of the RV, 3DE may be useful (C).

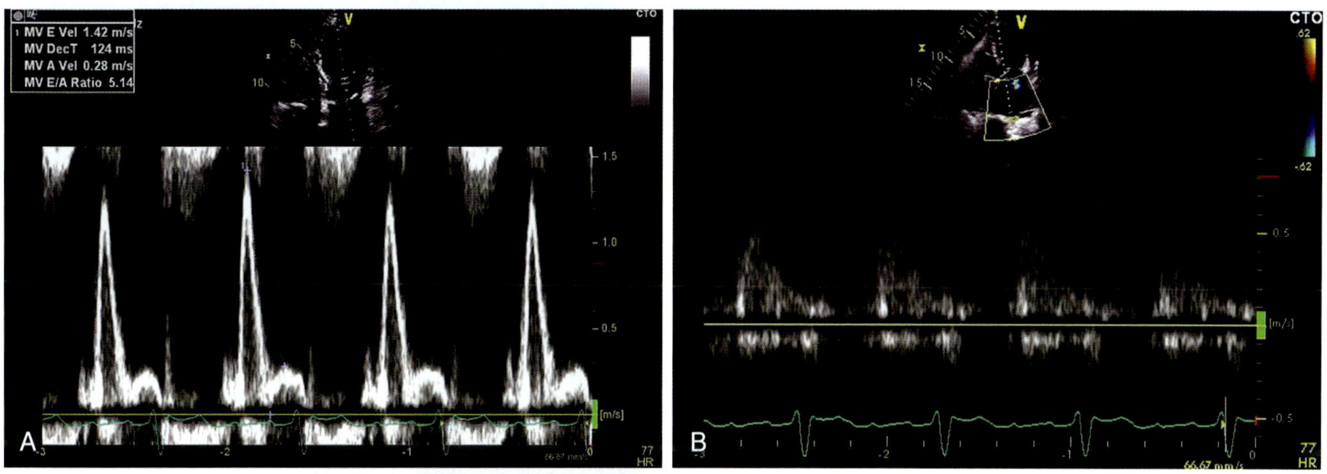

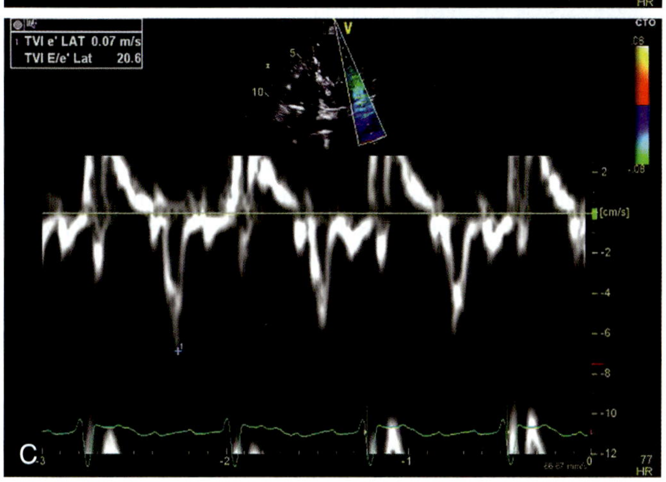

FIG. 15.15 Severe LV diastolic dysfunction after ACS. Restrictive LV filling after MI demonstrated by PWD interrogation of the (A) transmitral flow, (B) pulmonary venous flow and (C) Tissue Doppler examination of the lateral mitral anulus. *A*, Peak late diastolic trans-mitral flow velocity; *Am*, peak late diastolic mitral annulus velocity; *D*, peak diastolic pulmonary venous flow velocity; *Em*, peak early diastolic mitral anulus velocity; *MAV*, mitral anular velocity; *S*, peak systolic PVF velocity; *Sm*, systolic MAV.

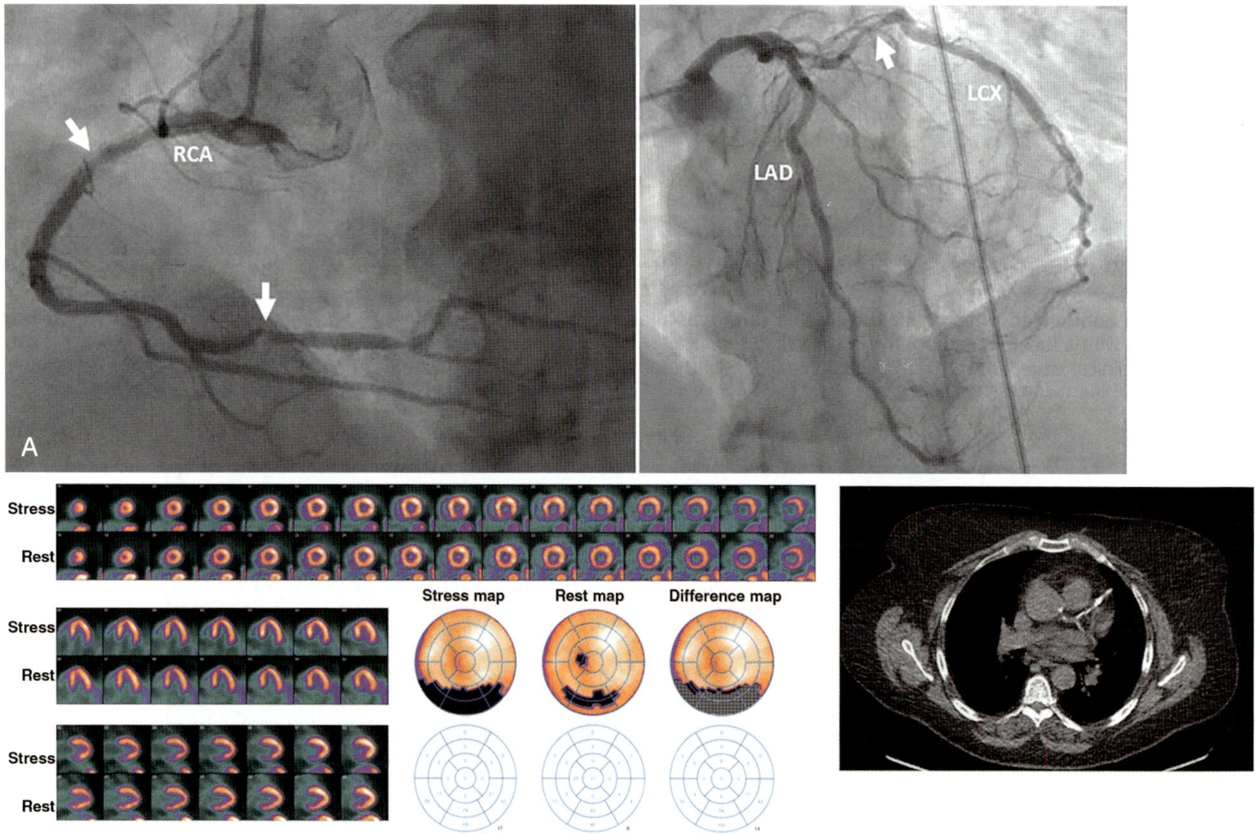

Territory	Stress	Rest	CFR
LAD	1.59	0.74	2.15
LCX	1.44	0.70	2.06
RCA	1.18	0.70	1.68
Global LV	1.39	0.71	1.96

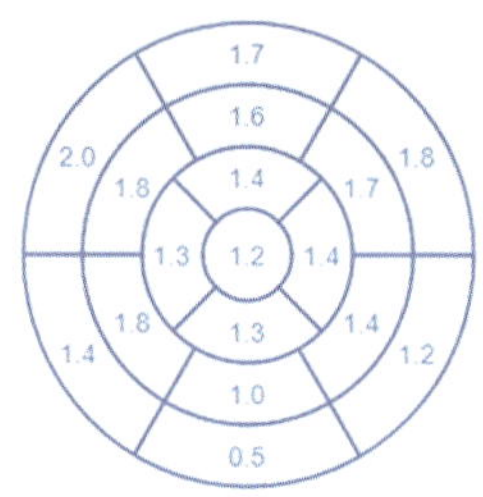

B

LAD RFR: 0.82
LCX RFR: 0.94

FIG. 16.11 Images for Case Vignette 2. (A) Coronary angiography images demonstrating obstructive disease in the right coronary artery (RCA) and the left circumflex artery (LCx) (*white arrows*) with nonobstructive disease in the left anterior descending artery (LAD). (B) Stress and rest 8^2-rubidium myocardial perfusion positron emission tomography/computed tomography (PET/CT) images. See text for details.

steps and therapeutic measures (see Chapters 10 and 14). The standard exercise electrocardiographic stress test may be reasonable for lower-risk patients with interpretable rest ECGs. For higher-risk patients, especially those with abnormal rest ECGs as in Case Vignette 2, stress imaging is more appropriate (see also Chapter 14).

The power of radionuclide myocardial perfusion imaging (SPECT and PET) for risk stratification is based on the fact that the major determinants of prognosis in patients with CAD are readily available from gated myocardial perfusion imaging. These risk indicators include the scintigraphic infarct size, the extent and severity of residual stress-induced ischemia, measurements of left ventricular volumes, and LVEF. Extensive evidence in stable patients after ACS supports the application of radionuclide perfusion imaging for risk assessment.[8] Exercise stress testing is a useful approach to risk stratification after ACS (see Chapter 14). Poor exercise effort (less than 4 METs), exercise-induced angina, ST-segment depression, ventricular arrhythmias, and hypotension during exercise identify high-risk patients. However, the frequency of such markers of risk is greatly diminished in the era of emergent coronary angiography and primary PCI because most high-risk patients (e.g., left main artery and/or multivessel CAD) are identified and treated before stress testing. Because most high-risk patients have been triaged at the time of presentation, noninvasive testing after ACS is most often used for the identification of residual stress-induced ischemia. In this regard, radionuclide imaging has improved sensitivity over that of stress ECG alone for identification of ischemia/viability with the infarct-related territory or in remote myocardium. Risk increases with the extent and severity of perfusion abnormalities and scintigraphic ischemia. For any given LVEF, a greater degree of scintigraphic ischemia identifies patients at higher clinical risk. This concept applies to all patient demographics and types of stress testing (exercise and pharmacologic stress). Data also support a potential role for perfusion imaging in guiding

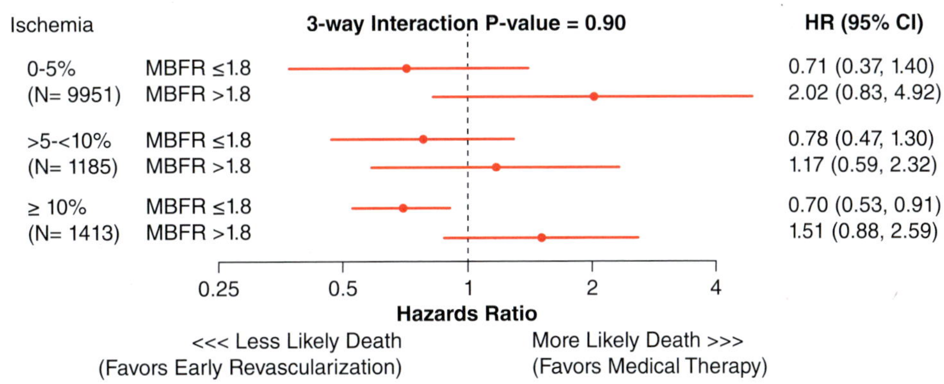

FIG. 16.12 Analysis of the interaction of myocardial blood flow reserve (MBFR, another term for coronary flow reserve (CFR)) with early revascularization versus medical therapy on long-term death, within levels of ischemia. Patients with low MBFR (CFR) appeared to have a survival benefit with revascularization compared to medical therapy across all ischemia strata; however, the confidence intervals (CIs) crossed 1.0 in the two lower strata of ischemia due to lower numbers of revascularization and less precision within those strata per the study investigators. (From Patel KK, Spertus JA, Chan PS et al. Myocardial blood flow reserve assessed by positron emission tomography myocardial perfusion imaging identifies patients with a survival benefit from early revascularization. *Eur Heart J.* 2020;41(6):759–768.)

revascularization. Propensity-matched observational data have supported an apparent benefit from revascularization for patients with a considerable extent of inducible ischemia (involving greater than 10% of left ventricular mass).[9]

As discussed in this chapter, CFR is a sensitive measure of myocardial ischemia and overall vascular health that is a unique and robust marker of clinical risk. As shown in Fig. 16.5, a severely reduced CFR (less than 1.5) is associated with a six-fold increased risk of cardiac death. Importantly, this information is incremental to other markers of clinical risk and to semiquantitative measures of myocardial ischemia and thus can refine risk estimates and potentially guide revascularization. Data suggest that global CFR may be able to modify the effect of revascularization, such that patients with low global CFR may benefit from early revascularization (Fig. 16.12).[10] These data also raise the possibility that revascularization in patients with relatively preserved CFR may not be associated with improved outcomes, which is consistent with the results observed in the FAME (FFR vs. Angiography for Multivessel Evaluation) trial.[11]

Finally, an increasingly recognized clinical entity where nuclear myocardial perfusion imaging has an importance is MI in the absence of obstructive CAD (MINOCA).[12] A large systematic review/meta-analysis of 28 publications found that MINOCA was found in approximately 6% of all patients with acute MI who are referred for coronary angiography. Specific causes of MINOCA include plaque erosion, coronary artery vasospasm, coronary thromboembolism, and coronary microvascular dysfunction.[13] Cardiac PET perfusion imaging with myocardial blood flow assessment can be utilized in cases of MINOCA to evaluate for the presence of coronary microvascular dysfunction.

Assessment of Nonculprit Vessels After Primary Percutaneous Coronary Intervention

Case Vignette 3

The patient was a 53-year-old man with a history of hypertension, dyslipidemia, diabetes, and tobacco use who presented with an anterior ST-elevation myocardial infarction (STEMI). Initial coronary angiography showed a 100% occluded LAD, 80% stenosis in a diagonal branch, and 80% stenosis in the RCA (Fig. 16.13A and Videos 16.7 and 16.8). At the time of the initial event, he underwent successful PCI to open the LAD (Video 16.9). His nonculprit CAD was managed medically (see also Chapter 11). One month later, he presented with recurrent chest pain. An exercise myocardial perfusion SPECT was performed to quantify residual ischemia to direct further management. He exercised for 7 minutes of a modified Bruce protocol, achieving 87% of the age-predicted maximal heart rate. The symptomatic response to this regimen was chest heaviness with exercise. The ECG response to exercise indicated no significant ST-T changes.

The myocardial perfusion SPECT images showed a severely dilated left ventricle with a large and severe perfusion defect throughout the LAD territory, without evidence of residual exercise-induced ischemia *(arrowheads)* (Fig. 16.13B). The polar maps confirmed the presence of a large area of scar throughout the LAD territory, with minimal evidence of ischemia. Increased radiotracer uptake was also evident in the right ventricular free wall, consistent with elevated pulmonary artery pressures. The ECG-gated images showed akinesis of the anterior, septal and apical walls, and an LVEF of 25% (Video 16.10). Based on these findings, the patient was managed conservatively because there was no objective evidence of significant ischemia to justify repeat angiography and revascularization.

This stepwise approach is particularly useful in symptomatic patients with residual angiographic disease in nonculprit coronary arteries, especially those in higher-risk groups (e.g., elderly persons or those with diabetes or renal disease) and patients with recurrent symptoms, as in Case Vignette 3, and is considered reasonable by current guidelines.

Evaluation of Patients with Heart Failure After Acute Coronary Syndrome

Case Vignette 4

The patient was an 88-year-old woman who presented with shortness of breath three days after severe chest pressure that had subsequently resolved. She had an elevated jugular venous pressure and had rales on examination. Her presenting ECG showed anterior Q-waves and

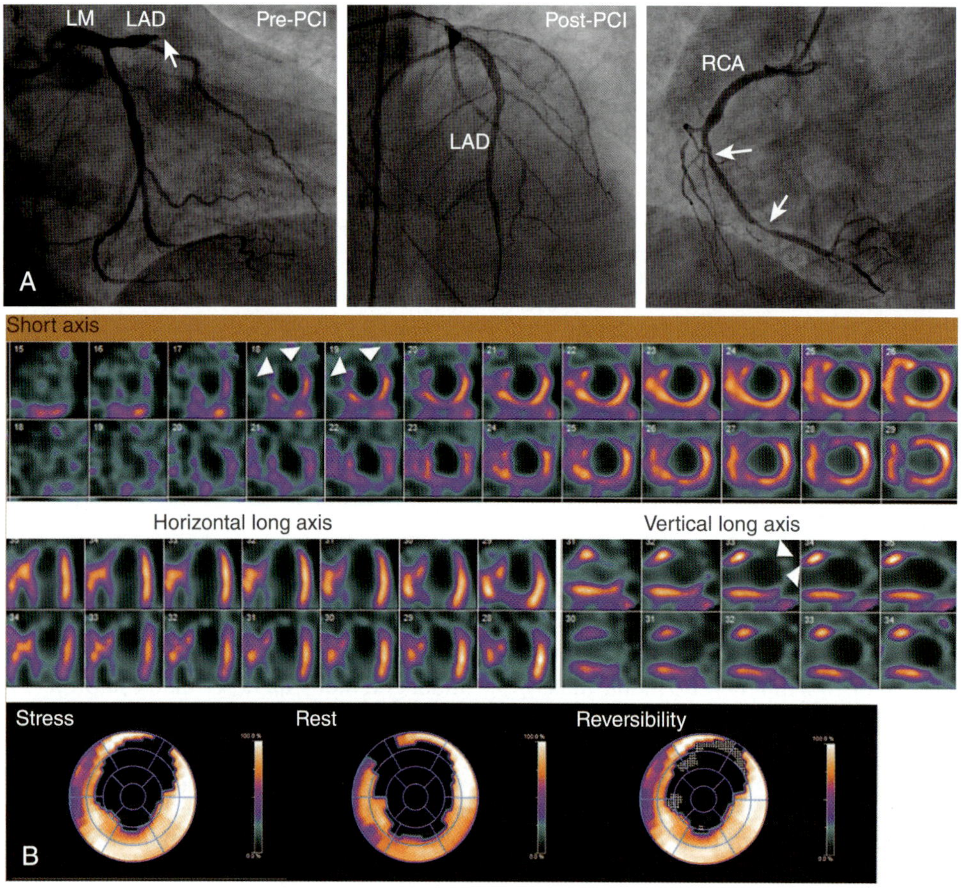

FIG. 16.13 Images for Case Vignette 3. (A) Coronary angiographic images. *Arrows* identify occluded LAD and serial 80% stenoses in the RCA. (B) Corresponding stress and rest[13]N-ammonia myocardial perfusion positron emission tomography (PET) images. See text for details. *LAD,* Left anterior descending artery; *LM,* left main artery; *PCI,* percutaneous coronary intervention; *RCA,* right coronary artery.

ST-segment elevations. Cardiac troponin T level was 1095 ng/L and a transthoracic echocardiogram showed apical hypokinesis and a LVEF of 40% (Video 16.11). She was referred for a myocardial PET/CT to evaluate the extent and magnitude of myocardial viability prior to potential revascularization.

The PET/CT images showed normal left ventricular cavity size with a large-sized perfusion defect of severe intensity involving the mid anterior and anteroseptal walls and the entire left ventricular apex with essentially preserved FDG uptake (perfusion-FDG mismatch) (Fig. 16.14A). This pattern was consistent with a large area of predominantly viable but hibernating myocardium through the mid-left anterior descending artery territory. Based on these findings, the patient underwent successful revascularization to a 99% stenosis of the mid to distal left anterior descending artery and a 90% stenosis of the first diagonal artery (Fig. 16.14B; Video 16.12).

Metabolic imaging with PET has an established role in the evaluation of myocardial viability (see also Chapter 14).[14] As discussed previously, specific abnormalities in myocardial metabolism reflecting viable and scarred myocardium have been described (see Fig. 16.3). Contractile dysfunction is predicted to be reversible after revascularization in regions with increased FDG uptake, or *perfusion-FDG mismatch*, and irreversible in those with reduced FDG uptake, or *perfusion-FDG match* pattern. Using these criteria, the average positive predictive value for predicting improved segmental function after revascularization is 76% (range, 52%–100%), whereas the average negative predictive value is 82% (range, 67%–100%). A clinically meaningful improvement in global left ventricular function can be expected after revascularization in patients with relatively large areas of hibernating and/or stunned myocardium (approximately 20% of the left ventricular mass). There is evidence that delineation of myocardial viability with FDG-PET is largely concordant with cardiac MRI but is more sensitive than dobutamine echocardiography and radionuclide perfusion SPECT imaging (see Fig. 14.3). Other relative advantages of radionuclide imaging over MRI relate to its improved ability to quantify peri-infarct ischemia, as well as its relative safety in patients with impaired renal function and cardiac devices (defibrillators and pacemakers).

The use of viability imaging also plays a role in determining the size and extent of scar in planning optimal implantable cardioverter-defibrillator (ICD)/cardiac resynchronization therapy (CRT) lead position in patients with ischemic cardiomyopathy. Studies have shown that cardiac resynchronization plus defibrillator therapy (CRT-D) devices are more successful when lead position is in an area of viable myocardium, with improved left ventricular systolic function and outcomes.[15]

Finally, MI and ischemia can lead to sympathetic denervation in both the infarct and the peri-infarct zone (Fig. 16.15). Viable but denervated myocardial regions show supersensitive shortening of the effective refractory

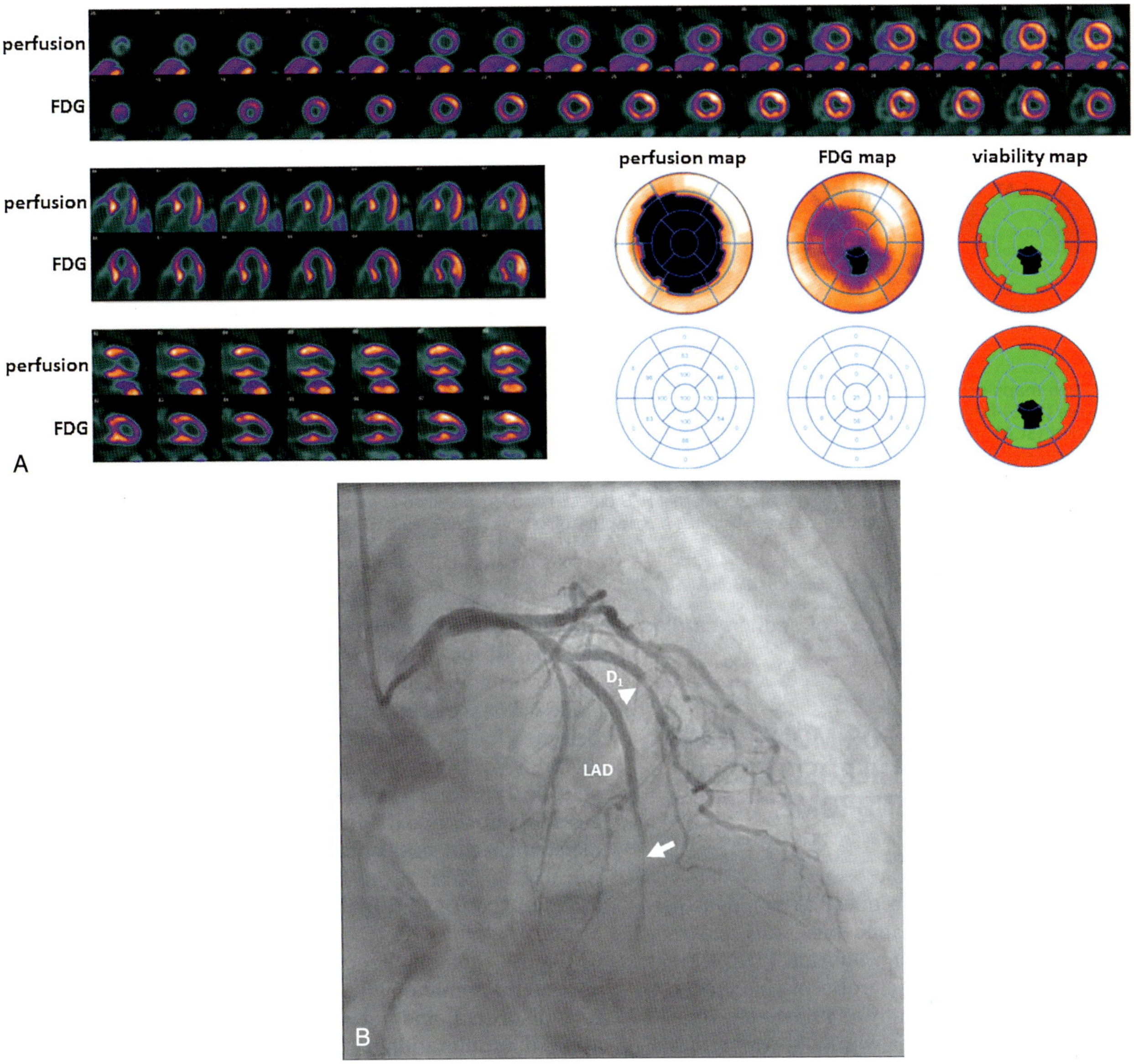

FIG. 16.14 Images for Case Vignette 4. (A) Corresponding N-13 ammonia rest perfusion and fluorodeoxyglucose (FDG) positron emission tomography/computed tomography (PET/CT) images. See text for details. (B) Coronary angiography images showing severe obstructive coronary artery disease in the left anterior descending artery (LAD) (*white arrow*) and the first diagonal artery (D_1) (*white arrowhead*).

period in response to the infusion of norepinephrine and are more vulnerable to ventricular arrhythmias. These observations suggest that direct imaging of cardiac sympathetic innervation may have an important clinical role in the risk stratification of patients after MI. The PAREPET (Prediction of ARrhythmic Events with Positron Emission Tomography) study was designed to test the hypothesis that the extent of inhomogeneity in myocardial sympathetic innervation and/or hibernating myocardium increased the risk of arrhythmic death independently of left ventricular function in patients with ischemic cardiomyopathy (LVEF of 35% or less). The study included 204 patients who were eligible for primary-prevention ICDs. PET imaging was used to quantify myocardial sympathetic denervation (with carbon-11 [^{11}C]-labeled hydroxyephedrine [HED]), perfusion, and metabolism. The primary endpoint was sudden cardiac arrest, defined as arrhythmia-related death or ICD discharge for ventricular fibrillation or ventricular tachycardia at a rate higher than 240 beats/min. Compared with patients in the lowest tertile of cardiac sympathetic denervation assessed by HED PET, patients in the highest tertile showed a greater than sixfold increase in the risk of sudden cardiac arrest. In multivariable analysis, the extent of PET-defined sympathetic denervation, left ventricular end-diastolic volume index, and serum creatinine were significantly associated with the risk of sudden cardiac arrest. Similar findings were reported in the ADMIRE-HF (ADreView Myocardial Imaging for Risk Evaluation in Heart Failure) study using iodine-123 metaiodobenzylguanidine (^{123}I-mIBG) imaging, in a more heterogeneous cohort of patients with ischemic and nonischemic heart failure. In this study, patients with a heart-to-mediastinum (H/M) count ratio below 1.6 had a relatively lower risk of death or of ventricular arrhythmias. Although none of the imaging approaches assessing autonomic innervation have been linked to therapeutics, including implantation of ICDs, the results of these clinical studies support the hypothesis that these techniques may be helpful in the identification

17 Cardiac Magnetic Resonance Imaging After Presentation With Acute Coronary Syndrome

JOHN D. GRIZZARD AND RAYMOND J. KIM

INTRODUCTION

The use of sensitive biomarkers has significantly improved the diagnosis of myocardial infarction (MI) and has been incorporated into the "Universal Definition" of MI (see Chapter 2).[1] However, the diagnosis of MI still can be difficult. There is significant overlap with other disorders that result in myocardial injury (see Chapter 4). For instance, disorders such as Takotsubo cardiomyopathy and myocarditis are associated with elevation of circulating cardiac troponin, and their clinical differentiation from acute MI can be problematic, often resulting in invasive diagnostic procedures (see Chapter 4). In other instances, patients may present late, after cardiac biomarkers have normalized, resulting in an "unrecognized" MI. Appreciating the value of cardiac imaging in such circumstances, the universal definition of MI incorporates imaging findings of a new loss of viable myocardium or new wall motion abnormality, in conjunction with other clinical criteria. Given its capacity for state-of-the-art imaging of both myocardial structure and wall motion, cardiac magnetic resonance (CMR) has emerged as an important method to confirm the diagnosis of MI in suspected cases, as well as to differentiate MI from other conditions.

Complementing its utility in the diagnosis of MI, CMR can provide substantial additional information in the patient with known or suspected MI, including the determination of the infarct-related artery (IRA), particularly in non-ST elevation MI (NSTEMI), the detection of inducible ischemia, and the determination of residual viability (see Chapter 14). Additionally, CMR can accurately assess various complications of MI such as thrombus formation, or the development of a ventricular aneurysm (see also Chapter 22). Lastly, given its accuracy and precision in determining infarct size, CMR is increasingly used as a research tool in population studies of MI, and as a surrogate endpoint in randomized trials of investigational MI therapies. In this chapter, we will examine the application of CMR in patients with known or suspected MI, with an emphasis on demonstrating modality-specific aspects and the possible implications for patient care.

CARDIAC MAGNETIC RESONANCE TECHNIQUE

CMR has undergone rapid evolution, and technical advances in scanner hardware and coil technology have resulted in the progressive expansion of clinical applications (Fig. 17.1). In particular, new pulse sequences have leveraged the inherently superior soft tissue contrast provided by MR to improve anatomic definition and the delineation of diseased from normal tissue. Overall, these advances have led to the recognition of CMR as the reference standard for the assessment of regional and global systolic function, imaging of MI and viability, and the differentiation of ischemic cardiomyopathy from various nonischemic etiologies. Although previously, CMR exams were lengthy (approximately 1 h) and many patients were not capable of completing a standard examination, accelerated imaging techniques are now sufficiently robust such that useful diagnostic information can be provided for patients with arrhythmias and/or limited ability to cooperate in 30 minutes or less. The multiplicity of techniques and the variety of information that can be obtained in a CMR exam can be exhaustive, but increasingly there has been a move toward standardization of imaging protocols tailored to specific indications, an effort spearheaded by the Society of Cardiovascular Magnetic Resonance.[2] Our suggested implementation and a timeline (Fig. 17.2) of a CMR protocol for a standard CMR exam is as follows:

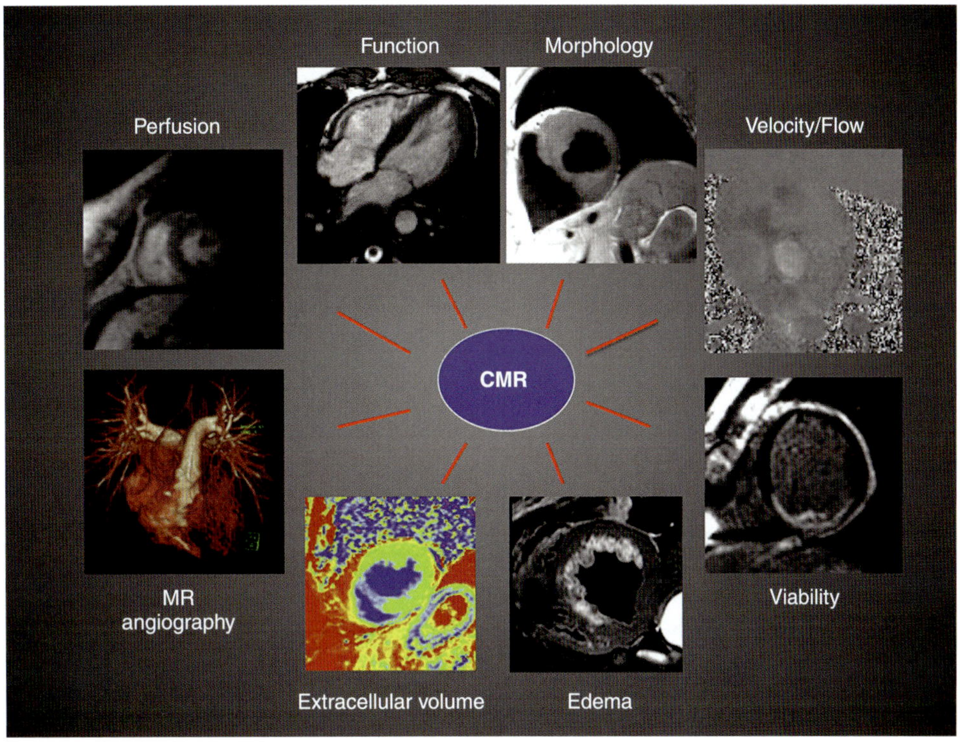

FIG. 17.1 Using different software programs to drive image acquisition, a variety of imaging is possible using a magnetic resonance (MR) scanner. As a result of innovations in pulse sequences, multiple parameters of cardiovascular structure and function can now be evaluated with cardiac (CMR). For an additional presentation of this image, click here.

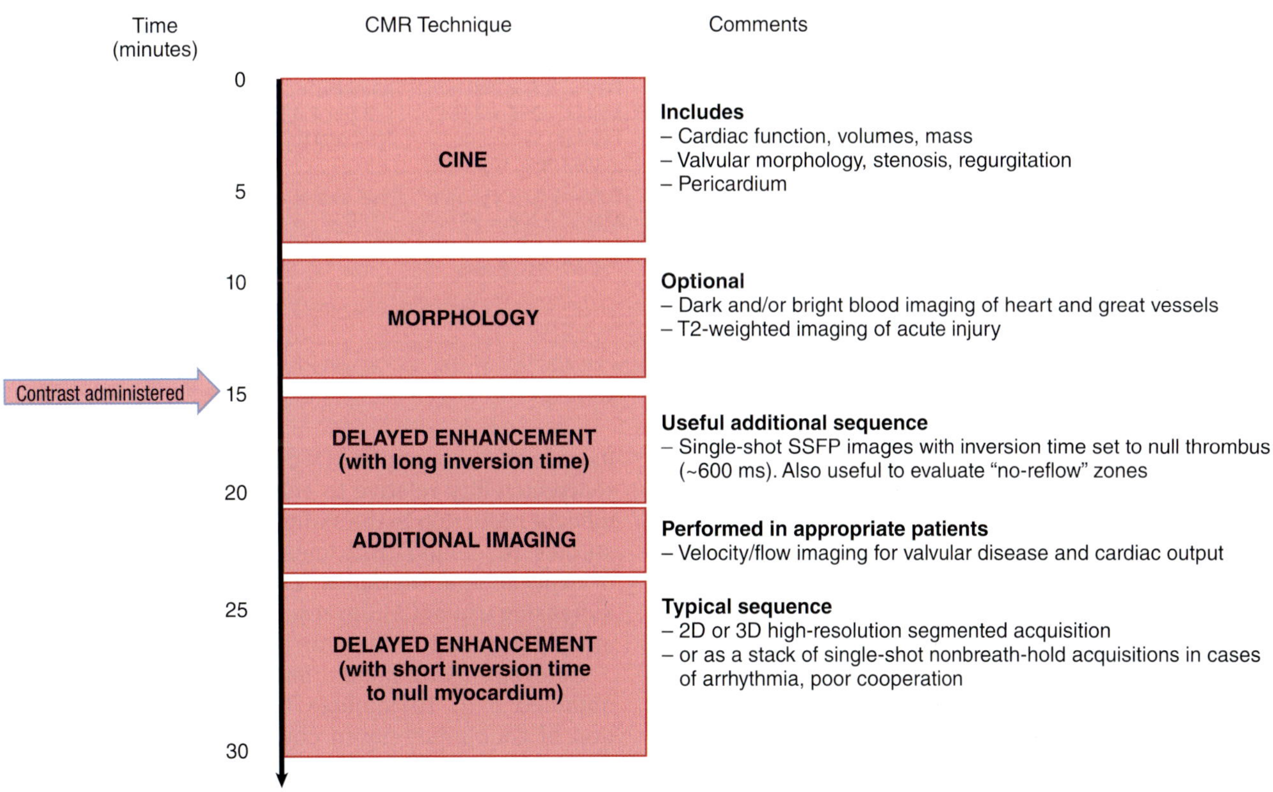

FIG. 17.2 Timeline of a standard cardiac magnetic resonance (CMR) examination. Note that the entire examination can be performed within 30 min. In cases in which the patient is unable to cooperate, the cine examination can be performed with real-time imaging and delayed enhancement with single-shot techniques. This technique will reduce artifacts in patients unable to perform a breath-hold, and total examination time will be shortened further. *SSFP*, Steady-state free-precession; *3D*, three-dimensional; *2D*, two-dimensional.

TABLE 17.1 Sequences and Imaging Parameters Used in a Typical Cardiac Magnetic Resonance Examination

IMAGING	SEQUENCE TYPE	LOCATION	IMAGING PARAMETERS	RESOLUTION	NOTES
Localizers	Single-shot SSFP images	Axial, sagittal, coronal	400-mm FOV	Low resolution	Allows scan planning for cardiac imaging
Cine SSFP (standard)	Segmented SSFP images obtained with retrospective gating	Short-axis images from base to apex; 2-, 3-, and 4-chamber long-axis views	FOV ≈ 360 × 290 mm Matrix ≈ 256 × 168 pixels; slice thickness, 6–8 mm	Pixel size ≈ 1.7 × 1.4 × 6 mm Temporal res. ≈ 40 ms	6–10 s breath-hold required
DE-CMR (standard)	Segmented gradient echo inversion recovery images with data obtained from every other heartbeat	Exactly matched to cines	FOV ≈ 360 × 290 mm Matrix ≈ 256 × 168 pixels; slice thickness, 6–8 mm	Pixel size ≈ 1.7 × 1.4 × 6 mm Temporal res. ≈ 160–200 ms	Inversion time chosen to null signal from myocardium
Modifications					
Cine SSFP (real-time)	Real-time images where each cine frame is obtained in single-shot fashion	Short-axis images from base to apex; 2-, 3-, and 4-chamber images	FOV ≈ 380 × 260 mm Matrix ≈ 192 × 84 pixels; slice thickness, 10 mm	Pixel size ≈ 3.1 × 2.0 × 10 mm Temporal res. ≈ 70 ms	Useful in uncooperative or severely arrhythmic patients
DE-CMR (single-shot)	Single-shot SSFP inversion recovery images	Short-axis stack from base to apex; long-axis stack(s) can also be obtained	FOV ≈ 360 × 290 mm Matrix ≈ 208 × 128 pixels; slice thickness, 8 mm	Pixel size ≈ 2.3 × 1.7 × 8 mm Temporal res. ≈ 160–200 ms	Useful in uncooperative or severely arrhythmic patients
Optional Sequences					
Morphologic images	Bright-blood imaging performed with single-shot SSFP; dark-blood imaging performed with HASTE	Stack of images obtained usually in the axial plane; can also obtain sagittal and coronal stacks	FOV ≈ 380 × 315 mm Matrix ≈ 256 × 152 pixels; slice thickness, 8 mm	Pixel size ≈ 2.0 × 1.5 × 8 mm Temporal res. ≈ 60–100 ms	Survey of heart and great vessels; aortic abnormalities, congenital defects
T2-weighted images	Gated T2 FSE or STIR images	Matched to short-axis cine and DE-MR images	FOV ≈ 360 × 290 mm Matrix ≈ 256 × 168 pixels; slice thickness, 6–8 mm	Pixel size ≈ 1.7 × 1.4 × 6 mm Temporal res. ≈ 60–80 ms	To evaluate for edema seen with acute disorders (AMI, myocarditis)
Flow sensitive images	Velocity-encoded gated images	Typically obtained through stenotic valves or proximal great vessels	FOV ≈ 360 × 240 mm Matrix ≈ 256 × 116 pixels; slice thickness, 6–8 mm	Pixel size ≈ 2.0 × 1.4 × 6 mm Temporal res. ≈ 45 ms	Used to measure peak gradients and flow
Perfusion imaging	Saturation recovery (T1-weighted) images to evaluate the transit of contrast through the myocardium	Typically obtained as a stack of 4 short-axis images to cover the LV	FOV ≈ 340 × 255 mm Matrix ≈ 208 × 98 pixels; slice thickness, 8 mm	Pixel size ≈ 2.6 × 1.6 × 8 mm Temporal res. ≈ 120 ms	Can be performed with pharmacologic stress to evaluate for inducible ischemia

AMI, Acute myocardial infarction; *DE-CMR*, delayed-enhancement cardiac magnetic resonance; *FOV*, field of view; *FSE*, fast spin echo; *HASTE*, half-acquisition turbo spin-echo; *LV*, left ventricular; *res*, resolution; *SSFP*, steady-state free-precession; *STIR*, short T1 inversion recovery.

Standard Cardiac Magnetic Resonance Exam

Cine images: Cine images are typically acquired in the short-axis plane from above the mitral valve through the LV apex along with standard 2-, 3-, and 4-chamber long-axis views (Fig. 17.e1). Typical parameters are shown in Table 17.1. The cine images have excellent spatial and temporal resolution and are not limited by acoustic windows. Therefore, they allow comprehensive evaluation of regional and global ventricular function and overall cardiac morphology. Visual evaluation of valvular function and morphology is also performed using these images.

Inter- and intra-observer reproducibility of cine CMR imaging for the quantification of LV volumes and function has been shown in multiple studies to be excellent, predominantly due to its high spatial and temporal resolution and its capacity for complete LV coverage. The improvement in reproducibility relative to echocardiography allows a significant reduction in the sample sizes required for research studies to demonstrate meaningful changes as a result of experimental therapies. This advantage has led to the increasing use of CMR in research studies that use cardiac morphology and/or function as an efficacy endpoint.

Delayed-enhancement images: These images are obtained 5 to 10 minutes following the IV administration of gadolinium-based contrast with 6 to 8 mm slices that are spatially matched to the cine images previously obtained (Fig. 17.e2). The delayed-enhancement sequence (DE-CMR) has been shown to be the most sensitive noninvasive imaging test for the detection of MI. It can accurately depict the presence, location, and extent of MI with

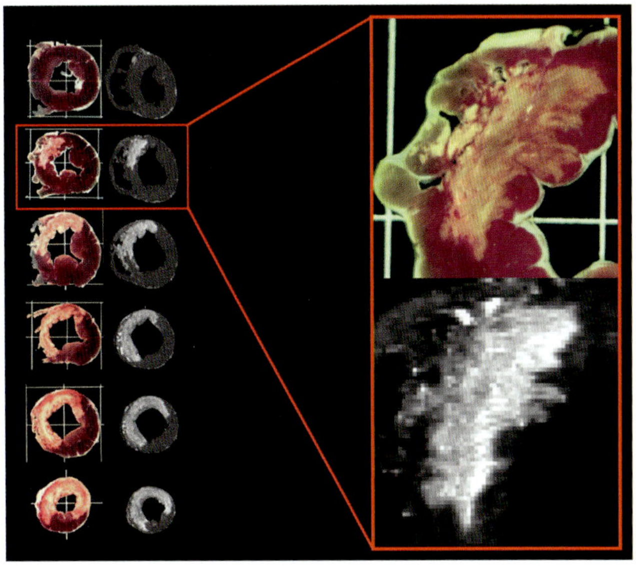

FIG. 17.3 **Comparison of high-resolution ex vivo delayed-enhancement cardiac magnetic resonance (*right*) with acute myocyte necrosis defined by histopathology (*left*).** The size and shape of the infarcted region (*yellowish-white region*) defined histologically by triphenyltetrazolium chloride (TTC) stain is nearly exactly matched by the size and shape of the hyper-enhanced (*bright*) region of delayed-enhancement cardiac magnetic resonance. For an additional presentation of this image, click here. (Adapted from Kim RJ, Fieno DS, Parrish TB, et al. Relationship of MRI delayed contrast enhancement to irreversible injury, infarct age, and contractile function. *Circulation*. 1999;100:1992–2002.)

high spatial resolution irrespective of infarct age. In animal models, DE-CMR has been shown to demonstrate acute and chronic MI with a near exact spatial match to histopathology specimens (Fig. 17.3). Additionally, these studies show that DE-CMR can distinguish between reversible and irreversible injury independent of wall motion, infarct age, and reperfusion status. Studies in humans have shown that infarct size measured by DE-CMR is associated with peak cardiac biomarker release (see Chapter 4) and measurements by positron emission tomography (see Chapter 16). Compared with SPECT imaging, the DE-CMR technique is significantly more sensitive for the detection of subendocardial infarction, over 40% of which are missed with SPECT (Fig. 17.4). With standard imaging parameters, DE-CMR is capable of demonstrating infarcts involving as little as one one-thousandth of total LV mass, and that is undetectable by techniques that assess myocardial perfusion or contractile function. The high spatial resolution of DE-CMR has been used to visualize microinfarctions, involving as little as 1g of tissue, which may occur during otherwise successful percutaneous coronary intervention.

The technique of DE-CMR has been extensively validated. Its ability to delineate viable from nonviable myocardium is based on the differential distribution of gadolinium contrast in diseased compared with normal tissue. It is important to note that all myocardium—normal, infarcted, or scarred—will demonstrate some contrast enhancement. However, conventional gadolinium contrast agents localize to the extracellular space since they are inert, and intact sarcolemmal membranes prevent them from entering the intracellular space. Normal myocardium, in which the myocytes are densely packed, thus has a limited extra-cellular volume of distribution (20%) and can be thought of as excluding the contrast agent. With acute necrosis (e.g., acute MI, myocarditis), there is membrane rupture, which allows gadolinium to diffuse into myocytes. This diffusion results in increased gadolinium concentration, shortened T1 relaxation, and thus hyperenhancement. In the chronic setting, the scar

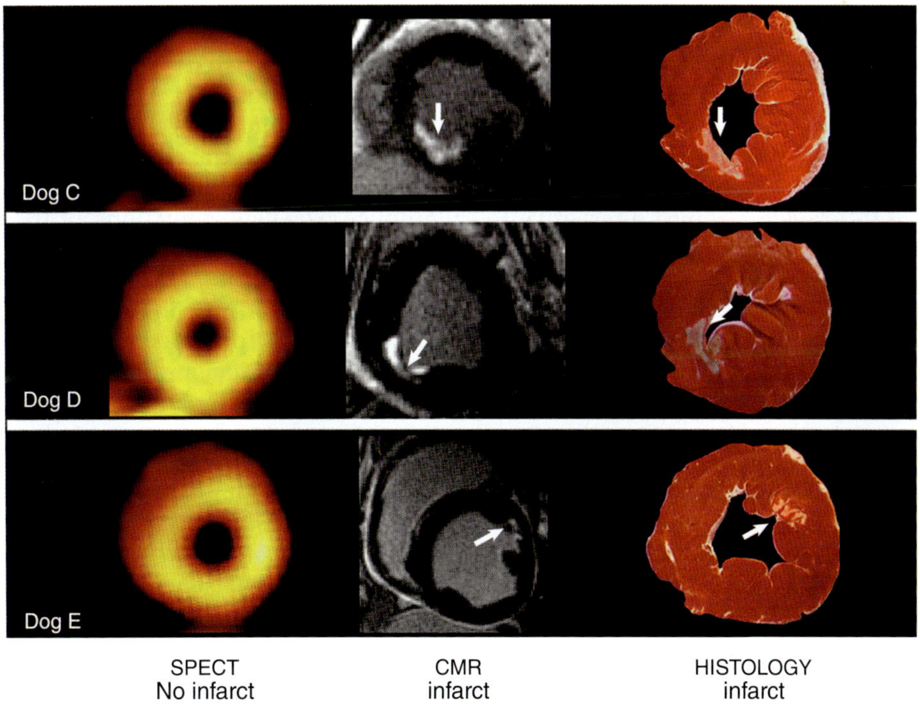

FIG. 17.4 **Short-axis views from three dogs that had subendocardial infarctions.** Unlike the single-photon emission computed tomography (SPECT) images, delayed-enhancement cardiac magnetic resonance (CMR) readily demonstrates the infarcted regions *(arrows)*. For an additional presentation of this image, click here. (Adapted from Wagner A, Mahrholdt H, Holly TA, et al. Contrast-enhanced MRI and routine single photon emission computed tomography [SPECT] perfusion imaging for detection of subendocardial myocardial infarcts: an imaging study. *Lancet*. 2003;361:374–379.)

has replaced necrotic tissue, and the interstitial space is expanded, leading to increased gadolinium concentration and hyperenhancement. In both acute and chronic settings (and all stages in between), one can consider viable myocytes as actively excluding gadolinium. Thus, the unifying mechanism of hyperenhancement appears to be the absence of viable myocytes rather than any inherent properties that are specific for acute necrosis, collagenous scar, or other forms of nonviable myocardium (Fig. 17.e3).

The standard delayed enhancement imaging sequence is a heavily T1-weighted segmented gradient echo sequence, in which an inversion pulse has been applied. The inversion pulse serves to flip the magnetization 180 degrees. The recovery of magnetization back to baseline by areas that have a higher gadolinium concentration such as infarcts or scar tissue will be more rapid (as they have a lower T1 value) than those with a lesser concentration of gadolinium such as normal myocardium. The time after the inversion pulse at which the magnetization of normal myocardium is at the zero-crossing line will result in maximum suppression of signal from normal myocardium (the myocardium is said to be "nulled") and will result in maximum conspicuity of the area of infarction (Fig. 17.e4). Because the magnetization of infarcted regions, by virtue of their increased contrast content, will recover above the baseline more rapidly (the contrast will accelerate the recovery back to baseline magnetization), infarctions will appear bright on these images.

The standard delayed enhancement sequences are segmented acquisitions, acquired at every other heartbeat in order to allow recovery of longitudinal magnetization in normal myocardium before the next inversion pulse is applied. They typically take approximately 8 to 12 seconds to acquire. For patients with significant arrhythmia or difficulty with breath holding, single-shot delayed enhancement images using an SSFP (steady-state free-precession) inversion recovery readout can provide comparable data in a fraction of the imaging time. These images have slightly worse spatial resolution and contrast-to-noise ratio but provide a satisfactory alternative in these circumstances. Motion-corrected DE-MR imaging has also been shown to provide a robust alternative to conventional scanning with preserved signal-to-noise even in patients with impaired ability to cooperate or with arrhythmia.[3] The delayed enhancement single-shot inversion recovery images may also be obtained with a long inversion time (550–600 ms at 1.5 T) and are quite useful in the detection of thrombi. In these images with a long inversion time, thrombi will appear dark in contrast to normal and infarcted myocardium, which will be medium to high in signal intensity. Since these do not require "washout" of contrast from the myocardium, these can be performed shortly after contrast administration while waiting for the appropriate delay for standard DE-CMR imaging (see Fig. 17.2).

Dark-blood delayed-enhancement imaging: While the DE-CMR imaging technique is widely recognized as the in vivo reference standard for the visualization of MI, a recognized limitation is that small subendocardial infarcts may be obscured by the adjacent bright signal of the blood pool. The uncertainty in identifying the border between the infarction and the blood pool is a primary source of variability in the quantification of MIs and has stimulated the development of a number of modifications of the DE-CMR sequence designed to produce a DE-CMR image with a dark blood pool. Multiple versions of such a sequence have been developed, including those with a T2 preparation pulse preceding the inversion pulse (T2 prep-IR) or following the inversion pulse (IR-T2 prep), which may be combined with phase-sensitive inversion recovery (PSIR) reconstruction.[4] A novel technique using a magnetization transfer (MT) prep followed by an inversion pulse with PSIR reconstruction (termed flow-independent dark-blood delayed enhancement [FIDDLE]) has been studied in animal models (with histologic validation) as well as in patients. Compared to the standard DE-CMR technique, FIDDLE has demonstrated superior overall sensitivity (96% vs. 85%) and accuracy (100% vs. 84%).[5] For purely subendocardial infarcts, its relative advantage was even more pronounced, as the sensitivity of the standard DE-CMR sequence declined to 80%, while that of the novel sequence remained high at 98% (see Fig. 17.5).[5] In some centers, dark-blood versions of DE-CMR are becoming part of the clinical routine, and promise to provide more accurate and reproducible measurements of infarct size, an increasingly important consideration as CMR measurements of infarct size become end-points in clinical trials.

Optional Sequences

Morphologic static images: In many cases, an overview of cardiac and great vessel anatomy is desirable and can be rapidly performed using single-shot dark blood and/or single-shot bright blood techniques such as HASTE (half-acquisition turbo spin-echo) and SSFP (steady-state free-precession) sequences, respectively. These techniques result in a stack of still-frame images and are usually acquired in the standard orthogonal imaging planes (axial, sagittal, or coronal). The rapidity of acquisition is such that breath-holding is not required. These produce excellent depictions of the overall myocardial structure, as well as the architecture of the great vessels (Fig. 17.e5).

T2 weighted images: In cases where the acuity of infarction is uncertain or in cases of suspected acute myocarditis, T2-weighted imaging may be useful in demonstrating the edema characteristically seen in the acute phase of these disorders. These sequences are performed prior to the administration of IV contrast as the presence of contrast may complicate image interpretation. These can be obtained via a double or triple inversion fast spin-echo black-blood sequence or with a T2-preparation SSFP bright-blood sequence. The T2-prep bright-blood sequence is far more resistant to artifacts than the black-blood sequence. However, the bright-blood sequence may be less sensitive for detecting regions with more moderate levels of edema, particularly if limited to the subendocardium. Increasingly, because of their greater resistance to artifacts and for the purposes of quantification, T2 mapping sequences are being used in those

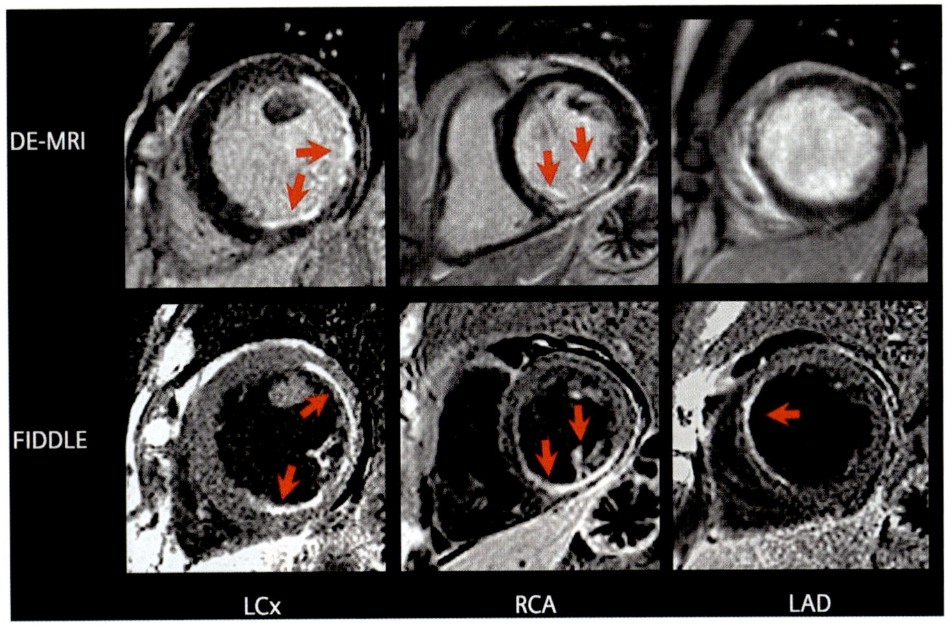

FIG. 17.5 Comparison of conventional DE-MR with FIDDLE images in three patients with myocardial infarctions (*red arrows*). In the first patient, a circumflex territory infarction is well seen in both images. In the second patient with a right coronary infarction, it is clear that abnormal enhancement is present, but the subendocardial border of the infarct is unclear. The third patient demonstrates an infarction in the left anterior descending coronary artery territory which is difficult to visualize on the standard DE-MR image but is well seen on the FIDDLE image.

circumstances where edema is suspected (see the section on mapping).[6]

Perfusion imaging: These sequences are designed to demonstrate contrast media passage through the myocardium in a manner that reliably reflects myocardial blood flow. The sequences used are heavily T1-weighted, in order to accurately depict the passage of a T1-shortening contrast agent, such as gadolinium, through the myocardium. It is most often used for the detection of obstructive coronary artery disease (CAD), where it is performed with pharmacologic vasodilation (e.g., adenosine or regadenoson).

The underlying principle is similar to that in nuclear perfusion imaging, where a vasodilator is used to accentuate regional differences in myocardial blood flow. However, as opposed to nuclear techniques, MR perfusion imaging is a first-pass imaging study that directly images the passage of contrast and therefore is performed using an abbreviated adenosine protocol (approximately 3 min). Also, MR perfusion imaging has a higher spatial resolution (>20-fold) than nuclear techniques and can depict a perfusion defect that is limited to the subendocardium. MR perfusion imaging has the additional advantage of providing a more linear depiction of myocardial blood flow in response to vasodilatation, without the plateau phenomenon seen with nuclear agents. A modification of the standard exam to include stress and rest perfusion imaging is shown in Fig. 17.e6.

Increasingly, stress and rest CMR perfusion imaging is being used to detect ischemia in patients with known or suspected coronary disease, and multiple studies have demonstrated excellent sensitivity and specificity, exceeding those of SPECT imaging. A study comparing stress CMR with invasive fractional flow reserve (FFR) for the detection of ischemia found that perfusion CMR was associated with a lower incidence of revascularization than FFR and was equivalent in the incidence of major adverse cardiac events or freedom from angina.[7] Stress perfusion CMR has also been shown to provide prognostic information beyond that of conventional clinical factors as demonstrated by two large multicenter registry studies.[8,9] Given the accumulating prognostic data validating the sensitive detection of ischemia by perfusion CMR combined with the superior delineation of infarction provided by DE-CMR, it is not surprising that the AHA/ACC guidelines now give stress CMR a class I indication for the evaluation of chest pain in intermediate-risk patients without known CAD.[10]

T1 and T2 mapping techniques: T1 and T2 mapping techniques are increasingly being investigated in a variety of myocardial disorders and can be performed before and/or after the administration of IV contrast. These sequences provide a quantitative assessment of regional myocardial T1 and T2 values and are not subject to surface coil sensitivity profiles that can result in variable image intensity for different regions of the heart. In the absence of gadolinium contrast, T1 and T2 values are increased in the setting of acute necrosis-related edema, and thus these sequences allow the depiction of edema and provide a metric, which may be useful for purposes of quantification and serial assessment (Fig. 17.6). A parametric map of extracellular volume fraction can be made by combining precontrast ("native") and postcontrast T1 mapping values. Extracellular volume fraction will be increased both in the setting of acute necrosis and chronic collagenous scar.

TYPICAL IMAGING FINDINGS IN MYOCARDIAL INFARCTION

Acute Ischemic Injury

Cine imaging–Acute ischemic injury of the myocardium usually results in myocardial dysfunction, with reduction

Chapter 28). While sometimes thought to have a benign prognosis, a recent CMR investigation of patients with a working diagnosis of MINOCA (MI without obstructed coronary arteries) found that prognosis was often guarded and varied with CMR diagnosis; with 10-year unadjusted MACE rates of 50% in nonischemic cardiomyopathy (predominantly Takotsubo cardiomyopathy), 47% in acute MI, and 24% in myocarditis. Patients with a normal CMR exam had a rate of 3.5%, similar to age-matched population-based cohorts completely free of clinical cardiovascular disease.[16] Thus, the prognosis in cases of MINOCA appears to vary with the underlying diagnosis and the syndrome may portend a significant risk of adverse events.

Characterization of Myocardial Infarction

DE-CMR may also allow assessment of gradations of injury within acute MI. Rather than simply identifying a region of acute infarction as nonviable, DE-CMR can distinguish acute infarcts with only necrotic myocytes from acute infarcts with necrotic myocytes and damaged microvasculature. The presence of a dark, nonenhancing central area contained within an area of hyperenhancement on DE-CMR is termed a "no-reflow zone," and represents an area of markedly delayed diffusion of contrast into the central core of what is usually an extensive infarction (Fig. 17.7C). These regions represent myocardium with compromised perfusion at the tissue level even after patency of the epicardial coronary artery has been restored. The presence of microvascular obstruction (MO) has been associated with worse outcome, including adverse ventricular remodeling, ventricular arrhythmia, and major adverse cardiac events (see Chapters 19 and 30). For example, among patients presenting with STEMI, the extent of no-reflow demonstrates a graded relationship between 1-year mortality and admissions for heart failure.[17] Unfortunately, the presence and extent of MO can also be quite variable within a given CMR exam since following contrast administration the spatial extent is greater at earlier time points, and it may disappear as contrast diffuses into the area of injury over time (Fig. 17.e14). Moreover, MO is a transient phenomenon since it disappears with infarct healing. Hence, there is likely a time window (approximately 4 weeks after AMI) beyond which the identification of no MO on CMR may not represent a marker of good prognosis since it may simply reflect its resolution. This issue is of particular relevance because acute MI is often clinically unrecognized, which precludes the precise determination of infarct age at the time of patient assessment. Given the transient nature of MO, it would be useful to identify clinical characteristics that are strongly associated with MO early after acute MI but are more stable and do not disappear with infarct healing. With this in mind, the novel concept of epicardial surface area of full-thickness infarction (EpiSA)—which can be quantified by delayed-enhancement imaging—has been introduced as a surrogate marker for MO. Smulders et al.[18] demonstrated that EpiSA accurately predicted the presence of MO in the early days following acute MI, but unlike MO, it remained stable over months and did not disappear with infarct healing.

Occasionally, circumstances arise where the patient may have more than one infarction, and the acuity of each is uncertain. In patients presenting with seemingly their first acute MI, the identification of a second infarct which is chronic—and which was clinically silent—was associated with poorer long-term clinical outcomes.[19] As noted previously, delayed enhancement imaging will demonstrate hyperenhancement in both acute and chronic MI, and thus by itself cannot distinguish between these possibilities. However, the presence of MO indicates an acute MI, and additional findings that suggest an area of hyperenhancement is likely acute include increased focal wall thickness on cine imaging and the presence of edema on T2 weighted imaging. The absence of all three features is suggestive but not specific for a chronic MI since in the setting of acute MI, these features may also be absent if the infarct is small and subendocardial.

Imaging of Acute Complications of Myocardial Infarction

Right ventricular MI (see Chapter 22): In patients with acute inferior MI, it has been shown that even when physical examination, ECG with right precordial leads, and echocardiography were negative, DE-CMR can detect right ventricular involvement in nearly 25% of patients. DE-CMR typically shows an extensive LV wall inferior MI with extension to involve the RV inferior wall and a variable portion of the RV free wall (Fig. 17.e15).[20,21] A recent CMR study of patients with AMI found a prevalence of RV MI of 12% and identified impaired RV global longitudinal strain as a predictor of adverse outcomes over and above established risk factors.[22]

Cardiac rupture (see Chapter 22): Free wall rupture has a high mortality rate (approaching 100%), and few patients come to imaging. Those surviving to imaging often have contained ruptures, but cine MR can demonstrate the focal loss of contractility in the affected segment, and the presence of intrapericardial fluid and blood products. DE-CMR demonstrates the causative infarction as an area of transmural enhancement.

Interventricular septal defects (see Chapter 22): Although usually assessed adequately by echo, MR can demonstrate the septal defect, the trans-septal flow, and the underlying MI (Fig. 17.e16). Importantly, MR can also noninvasively measure the pulmonary to systemic flow ratio (Qp/Qs), a parameter that may be useful in follow-up imaging of smaller defects or those treated with septal occlusion devices.

Pericarditis/pericardial effusion (see Chapter 22): Up to 31% of acute STEMI patients are found to have evidence of pericardial inflammation on CMR, manifested by pericardial effusions or abnormal enhancement on DE-CMR. Effusions are easily recognized as high-signal fluid in the pericardial space and are readily depicted with cine MR. Complicating hemorrhage is usually identifiable owing to the increased complexity of the pericardial fluid (Fig. 17.e17). Thickening of the pericardium can also clearly be seen. Postcontrast imaging can be helpful in assessing the presence of enhancement, signifying inflammatory pericarditis, and distinguishing it from chronic fibrous thickening, which often does not enhance.[23]

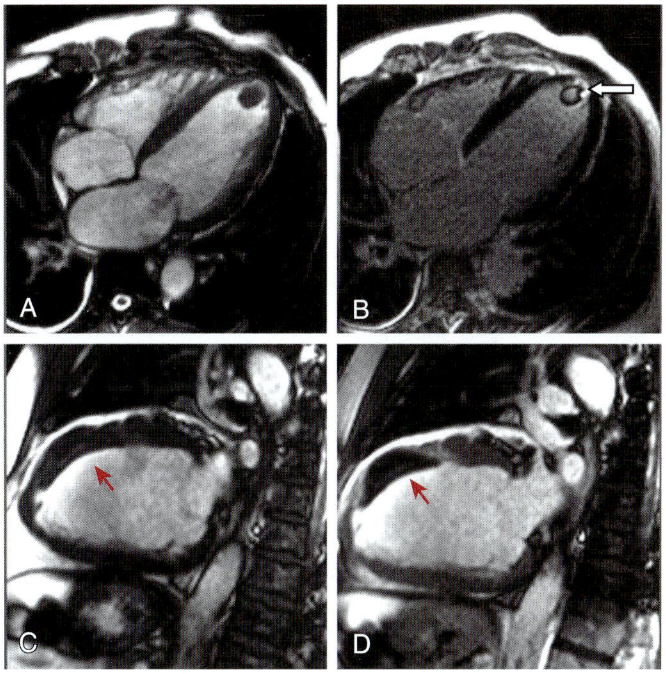

FIG. 17.10 Intracavitary thrombus is recognized as a filling defect separate from papillary muscles and trabeculae on the four-chamber cine view (A) and is noted on the delayed enhancement image (B) to be adherent to a site of previous apical infarction (*white arrow*). Thrombus may sometimes have an "etched" appearance on delayed-enhancement cardiac magnetic resonance images obtained with a standard inversion time but will be homogenously dark on images with a long inversion time (550–600 ms). In another patient with a mural thrombus lining a true aneurysm of the anterior wall, the precontrast two-chamber cine steady-state free-precession image (C) does not clearly differentiate the thrombus (*red arrow*) from the myocardium because their signal intensities are similar. (D) The postcontrast inversion-recovery steady-state free-precession image with a long inversion time (600 ms) allows clear differentiation of thrombus from myocardium. Echocardiography did not detect this thrombus. For an additional presentation of this image, click here.

Imaging of Chronic Complications of Myocardial Infarction

Thrombus (see Chapter 22): A meta-analysis of 10 studies involving STEMI patients treated with primary PCI found that the overall incidence of LV thrombus was 6.3%, with 96% occurring in patients with an anterior STEMI (12.2% incidence).[24] DE-CMR was used in these studies as it is the most sensitive imaging technique for the detection of LV thrombus and picks up approximately twice as many ventricular thrombi as cine-CMR and transthoracic echocardiography.

Thrombus is recognized on cine-CMR and echocardiography when it presents as an intracavitary structure that is discernible from adjacent trabeculations and papillary muscles (Fig. 17.10A and B). Recognition of mural thrombus, however, can be quite difficult, and the ability of DE-CMR to identify thrombus based on tissue characteristics rather than just anatomical appearance likely explains its improved performance compared with cine-CMR or echocardiography. The basic underlying principle is that thrombi are avascular and have essentially no gadolinium uptake. Thus, thrombus can be identified as a nonenhancing defect surrounded by bright ventricular blood and contrast-enhanced myocardium. Image intensity differences between normal myocardium and thrombus can be accentuated by using a DE-CMR sequence in which the inversion time is increased to null avascular tissue such as thrombus (500–600 ms at 1.5 T). With long-inversion-time imaging, regions with contrast uptake such as viable myocardium increase in image intensity, whereas thrombus appears homogeneously black, and there is improved delineation, particularly of mural thrombus (Fig. 17.10C and 10D). This long-inversion recovery variation of DE-CMR can be acquired using a single-shot inversion-recovery SSFP sequence in multiple planes to rapidly screen for thrombus, even in patients with arrhythmias or who are uncooperative.

Clinically, it is frequently noted that ventricular thrombi are found adherent to sites of prior infarction, where wall motion abnormalities and possibly denudation of the endothelium produced by prior infarction result in a nidus for thrombus formation. The latter mechanism is suggested given that CMR data demonstrate that patients with ischemic cardiomyopathy have an approximately fivefold increased risk relative to those with nonischemic systolic dysfunction of similar extent, and the presence of regions with >50% transmural infarction appears to be an additional risk factor for thrombus development. In particular, thrombi are often noted along the endocavitary aspect of ventricular aneurysms (Fig. 17.10C and 10D).

Ventricular aneurysms (see Chapter 22): Certain imaging characteristics have been noted to provide differentiation in most cases between true aneurysms (intact thinned myocardium) and false aneurysms (contained rupture). True aneurysms are said to have a wide neck that is similar in diameter to the base of the aneurysm, while false aneurysms, representing a contained rupture, typically have a narrow neck with a broad base (Fig. 17.e18). Ultimately, however, the real distinction between the two is the presence of residual myocardium forming the boundary of the lesion in the case of a true aneurysm or the lack thereof in a false aneurysm. Visualization of the wall of the aneurysm as separate and distinct from the pericardium is usually possible with cine MR imaging. Conversely, if the pericardium appears to make up the boundary of the aneurysm without residual myocardium, the lesion should be deemed a false aneurysm. Delayed enhancement imaging is also helpful in that pericardial enhancement has been described as occurring frequently in false aneurysms with a much lower incidence in true aneurysms. Both may have associated mural thrombus.

The "myocardial cut-off" sign has recently been proposed to aid in this distinction. It involves measurement of the thickness of the aneurysm wall relative to the normal myocardium. A >50% decrease at a point 1 cm from the aneurysm neck is termed a positive "cut-off sign" for pseudoaneurysm and was 91% sensitive and 97% specific. Subjective assessment of the myocardium appearing "cut-off" also had high sensitivity (94%–100%).[25]

PREDICTING FUNCTIONAL RECOVERY AND OUTCOMES

Predicting Left Ventricular Recovery

In the setting of acute MI, prompt restoration of coronary blood flow has been shown to result in salvage of

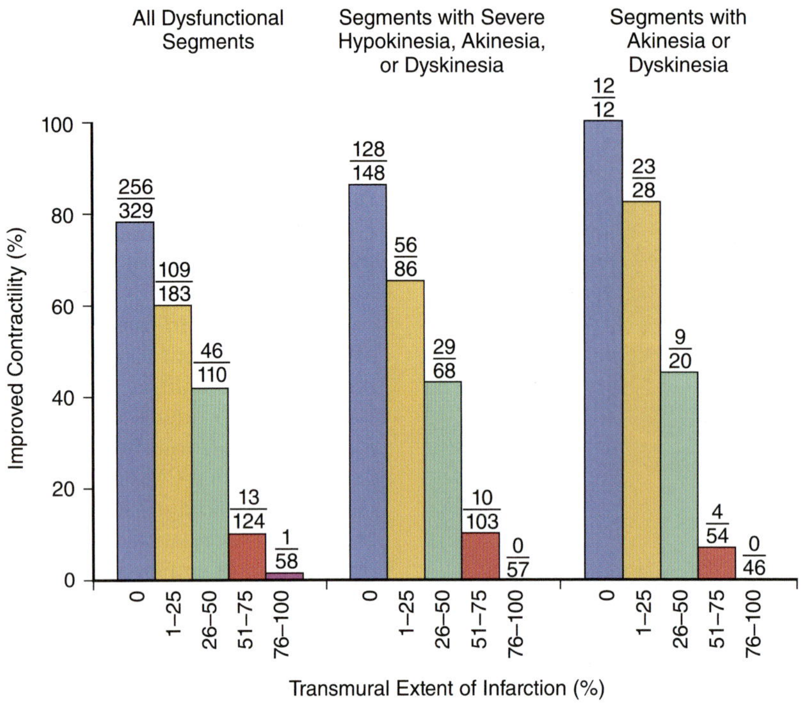

FIG. 17.11 The likelihood of recovery of wall motion following revascularization is inversely related to the transmural extent of infarction (hyperenhancement) on delayed enhancement imaging, even in severely hypokinetic, akinetic, or dyskinetic segments. (From Kim RJ, Wu E, Rafael A, et al. The use of contrast-enhanced magnetic resonance imaging to identify reversible myocardial dysfunction. *N Engl J Med.* 2000;343:1445–1453.)

viable myocardium, improvement in LV ejection fraction, and long-term improvement in survival (see Chapter 8). However, early after successful coronary reperfusion, myocardial dysfunction may persist, and it is important to distinguish whether it is due to myocardial necrosis or stunning (see Chapter 19). In the setting of acute MI, the TEI as measured on DE-CMR has been shown by multiple studies to be highly predictive of later improvement in wall motion (Fig. 17.e19). That is, the greater the TEI in a given segment, the lower the likelihood of recovery of function.

For instance, in one representative study, almost 80% of segments without infarction showed improvement, whereas only 5% of segments with greater than 75% TEI showed improvement. Areas of intermediate TEI demonstrated intermediate levels of recovery. In addition to predicting segmental functional recovery, DE-CMR also predicted improvement in global function. On a per-patient basis, the total number of segments that were dysfunctional but viable (<25% TEI) was directly related to the change in LV ejection fraction. Multiple other studies have subsequently confirmed that the transmural extent of enhancement on DE-CMR predicts functional improvement following MI.[26]

Predicting the Impact of Revascularization

In patients who have severe myocardial dysfunction in the setting of chronic CAD and are incompletely revascularized or not yet revascularized, a common clinical question centers on whether to proceed with coronary revascularization. In this setting, improvement in LVEF following revascularization will likely improve symptoms and outcomes, but such recovery requires viable myocardium. Multiple studies have demonstrated that among patients with chronic CAD, the likelihood of functional improvement is inversely related in a progressive stepwise fashion to the TEI as depicted by DE-CMR. That is, the greater the TEI, the lower the likelihood of recovery of wall motion in any given segment. Alternatively, minimal or no enhancement is associated with a high probability of improvement following revascularization (Fig. 17.11). This observation is true even in segments that are akinetic or dyskinetic prior to revascularization.

When interpreting the information that DE-CMR can provide in this setting, it is important to take advantage of the high spatial resolution it affords; DE-CMR allows the visualization of the transmural extent of viability/infarction and thus changes the assessment of viability from a binary "yes/no" characterization to that of a continuum, which better reflects reality. This ability to grade myocardial viability along a continuum is one of the great strengths of DE-CMR. As such, the use of a single cutoff value on which to base predictions of functional improvement would not have a physiologic basis and would be suboptimal. Again, areas demonstrating intermediate levels of viability are likely to predict intermediate levels of functional improvement rather than a 50% likelihood of either complete recovery or zero recovery.

It should be noted that the value of viability imaging in guiding revascularization is controversial. The landmark STICH trial found that at a median follow-up of 5.1 years, there was no significant interaction between viability status (as determined by SPECT or dobutamine echocardiography) and medical therapy with or without coronary artery bypass grafting (CABG) with respect to the primary endpoint of all-cause mortality, as well as the secondary endpoints of cardiovascular death or a composite of death or hospitalization for cardiovascular causes. This observation was also true at the subsequent 10-year follow-up, when, despite a statistically significant decrease in all-cause mortality in the CABG group, no significant interaction was observed between the presence or absence of myocardial viability and the beneficial effect of CABG plus medical therapy over medical therapy alone ($P = .34$ for interaction). However, analysis of the data reveals that in the group deemed to have viability, all-cause mortality was reduced in those undergoing surgical revascularization (hazard ratio, 0.70; 95% confidence intervals, 0.56–0.88). For the patients found to lack viability, the mortality hazard ratio was higher (0.81; 0.5–1.31), but the difference in the interaction between viability status and outcomes lacked statistical significance, likely because the group with no viability was so small. Only 19% of patients (114 total) were deemed to have no viability, resulting in a study that was limited in its ability to show whether the beneficial effect of CABG was reliably different in those with versus those without viability.

Other Aspects of Viability Assessment

Delayed enhancement imaging provides significantly better spatial resolution than the competing modality of SPECT imaging. However, even if SPECT imaging had similar spatial resolution, DE-CMR would still have a significant advantage in that it allows the assessment of the amount of viability and the amount of infarction *simultaneously*. This property of DE-CMR is particularly important in the differentiation of possibly hibernating myocardium from myocardium that is significantly thinned as a result of extensive scar. As an example of this principle, consider the evaluation of a patient with a region of thinned (<5.5 mm in diastole), dysfunctional myocardium (Fig. 17.e20). Classic echo teaching would infer that such areas are invariably reflective of transmural infarction, and nuclear perfusion imaging would indicate that such areas are nonviable, simply based on the significant reduction of counts in the thinned area relative to remote, normal myocardium. However, CMR provides evidence that this assertion is not always the case. Shah and colleagues found that 19% of a group of 1055 patients undergoing CMR had regional wall thinning (≤5.5 mm) involving an average of 34% of the LV. Of those regions with thinning, 18% were found to have a limited scar burden (defined as <50% hyperenhancement), and such patients undergoing revascularization uniformly demonstrated significant improvement in contractile function (Fig. 17.12). Also notable was that in regions with limited scar burden, there was substantial reverse remodeling of the myocardial wall and disappearance of thinned regions since diastolic wall thickness increased from a mean of 4.4 mm to a mean of 7.5 mm (Fig. 17.12). Hence, it appears for a given myocardial region that the amount of scar in relation to the amount of viability is more important than just the absolute amount of viability in predicting contractile improvement and reverse remodeling following revascularization.

USE IN CLINICAL TRIALS

The ultimate goal of a new therapy for acute MI is a reduction in mortality. In the current era, treatment of acute MI is quite effective; therefore, demonstrating a further reduction in mortality with novel treatments is increasingly difficult and necessitates studies with large sample sizes with corresponding logistical and financial barriers. As such, there is considerable interest in using surrogate endpoints to assess the efficacy of acute MI therapies. Several investigations have reported that infarct size measured by DE-CMR is a stronger predictor of outcome than LVEF and LV volumes. Moreover, Stone et al. in a patient-level analysis of 10 randomized PCI trials found a strong graded response between infarct size and mortality as well as hospitalizations for heart failure; for every 5% increase in infarct size the mortality hazard ratio increased 1.19 and for hospitalization 1.20.

Infarct size is a particularly attractive surrogate endpoint for several reasons. First, it is useful in early screening studies to test whether a new therapy is biologically active. Second, it can serve as an endpoint for phase 2 dose-ranging studies to test efficacy and/or safety; more recently it is being used in several phase 3 trials as a primary endpoint. Third, it may indicate a late mortality benefit, and thus rationale for performing a longer-term study, even if an early benefit is not seen. For instance, a reduction in infarct size may lead to a long-term improvement in ventricular remodeling, a benefit that may not be manifest in 30-day mortality rates. Fourth, it can provide a mechanism for improvement in outcome, because prognosis after acute MI is strongly determined by infarct size.

Care should be taken in planning the timing of the CMR acquisition, as MIs are known to demonstrate what Reimer and Jennings have termed "a changing anatomic reference base." That is, the size of infarction can show dramatic changes over time, with edema and swelling resulting in near-doubling of infarct size in the acute phase, and significant shrinkage (up to 75% reduction of infarct size)

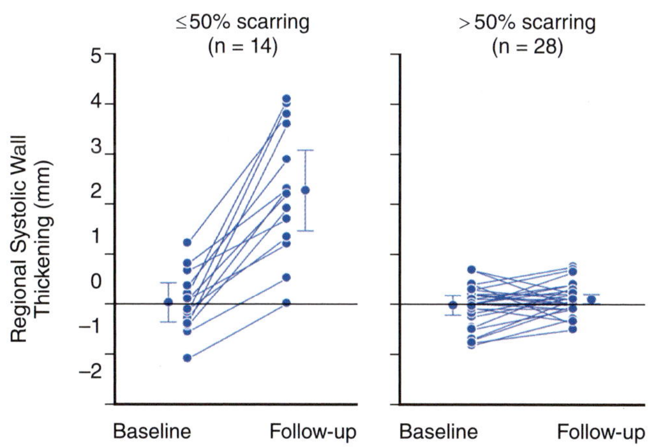

FIG. 17.12 In patients with regional left ventricular wall thinning and akinesis, significant improvement in contractile function can be seen postrevascularization. However, contractile function (e.g., systolic wall thickening) improved only in those with limited scarring (<50% transmural scar). (Modified from Shah DJ, Kim HW, James O, et al: Prevalence of regional myocardial thinning and relationship with myocardial scarring in patients with coronary artery disease. *JAMA*. 2013;309:909–918.)

occurring in the chronic phase as necrosis is replaced by collagenous scar. These findings have been confirmed in CMR studies of the evolution of infarct size over time; Fieno and colleagues demonstrated that terminal infarct size at 4 to 8 weeks in a canine model averaged 24% of that found at 3 days. Moreover, the mass of viable myocardium increased systematically with time, although the time course of hypertrophy was different from that of infarct resorption. Importantly, measurements of total LV mass did not reflect the changes occurring separately in infarcted and viable regions. These results highlight the capability of DE-CMR to improve the assessment of postinfarction ventricular remodeling by allowing evaluation of concurrent changes such as resorption of infarcted tissue and hypertrophy of viable myocardium at an early time point before measurements of ventricular volumes and mass have changed.

Another important implication of the "changing anatomic reference base" is that a reduction in hyperenhancement size from an acute scan to a chronic scan should not lead to confusion regarding the interpretation of hyperenhancement zones. Some previous studies have suggested that hyperenhancement in the acute phase represents both infarcted myocardium and a rim of surrounding viable myocardium whereas hyperenhancement in the chronic phase solely represents infarcted myocardium in an effort to explain the differences in hyperenhancement size. This interpretation is incorrect. In both acute and chronic settings, hyperenhancement depicts infarction, however, infarct size itself is dynamic (see Chapter 19).

Several studies have shown that the measurement of infarct size by DE-CMR is highly reproducible. The implication of high reproducibility is that DE-CMR may enable robust detection of small changes in infarct size, and potentially allow substantial reduction in sample size for clinical trials using infarct size as an efficacy endpoint. Because of its accuracy and reproducibility, CMR quantification of MI has increasingly been used in a variety of clinical trials, most notably in the evaluation of cardioprotective interventions. However, the complex evolution of histologic changes in acute MI could result in significant variability in infarct size measurements over time, suggesting a need for standardization of imaging techniques and scan timing. To this end, a panel of scientific experts was assembled to develop a consensus regarding the utility of various CMR techniques and their appropriate implementation for use in clinical trials.[11] Their recommendations are summarized in Table 17.2.

Few studies have directly compared infarct size measurements by DE-CMR to those by technetium-99m SPECT, although the latter is considered one of the best available techniques for the quantification of infarct size. An early study by Mahrholdt and colleagues reported that the SD of infarct size was 6% by DE-CMR and 7.5% by SPECT in a population with chronic MI. Because DE-CMR led to a 20% reduction in variability (1.5 of 7.5), the improved precision would result in a nearly 40% reduction in sample size. Similarly, Lunde and colleagues evaluated infarct size in STEMI patients randomized to intracoronary injection of mononuclear bone marrow cells at both acute and chronic time points. In the control group, both early and late after MI, the SD of infarct size was lower by DE-CMR than by SPECT (14.0 vs. 21.1 and 12.5 vs. 20.9, respectively). Although the variability of infarct size will change with the population being studied (e.g., cohorts with a high prevalence of anterior MI will have larger mean infarct size and larger SD), these data suggest that total variability is smaller when utilizing DE-CMR and will lead to appreciable differences in sample size. As a result, interest in DE-CMR for infarct size quantification is rapidly growing. General strengths and weaknesses of CMR for clinical trials are shown in Table 17.e1.

SUMMARY

In patients with known or suspected MI, CMR provides a comprehensive, multifaceted view of the heart. The data, including those from a multicenter clinical trial, indicate that DE-CMR is a well-validated, robust technique that

TABLE 17.2 Consensus Recommendations Related to CMR Endpoints in Experimental and Clinical Studies of Myocardial Infarction

It is recommended that the index CMR scan be performed 5 ± 2 days after reperfusion. At this time point, several key parameters have been shown to be relatively stable.
LGE extent, expressed both in absolute (grams) and relative (percentage of LV mass) terms, is the recommended CMR primary endpoint.
In experimental studies, if LGE extent is expressed as a ratio to AAR, the latter should not rely on edema and ideally, both AAR and LGE have to be obtained on the same day post-MI (e.g., perfusion imaging during coronary occlusion by MDCT) and LGE by CMR).
LVEF (%) and MVO (areas of hypoenhancement within LGE, in grams or as % of LV) are recommended as main secondary endpoints.
Edema extent (T2 mapping) may be used as secondary endpoint to assess the effect of cardioprotective therapies.
LV volumes (mL; mL/m^2), RVEF (%), RV LGE (presence), and IMH (% of LV) can be included as secondary endpoints.
Myocardial mapping indexes (T1 [ms]; T2 [ms]; ECV [percentage of LV mass]), and strain (feature tracking) may be considered as exploratory endpoints.
The use of edema-sensitive CMR sequences as a surrogate for AAR (as well as edema-based MSI) is not recommended because edema is not stable in the days following MI and is potentially affected by duration of ischemia and by cardioprotective strategies.[a]
Due to its easy implementation, ESL-based salvage index may be used as an exploratory outcome but not in cases with small amounts of LGE or aborted infarction, i.e., when a high degree of cardioprotection is expected.[a]
For LGE postprocessing, automated techniques using signal-intensity thresholding, manual delineation, and visual scoring (the two latter at intermediate signal intensities) have similar good accuracy and reproducibility. For delineation of edema, T2 mapping (automated >2SD thresholding with manual correction) showed greater intraobserver and interobserver agreement. For MVO quantification, the most widely used is the manual delineation of dark areas within LGE region.

[a]Controversial topic (majority but not all panelists in agreement).
AAR, Area at risk; *ECV*, extracellular volume; *ESL*, endocardial surface length; *LVEF*, left ventricular ejection fraction; *MSI*, myocardial salvage index; *RV*, right ventricle/ventricular.
Adapted from Ibanez B, Aletras AH, Arai AE, et al. Cardiac MRI endpoints in myocardial infarction experimental and clinical trials: JACC scientific expert panel. *J Am Coll Cardiol*. 2019;74:238–256.

can be easily implemented on scanners that are commonly available worldwide, with an effectiveness that rivals the best available imaging techniques for the detection and assessment of acute and chronic MI. CMR may be especially useful when patients present outside the diagnostic window of cardiac biomarkers. Moreover, because CMR can uniquely differentiate between ischemic and various nonischemic forms of injury, it may be helpful in cases of diagnostic uncertainty, such as in patients with classical features of MI in whom coronary angiography does not show a culprit lesion. Even after the diagnosis of MI has been made, CMR can provide clinically relevant information with regard to identification of post-MI sequelae and further infarct characterization. The high accuracy and reproducibility of DE-CMR have led to the increasing use of this technique as the preferred method for quantification of infarct size in many clinical trials.

CLASSIC REFERENCES

Fieno DS, Hillenbrand HB, Rehwald WG, et al. Infarct resorption, compensatory hypertrophy, and differing patterns of ventricular remodeling following myocardial infarctions of varying size. *J Am Coll Cardiol*. 2004;43:2124–2131.

Kim RJ, Fieno DS, Parrish TB, et al. Relationship of MRI delayed contrast enhancement to irreversible injury, infarct age, and contractile function. *Circulation*. 1999;100:1992–2002.

Kim RJ, Wu E, Rafael A, et al. The use of contrast-enhanced magnetic resonance imaging to identify reversible myocardial dysfunction. *N Engl J Med*. 2000;343:1445–1453.

Shah DJ, Kim HW, James O, et al. Prevalence of regional myocardial thinning and relationship with myocardial scarring in patients with coronary artery disease. *JAMA*. 2013;309:909–918.

Simonetti OP, Kim RJ, Fieno DS, et al. An improved MR imaging technique for the visualization of myocardial infarction. *Radiology*. 2001;218:215–223.

Stone GW, Selker HP, Thiele H, et al. Relationship between infarct size and outcomes following primary PCI: patient-level analysis from 10 randomized trials. *J Am Coll Cardiol*. 2016;67:1674–1683.

Velazquez EJ, Lee KL, Deja MA, et al. Coronary-artery bypass surgery in patients with left ventricular dysfunction. *N Engl J Med*. 2011;364:1607–1616.

Velazquez EJ, Lee KL, Jones RH, et al. Coronary-artery bypass surgery in patients with ischemic cardiomyopathy. *N Engl J Med*. 2016;374:1511–1520.

Wagner A, Mahrholdt H, Holly TA, et al. Contrast-enhanced MRI and routine single photon emission computed tomography (SPECT) perfusion imaging for detection of subendocardial myocardial infarcts: an imaging study. *Lancet*. 2003;361:374–379.

Weinsaft JW, Kim HW, Crowley AL, et al. LV thrombus detection by routine echocardiography: insights into performance characteristics using delayed enhancement CMR. *JACC Cardiovasc Imaging*. 2011;4:702–712.

REFERENCES

1. Thygesen K, Alpert JS, Jaffe AS, et al. Fourth universal definition of myocardial infarction (2018). *Eur Heart J*. 2019;40:237–269.
2. Kramer CM, Barkhausen J, Bucciarelli-Ducci C, et al. Standardized cardiovascular magnetic resonance imaging (CMR) protocols: 2020 update. *J Cardiovasc Magn Reson*. 2020;22:17.
3. Captur G, Lobascio I, Ye Y, et al. Motion-corrected free-breathing LGE delivers high quality imaging and reduces scan time by half: an independent validation study. *Int J Cardiovasc Imaging*. 2019;35:1893–1901.
4. Holtackers RJ, Van De Heyning CM, Chiribiri A, et al. Dark-blood late gadolinium enhancement cardiovascular magnetic resonance for improved detection of subendocardial scar: a review of current techniques. *J Cardiovasc Magn Reson*. 2021;23:96.
5. Kim HW, Rehwald WG, Jenista ER, et al. Dark-blood delayed enhancement cardiac magnetic resonance of myocardial infarction. *JACC Cardiovasc Imaging*. 2018;11:1758–1769.
6. O'Brien AT, Gil KE, Varghese J, et al. T2 mapping in myocardial disease: a comprehensive review. *J Cardiovasc Magn Reson*. 2022;24:33.
7. Nagel E, Greenwood JP, McCann GP, et al. Magnetic resonance perfusion or fractional flow reserve in coronary disease. *N Engl J Med*. 2019;380:2418–2428.
8. Kwong RY, Ge Y, Steel K, et al. Cardiac magnetic resonance stress perfusion imaging for evaluation of patients with chest pain. *J Am Coll Cardiol*. 2019;74:1741–1755.
9. Heitner JF, Kim RJ, Kim HW, et al. Prognostic value of vasodilator stress cardiac magnetic resonance imaging: a multicenter study with 48,000 patient-years of follow-up. *JAMA Cardiol*. 2019;4:256–264.
10. Gulati M, Levy PD, Mukherjee D, et al. 2021 AHA/ACC/ASE/CHEST/SAEM/SCCT/SCMR guideline for the evaluation and diagnosis of chest pain: executive summary: a report of the American College of Cardiology/American Heart Association joint committee on clinical practice guidelines. *Circulation*. 2021;144:e368–e454.
11. Ibanez B, Aletras AH, Arai AE, et al. Cardiac MRI endpoints in myocardial infarction experimental and clinical trials: JACC scientific expert panel. *J Am Coll Cardiol*. 2019;74:238–256.
12. Kaolawanich Y, Azevedo CF, Kim HW, et al. Native T1 mapping for the diagnosis of myocardial fibrosis in patients with chronic myocardial infarction. *JACC cardiovasc imaging*. 2022;15:2069–2079.
13. Hundley WG, Bluemke DA, Bogaert J, et al. Society for cardiovascular magnetic resonance (SCMR) guidelines for reporting cardiovascular magnetic resonance examinations. *J Cardiovasc Magn Reson*. 2022;24:29.
14. Heitner JF, Senthilkumar A, Harrison JK, et al. Identifying the infarct-related artery in patients with non-ST-segment-elevation myocardial infarction. *Circ Cardiovasc Interv*. 2019;12:e007305.
15. Smulders MW, Kietselaer B, Wildberger JE, et al. Initial imaging-guided strategy versus routine care in patients with non-ST-segment elevation myocardial infarction. *J Am Coll Cardiol*. 2019;74:2466–2477.
16. Konst RE, Parker M, Bhatti L, et al. Prognostic value of cardiac magnetic resonance imaging in patients with a working diagnosis of MINOCA-An outcome study with up to 10 Years of follow-up. *Circ Cardiovasc Imaging*. 2023;16(8):e014454. doi:10.1161/CIRCIMAGING.122.014454.
17. de Waha S, Patel MR, Granger CB, et al. Relationship between microvascular obstruction and adverse events following primary percutaneous coronary intervention for ST-segment elevation myocardial infarction: an individual patient data pooled analysis from seven randomized trials. *Eur Heart J*. 2017;38:3502–3510.
18. Smulders MW, Van Assche LMR, Bekkers S, et al. Epicardial surface area of infarction: a stable surrogate of microvascular obstruction in acute myocardial infarction. *Circ Cardiovasc Imaging*. 2021;14:e010918.
19. Amier RP, Smulders MW, van der Flier WM, et al. Long-term prognostic implications of previous silent myocardial infarction in patients presenting with acute myocardial infarction. *JACC Cardiovasc Imaging*. 2018;11:1773–1781.
20. Jensen CJ, Jochims M, Hunold P, et al. Right ventricular involvement in acute left ventricular myocardial infarction: prognostic implications of MRI findings. *Am J Roentgenol*. 2010;194:592–598.
21. Albulushi A, Giannopoulos A, Kafkas N, et al. Acute right ventricular myocardial infarction. *Expert Rev Cardiovasc Ther*. 2018;16:455–464.
22. Stiermaier T, Backhaus SJ, Matz J, et al. Frequency and prognostic impact of right ventricular involvement in acute myocardial infarction. *Heart*. 2020;563–570.
23. Chiabrando JG, Bonaventura A, Vecchie A, et al. Management of acute and recurrent pericarditis: JACC state-of-the-art review. *J Am Coll Cardiol*. 2020;75:76–92.
24. Bulluck H, Chan MHH, Paradies V, et al. Incidence and predictors of left ventricular thrombus by cardiovascular magnetic resonance in acute ST-segment elevation myocardial infarction treated by primary percutaneous coronary intervention: a meta-analysis. *J Cardiovasc Magn Reson*. 2018;20:72.
25. Ballard DH, Jokerst C, Raptis CA, et al. Myocardial cut-off sign is a sensitive and specific cardiac computed tomography and magnetic resonance imaging sign to distinguish left ventricular pseudoaneurysms from true aneurysms. *J Thorac Imaging*. 2022;37:58–65.
26. Holtackers RJ, Emrich T, Botnar RM, et al. Late gadolinium enhancement cardiac magnetic resonance imaging: from basic concepts to emerging methods. *Rofo*. 2022;194:491–504.

18 Optical Coherence Tomography and Other Intracoronary Diagnostic Procedures

YOSHIYASU MINAMI, DANIEL S. ONG, AND IK-KYUNG JANG

INTRODUCTION

Outcomes after percutaneous coronary intervention (PCI) have improved over the past few decades, in large part due to newer stent platforms, better implantation techniques, and improved adjunctive medical therapy. However, the optimization and personalization of both interventional and pharmacological therapy in patients with acute coronary syndrome (ACS) continue to be explored; balancing the risk of bleeding events with antithrombotic therapy versus the high incidence of recurrent events caused by residual vulnerable plaques at nonculprit sites.[1] Intracoronary imaging techniques may be able to inform such optimization by providing insight into the dominant coronary pathology of the individual patient.

Pathology studies have revealed three main patterns observed in thrombotic culprit lesions among patients with sudden cardiac death: plaque rupture, plaque erosion, and calcified nodules (see also Chapter 32). Ruptured plaques are the most common, accounting for approximately 50% of cases, and are characterized by fibrous cap disruption with an overlying thrombus that is in continuity with an underlying necrotic core. In contrast, eroded plaques are found in approximately 35% of cases and are characterized by coronary thrombus with an intact fibrous cap. The endothelial lining is commonly absent, exposing the intima which is primarily composed of smooth muscle cells and proteoglycan. Calcified nodules comprise approximately 5% of cases and are identified by fibrous cap disruption and thrombus overlying a fractured calcified plate. In addition to these three main underlying mechanisms, other morphological and functional coronary characteristics causing the onset of ACS have been reported, including spontaneous coronary dissection, severely calcified lesions, vasospasm, tight stenosis, and thromboembolism. Importantly, pathology studies are limited to the retrospective identification of features prevalent in culprit plaques. The development of intravascular imaging modalities, however, has enabled the study of these same features in vivo and prospectively. Moreover, the use of intracoronary imaging modalities facilitates the differential diagnosis of underlying mechanisms of ACS and more tailored therapeutic approaches for managing both culprit and nonculprit lesions.[2]

Clinical risk models can estimate the risk of recurrent events but do not provide anatomic information, and angiographic parameters have poor predictive value in identifying the specific high-risk lesions responsible for future coronary events. Early angiographic studies suggested that the culprit lesions for these recurrent events were often only mildly stenotic at the time of index angiography, whereas pathology studies of patients with fatal cardiac events found that the majority of acute occlusive thromboses occur at sites with large plaque burden and severe luminal narrowing. A significant amount of research has therefore been devoted to exploring the risk factors for individual plaque progression and thrombosis. Although each of the intravascular imaging modalities has unique advantages and disadvantages, they can be broadly grouped as modalities that provide primarily anatomic or compositional information, such as optical coherence tomography (OCT), intravascular ultrasound (IVUS), and near-infrared spectroscopy (NIRS). In this chapter, we will explore the contribution of intravascular imaging, in particular OCT, toward extending our understanding of the underlying mechanisms of ACS and vulnerable plaques. Other techniques such as angioscopy, thermography, elastography, intravascular near-infrared fluorescence are no longer used in research or clinically and are thus no longer discussed in this chapter.

OCT ASSESSMENT OF CORONARY PLAQUE ANATOMY OR COMPOSITION

OCT is a high-resolution intravascular imaging modality that enables the detailed characterization of plaque

Disclosure: Dr. Jang received a research grant and honorarium from St. Jude Medical and research grants from Medtronic and Boston Scientific Corp. Dr. Minami received an honorarium from Abbott.

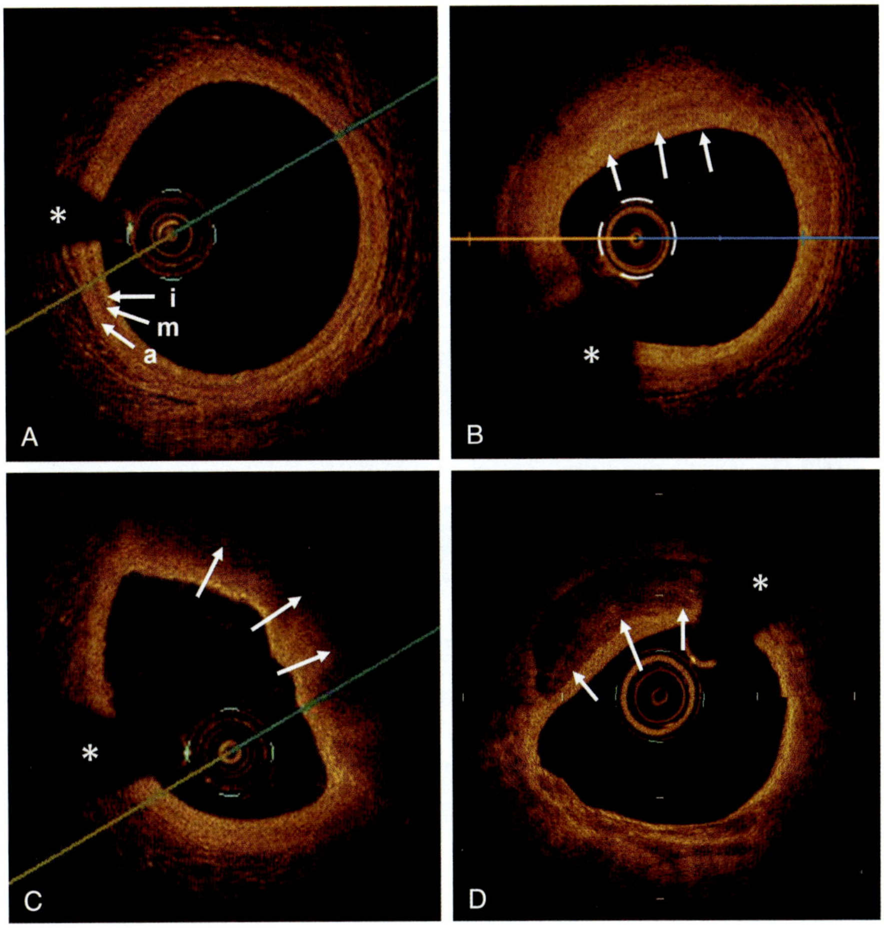

FIG. 18.1 Plaque characterization using optical coherence tomography. (A) Cross-sectional optical coherence tomography image of a normal coronary artery with a three-layered structure, corresponding to the intima (i), media (m), and adventitia (a). (B) Fibrous tissue (*arrows*) appears as a homogenous area with high signal intensity and low signal attenuation. (C) Lipid (*arrows*) appears as a homogenous area with low signal intensity and high signal attenuation. (D) Calcium (*arrow*) appears as a heterogeneous area of high and low signal intensity with low signal attenuation and a sharp demarcating border. The asterisks denote guidewire shadow artifact.

morphology in vivo.[3] In a manner analogous to the use of sound waves in ultrasonography, OCT measures the magnitude and time delay of backscattered light waves to produce images resembling an "optical biopsy," with 15 to 20 μm resolution. This resolution represents a 10-fold improvement compared with IVUS and allows for the in vivo differentiation of fibrous, lipid, and calcific plaques (Fig. 18.1). Additionally, OCT can be used to detect intraluminal thrombi and identify the pathogenesis of ACS, including plaque rupture, plaque erosion, and calcified plaques (Fig. 18.2).[2]

Plaque Rupture

Plaque rupture is the most common underlying mechanisms of ACS. On OCT images, plaque rupture is characterized by the presence of a thrombus concomitant with the abrupt disruption of fibrous cap overlying lipid-rich plaques (Fig. 18.3A). Since the presence of a thrombus frequently obstructs clear visualization of the ruptured site, thrombectomy and/or balloon dilatation before OCT is recommended. Plaque rupture mostly occurs in the thin-cap fibroatheroma (TCFA), which is defined as a fibrous cap <65 μm overlying a lipid-rich plaque.[3] Luminal narrowing, larger residual thrombus, and higher frequency of coexistent small plaque components, including microchannels, spotty calcification, and cholesterol crystals, are also characteristics of plaque rupture on OCT images.[4] Although its exact role has not been clarified, spotty calcification and/or cholesterol crystals may facilitate the deterioration of the fibrous cap through physical stimulation.[5] Several OCT studies have reported worse outcomes in both acute and chronic phases in patients with plaque rupture than in patients with other causes of ACS.[4]

Plaque Erosion

Plaque erosion is the second major pathogenesis of ACS.[6] If there is no lipid plaque with a ruptured fibrous cap or substantial calcification at the culprit lesion, plaque erosion is the underlying cause of ACS.[2] The term "OCT-erosion" or "intact fibrous cap" is also used as an alternative to "plaque erosion" diagnosed based on OCT findings.[4] On OCT images, plaque erosion is characterized by the presence of a mural thrombus and/or irregularity of the luminal surface, suggesting the presence of a platelet-rich thrombus (Fig. 18.3B). Although approximately half of the culprit plaques in cases of plaque erosion contain lipids, the presence of vulnerable characteristics, including TCFA, microphages, and microchannels, is less frequent than in

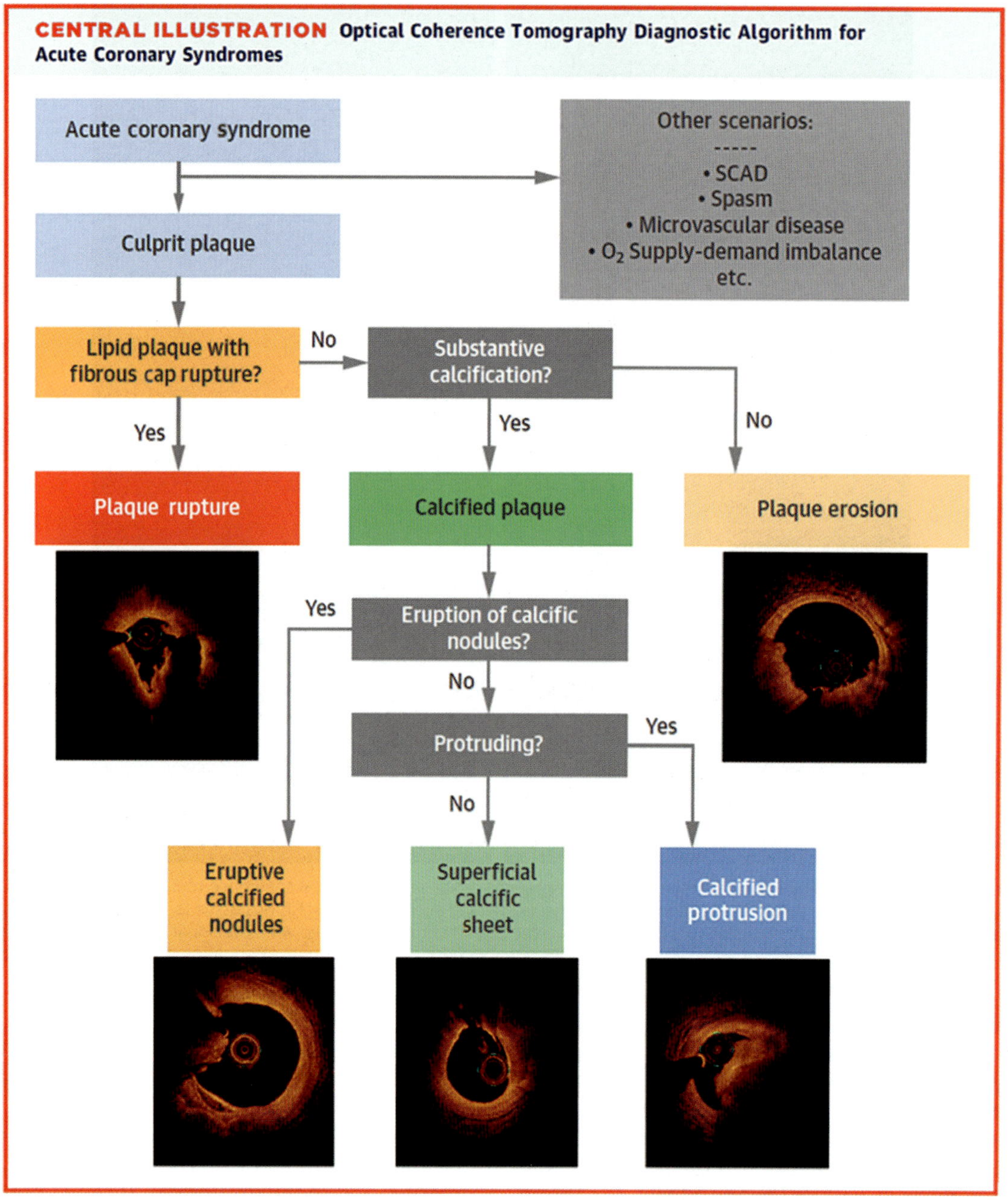

FIG. 18.2 Optical coherence tomography diagnostic algorithm for acute coronary syndrome. The presence or absence of rupture of a lipid plaque is the most distinguishing finding. In plaques with the absence of a ruptured lipid core, calcified plaques are characterized by the presence of substantive superficial calcification. Depending on the morphology of calcification, calcified culprit plaques are categorized into three groups. Plaque erosion is a diagnosis of exclusion. *SCAD*, spontaneous coronary artery dissection. (Adapted from Sugiyama T, Yamamoto E, Fracassi F, et al. *JACC Cardiovasc Interv.* 2019;12:531–540.)

plaque rupture.[6] Because the diagnosis of plaque erosion on OCT images is primarily based on exclusion criteria, it is sometimes difficult to make a definitive diagnosis. Automated algorithms for the diagnosis of plaque erosion on OCT images have been explored for diagnostic support.[7] The EROSION study tested the feasibility of antiplatelet agents without stenting to manage the thrombus at the culprit segment and reported a significant reduction in thrombus volume at 1 month.[8] Although a limited incidence of adverse events up to 4 years has been reported, gradual liminal narrowing has also been reported in a sub-study.[8,9] Because the EROSION study was a small proof-of-concept study focusing on the reduction of thrombus volume without aiming to show its clinical relevance, further studies are required to explore the possibility of precision medicine based on the diagnosis of plaque erosion on OCT images.

Calcification-Related ACS

Several types of calcified plaques may be the cause of ACS (Fig. 18.3C–F). An OCT study of 1241 patients with ACS reported that 12.7% of patients were found to have a calcified plaque at the culprit lesion and that there were three distinct types of calcification: superficial calcific sheet (67.4%), eruptive calcified nodule (25.5%), and calcified protrusion (7.1%).[2] Although the exact mechanism of thrombus formation in lesions with superficial calcific sheets has not been

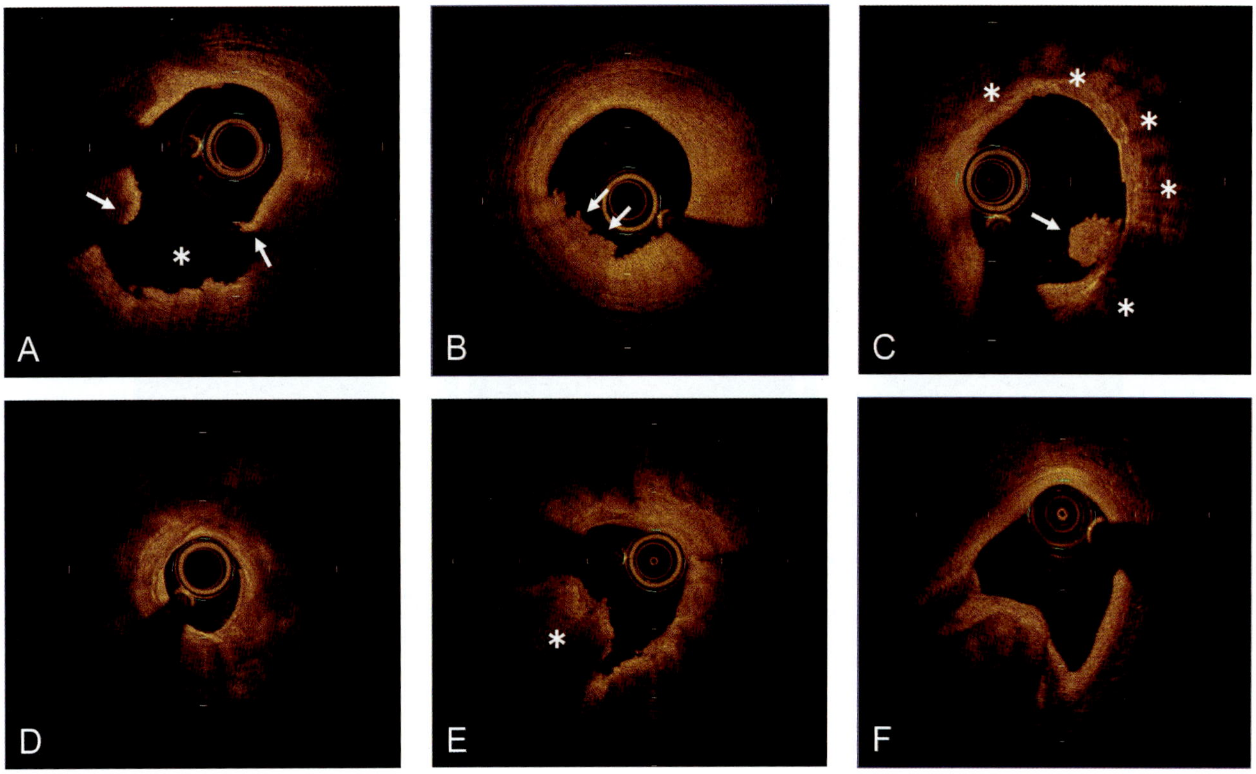

FIG. 18.3 Representative optical coherence tomography images of culprit lesion in patients with acute coronary syndrome. (A) Plaque rupture is identified as lipid plaque with fibrous cap discontinuity (*arrow*) and cavity formation (*asterisk*) inside the plaque. (B) Plaque erosion is confirmed by the presence of an attached thrombus (*arrows*) overlying an intact and visualized plaque. (C) Calcified plaque is characterized by heterogeneous areas of high- and low-signal intensity with low-signal attenuation and a sharp demarcating border (*asterisk*). An arrow represents an attached thrombus. (D) A superficial calcific sheet appears as a sheet-like calcific plate with luminal narrowing without apparent disruption of overlying fibrous tissue. (E) The eruptive calcified nodule is a site of intimal disruption and protruding irregular mass (*asterisk*) with high signal attenuation. (F) Calcified protrusion represents protruding calcific mass with overlying smooth tissue without apparent intimal disruption.

fully elucidated, the smaller lumen area in addition to the abundant collagenous matrix in the lesions can be considered the cause of local high shear stress environment and subsequent thrombus formation.[2] The discrepant results in pathological studies not showing superficial calcific sheets as the major cause of sudden death may be due to selection bias. Eruptive calcified nodules are unique entities composed of disrupted luminal surfaces with fibrin-rich thrombi, multiple nodular masses protruding into the lumen, and sheet-like calcifications in peripheral segments.[10] Mechanical stress according to the cardiac cycle is considered a pathogenesis because the mid-portion of the right coronary artery is reported to be the dominant location.[10] On OCT images, the eruptive calcified nodules were characterized by an irregular protruding mass with high signal attenuation (Fig. 18.3E). Although the peripheral area appears severely calcified, the opposite site of the eruptive calcified nodule may be almost normal, with preserved three layers of the vessel wall. Because patients with eruptive calcified nodules have worse clinical outcomes than those with other types of calcification after conventional stent-based PCI, exploring alternative therapeutic strategies using excimer laser, lithotripsy, and drug-coated balloons may be required.[11,12] In contrast, little is known about calcified protrusions. A calcified protrusion is characterized by a smooth leading edge of the local protruding calcification, in contrast to the irregular leading edge in eruptive calcified nodules on OCT images (Fig. 18.3F). This morphology may cause thrombus formation through flow disturbance and/or local instability of the shear stress due to the eccentric and protruding shape. Further studies are required to elucidate the pathogenesis of this unique morphology.

OCT DEFINITION OF VULNERABLE PLAQUE

Vulnerable plaques have been defined as those at a high risk of disruption (rupture or erosion) resulting in occlusive thrombosis. The framework for studying vulnerable plaque features was established using data from autopsy studies examining the culprit lesions in patients with sudden coronary death. The high resolution of OCT imaging has enabled the identification of many features suggested by pathological studies to be associated with plaque vulnerability. Given the high prevalence of plaque rupture as the underlying mechanism for coronary thrombus formation, the features and risk factors associated with plaque vulnerability to rupture are the most commonly studied. These features include large extracellular lipid pools, thin fibrous caps, small calcifications, macrophage accumulation, microchannels, and cholesterol crystals (Fig. 18.4). However, these characteristics may differ, depending on the features and risk factors associated with plaque erosion and calcified nodules.

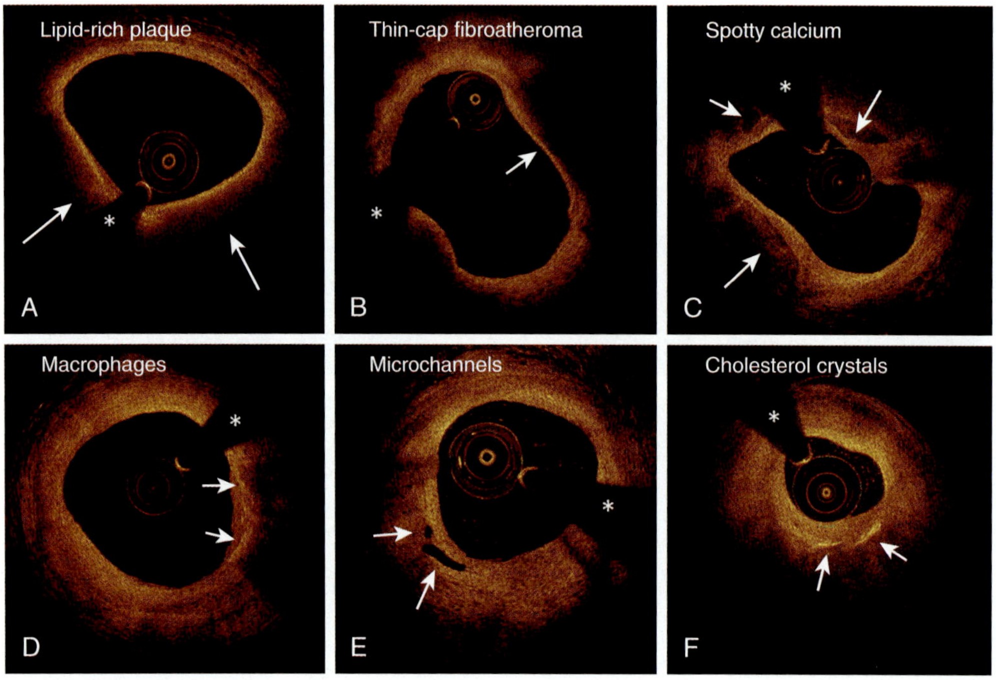

FIG. 18.4 Vulnerable plaque features were identified using optical coherence tomography. (A) Lipid-rich plaques are defined as those with a lipid arc >90 degrees (*arrows*). (B) Thin-cap fibroatheroma are identified as lipid-rich plaques with an overlying fibrous cap measuring less than 65 μm (*arrow*). (C) Spotty calcium deposits are defined as small calcifications with an arc ≤90 degrees (*arrows*). (D) Macrophages/bright spots appear as linear series of signal-rich (*bright*) spots with high signal attenuation (*arrows*). (E) Microchannels/neovascularization are identified as small black holes or tubes (*arrows*) measuring 50 to 300 μm in diameter and spanning at least three consecutive cross-sectional frames on pullback imaging. (F) Cholesterol crystals appear as thin, linear, signal-rich structures with low signal attenuation (*arrows*). The asterisks denote guidewire shadow artifact.

Extracellular Lipid Pools

Autopsy studies have identified large lipid cores as a common feature of culprit plaques in patients with sudden coronary death. On OCT imaging, lipids appear as homogeneous areas with low signal intensity (dark) and high signal attenuation (significant shadowing), in contrast to fibrous tissue, which appears as homogeneous areas with high signal intensity (bright) and low signal attenuation (no significant shadowing). Lipid-rich plaques are defined as those with a lipid arc of >90 degrees on cross-sectional imaging (Fig. 18.4A). OCT studies have shown that lipid-rich plaques are more prevalent in the culprit lesions of patients with acute unstable presentations, such as ST-segment elevation myocardial infarction (STEMI) or non–ST-segment elevation MI (NSTEMI) than in those presenting with stable angina pectoris (SAP).[4] Furthermore, lipid pools are associated with poor clinical outcomes and the presence of OCT-defined lipid-rich plaques can serve as a surrogate for future adverse events. In a study of 1474 patients from 20 sites across six countries who underwent OCT imaging of the target vessel for PCI, patients with lipid-rich plaques had a higher incidence of nonculprit lesion-related adverse events over 48 months compared with those without lipid-rich plaque (7.2% vs. 2.6%, $P = .033$).[13]

Thin-Cap Fibroatheroma

TCFA is postulated to be a vulnerable precursor lesion for plaque rupture given its morphological similarity. On pathology examination, most ruptured coronary plaques have fibrous caps measuring <65 μm and this threshold has therefore been used to define thick- versus TCFA. The sharp contrast in appearance between lipid and fibrous tissues on OCT imaging, coupled with its high resolution, makes it an ideal intravascular imaging modality for measuring the fibrous cap thickness and thereby identifying TCFA (Fig. 18.4B). Multiple OCT studies have shown a higher prevalence of TCFA at culprit sites in patients with acute or unstable clinical presentations than in those with SAP.[4] Moreover, the presence of TCFA was demonstrated to be an independent predictor of subsequent rapid plaque progression in an OCT study of 517 nonculprit lesions, including 50 lesions with subsequent rapid plaque progression.[14]

The clinical significance of TCFA has also been demonstrated in multiple OCT studies. In a study of 3533 nonculprit plaques in 1378 patients who underwent OCT, a higher incidence of ACS for a median of 6 years was shown in patients with both lipid-rich plaques and TCFA than in those with lipidic plaques without these two characteristics (33% vs. 2%, $P < .001$).[15] It is important to note that TCFA is a signature of panvascular vulnerability and is not necessarily a culprit lesion for future development of ACS. Intensive lipid-lowering therapies, including statins, ezetimibe, and proprotein convertase subtilisin kexin 9 (PCSK9) inhibitors, have been shown to increase fibrous cap thickness, suggesting that one of the mechanisms underlying the clinical benefit is the stabilization of vulnerable TCFA plaques (Fig. 18.5).[16–18]

Macrophages

Inflammation plays an important role in atherosclerosis. Lipid-laden macrophages constitutively produce

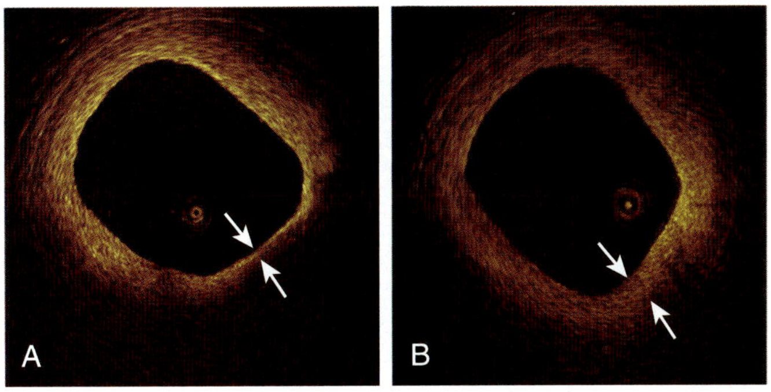

FIG. 18.5 Matching optical coherence tomography cross-sections of a lipid-rich plaque at (A) baseline and (B) 12-month follow-up in a patient receiving 20 mg/day of atorvastatin, showing thickening of the fibrous cap (*arrows*). (Reproduced from Komukai K, Kubo T, Kitabata H, et al. *J Am Coll Cardiol.* 2014;64(21):2207–2217.)

extracellular matrix-degrading enzymes promoting plaque vulnerability.[19] Macrophage accumulations can be identified on OCT imaging as a linear series of signal-rich (bright) spots with high signal attenuation (Fig. 18.4D). Semi-quantitative assessment of macrophages on OCT images has been used to characterize the grade of focal inflammation in the coronary plaques. Studies of intensive lipid-lowering therapy, including high-intensity statins and PCSK9 inhibitors, reported the efficacy of reducing macrophage grade on serial OCT images.[20] Caution should be exercised when evaluating macrophages on OCT images. OCT bright spots correlate with the interface of plaque components with different optical indices of refraction, including not only macrophages but also cholesterol clefts in necrotic cores and the interfaces between old and new fibrous tissue, calcium and lipid or fibrous tissue, fibrous cap and lipid pools, and neovascularization and media. Additionally, not all macrophage accumulations identified histologically are visible as bright spots on OCT imaging, which may be related to differences in the backscattering properties of the different types of macrophages present (e.g., M1 vs. M2 macrophages).

Microchannels/Neovascularization

Mechanistically, the development of microchannels (neovascularization) within plaques is thought to facilitate inflammatory cell infiltration and necrotic core formation. These factors, along with a greater risk of intraplaque hemorrhage, may contribute to more rapid plaque progression. On OCT imaging, microchannels are identified as small black holes or tubes measuring 50 to 300 μm in diameter and spanning at least three consecutive cross-sectional frames on pullback imaging (Fig. 18.4E). Some results in previous studies imply that the number of microchannels increases with the development of lipid-rich plaque; however, intraplaque microchannels themselves may not facilitate plaque progression.[14]

Cholesterol Crystals

In pathology studies, cholesterol crystal content is an independent predictor of thrombus formation and clinical events. Volume expansion during cholesterol crystallization is hypothesized to cause the disruption and perforation of neighboring fibrous tissues, thereby contributing to plaque vulnerability to rupture. On OCT imaging, cholesterol crystals appear as thin, linear, signal-rich structures with low-signal attenuation (Fig. 18.4F). Although few OCT studies have directly investigated the potential role of cholesterol crystals in plaque vulnerability, the presence of cholesterol crystals is associated with more vulnerable features of coronary plaques in patients with ACS.[21] Intraplaque cholesterol crystals are more prevalent in patients with STEMI than in those with NSTEMI.[21] Moreover, in a study of 340 patients who underwent OCT imaging of the culprit lesions, compared with patients without cholesterol crystals, patients with cholesterol crystals had a higher incidence of 1-year major adverse cardiac events.[22] The data related to cholesterol crystals should be interpreted with caution, as cholesterol crystals have never been systematically validated against histology as the gold standard.

Calcifications

The coronary artery calcium score, as assessed using cardiac computed tomography, correlates with total atherosclerotic burden and risk of future events.[23] Biomechanical models and pathological studies have suggested that the pattern of vascular calcification may be a more important determinant of local plaque vulnerability than the total calcium burden.[24] In contrast to ultrasound signals, which are highly attenuated by calcium, the light waves used in OCT imaging can penetrate calcium, thereby allowing for a more detailed characterization of calcium deposits and better visualization of structures deep in those deposits than is possible with IVUS. OCT imaging, calcium deposits appear as heterogeneous areas of high- and low-signal intensities with low-signal attenuation and a sharp demarcating border. Although scattered microcalcifications located within the fibrous cap may be visualized by OCT as bright spots with high backscattering, it may be difficult to differentiate them from other plaques, including macrophages and TCFAs. Spotty calcification is the smallest calcium deposit that can be clearly identified using OCT. It is defined as small calcifications with an arc of ≤90 degrees on at least 3 consecutive cross-sectional images (Fig. 18.4C). In a study of 282 patients with ACS who underwent culprit lesion OCT imaging, the percentage of coexisting spotty calcium deposition and lipidic plaques was significantly higher in patients with ruptured fibrous caps than in those with intact fibrous cap.[5] In contrast, in another study, the prevalence of spotty calcification at the culprit plaque did not differ between patients with STEMI mediated by plaque rupture and those with SAP.[24] Collectively, a mechanistic hypothesis that small calcifications increase the vulnerability of plaques to rupture is still unsettled.

Layered Plaque

Layered plaque is characterized by the presence of one or more layers of different optical densities and a clear demarcation from underlying components on OCT images

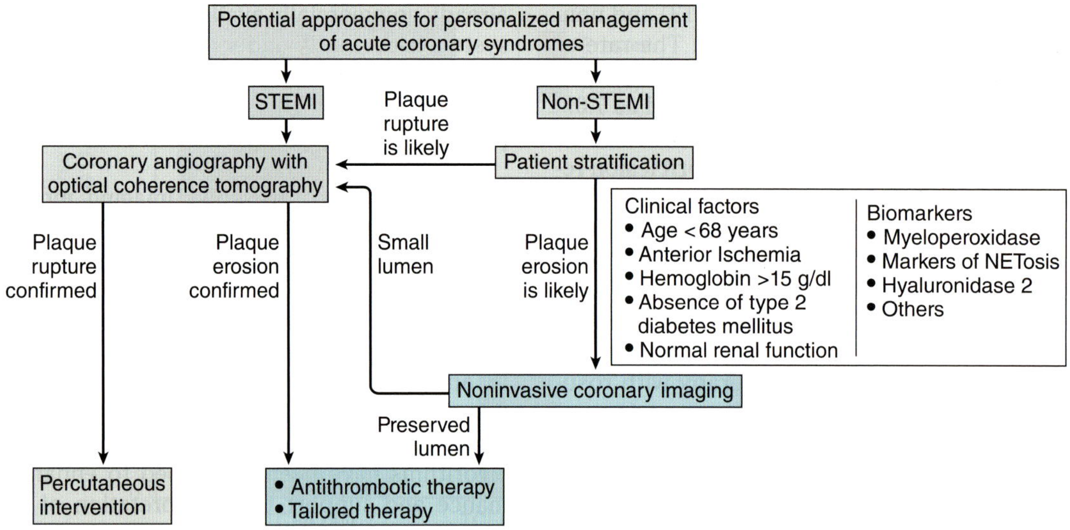

FIG. 18.11 **The potential future paradigm for tailored management of acute coronary syndrome. Flow diagram showing the proposed future tailored management of acute coronary syndrome.** Patients with ST-segment elevation myocardial infarction (STEMI) would undergo emergency catheterization with optical coherence tomography imaging of the culprit lesion. Patients with confirmed plaque rupture should undergo treatment with percutaneous coronary intervention. In those with plaque erosion, pharmacological management without mechanical stenting would become an option. Patients with non-STEMI would undergo risk stratification first. If the patient has a high probability of plaque erosion on the basis of clinical and laboratory characteristics (such as markers of NETosis), noninvasive coronary imaging would be performed after stabilization of the plaque with pharmacological treatment. If the presence of a large residual lumen is confirmed by the imaging, the patient could potentially be treated pharmacologically without the need for an invasive procedure and mechanical intervention. Pharmacological treatments could include, in addition to current antiplatelet and anticoagulant therapies, specific therapies targeted at the mechanisms involved in plaque erosion, such as inhibition of myeloperoxidase, anticytokine therapy or inhibition of peptidyl arginine deiminase four. This diagram is hypothetical and serves as a roadmap to inform future research priorities in plaque erosion. (Reproduced from Fahed AC, Jang IK. *Nat Rev Cardiol*. 2021;18(10):724–734.)

Indeed, the focus on individual lesion vulnerability has been criticized in favor of shifting our attention back to the assessment of risk related to overall atherosclerotic burden. Certainly, the isolated assessment of local plaque vulnerability without consideration of the overall clinical context runs the risk of "missing the forest for the trees." Therefore, future investigations should integrate the assessment of vulnerable plaque features using noninvasive imaging with the assessment of vulnerable patient features including clinical risk factors, systemic inflammation, and hypercoagulability using various biomarkers. Additionally, given the invasive nature of intravascular imaging, its future clinical utility requires evidence from prospective studies, without which it will be impossible to determine whether pharmacological or device-based treatment of vulnerable plaques can improve clinical outcomes in a cost-effective manner.

SUMMARY

Intravascular imaging has advanced our understanding of the mechanisms underlying coronary events and vulnerable plaques. Although approximately half of ACS cases are caused by intimal rupture of lipidic plaques, the recognition of other causes provides an opportunity to realize precision therapeutic approaches. Because approximately one-third of recurrent events in patients with ACS are related to an initially nonculprit lesion, the assessment of plaque characteristics in nonculprit segments is important. The high resolution of OCT makes it a robust tool for identifying microscopic anatomical features associated with plaque vulnerability. However, OCT has limited utility in assessing plaque burden, arterial remodeling, and plaque functional activity or biomechanics. In addition to the presence of lipid-rich plaque and TCFA assessed by OCT, plaque burden ≥70%, a minimum lumen area ≤4.0 mm^2, and a greater $maxLCBI_{4mm}$ assessed using gray-scale IVUS and NIRS are independent predictors of future events related to initially nonculprit lesions. Appropriate use of these intracoronary imaging modalities is required to assess both culprit and nonculprit lesions for risk stratification and the future development of precision therapeutic approaches.

REFERENCES

1. Erlinge D, Maehara A, Ben-Yehuda O, et al. Identification of vulnerable plaques and patients by intracoronary near-infrared spectroscopy and ultrasound (PROSPECT II): a prospective natural history study. *Lancet*. 2021;397(10278):985–995. https://doi.org/10.1016/S0140-6736(21)00249-X.
2. Sugiyama T, Yamamoto E, Fracassi F, et al. Calcified plaques in patients with acute coronary syndromes. *JACC Cardiovasc Interv*. 2019;12(6):531–540. https://doi.org/10.1016/j.jcin.2018.12.013.
3. Araki M, Park S-J, Dauerman HL, et al. Optical coherence tomography in coronary atherosclerosis assessment and intervention. *Nat Rev Cardiol*. 2022;19(10):684–703. https://doi.org/10.1038/s41569-022-00687-9.
4. Aguirre AD, Arbab-Zadeh A, Soeda T, Fuster V, Jang I-K. Optical coherence tomography of plaque vulnerability and rupture: JACC focus seminar part 1/3. *J Am Coll Cardiol*. 2021;78(12):1257–1265. https://doi.org/10.1016/j.jacc.2021.06.050.
5. Abdelwahed YS, Nelles G, Frick C, et al. Coexistence of calcified- and lipid-containing plaque components and their association with incidental rupture points in acute coronary syndrome-causing culprit lesions: results from the prospective OPTICO-ACS study. *Eur Hear J Cardiovasc Imaging*. 2022;23(12):1598–1605. https://doi.org/10.1093/ehjci/jeab247.
6. Kolte D, Yonetsu T, Ye JC, Libby P, Fuster V, Jang I-K. Optical coherence tomography of plaque erosion: JACC focus seminar part 2/3. *J Am Coll Cardiol*. 2021;78(12):1266–1274. https://doi.org/10.1016/j.jacc.2021.07.030.
7. Park S, Araki M, Nakajima A, et al. Enhanced diagnosis of plaque erosion by deep learning in patients with acute coronary syndromes. *JACC Cardiovasc Interv*. 2022;15(20):2020–2031. https://doi.org/10.1016/j.jcin.2022.08.040.
8. He L, Qin Y, Xu Y, et al. Predictors of non-stenting strategy for acute coronary syndrome caused by plaque erosion: four-year outcomes of the EROSION study. *EuroIntervention*. 2021;17(6):497–505. https://doi.org/10.4244/EIJ-D-20-00299.

9. Yin Y, Fang C, Jiang S, et al. In vivo evidence of atherosclerotic plaque erosion and healing in patients with acute coronary syndrome using serial optical coherence tomography imaging. *Am Heart J*. 2022;243:66–76. https://doi.org/10.1016/j.ahj.2021.09.007.
10. Torii S, Sato Y, Otsuka F, et al. Eruptive calcified nodules as a potential mechanism of acute coronary thrombosis and sudden death. *J Am Coll Cardiol*. 2021;77(13):1599–1611. https://doi.org/10.1016/j.jacc.2021.02.016.
11. Iwai S, Watanabe M, Okamura A, et al. Prognostic impact of calcified plaque morphology after drug eluting stent implantation - an optical coherence tomography study. *Circ J*. 2021;85(11):2019–2028. https://doi.org/10.1253/circj.CJ-20-1233.
12. Nagata T, Minami Y, Katsura A, et al. Optical coherence tomography factors for adverse events in patients with severe coronary calcification. *Int J Cardiol*. 2023;376:28–34. https://doi.org/10.1016/j.ijcard.2023.02.027.
13. Gaba P, Gersh BJ, Muller J, Narula J, Stone GW. Evolving concepts of the vulnerable atherosclerotic plaque and the vulnerable patient: implications for patient care and future research. *Nat Rev Cardiol*. 2023;20(3):181–196. https://doi.org/10.1038/s41569-022-00769-8.
14. Araki M, Yonetsu T, Kurihara O, et al. Predictors of rapid plaque progression: an optical coherence tomography study. *JACC Cardiovasc Imaging*. 2021;14(8):1628–1638. https://doi.org/10.1016/j.jcmg.2020.08.014.
15. Kubo T, Ino Y, Mintz GS, et al. Optical coherence tomography detection of vulnerable plaques at high risk of developing acute coronary syndrome. *Eur Hear J Cardiovasc Imaging*. 2021;22(12):1376–1384. https://doi.org/10.1093/ehjci/jeab028.
16. Nicholls SJ, Kataoka Y, Nissen SE, et al. Effect of evolocumab on coronary plaque phenotype and burden in statin-treated patients following myocardial infarction. *JACC Cardiovasc Imaging*. 2022;15(7):1308–1321. https://doi.org/10.1016/j.jcmg.2022.03.002.
17. Dawson LP, Lum M, Nerleker N, Nicholls SJ, Layland J. Coronary atherosclerotic plaque regression: JACC state-of-the-art review. *J Am Coll Cardiol*. 2022;79(1):66–82. https://doi.org/10.1016/j.jacc.2021.10.035.
18. Di Giovanni G, Kataoka Y, Bubb K, Nelson AJ, Nicholls SJ. Impact of lipid lowering on coronary atherosclerosis moving from the lumen to the artery wall. *Atherosclerosis*. 2023;367:8–14. https://doi.org/10.1016/j.atherosclerosis.2023.01.017.
19. Jinnouchi H, Guo L, Sakamoto A, et al. Diversity of macrophage phenotypes and responses in atherosclerosis. *Cell Mol Life Sci*. 2020;77(10):1919–1932. https://doi.org/10.1007/s00018-019-03371-3.
20. Räber L, Ueki Y, Otsuka T, et al. Effect of alirocumab added to high-intensity statin therapy on coronary atherosclerosis in patients with acute myocardial infarction: the PACMAN-AMI randomized clinical trial. *JAMA*. 2022;327(18):1771–1781. https://doi.org/10.1001/jama.2022.5218.
21. Nidorf SM, Fiolet A, Abela GS. Viewing atherosclerosis through a crystal lens: how the evolving structure of cholesterol crystals in atherosclerotic plaque alters its stability. *J Clin Lipidol*. 2020;14(5):619–630. https://doi.org/10.1016/j.jacl.2020.07.003.
22. Fujiyoshi K, Minami Y, Ishida K, et al. Incidence, factors, and clinical significance of cholesterol crystals in coronary plaque: an optical coherence tomography study. *Atherosclerosis*. 2019;283:79–84. https://doi.org/10.1016/j.atherosclerosis.2019.02.009.
23. Bianchini E, Lønnebakken MT, Wohlfahrt P, et al. Magnetic resonance imaging and computed tomography for the noninvasive assessment of arterial aging: a review by the VascAgeNet cost action. *J Am Heart Assoc*. 2023;12(10):e027414. https://doi.org/10.1161/JAHA.122.027414.
24. Jinnouchi H, Sato Y, Sakamoto A, et al. Calcium deposition within coronary atherosclerotic lesion: implications for plaque stability. *Atherosclerosis*. 2020;306:85–95. https://doi.org/10.1016/j.atherosclerosis.2020.05.017.
25. Fracassi F, Crea F, Sugiyama T, et al. Healed culprit plaques in patients with acute coronary syndromes. *J Am Coll Cardiol*. 2019;73(18):2253–2263. https://doi.org/10.1016/j.jacc.2018.10.093.
26. Araki M, Yonetsu T, Kurihara O, et al. Predictors of rapid plaque progression: an optical coherence tomography study. *JACC Cardiovasc Imaging*. 2021;14(8):1628–1638. https://doi.org/10.1016/j.jcmg.2020.08.014.
27. Nishi T, Kume T, Yamada R, et al. Layered plaque in organic lesions in patients with coronary artery spasm. *J Am Heart Assoc*. 2022;11(7):e024880. https://doi.org/10.1161/JAHA.121.024880.
28. Hoshino M, Yonetsu T, Kanaji Y, et al. Impact of baseline plaque characteristic on the development of neoatherosclerosis in the very late phase after stenting. *J Cardiol*. 2019;74(1):67–73. https://doi.org/10.1016/j.jjcc.2019.01.002.
29. Okada K, Hibi K. Intravascular ultrasound in vulnerable plaque and acute coronary syndrome. *Interv Cardiol Clin*. 2023;12(2):155–165. https://doi.org/10.1016/j.iccl.2022.10.003.
30. Legutko J, Bryniarski KL, Kaluza GL, et al. Intracoronary imaging of vulnerable plaque-from clinical research to everyday practice. *J Clin Med*. 2022;11(22):6639. https://doi.org/10.3390/jcm11226639.
31. Kitahara S, Kataoka Y, Sugane H, et al. In vivo imaging of vulnerable plaque with intravascular modalities: its advantages and limitations. *Cardiovasc Diagn Ther*. 2020;10(5):1461–1479. https://doi.org/10.21037/cdt-20-238.
32. Waksman R, Di Mario C, Torguson R, et al. Identification of patients and plaques vulnerable to future coronary events with near-infrared spectroscopy intravascular ultrasound imaging: a prospective, cohort study. *Lancet*. 2019;394(10209):1629–1637. https://doi.org/10.1016/S0140-6736(19)31794-5.
33. Li J, Montarello NJ, Hoogendoorn A, et al. Multimodality intravascular imaging of high-risk coronary plaque. *JACC Cardiovasc Imaging*. 2022;15(1):145–159. https://doi.org/10.1016/j.jcmg.2021.03.028.
34. Kakizaki S, Otake H, Seike F, et al. Optical coherence tomography fractional flow reserve and cardiovascular outcomes in patients with acute coronary syndrome. *JACC Cardiovasc Interv*. 2022;15(20):2035–2048. https://doi.org/10.1016/j.jcin.2022.08.010.
35. Baruah V, Zahedivash A, Hoyt T, et al. Automated coronary plaque characterization with intravascular optical coherence tomography and smart-algorithm approach: virtual histology OCT. *JACC Cardiovasc Imaging*. 2020;13(8):1848–1850. https://doi.org/10.1016/j.jcmg.2020.02.022.
36. Fahed AC, Jang I-K. Plaque erosion and acute coronary syndromes: phenotype, molecular characteristics and future directions. *Nat Rev Cardiol*. 2021;18(10):724–734. https://doi.org/10.1038/s41569-021-00542-3.

19 Reperfusion Injury: Prevention and Management

ROBERT A. KLONER AND SHARON L. HALE

INTRODUCTION

The term "reperfusion injury" refers to cellular damage that occurs during the reperfusion phase following an episode of ischemia. If reperfusion occurs after a short period of ischemia, all cells are salvaged (Fig. 19.1A). However, as the duration of ischemia increases, cells become irreversibly injured, and the territory of cell death increases in size over time (Fig. 19.1B). Sorting out the damage that occurs primarily due to reperfusion rather than during the preceding ischemic phase can be difficult because it is impossible to have reperfusion without ischemia. For this reason, the resulting myocardial damage is often referred to as ischemia/reperfusion injury. Evidence that reperfusion itself is harmful to the heart comes from studies showing that certain phenomena first manifest during the reperfusion phase (no-reflow, reperfusion ventricular arrhythmias, stunned myocardium) and then worsen as the phase of reperfusion progresses. In addition, studies of therapies administered only at the time of or solely during the reperfusion phase that result in some benefit also provide evidence that reperfusion itself has detrimental effects. Examples include the administration of oxygen radical scavengers at reperfusion, resulting in improved function of stunned myocardium, the initiation of hypothermia at 30 minutes after reperfusion, resulting in a reduction of the zone of no-reflow, and administering a pharmacologic agent or postconditioning at reperfusion resulting in myocardial infarct size reduction. In this chapter, we will describe the pathobiology and clinical manifestations of reperfusion injury as well as therapeutic strategies for which studies are completed or ongoing. The pathobiology of infarct healing and adverse remodeling of the myocardium after myocardial infarction (MI) are described in Chapter 32.

Conflict of Interest: Dr. Kloner is a paid consultant for Sanofi, Nervimed, a non-paid consultant to ABIOMED, and receives grant support from Sanofi, Young Inc., Stealth Biotherapeutics, and Pulse/Euphrates Therapeutics Inc.

PATHOLOGICAL AND CLINICAL COMPONENTS OF REPERFUSION INJURY

There are four basic components of "reperfusion injury": (1) stunned myocardium, (2) reperfusion arrhythmias, (3) no-reflow phenomenon, also known as microvascular obstruction, and (4) lethal myocardial cell injury due to reperfusion (Fig. 19.2). In our opinion, there is little doubt that the first three phenomena are due to reperfusion itself. However, we still question the significance and importance of lethal myocardial cell injury due to reperfusion and will address this uncertainty later in this chapter (see Lethal Myocardial Cell Injury Due to Reperfusion).

Stunned Myocardium

Stunned myocardium refers to the myocardium that has been subjected to a period of ischemia resulting in reversible injury (meaning that the cells become ischemic, but not necrotic) in which following reperfusion there is prolonged but transient contractile dysfunction.[1] In early studies in canine models of proximal coronary artery occlusion followed by reperfusion, 5 to 15-minute episodes of ischemia resulted in regional wall motion abnormalities that persisted for several hours to days, despite the absence of cell death. Hence, in such experiments, the myocardium behaved as if it were "stunned" by a brief episode of ischemia followed by reperfusion. The entire hypoperfused area of myocardium is described as the area at risk (Fig. 19.1A), and may demonstrate stunning when reperfusion occurs shortly after occlusion. Whereas, when occlusion of the coronary artery is prolonged, irreversible cellular injury occurs resulting in infarction within that area at risk (Fig. 19.1B).

The mechanism of stunning is thought to involve damage from the release of reactive oxygen species and from calcium overload that occurs in the early stages of reperfusion, resulting in reduced responsiveness of the contractile

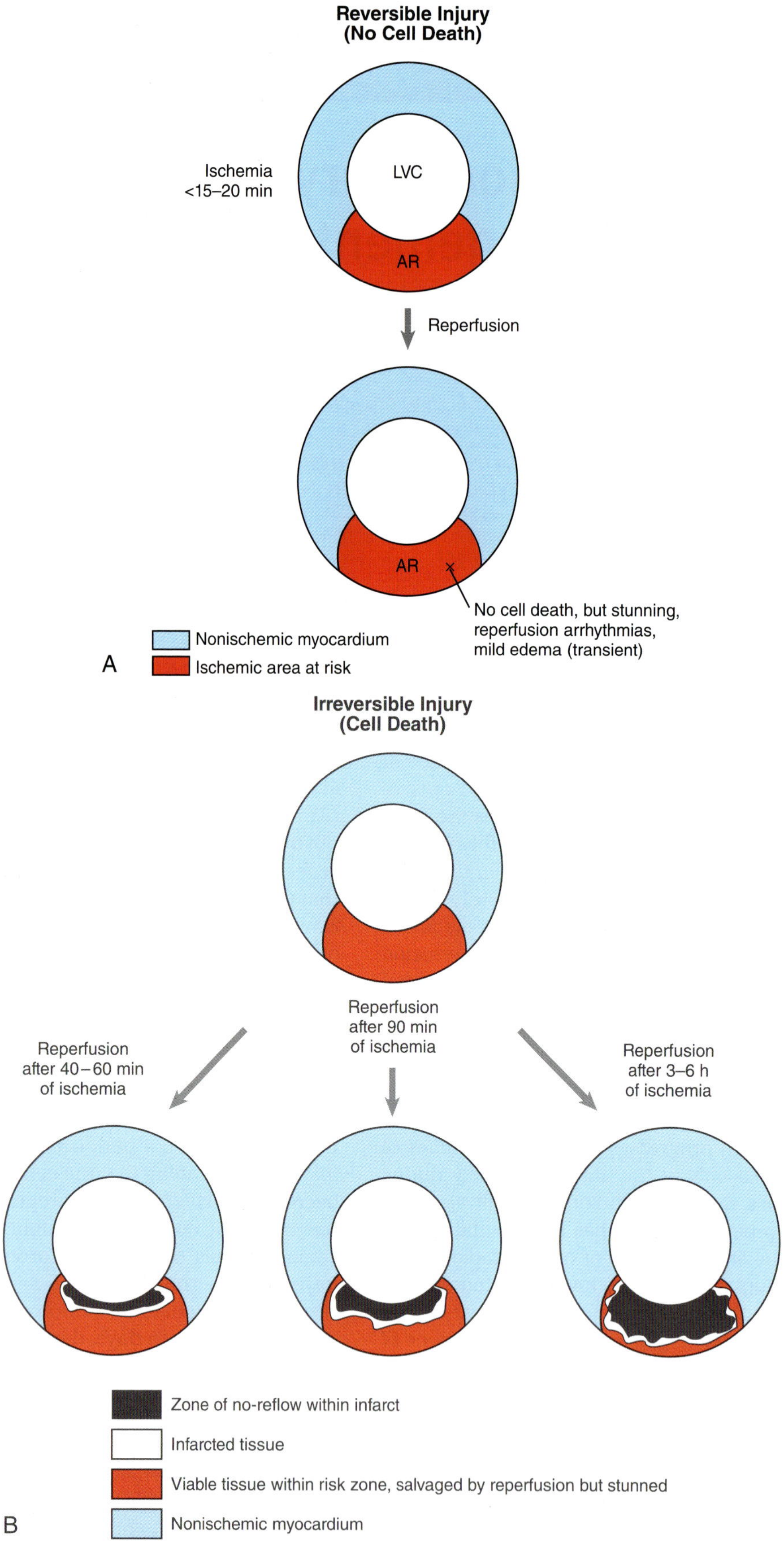

FIG. 19.1 (A) Schematic of a transmural section of the heart after a short period of ischemia (≤20 min). Cell death does not occur (reversible injury), but tissue is stunned and reperfusion arrhythmias might ensue. *AR*, Area at risk; *LVC*, left ventricular cavity. (B) Schematic of a transmural section of the left ventricle derived from studies in the anesthetized canine model of proximal coronary occlusion and reperfusion. After 40 to 60 minutes of ischemia, irreversible cell damage is confined to the subendocardium. A smaller area of no-reflow is present within the necrotic region. If reperfusion is delayed to 90 minutes, the necrotic region expands from subendocardium to mid-myocardium within the ischemic risk zone, accompanied by an expansion of the no-reflow region. After 3 to 6 hours of ischemia, necrosis becomes nearly transmural, and the no-reflow region, although contained within the necrotic area, becomes larger.

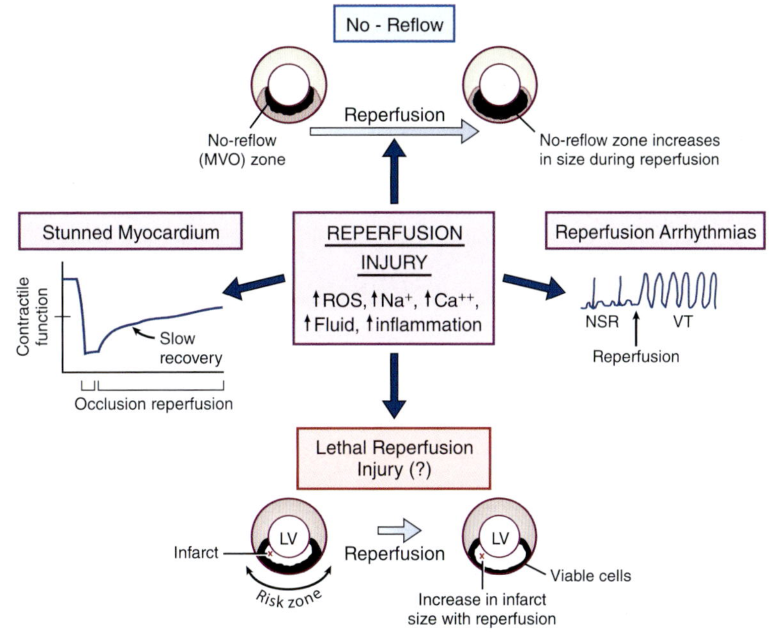

FIG. 19.2 There are four general manifestations of reperfusion injury. Following reperfusion of a myocardial infarction, one form of reperfusion injury is the no-reflow phenomenon, in which there is damage to the microvasculature including microvascular obstruction (MVO) that prevents full reperfusion of the myocardium. Hemorrhage into the myocardium may also contribute to impeded scar healing due to iron deposits leading to fatty infiltration of the myocardium. The size of the no-reflow zone expands during the first few hours of reperfusion of the infarct-related coronary artery. Another manifestation of reperfusion injury is stunned myocardium, whereby contractile function of regional areas of the myocardium remains depressed following restoration of flow. Even after only a 15-minute episode of ischemia in a model where the myocardial cells do not die, the return to normal function may take hours to days. Reperfusion ventricular arrhythmias may be observed right at the time of reperfusion and include ventricular premature beats, forms of ventricular tachycardia, and ventricular fibrillation. In our experimental models, postconditioning protocols limit this form of reperfusion injury. These arrhythmias are usually amenable to treatment. The big question remains: does reperfusion itself kill myocardial cells that are viable at the end of a period of ischemia and contribute to an increase in infarct size? In our models, reperfusion may contribute to scattered apoptosis, but most likely does not result in large swaths of additional infarcted tissue. This concept in our opinion remains controversial, whereas other investigators are convinced that reperfusion contributes to large areas of additional cell death. However, at the time of this writing, the only accepted and standard way of reducing myocardial infarct size is early and persistent reperfusion, and the sooner that reperfusion is instituted following coronary artery occlusion, the greater the myocardial salvage will be. *Ca^{++}*, calcium; *MVO*, microvascular obstruction; *Na^{+}*, sodium; *NSR*, normal sinus rhythm; *ROS*, reactive oxygen species; *VT*, ventricular tachycardia.

apparatus to calcium. Calcium uptake by the sarcoplasmic reticulum appears to be impaired in stunned myocardium and might contribute to contractile dysfunction. The observation that therapy with oxygen radical scavengers at reperfusion improves function supports the concept that stunning is a form of functional reperfusion injury. Clinical examples of stunned myocardium include: (1) slow recovery of salvaged myocardium in the outer wall of the ventricle following thrombolytic therapy or percutaneous coronary intervention (PCI) therapy for ST elevation MI (STEMI)[1]; (2) slow recovery of ventricular function following cardiopulmonary bypass procedures; (3) persistent regional wall motion abnormalities following exercise-induced ischemia or prolonged angioplasty balloon inflation during PCI; and (4) slow recovery of function with Takotsubo cardiomyopathy.

Reperfusion Arrhythmias

Our laboratory and others have observed that reperfusion, following a brief period of ischemia (only 5 min in the anesthetized rat model), results in a barrage of ventricular arrhythmias, including polymorphic ventricular tachycardia, and ventricular fibrillation. The release of toxic oxygen radicals at the time of reperfusion as well as electrolyte disturbances, including sodium and calcium overload of cardiomyocytes, may contribute to the onset of these arrhythmias. In addition, during the first seconds of reperfusion, inhomogeneity of action potential amplitude and duration in the previously ischemic zone and border zone might contribute to reentry-related arrhythmias. Certain therapies introduced at the time of reperfusion, such as postconditioning (transient episodes of brief coronary reocclusion and reperfusion) markedly diminish reperfusion-induced arrhythmias. In patients, reperfusion arrhythmias, including accelerated idioventricular rhythms, ventricular tachycardia, and ventricular premature beats, have been observed following reperfusion therapy for STEMI (see Chapter 23). The incidence of ventricular arrhythmias during acute MI has declined with adoption of early revascularization and medical therapy but still may occur in up to 6% of patients with acute coronary syndromes.[2] Bursts of reperfusion-induced ventricular arrhythmias may be associated with larger infarcts and might represent a biomarker of reperfusion injury. Reperfusion arrhythmias may also pose a potentially unrecognized problem in the setting of reversal of coronary vasospasm (such as in Prinzmetal angina), which is, on rare occasions, followed by sudden death.

The No-Reflow Phenomenon and Microvascular Obstruction

Pathobiology

No-reflow phenomenon refers to the inability to perfuse portions of the myocardium due to microvascular obstruction following successful reopening of an occluded proximal epicardial coronary artery (Fig. 19.3). The fluorescent dye, thioflavin S, is used in animal models to show the anatomic no-reflow zone (Fig. 19.3).[3] In a study performed in anesthetized canines

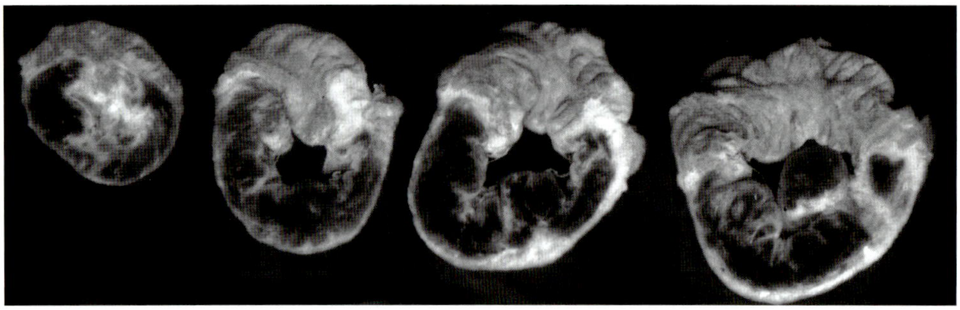

FIG. 19.3 Thioflavin S-stained sections of rabbit heart subjected to 30 minutes ischemia plus reperfusion. The fluorescent white represents areas within the risk zone that received blood flow during reperfusion. Dark areas did not receive blood flow containing the fluorescent dye thioflavin S, even after reperfusion of the epicardial coronary artery and represent the anatomic zone of no-reflow. Grey areas at the top contain an overlap of blue dye used to delineate the nonischemic risk zone during coronary artery occlusion plus thioflavin S.

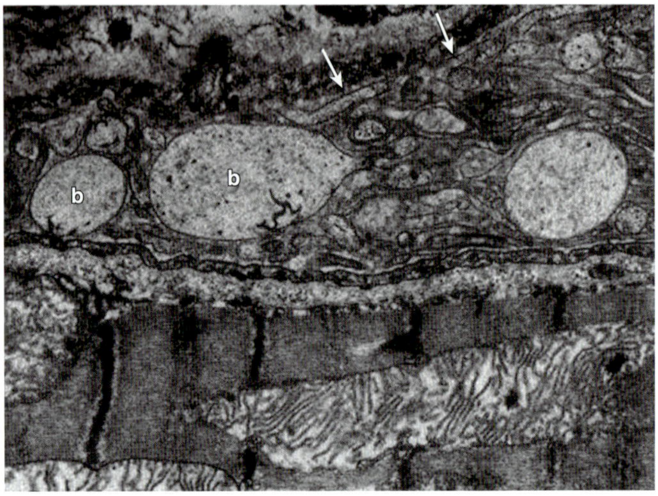

FIG. 19.4 Posterior papillary region of the heart from a canine model made temporarily ischemic for 90 minutes with 10 to 12 s of coronary blood reperfusion (from area of no reflow). Endothelial pinocytotic vesicles are sparse. The capillary lumen is full of endothelial protrusions (*arrows*) and membrane-bound bodies (b), some of which might represent degranulated platelets. Mitochondria are swollen with amorphous matrix dense bodies. I bands and intermyofibrillar edema are present, ×22,640. (Reproduced with permission from Kloner RA, et al: The "no-reflow" phenomenon after temporary coronary occlusion in the dog. *J Clin Invest* 56:1496, 1974; Fig 8a.)

in the mid-1970s, we observed that when the proximal circumflex coronary artery was occluded for 90 minutes followed by reperfusion, that thioflavin S, when injected into the vasculature, failed to penetrate the subendocardium of the posterior LV wall. An electron microscopic examination (Fig. 19.4) of these non-fluorescent zones of no-reflow revealed capillaries with focal endothelial swelling, or "blebs" that appeared to be obstructing blood flow.[3] Areas of microvascular hemorrhage with extrusion of red blood cells into the interstitial space adjacent to endothelial gaps were also observed. Occasionally, capillaries appeared to be compressed by adjacent swollen cardiomyocytes and damaged vessels appeared plugged by fibrin tactoids, platelets, and neutrophils. It is likely that the cause of no-reflow is structural damage to the microvasculature within the zone of MI (Fig. 19.5). Emerging data also suggests that pericyte contraction causes capillary constriction contributing to the mechanism of no-reflow.[4] Although the size of the zone of no-reflow within the infarct is correlated with the duration of coronary occlusion (Fig. 19.1B), we showed that neither streptokinase, tissue plasminogen activator, nor dabigatran could prevent no-reflow. Studies have shown that the size of the no-reflow zone expanded over several hours after reperfusion of the proximal, patent coronary artery. The growth of the anatomic no-reflow zone, assessed by injecting fluorescent dye into the vasculature, was accompanied by a

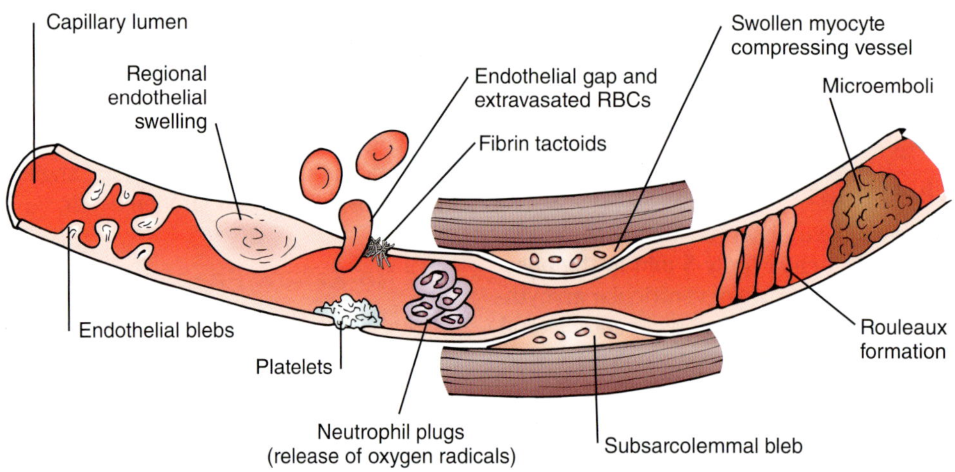

FIG. 19.5 Schematic figure, summarizing different mechanisms, involved in the development of no-reflow, and accompanying ultrastructural alterations of the microvascular bed. *RBC*, red blood cell. (Reproduced with permission from Reffelmann T, Kloner RA: The "no-reflow" phenomenon: basic science and clinical correlates. *Heart* 87:162, 2002; Figure 2.)

deterioration of regional myocardial blood flow within this zone. These findings suggest that whatever damage is occurring to the microvasculature occurs in part during the reperfusion phase and therefore no-reflow is a form of reperfusion injury. Hemorrhage into the infarcted myocardium also may be a manifestation of reperfusion injury and residual iron deposits may contribute to fatty degeneration.[5]

An influx of electrolytes, fluid, calcium, and reactive oxygen species during the early minutes of reperfusion might result in damage to endothelial cells, including focal and diffuse edema and eventual rupture of endothelial cells that then blocks flow. The zone of no-reflow rapidly expands outward within the infarcted region, finally leveling off at about 2 to 8 hours. In general, we have observed that the zone of no-reflow is contained within the zone of MI (myocyte cell death). We do not believe that no-reflow contributes directly to myocyte cell death. However, experimental and clinical studies increasingly suggest that the no-reflow phenomenon is an important marker of prognosis. The larger the extent of no-reflow, the more myocardial infarct expansion and LV remodeling are likely to occur. This observation makes intrinsic sense: if blood elements cannot access the zone of necrotic debris, healing of the scar is impaired.

Clinical Manifestations

No-reflow is now well documented in patients and is clinically manifest in about a third of patients undergoing reperfusion therapy for acute MI. Several imaging techniques, including nuclear imaging (Chapter 16), echo-contrast (Chapter 15) and magnetic resonance imaging (Chapter 17) have visualized anatomic zones of no-reflow or microvascular obstruction in patients. Similar to the findings in experimental animal studies, in humans, the zones of no-reflow observed are typically subendocardial to midmyocardial and appear confined to the necrotic zone. As in animal studies, the presence of no-reflow in patients is associated with greater LV dilatation and adverse LV remodeling, as well as a worse clinical outcome, including higher mortality rates and more heart failure.[6] Some studies have now shown that the size of the no-reflow zone is a marker of poor clinical outcome, independent of the size of the MI.

No-reflow in humans is complicated by the fact that during PCIs, atherosclerotic fragments and thrombi can break off and cause distal embolization, contributing to additional distal microvascular obstruction (Fig. 19.5). No-reflow may be observed in the catheterization laboratory even during routine, nonemergent, coronary angioplasties or stenting procedures. In the catheterization laboratory, sluggish flow in an otherwise patent epicardial coronary artery and reduced myocardial blush grade are signs of low or no-reflow and predict a poor outcome. There are a number of recent studies that have assessed clinical markers that predict no-reflow in patients as shown in Table 19.1.[7–19]

TABLE 19.1 Predictors of No-Reflow in Patients with STEMI

Demographics That Correlate with No-Reflow
Divided evidence on males vs. females
Smoking
High BMI; Weight <78 kg
Advanced age
Diabetes
Laboratory Findings That Correlate with No-Reflow
Increased: Neutrophil to lymphocyte ratio, mean platelet volume, platelet count, platelet distribution width, platelet to lymphocyte ratio
Increased blood glucose
Increased total cholesterol; increased LDL cholesterol
Increased blood viscosity
Elevation of certain plasma lipids: phosphatidyl choline, alkyl phosphatidyl choline, sphingomyelin
Decreased eosinophil count
Higher peak troponin levels
Increased serum uric acid
Increased serum creatinine
Increased preintervention soluble suppression of tumorigenicity 2 (sST2)
Findings on Presentation That Correlate with No-Reflow (Physical, Angiographic, and Imaging)
Cardiac arrest at presentation
Systolic hypertension or hypotension
Killip Class for heart failure ≥3.
Lengthy reperfusion time (greater than 6–8 h)
Heart rate ≥89 beats/min.
Increased lesion complexity on angiogram
Reduced left ventricular ejection fraction (≤30%–35%)
High thrombus burden
R2-CHA2DS2-VASc score of ≥3
Higher Syntax and Gensini coronary artery angiographic score
Diastolic dysfunction (higher H2FPEF score)
Higher left ventricular end-diastolic pressure (≥24 mmHg)
Culprit proximal left anterior descending coronary artery disease
Multivessel involvement
Long lesion length (≥35 mm)
Preprocedure TIMI score of 0
Cholesterol crystals in lipid core by optical coherence tomography
Lower brachial artery flow-mediated vasodilatation

Lethal Myocardial Cell Injury Due to Reperfusion

The fourth, most important, but still controversial (in our opinion) component of reperfusion injury is lethal myocardial cell injury due to reperfusion itself. In this construct, cardiomyocytes are injured but still alive at the end of ischemia. However, once reperfusion occurs, the cardiomyocytes become irreversibly injured and die due to the act of reperfusion. Potential mechanisms whereby reperfusion could cause a reversibly injured cardiomyocyte to become irreversibly injured (dead) are listed in Table 19.2. In particular, the generation of oxygen-free radicals and the opening of mitochondrial permeability transition pore during reperfusion are believed to be important contributors to ischemia/reperfusion injury and have become targets for therapy (see Prevention and Management of Ischemia/Reperfusion Injury). The mitochondrial permeability transition pore is a large-conductance mega-channel that is closed under physiological conditions but opens in response to changes in mitochondrial membrane potential, reactive oxygen species, and increased calcium concentration. Opening of the pore is believed to be a key event in the initiation of apoptotic cell death.

TABLE 19.2

Potential Mechanisms of Lethal Myocyte Injury Due to Reperfusion
1. An influx of sodium, calcium, or water into myocytes with leaky sarcolemmal membranes, resulting in volume and calcium overload of the cells and cellular organelles such as mitochondria
2. Damage to cellular membranes and structures due to the generation of reactive oxygen species at the time of reperfusion
3. Opening of the mitochondrial permeability transition pore during reperfusion
4. Hypercontracture of myocytes due to calcium overload with the formation of contraction bands
5. Changes in pH that occur with reperfusion
6. Damage due to the presence of inflammatory cytokines and neutrophil infiltration into the previously ischemic reperfused zone

Support for the concept that lethal cardiomyocyte reperfusion injury is a real phenomenon comes largely from studies in which therapies given at the time of or very shortly before reperfusion further reduce MI size above and beyond reperfusion alone.[20] However, very few clinical trials have shown such benefits.[21] Worsening of chest pain or re-elevation of ST segments on the electrocardiogram at reperfusion are sometimes interpreted as a clinical manifestation of reperfusion injury.

PREVENTION AND MANAGEMENT OF ISCHEMIA/REPERFUSION INJURY

The prevention and management of ischemia/reperfusion injury are discussed below. Interventions to achieve these goals may be divided into those that are directed at managing the clinical manifestations of ischemia/reperfusion injury, such as supporting contractility in the setting of myocardial stunning, treating reperfusion arrhythmias, reducing no-reflow, and those interventions that are aimed at the prevention of lethal reperfusion injury itself (reduction of infarct size). At present, most therapies in this latter category are investigational only.

General Interventions to Manage Complications of Ischemia-Reperfusion Injury

Stunned myocardium

Stunned myocardium can be prevented by avoiding the initial episode of ischemia. Stunning has been successfully treated by administering oxygen radical scavenging agents at the time of reperfusion. In addition, stunned myocardium can be managed by using inotropic drugs. Since stunned myocardium is a transient phenomenon and responds to inotropic drugs, it can usually be managed in the clinical setting with appropriate titration of such therapy.

Reperfusion arrhythmias

In general, reperfusion arrhythmias that occur in the setting of MI are amenable to therapy, and, in most instances, are not a major clinical problem. Studies in our laboratory have shown that reperfusion-induced ventricular arrhythmias are responsive to treatment with lidocaine, sotalol, ranolazine, and postconditioning.

Interventions Aimed at Reducing Microvascular Obstruction

In general, we have observed that most agents that reduce MI size also reduce the size of the no-reflow zone within the ischemic risk zone. A few therapies have been notable for their ability to reduce no-reflow, even when administered relatively late during the occlusion or even after reperfusion has begun.

Hypothermia

When hypothermia was introduced early during a coronary artery occlusion/reperfusion protocol in the rabbit, it reduced both MI size and the extent of the anatomic zone of no-reflow. When hypothermia was introduced 5 minutes before or 5 minutes after reperfusion it failed to reduce MI size but still reduced no-reflow. In one study, we introduced hypothermia as late as 30 minutes after reperfusion. Again, it had no effect on MI size but still reduced the area of no-reflow.

Agents Influencing Free Radicals

The oxygen radical scavenging agents, superoxide dismutase plus catalase, given at reperfusion in our canine model of 2 hours of proximal coronary artery occlusion and 4 hours of reperfusion did not reduce MI size but did reduce microvascular injury and reduced low reflow. This shows that administering therapy at, or close to the time of reperfusion, or even after reperfusion reduces no-reflow and microvascular injury, providing additional support for the concept that no-reflow is a true form of reperfusion injury.

The no-reflow phenomenon is commonly treated in the catheterization laboratory.[22–26] Various therapies that have shown some success in improving low or no-reflow after cardiac catheterization include vasodilators such as nitroprusside, adenosine, and calcium channel blockers including verapamil, diltiazem; epinephrine, and others.[23–27]

Interventions Aimed at Preventing Reperfusion Injury Due to Cellular Necrosis

The primary treatment of acute STEMI should be early and complete reperfusion of the occluded culprit epicardial coronary artery (see Chapter 1). Reperfusion salvages tissue, has a substantial impact on infarct size, and improves clinical outcomes. However, if the act of reperfusion also kills some population of cardiomyocytes that are hovering between life and death, then efforts to reduce this reperfusion injury might further improve outcome (Fig. 19.6). Numerous clinical trials have attempted to further reduce MI size by administering adjunctive therapies near the time of reperfusion in order to mitigate reperfusion injury.[24–45] There is a long list of agents that showed promise in preclinical trials but failed in clinical trials. We have previously described these trials and discussed reasons why these trials may have failed.

Therapies that have been used clinically in an attempt to reduce MI size by inhibiting reperfusion injury have included oxygen radical scavengers, calcium blockers, and anti-inflammatory agents. Early studies with these and other agents primarily yielded negative results. One reason for the failure of early studies is likely that therapy was administered too late after reperfusion. In general, we have observed that most therapies aimed at reducing MI size work only when they are present early enough to protect the myocardium during at least a portion of the ischemic phase and are present at the moment of reperfusion. Since oxygen radical generation, sodium and calcium overload and myocardial edema occur within seconds of the release of a coronary artery occlusion, therapies aimed at these adverse reperfusion phenomena must be present in the very early phase of reperfusion in order to confer a benefit. Despite the substantial number of clinical trials that failed to show the benefit of strategies to reduce reperfusion injury, some studies have had more promising results.

There are some studies that have shown promise in reducing myocardial infarct size beyond reperfusion. These include IV infusions of adenosine, hypothermia when instituted prior to reperfusion, supersaturated oxygen, the potassium channel activator and vasodilator nicorandil.

However, it is important to point out that in most studies, it is not possible to determine whether the benefits observed were due to a reduction in initial ischemic damage, a reduction in reperfusion injury, or some combination of the two. In many of these studies, therapies were started prior to reperfusion (Table 19.3); thus, therapies given during the later phase of an episode of ischemia might have conferred benefit by protecting the heart during critical phases of the ischemic insult rather than by protecting the heart during the reperfusion phase alone. There are a few exceptions in which therapy did not commence until after reperfusion had begun. Selected interventions of particular interest in the evolution of this field are discussed below and recent studies that have attempted to treat ischemia/reperfusion damage in STEMI published since the last edition of this book are shown in Table 19.3.

Postconditioning and Remote Ischemic Conditioning

The effectiveness of postconditioning (stuttering reperfusion) in clinical trials of myocardial infarct size reduction has been mixed. In one recent study, postconditioning did improve blush grade and enzymatic infarct size.[28] Some studies now suggest that postconditioning only is effective in those patients who do not also undergo thrombectomy.[29,30] Because of the timing of the intervention, postconditioning is plausibly working only during the reperfusion phase. In our laboratory, whereas postconditioning was very effective at reducing reperfusion-induced ventricular arrhythmias, it was ineffective at reducing MI size.

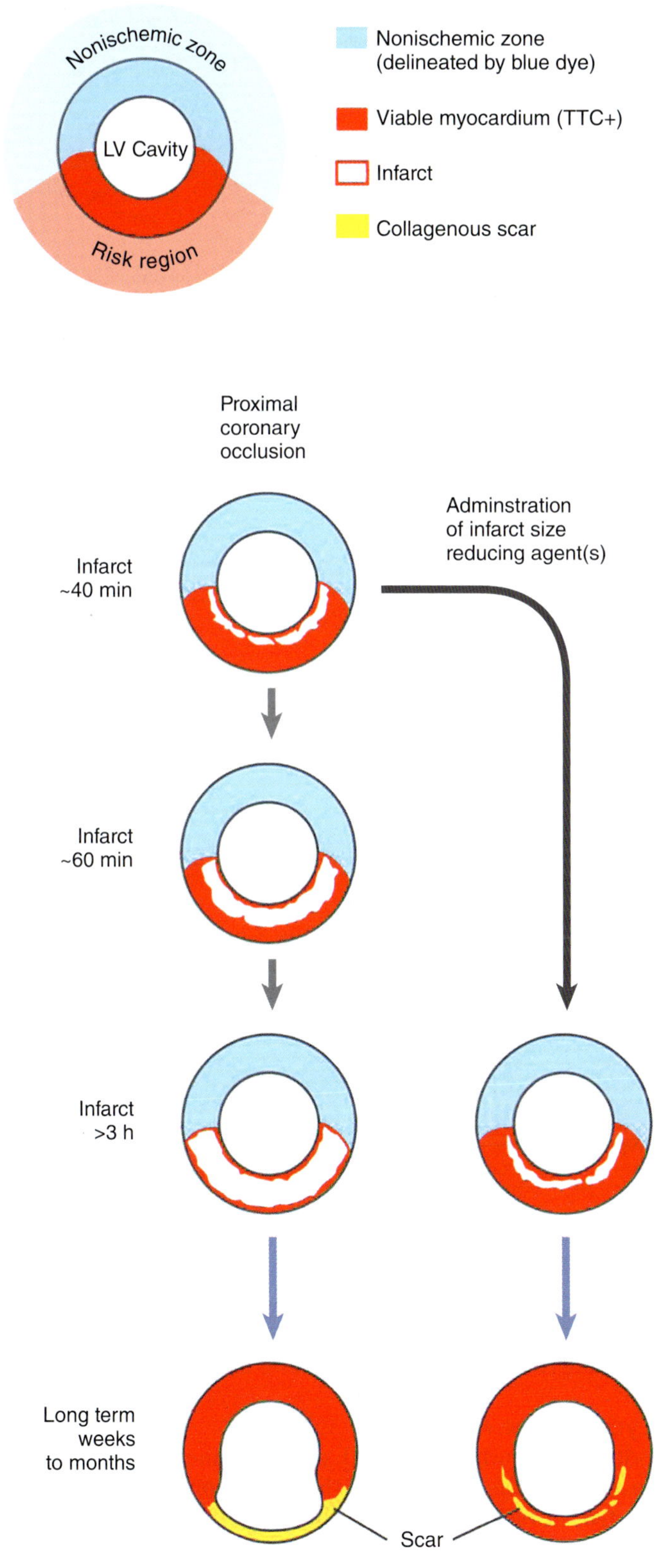

FIG. 19.6 Schematic showing how reducing myocardial infarct size early could have benefits on long-term structure of the heart. The left-hand drawings show a schematic derived from the wavefront concept of Reimer and Jennings. After proximal coronary occlusion, a portion of the left ventricle (LV) becomes ischemic, defined as the ischemic risk region. When a blue dye is injected into the vasculature the blue dye circulates to areas receiving blood flow and fails to penetrate the ischemic zone. If reperfusion occurs after ≈40 min of ischemia, irreversible myocardial damage–that is necrosis (*pale white area*) is confined to the subendocardial myocardium. Viable myocardium within the risk zone is stained red by triphenyltetrazolium chloride (TTC). If reperfusion is delayed (after 60 min) or after 3 to 6 hours of coronary artery occlusion, the extent of necrosis expands from subendocardium to midmyocardium to subepicardium within the ischemic risk zone. This march of necrosis becomes transmural or nearly transmural if reperfusion is not instituted within about 3 to 6 hours or if reperfusion does not occur. Large transmural infarcts may then go on to result in severe LV remodeling with infarct expansion, LV cavity dilation, LV aneurysm formation, and eccentric hypertrophy of the noninfarcted tissue. If agents are administered to reduce infarct size or if very early reperfusion is instituted the size of the infarct can be limited (first transverse LV slice shown in right column). During the long term, this smaller infarct will shrink in size with a minimum of subendocardial scar tissue and substantial viable tissue remaining in the midmyocardial wall. LV remodeling will be minimized with less infarct wall thinning, less LV dilation, and less eccentric hypertrophy. In addition, LV function will be better preserved. (Reproduced with permission from Kloner RA: Current state of clinical translation of cardioprotective agents for acute myocardial infarction. *Circ Res* 113:451, 2013.)

TABLE 19.3 **Selected Studies Aimed at Reducing Myocardial Infarct Size**

INTERVENTION	TIME TREATMENT INITIATED	OUTCOME	TOTAL PTS.	REFERENCES
Ciclosporin	Before PCI	Single ciclosporin bolus did not affect IS or left ventricular remodeling	52	Cormack et al.[36]
Nicorandil	Bolus before PCI, 6 h infusion	Nicorandil before PCI led to improved myocardial perfusion grade, increased LV ejection fraction, and reduced IS	238	Qian et al.[25]
Nicorandil	During PCI	Administering nicorandil distal to the vascular lesion during PCI in STEMI patients may reduce the incidence of reperfusion injury, improve short-term clinical outcomes, and improve MVO	170	Feng et al.[37]
Everolimus	Oral treatment peri-PCI	Early mTOR inhibition with everolimus did not reduce MI size or MVO at 30 days	150	Stähli et al.[38]
Lecithin-cholesterol acyltransferase	Treatment for 12 weeks post PCI	No reduction in MI size or MVO at 30 days	593	Bonaca et al.[39]
Allogenic heart stem cells	4–12 weeks after MI	Did not reduce scar size relative to placebo at 6 months	134	Makkar et al.[40]
Postconditioning	After PCI	Postconditioning significantly improved blush grade and enzymatic infarct size reduction with a trend toward significant reduction of mean ST-segment deviation.	43	Mukherjee and Jain[28]
Remote ischemic conditioning	Within 48 h post PCI	After one year, single-cycle RIC was associated with LV end-systolic volume reduction	270	Ikonomidis et al.[32]
Remote ischemic conditioning	Before PCI	Remote ischemic conditioning did not improve clinical outcomes (cardiac death or hospitalization for heart failure) at 12 months	5401	Hausenloy et al.[31]
Colchicine	Before PCI; daily until discharge	No difference in MVO or MACE	321	Hosseini et al.[41]
Colchicine	Pts. with acute AMI treated for 5 days after PCI	Reduced IS and inflammatory response	150	Deftereos et al. 2015 (Classic references)
Colchicine	Pts. with AMI within 30 days treated orally with low dose	Colchicine daily led to a significantly lower risk of ischemic cardiovascular events than placebo	4745	Tardif et al.[42]
Colchicine	At PCI, pts received oral colchicine dose followed by 5-day treatment	No difference in MI size assessed by cardiac MRI	192	Mewton et al.[43]
IL-6 inhibition	Meta-analysis of preclinical studies and MI patients	No difference in cardiac function in preclinical models; modest effect on cardiac remodeling	NS	Duddu et al.[44]
IL-6 inhibition	Pts. received tocilizumab within 6 h of symptom onset	Myocardial salvage greater in treated group, and MVO less. No difference in final IS.	199	Broch et al.[45]
Intravenous Metoprolol	Before PCI	Reduced arrhythmias; no effect on IS	683	Roolvink et al. 2016 (Classic reference)
Intravenous Metoprolol	Before PCI plus orally within 24 h	Decreased IS and improved EF	270	Ibanez et al. 2013 (Classic reference)
Unloading LV	Unloading of LV followed by immediate reperfusion vs. 30 min unloading and delayed reperfusion	Unloading for 30 min followed by delayed reperfusion did not increase infarct size or worsen clinical outcome, suggesting that unloading could extend the window of protection	50	Kapur et al.[35]

EF, Ejection fraction; *IS*, infarct size; *LV*, left ventricle; *MACE*, major adverse cardiac events; *MI*, myocardial infarction; *MRI*, magnetic resonance imaging; *min*, minutes; *MVO*, microvascular obstruction; *NS*, not specified; *PCI*, percutaneous coronary intervention; *pts*, patients; *RIC*, remote ischemic conditioning; *STEMI*, ST-elevation myocardial infarction.

Remote ischemic preconditioning was shown to reduce myocardial infarct size in animal studies; but the preconditioning aspect of this is not feasible in humans, since the onset of MI is not predictable. Initial studies of remote ischemic per-conditioning, where brief episodes of ischemia were instituted by inflating and deflating an arm cuff during ischemia, often in the setting of an ambulance, initially looked promising and appeared to salvage myocardium. A larger subsequent study did not show any clinical benefit on reduction of cardiac death or heart failure; although the patients recruited for this study were likely very low risk.[31] However, in another study, remote ischemic conditioning did facilitate reverse LV remodeling after acute MI.[32]

Cyclosporine A

Both postconditioning and cyclosporine A are thought to prevent the opening of the mitochondrial permeability transition pore during the early phase of reperfusion (see Lethal Myocardial Cell Injury Due to Reperfusion). The opening of this pore has been linked to mitochondrial damage and reperfusion injury (Table 19.2). Early small studies with cyclosporine A suggested that administration of cyclosporine A at reperfusion reduced MI size assessed both by serial cardiac biomarkers of necrosis and by magnetic resonance imaging. However, in a study in which cyclosporine A was administered just before fibrinolytic therapy in 101 patients with STEMI, no benefit was observed. A large randomized trial of cyclosporin A in patients with STEMI named CIRCUS (Cyclosporine and Prognosis in Acute Myocardial Infarction Patients; NCT01502774) was neutral with no evidence that cyclosporine A altered the endpoints of death, hospitalization for heart failure, or LV remodeling at 1 year.

Nicorandil

Nicorandil is a potassium channel activator that also is a vasodilator and is used to treat angina. Several reports suggest that nicorandil both reduces acute myocardial infarct size in humans as well as reduces the no-reflow when given prior to PCI.[33] In one study, LV ejection fraction was found to be greater in the nicorandil group versus the placebo group at both 5 to 7 days after the MI as well as 6 months after MI. Nevertheless, available data are insufficient for professional society guidelines to include recommendations for the clinical use of nicorandil for amelioration of reperfusion injury.

Other Therapeutic Approaches

Hyperoxemia and ANP

Therapeutic hyperoxemia in the AMIHOT trial and atrial natriuretic peptide (ANP) have been studied with initiation *after* reperfusion had commenced and demonstrated favorable effects. Therefore, the reported benefits of these agents may represent a reduction in lethal myocardial cell injury; although supersaturated oxygen may allow oxygenation of areas that red blood cells cannot reach within the microvasculature, thus actually treating ischemic injury.[21]

Hypothermia

Therapeutic hypothermia has consistently reduced MI size in our laboratory. However, it must be present during the ischemic phase, and an adequate degree of temperature reduction must be achieved prior to reperfusion for the intervention to be effective.[20] Studies in humans also suggest that reducing core temperature to <35°C in anterior infarcts, coupled with timely reperfusion, may reduce MI size. The issue has been how to achieve rapid hypothermia. A technique called the Thermosuit (already approved by the FDA to treat hyperthermia) uses immersion-convection cooling and is able to reduce core temperature to desired levels in humans in about 20 minutes. Therapeutic hypothermia attained using the Thermosuit technique remains the single most effective therapy for reducing infarct size in our laboratory. Clinical trials testing hypothermia for reducing myocardial infarct size have been mixed, in part due to difficulty achieving optimal temperatures prior to reperfusion, delays in reperfusion, and other adverse events.[34] One analysis did show that effective hypothermia with endovascular cooling could reduce both infarct size and heart failure predominantly in patients with large areas at risk.

Left Ventricular Unloading

Preclinical study suggested that unloading the LV prior to reperfusion could reduce myocardial infarct size. The door-to-unload in STEMI Pilot study tested whether unloading the LV with the Impella LV assist device and delaying reperfusion in patients with STEMI but without cardiogenic shock is safe. Investigators assigned 50 patients with anterior STEMI to LV unloading followed by immediate reperfusion versus 30 minutes of unloading followed by delayed reperfusion. Thirty-day mean infarct size did not differ between the groups and there were no significant differences in cardiovascular or cerebrovascular events between groups. The study suggested that delaying reperfusion while the LV was unloaded was safe and did not increase infarct size suggesting that the window for protecting the myocardium could be extended by unloading the left ventricle.[35] Larger studies are further exploring this phenomenon.

Importance of Timing of Administration

Despite the few apparent successes described above, our group has observed less evidence for the ability of agents to reduce MI size when administered *only* at the time of reperfusion. Most cardioprotective agents that we have tested have required that the agent be present for at least a portion of the ischemic phase. We have been unable to verify that postconditioning or oxygen radical scavengers given at reperfusion reduce MI size. Hypothermia reduced infarct size when present during at least the last third of the ischemic time, but when initiated after reperfusion had commenced, it failed to reduce infarct size; although, it did reduce the zone of no-reflow. Reports from a randomized, blinded, multicenter study, showed that sodium nitrite and the phosphodiesterase 5 inhibitor, sildenafil, failed to reduce MI size when administered shortly before reperfusion.

Lessons Learned from Previous Studies

Whether adjunctive agents work only during ischemia, during reperfusion, or during both may not be such a crucial question. Therapies can be started either in the catheterization laboratory or emergency department before the infarct-related coronary artery is opened, ensuring that a portion of the ischemic period is treated. Some studies, such as those evaluating remote ischemic perconditioning and glucose-insulin-potassium, have shown the feasibility of starting therapy even before a patient with acute MI is admitted to the hospital. Hence, adjunctive therapies could be instituted during the ischemic phase, the reperfusion phase, or both, protecting the patient from "ischemia-reperfusion injury." In addition, it might be naïve to think that only one adjunctive agent need be given to further protect against ischemia/reperfusion injury. For example, perhaps an intervention such as hypothermia or metoprolol, which can reduce oxygen demand during ischemia should be administered during the ischemic phase, and then a mitochondrial permeability transition pore closing agent, such as cyclosporine, or a mitochondrial protective agent that reduces generation of reactive oxygen species should be given during the reperfusion phase. In other words, a cocktail of compounds might be needed to optimally reduce MI size. To this point, we observed that a combination of hypothermia, preconditioning, and sodium-hydrogen exchange inhibition profoundly reduced MI size to levels greater than what would have been expected with any of these agents given alone.

SUMMARY

Reperfusion injury in the setting of acute MI consists of four main components: (1) stunned myocardium, (2) reperfusion-induced arrhythmias, (3) no-reflow phenomenon (microvascular obstruction), and (4) lethal myocardial cell injury (Fig. 19.2). Data supporting stunned myocardium, reperfusion-induced arrhythmias, and no-reflow as a form of reperfusion injury are solid. The importance of lethal myocardial cell injury due to reperfusion remains, in our opinion, controversial. However, despite improvements in reperfusion therapy, morbidity and mortality from MI are still unacceptable. There is still a need to further reduce MI size and no-reflow, which are both determinants of poor outcome following MI (see Chapter 1). The search for agents and therapies that reduce ischemic damage, reperfusion injury, or some combination of the two should continue to be of high priority to optimize outcome following MI.

CLASSIC REFERENCES

Braunwald E, Kloner RA. Myocardial reperfusion: a double-edged sword? *J Clin Invest.* 1985;76:1713–1719.

Braunwald E, Kloner RA. The stunned myocardium: prolonged postischemic ventricular dysfunction. *Circulation.* 1982;66:1146–1149.

Deftereos S, Giannopoulos G, Angelidis C, et al. Anti-inflammatory treatment with colchicine in acute myocardial infarction: a pilot study. *Circulation.* 2015;132:1395–1403.

Elllis SG, Henschke CI, Sandor T, Wynne J, Braunwald E, Kloner RA. Time course of functional and biochemical recovery of myocardium salvaged by reperfusion. *J Am Coll Cardiol.* 1983;1:1047–1055.

Erlinge D, Götberg M, Noc M, et al. Therapeutic hypothermia for the treatment of acute myocardial infarction-combined analysis of the RAPID MI-ICE and the CHILL-MI trials. *Ther Hypothermia Temp Manag.* 2015;5:77–84.

Ibáñez B, Heusch G, Ovize M, Van de Werf F. Evolving therapies for myocardial ischemia/reperfusion injury. *J Am Coll Cardiol.* 2015;65:1454–1471.

Ibanez B, Macaya C, Sánchez-Brunete V, et al. Effect of early metoprolol on infarct size in ST-segment-elevation myocardial infarction patients undergoing primary percutaneous coronary intervention: the Effect of Metoprolol in Cardioprotection During an Acute Myocardial Infarction (METOCARD-CNIC) trial. *Circulation.* 2013;128:1495–1503.

Kloner RA, Ganote CE, Jennings RB. The "no reflow" phenomenon after temporary coronary occlusion in the dog. *J Clin Invest.* 1974;54:1496–1508.

Kloner RA, Hale SL, Dai W, Shi J. Cardioprotection: where to from here? *Cardiovasc Drugs Ther.* 2017;31:53–61.

Kloner RA, Schwartz Longacre L. State of the Science of Cardioprotection: challenges and opportunities—proceedings of the 2010 NHLBI workshop on cardioprotection. *J Cardiovasc Pharmacol Ther.* 2011;16:223–232.

Kloner RA. Current state of clinical translation of cardioprotective agents for acute myocardial infarction. *Circ Res.* 2013;113:451–463.

Murry CE, Jennings RB, Reimer KA. Preconditioning with ischemia: a delay of lethal cell injury in ischemic myocardium. *Circulation.* 1986;74:1124–1136.

Reimer KA, Jennings RB. The "wavefront" phenomenon of myocardial ischemic cell death II. Transmural progression of necrosis within the framework of ischemic bed size (myocardium at risk) and collateral flow. *Lab Invest.* 1979;40:633–644.

Roolvink V, Ibáñez B, Ottervanger JP, et al. Early Intravenous Beta-blockers in patients with ST-segment elevation myocardial infarction before primary percutaneous coronary intervention. *J Am Coll Cardiol.* 2016;67:2705–2715.

Schwartz Longacre L, Kloner RA, Arai AE, et al. New horizons in cardioprotection: recommendations from the 2010 National Heart, Lung, and Blood Institutes Workshop. *Circulation.* 2011;124:1172–1179.

Stone GW, Martin JL, de Boer MJ, et al. Effect of supersaturated oxygen delivery on infarct size after percutaneous coronary intervention in acute myocardial infarction. *Circ Cadiovasc Intev.* 2009;2:366–375.

Yellon DM, Hausenloy Dj. Myocardial reperfusion injury. *N Engl J Med.* 2007;357:1121–1135.

REFERENCES

1. Kloner RA. Stunned and hibernating myocardium: where are we nearly 4 decades later? *J Am Heart Assoc.* 2020;9:e015502.
2. Kalarus Z, Svendsen JH, Capodanno D, et al. Cardiac arrhythmias in the emergency settings of acute coronary syndrome and revascularization: an European Heart Rhythm Association (EHRA) consensus document, endorsed by the European Association of Percutaneous Cardiovascular Interventions (EAPCI), and European Acute Cardiovascular Care Association (ACCA). *Europace.* 2019;21:1603–1604.
3. Kloner RA, King KS, Harrington MG. No-reflow phenomenon in the heart and brain. *Am J Physiol Heart Circ Physiol.* 2018;315:H550–H562.
4. Methner C, Cao Z, Mishra A, Kaul S. Mechanism and potential treatment of the "no reflow" phenomenon after acute myocardial infarction: role of pericytes and GPR39. *Am J Physiol Heart Circ Physiol.* 2021;321:H1030–H1041.
5. Cokic I, Chan SF, Guan X, et al. Intramyocardial hemorrhage drives fatty degeneration of infarcted myocardium. *Nat Commun.* 2022;13:6394.
6. Allencherril J, Jneid H, Atar D, et al. Pathophysiology, diagnosis, and management of the no-reflow phenomenon. *Cardiovasc Drugs Ther.* 2019;33:589–597.
7. Aggarwal P, Rekwal L, Sinha SK, et al. Predictors of no-reflow phenomenon following percutaneous coronary intervention for ST-segment elevation myocardial infarction. *Ann Cardiol Angeiol (Paris).* 2021;70:136–142.
8. Badran HM, Fatah AA, Soltan G. Platelet/lymphocyte ratio for prediction of no-reflow phenomenon in ST-elevation myocardial infarction managed with primary percutaneous coronary intervention. *J Clin Transl Res.* 2020;6:20–26.
9. Katayama Y, Taruya A, Kashiwagi M, et al. No-reflow phenomenon and in vivo cholesterol crystals combined with lipid core in acute myocardial infarction. *Int J Cardiol Heart Vasc.* 2022;38:100953.
10. Li Z, Yin H, Wang D, et al. Prediction of microvascular obstruction by coronary artery angiography score after acute ST-segment elevation myocardial infarction: a single-center retrospective observational study. *BMC Cardiovasc Disord.* 2022;22:410.
11. Namazi M, Mahmoudi E, Safi M, et al. The no-reflow phenomenon: Is it predictable by demographic factors and routine laboratory data? *Acta Biomed.* 2021;92:e2021297.
12. Rossington JA, Sol E, Masoura K, et al. No-reflow phenomenon and comparison to the normal-flow population postprimary percutaneous coronary intervention for ST elevation myocardial infarction: case-control study (NORM PPCI). *Open Heart.* 2020;7(2):e001215.
13. Seyyed Mohammadzad MH, Khademvatani K, Gardeshkhah S, Sedokani A. Echocardiographic and laboratory findings in coronary slow flow phenomenon: cross-sectional study and review. *BMC Cardiovasc Disord.* 2021;21:230.
14. Søndergaard FT, Beske RP, Frydland M, et al. Soluble ST2 in plasma is associated with post-procedural no-or-slow reflow after primary percutaneous coronary intervention in ST-elevation myocardial infarction. *Eur Heart J Acute Cardiovasc Care.* 2023;12:48–52.
15. Stajic Z, Milicevic D, Kafedzic S, et al. Predicting no-reflow phenomenon prior to primary percutaneous coronary intervention using a novel probability risk score derived from clinical and angiographic parameters. *Eur Rev Med Pharmacol Sci.* 2022;26:759–770.
16. Surendran A, Ismail U, Atefi N, et al. Lipidomic predictors of coronary no-reflow. *Metabolites.* 2023;13(1):79.
17. Yildirim A, Kucukosmanoglu M, Koyunsever NY, et al. Relationship between blood viscosity and no-reflow phenomenon in ST-segment elevation myocardial infarction performed in primary percutaneous coronary interventions. *Biomark Med.* 2021;15:659–667.
18. Zhang Q, Hu M, Ma S, Niu T. New R(2)-CHA(2)DS(2)-VASc score predicts no-reflow phenomenon and long-term prognosis in patients with ST-segment elevation myocardial infarction after primary percutaneous coronary intervention. *Front Cardiovasc Med.* 2022;9:899739.
19. Zhang Q, Hu M, Sun J, Ma S. The combination of neutrophil-to-lymphocyte ratio and platelet correlation parameters in predicting the no-reflow phenomenon after primary percutaneous coronary intervention in patients with ST-segment elevation myocardial infarction. *Scand Cardiovasc J.* 2020;54:352–357.
20. Heusch G. Myocardial ischaemia-reperfusion injury and cardioprotection in perspective. *Nat Rev Cardiol.* 2020;17:773–789.
21. Kloner RA, Creech JL, Stone GW, et al. Update on cardioprotective strategies for STEMI: focus on supersaturated oxygen delivery. *JACC Basic Transl Sci.* 2021;6:1021–1033.
22. Kloner RA, Dai W, Hale SL. No-reflow phenomenon. A new target for therapy of acute myocardial infarction independent of myocardial infarct size. *J Cardiovasc Pharmacol Ther.* 2018;23:273–276.
23. Darwish A, Frere AF, Abdelsamie M, et al. Intracoronary epinephrine versus adenosine in the management of refractory no-reflow phenomenon: a single-center retrospective cohort study. *Ann Saudi Med.* 2022;42:75–82.
24. Geng N, Ren L, Xu L, et al. Clinical outcomes of nicorandil administration in patients with acute ST-segment elevation myocardial infarction undergoing primary percutaneous coronary intervention: a systematic review and meta-analysis of randomized controlled trials. *BMC Cardiovasc Disord.* 2021;21:488.
25. Qian G, Zhang Y, Dong W, et al. Effects of nicorandil administration on infarct size in patients with ST-Segment-Elevation myocardial infarction undergoing primary percutaneous coronary intervention: the CHANGE trial. *J Am Heart Assoc.* 2022;11:e026232.
26. Sadeghian M, Mousavi SH, Aamaraee Z, Shafiee A. Administration of intracoronary adenosine before stenting for the prevention of no-reflow in patients with ST-elevation myocardial infarction. *Scand Cardiovasc J.* 2022;56:23–27.

27. Zhou J, Xu J, Cheng A, et al. Effect of nicorandil treatment adjunctive to percutaneous coronary intervention in patients with acute myocardial infarction: a systematic review and meta-analysis. *J Int Med Res*. 2020;48:300060520967856.
28. Mukherjee P, Jain M. Effect of ischemic postconditioning during primary percutaneous coronary intervention for patients with ST-segment elevation myocardial infarction: a single-center cross-sectional study. *Ann Card Anaesth*. 2019;22:347–352.
29. Madsen JM, Glinge C, Jabbari R, et al. Comparison of effect of ischemic postconditioning on cardiovascular mortality in patients with ST-segment elevation myocardial infarction treated with primary percutaneous coronary intervention with versus without thrombectomy. *Am J Cardiol*. 2022;166:18–24.
30. Nepper-Christensen L, Høfsten DE, Helqvist S, et al. Interaction of ischaemic postconditioning and thrombectomy in patients with ST-elevation myocardial infarction. *Heart*. 2020;106:24–32.
31. Hausenloy DJ, Kharbanda RK, Møller UK, et al. Effect of remote ischaemic conditioning on clinical outcomes in patients with acute myocardial infarction (CONDI-2/ERIC-PPCI): a single-blind randomised controlled trial. *Lancet*. 2019;394:1415–1424.
32. Ikonomidis I, Vlastos D, Andreadou I, et al. Vascular conditioning prevents adverse left ventricular remodelling after acute myocardial infarction: a randomised remote conditioning study. *Basic Res Cardiol*. 2021;116:9.
33. Ilyas M, Noor M, Khan HS, et al. Cardio protective effect of nicorandil in reperfusion injury among patients undergoing primary percutaneous coronary intervention. *Pak J Med Sci*. 2023;39:177–181.
34. Bashtawi Y, Almuwaqqat Z. Therapeutic hypothermia in STEMI. *Cardiovasc Revasc Med*. 2021;29:77–84.
35. Kapur NK, Alkhouli MA, DeMartini TJ, et al. Unloading the left ventricle before reperfusion in patients with anterior ST-segment-elevation myocardial infarction. *Circulation*. 2019;139:337–346.
36. Cormack S, Mohammed A, Panahi P, et al. Effect of ciclosporin on safety, lymphocyte kinetics and left ventricular remodelling in acute myocardial infarction. *Br J Clin Pharmacol*. 2020;86:1387–1397.
37. Feng C, Liu Y, Wang L, et al. Effects of early intracoronary administration of nicorandil during percutaneous coronary intervention in patients with acute myocardial infarction. *Heart Lung Circ*. 2019;28:858–865.
38. Stähli BE, Klingenberg R, Heg D, et al. Mammalian target of rapamycin inhibition in patients with ST-segment elevation myocardial infarction. *J Am Coll Cardiol*. 2022;80:1802–1814.
39. Bonaca MP, Morrow DA, Bergmark BA, et al. Randomized, placebo-controlled phase 2b study to evaluate the safety and efficacy of recombinant human lecithin cholesterol acyltransferase in acute ST-Segment-Elevation myocardial infarction: results of REAL-TIMI 63B. *Circulation*. 2022;146:907–916.
40. Makkar RR, Kereiakes DJ, Aguirre F, et al. Intracoronary ALLogeneic heart STem cells to Achieve myocardial Regeneration (ALLSTAR): a randomized, placebo-controlled, double-blinded trial. *Eur Heart J*. 2020;41:3451–3458.
41. Hosseini SH, Talasaz AH, Alidoosti M, et al. Preprocedural colchicine in patients with acute ST-elevation myocardial infarction undergoing percutaneous coronary intervention: a randomized controlled trial (PodCAST-PCI). *J Cardiovasc Pharmacol*. 2022;80:592–599.
42. Tardif JC, Kouz S, Waters DD, et al. Efficacy and safety of low-dose colchicine after myocardial infarction. *N Engl J Med*. 2019;381:2497–2505.
43. Mewton N, Roubille F, Bresson D, et al. Effect of colchicine on myocardial injury in acute myocardial infarction. *Circulation*. 2021;144:859–869.
44. Duddu S, Agrawal M, Chakrabarti R, et al. Meta-analysis reveals inhibition of the inflammatory cytokine IL-6 affords limited protection post-myocardial ischemia/infarction. *Heliyon*. 2022;8:e10435.
45. Broch K, Anstensrud AK, Woxholt S, et al. Randomized trial of Interleukin-6 receptor inhibition in patients with acute ST-segment elevation myocardial infarction. *J Am Coll Cardiol*. 2021;77:1845–1855.

20 Recurrent Ischemia: Detection, Diagnosis, and Outcomes

HARVEY D. WHITE

INTRODUCTION

According to the Global Burden of Disease study, ischemic heart disease is the number one cause of death and is increasing with the number of years of life lost increasing by 17.3% from 2007 to 2017[1] with 8.93 million (8.79–9.14) deaths in 2017. Although the incidence of myocardial infarction (MI) in the developed world has declined, with the proportion of ST-elevation MI (STEMI) decreasing and the proportion of non–ST-elevation MI (NSTEMI) increasing (see Chapter 31), the incidence of MI has been increasing in the developing world. As survival following an acute coronary syndrome (ACS) improves, more survivors are candidates for recurrent ischemic events, including recurrent MI.

In the developed world, improvements in secondary prevention, such as for hypertension, dyslipidemia, and stopping smoking, and the shift toward invasive management of the initial ACS have contributed to a relative reduction in recurrent ischemic events. For example, in patients with STEMI, recurrent MI is less frequent after primary percutaneous coronary intervention (see Chapter 11) than after fibrinolytic therapy.

Other changes in clinical practice have also affected the epidemiology of recurrent ischemic events, with sometimes competing directions. Recurrent MI rates are sensitive to changes in MI definitions, and after the introduction of the Universal Definition of MI in 2000 updated in the 4th edition of the Universal Definition in 2018,[2] the number of MIs increased (see Chapter 2). Moreover, the use of biomarkers with increased sensitivity (e.g., high-sensitivity troponin assays) has greatly increased the detection of recurrent MI. Increased use of revascularization whether with percutaneous coronary intervention (PCI) (type 4) or coronary artery bypass grafting (CABG) (type 5) will increase the incidence of periprocedural MIs.

Although mortality rates have decreased in registries and clinical trials, 30-day recurrent MI rates have remained relatively stable up until recently ([1994–1998] 9.2% [2004–2008] 10% whereas from [2008–2023] rates have markedly decreased at 30 days 3.7%,[3] at 90 days 3.9%,[4] at 1 year 1.9%[5]–7.8%,[4] at 3 years 5.2%[6]–7.9%,[7] at 5 years 10.3%,[8] and at 9.6 years 30.6%) (Table 20.1).[9] Over the same period, the incidence of periprocedural MIs (types 4a and 5) has increased, whereas that for type 1 MIs has decreased.

An incident MI is defined as the individual's first MI. The term re-infarction is used clinically for an acute MI that occurs within 28 days of an incident MI. When features of MI occur in the first 28 days after an incident event, the second event is not counted as a new MI for epidemiological purposes. If an MI occurs after 28 days following an incident MI, it is deemed a recurrent MI.

TABLE 20.1 **Incidence of Recurrent Myocardial Infarction in Contemporary Registries and Trials**

NAME OF STUDY (PUBLICATION DATE)	YEARS OF ENROLMENT	PATIENTS	MYOCARDIAL INFARCTION RATE	FOLLOW UP
Registries				
Wang (2022)[17]	2008–2010	15,069	35%	5
Schmitz (2022)[8]	2000–2017	11,871	MI 10.3%, 2nd MI 1.7%	5.3 years
Chen (2019)[6]	2008–2009	11,183	5.8%	3 years
Mai (2010)[18]	2018–2018	243	6.9%	In-hospital
Minana (2020)[9]	2000–2003	435	30.6%	9.6 years
Kedhi (2021)[14]	2015–2018	390	8.2% TCFA 1.0% no TCFA	18 months
Galasso (2021)[30]	2013–2019	724	10.1%	803 days
Nedkoff (2023)[4]	2011–2016	8024	3.9% 8.0%	90 days 1 year
Virgo (2023)[11]	2008–2012	2999	30.9 female, 25.3 male (per 1000 person-years)	1 year
Randomized Clinical Trials				
CANTOS (2017)[20]	2011–2017	10,061	Rates per 100 person-years placebo 2.43, Canakinumab 2.06	3.7 years
SECURE-PCI (2018)[3]	2012–2017	4191	3.7% placebo, 2.9% atorvastatin Non-PCI related, 1.2% placebo, 1.0% atorvastatin	30 days
COMPLETE (2019)[24]	2013–2017	4041	Complete revascularization 5.4%, culprit lesion only 7.9%	3 years
ISAR-REACT 5 (2019)[10]	2013–2018	4018	4.8% ticagrelor, 3.0% prasugrel	1 year
ODYSSEY (2019)[7]	2012–2017	18,924	7.9% placebo, 6.8% alirocumab	2.8 years
COLCOT (2019)[21]	2015–2018	4745	4.1% placebo, 3.8% colchicine	22.6 months
COPS (2020)[22]	2018–2018	795	3.8% placebo, 2.8% colchicine	24 months
PEGASUS (2120)[12]	2010–2013	21,162	With stenting 5.6% placebo, 4.8% ticagrelor Without stenting 5.2% placebo, 4.4% ticagrelor	3 years
BIOVASC (2023)[5]	2018–2021	764	1.9% immediate, 4.5% staged PCI	1 year

PCI, Percutaneous coronary intervention; *TCFA*, thin-cap fibroatheroma.

Recurrent Myocardial Infarction in Registry Studies

In a population-based linked data study from 1 November 2011 to 31 October 2016 in Western Australia, 8024 high-risk MI patients were identified as having survived ≥ 3 days, had no acute kidney injury, and had ≥1 of: age ≥65 years, prior MI, diabetes or peripheral arterial disease.[4] Half of the risk of major adverse cardiovascular (CV) events (MACE - composite of CV death, MI, or stroke) occurred early in the first 90 days, post-MI (Fig. 20.1). At 90 days, the incidence of recurrent MI was 3.9%. At 1-year MACE (12.6%) was dominated by the risk of recurrent MI (8.0%) (Table 20.1). On multivariable analysis, a history of hypertension was associated with a 42% higher risk of recurrent MI at 90 days (HR, 1.42 95% CI, 1.07, 1.88) while female sex was associated with a 33% lower risk of MI (HR, 0.67, 95% CI 0.52, 0.86). At 1 year, there was no sex difference in the incidence of recurrent MI (8.0% female vs. 8.0% male).

Recurrent Myocardial Infarction in Randomized Clinical Trials

In the Intracoronary Stenting and Antithrombotic Regimen: Rapid Early Action for Coronary Treatment 5 trial, 4018 patients with ACS were randomized between 2015 and 2018 in an open-labeled trial to receive either ticagrelor or prasugrel.[10] MI rates were 4.8% in the ticagrelor group and 3.0% in the prasugrel group (HR, 1.63; 95% CI, 1.18–2.25) (Fig. 20.2, Tables 20.1 and 20.2). Type 1 MIs occurred in 2.5% ticagrelor and 1.7% prasugrel and type 2 MIs occurred in 0.2% ticagrelor and 0.1% prasugrel patients.

In the Variation in Recovery: Role of Gender on Outcomes of Young AMI Patients study in 2999 patients aged 18 to 55 years, from 2008 to 2012, women after MI experienced more hospitalizations than men 444.3 per 1000 person-years (412.1–478.9) versus 269.5 (236.0–307.7), $P < .001$, and more deaths 25.3 per 1000 person-years (19.2–33.4) among women versus 11.4 (6.3–20.5) among men, $P = .01$.[11] However, the incidence rate per 1000 person-years for recurrent MI in the first year was similar for women 30.0 (24.0–39.8) and men 25.3 (17.0–0.378) (Fig. 20.3). In this study, MI with nonobstructive coronary arteries (MINOCA) occurred in 12.8% of women and 2.9% of men, $P = .34$. Recurrent MI in women with MINOCA occurred in 20.6 (7.7–54.9) per 1000 person-years with an incidence ratio compared to recurrent MIs in women with MI and coronary artery disease (CAD) of 0.53 (0.26–1.05). Data were not available for men.

In a substudy of the Prevention of Cardiovascular Events in Patients with Prior Heart attacks using Ticagrelor compared to Placebo on the background of Aspirin–Thrombolysis in MI, 21,162 patients were randomized to ticagrelor versus placebo in patients with prior MI (1–3 years) with or

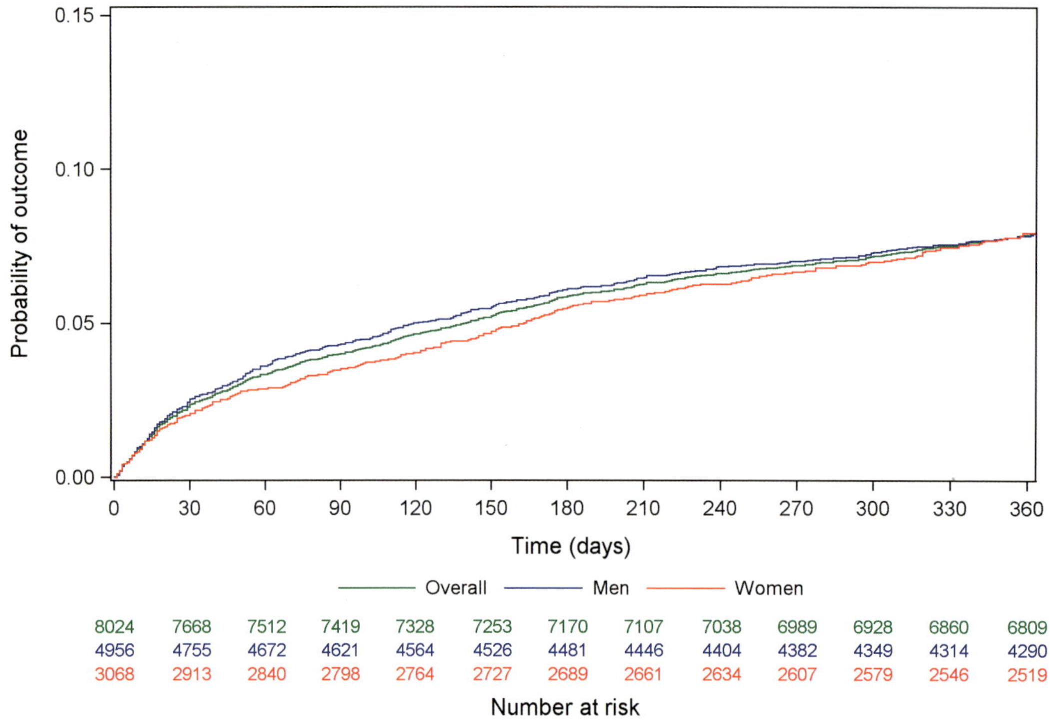

FIG. 20.1 Recurrent myocardial infarction.[4] Kaplan-Meier curves for recurrent MI following incident MI in men and women. At least 50% of recurrent MIs occur within the first 90 days. There was no difference between males and females. (Reproduced from Nedkoff L, Briffa T, Murray K, et al. Risk of early recurrence and mortality in high-risk myocardial infarction patients: a population-based linked data study. *Int J Cardiovasc Risk Prev*. 2023:17;200185. Fig. 1 (graph on MI only).)

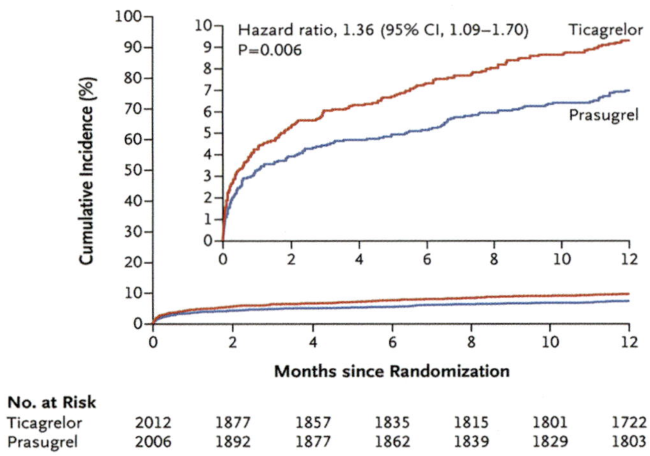

FIG. 20.2 Ticagrelor or prasugrel in patients with acute coronary syndromes: Cumulative incidence of the primary end point at one year.[10] Primary endpoint = the primary composite of death, MI or stroke at 1 year occurred in 9.3% in the prasugrel group and 6.9% in the ticagrelor group (HR, 1.36; 95% CI, 1.09–1.70; *P* = .006). The Kaplan–Meier curves show the cumulative incidence of the primary end point. The inset shows the same data on an enlarged y axis. (Reproduced from Schüpke S, Neumann FJ, Menichelli M, et al. Ticagrelor or prasugrel in patients with acute coronary syndromes. *N Engl J Med*. 2019;381:1524–1534. Fig. 2 page 1531.)

without (n = 4199) a history of coronary artery stenting.[12] Recurrent MI rates without prior stenting were 4.4% ticagrelor and 5.2% placebo and with prior stenting 4.8% ticagrelor and 5.6% placebo (Table 20.1).[12]

In the Statins Evaluation in Coronary Procedures and Revascularization (SECURE-PCI) randomized clinical trial, 4191 patients with ACS were randomized between 2012 and 2017 to receive two loading doses of 80 mg of atorvastatin (n = 2087) or matching placebo (n = 2104) before and

TABLE 20.2 Effect of Ticagrelor Compared with Prasugrel on Types of Myocardial Infarction at 1 Year[10]

END POINT	TICAGRELOR GROUP (N = 2012)	PRASUGREL GROUP (N = 2006)	HAZARD RATIO (95% CI)
Myocardial Infarction Type – no (% of MIs)	96 (4.8%)	60 (3.0%)	1.63 (1.18–2.25)
Type 1	52 (54.2%)	35 (58.3%)	
Type 2	4 (4.2%)	3 (5.0%)	
Type 4a	19 (19.8%)	11 (18.3%)	
Type 4b	20 (20.8%)	11 (18.3%)	
Type 5	1	0	

The data reported for the individual types of MI are the number and the proportion of total MIs represented by the MI subtype. *CI*, Confidence interval; *MI*, myocardial infarction.
Adapted Table 2 on Page 1532 from Schüpke S, Neumann FJ, Menichelli M, et al. Ticagrelor or prasugrel in patients with acute coronary syndromes. *N Engl J Med*. 2019; 381:1524–1534.

24 hours after a planned PCI. Among patients with planned invasive management with PCI, periprocedural loading doses of atorvastatin did not reduce the rate of MACE at 30 days.[3] MIs including type 4a MIs occurred in 3.7% placebo and 2.9% atorvastatin, HR 0.80 (0.57–1.11), *P* = .18 (Table 20.1).

DETECTION OF RECURRENT ISCHEMIA

Recurrent ischemia after presentation with ACS portends an unfavorable outcome for patients with increased MACE and major implications for the use of health care resources. Ischemic symptoms at rest carry a worse prognosis than ischemia with exercise. Ischemia is often silent and can be

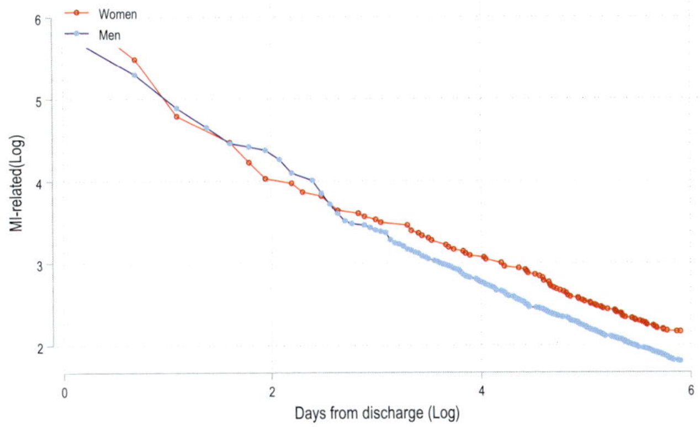

FIG. 20.3 Sex difference in outcomes of acute myocardial infarction in young patients.[11] Myocardial infarction related hospitalization. Log plot of survival after Cox regression analysis. (Reproduced from Sawano M, Lu Y, Caraballo C, et al. Sex difference in outcomes of acute myocardial infarction in young patients. *J Am Coll Cardiol*. 2023;81(18):1797–1806. Fig. 1B in supplement.)

detected on 24-hour continuous ECG monitoring. The frequency and duration of silent ischemia have a direct relationship to prognosis and may result in silent recurrent MI. Because of the adverse prognosis of recurrent ischemia, clinical practice may incorporate monitoring for recurrent ischemia, and in some centers, continuous ST-segment monitoring is used. With early invasive management of STEMI and NSTEMI, the incidence of early recurrent ischemia has decreased substantially (see Chapter 11).

In patients who have typical ischemic pain at rest, a stress test is not necessary to define the need for further investigation and additional therapy. Exercise stress or pharmacologic stress test for inducible ischemia may be considered before hospital discharge in patients who have not been revascularized or who are not fully revascularized to help determine whether coronary angiography should be performed and whether initial or further revascularization should be undertaken (see Chapter 14).

DIAGNOSIS OF RECURRENT MYOCARDIAL INFARCTION

The diagnosis of the initial MI is discussed in Chapters 2 and 4. This section focuses on the diagnosis of recurrent MI as a complication in patients who have presented with an initial MI. The criteria for the diagnosis of recurrent MI should be according to the Fourth Universal Definition of MI (Chapter 2).[2] MIs are a heterogeneous group of events and are classified by the Universal Definition of MI into five types that differ according to pathophysiology, prognosis, and treatment.

Myocardial Infarction (Type 1 and Type 2)

Type 1 MIs are the most commonly observed MIs in clinical practice, and they are also the most common type of recurrent MI during the long term. Clinical judgment is required to distinguish type 2 (supply/demand imbalance) MIs from type 1 MIs by taking into account the contribution of increased myocardial demand and decreased supply and the likely absence of acute plaque rupture based on all of the clinical information available.

Myocardial Infarction Related to Percutaneous Coronary Intervention (Type 4a)

Myocardial necrosis associated with PCI is a frequent cause of early recurrent MI and may be caused by several mechanisms, including distal embolization of plaque and/or thrombus with resultant microvascular plugging, occlusion of a side branch or a major coronary artery, coronary dissection, spasm, or endothelial dysfunction. The association between type 4a MI and mortality is controversial and less important than the relationship of mortality with spontaneous MI.[13]

Myocardial Infarction Caused by Stent Thrombosis (Type 4b)

Stent thrombosis after PCI for STEMI and NSTEMI is infrequent but an important event because of its adverse prognosis. This risk is higher with drug-eluting stents (DES) than MI caused by restenosis with bare metal stents and is associated with MI and death. MI may also occur that is unrelated to the stent. The risk of stent thrombosis is less with the new generation DES.

Myocardial Infarction Caused by Restenosis (Type 4c)

Type 4c MI is related to restenosis after balloon angioplasty without stenting or with stenting.

Myocardial Infarction with Coronary Artery Bypass Grafting (Type 5)

During CABG, numerous factors can lead to periprocedural myocardial injury with necrosis. These include direct myocardial injury from (1) suture placement or manipulation of the heart, (2) coronary dissection, (3) global or regional ischemia related to inadequate intraoperative cardiac protection, (4) microvascular events related to reperfusion, (5) myocardial injury induced by oxygen free radical generation, or (6) failure to reperfuse areas of the myocardium that are not subtended by graftable vessels.

Silent Myocardial Infarction

Asymptomatic patients who develop new Q wave criteria for MI detected during routine ECG follow-up, or who have evidence of MI by cardiac imaging should be classified as having silent MIs. In studies where serial ECG analysis has been used, silent MIs have accounted for 9% to 37% of nonfatal MIs and have been associated with increased mortality.[2] An annual ECG is reasonable in clinical trials to monitor for silent Q wave MIs.

RECURRENT MYOCARDIAL INFARCTION AND THE ELECTROCARDIOGRAM

The ECG diagnosis of recurrent MI following the initial MI may be confounded by the initial evolutionary ECG changes. Recurrent MI can be diagnosed when ST-segment elevation of ≥0.1 mV recurs or new pathologic Q waves appear in at least two contiguous leads.

BIOMARKERS AND RECURRENT MYOCARDIAL INFARCTION

Because of the persistent elevation of biomarkers of necrosis in the first days to weeks after an initial MI, the diagnosis of recurrent MI can be challenging and is dependent on identifying a dynamic pattern of biomarker values separate from the initial MI, rather than simply elevation above the 99th percentile alone. In patients in whom recurrent MI is suspected from clinical signs or symptoms following the initial MI, an immediate measurement of cardiac troponin is recommended. A second sample should be obtained 3 to 6 hours later. Recurrent MI can be diagnosed if there is a more than 20% increase in the cardiac troponin value in the second sample. Two cardiac troponin values are considered to be analytically different if they are separated by more than 3 SDs of the variance. For most assays, the SD is 5% to 7% at the levels involved with recurrent MI. Therefore, a 20% change should be considered significant. This value should also exceed the 99th percentile upper reference limit (URL). If the initial cardiac troponin concentration is normal, the criteria for diagnosing a new acute MI apply.

Recurrent Myocardial Infarction in the Culprit or Nonculprit Arteries

Recurrent MI may occur in the territory of the culprit artery or in different arteries from the culprit artery. If recurrent MI occurs in the culprit artery territory after administration of fibrinolytic therapy, it is likely caused by reocclusion or spasm, and after PCI, it may be the result of stent thrombosis, spasm, or restenosis. Plaque rupture can also occur proximally or distally to the previous culprit stenosis or in a nonculprit artery.

Frequency of Recurrent Myocardial Infarction

Table 20.1 shows the frequency of recurrent MI types in registries and contemporary clinical trials. The rates from in-hospital and at 30-day range from 3.9%[5] to 6.9%[4] at 1 year 1.9%[5] to 4.8%,[10] and at 3 years 4.4%[6] to 7.9%.[7] Longer follow-up has been associated with a rate of MI of 30.6% at 9.6 years.[8] Type 1 MIs are the most common type of recurrent MI.

In ODYSSEY, the proportion of MIs through 2.8 years follow-up that were type 2 was 20.8% compared with the proportion that were type 1 MI of 65.8% and type 4 MI of 13.1%.[7] In ISAR REACT-5 type 1 MI made up 56%, type 2 MI 4.5%, type 4a 19.2%, type 4b 19.8% of MIs (Table 20.2).[10]

Comparison of Characteristics Between Incident Myocardial Infarction and Recurrent Myocardial Infarction

A study of 13,276 patients between 2000 and 2017 in the city of Augsburg and two adjacent counties in Germany compared characteristics of incident acute MI (11,817), first recurrent MI (1217), and second recurrent MIs (202). The median follow-up was 5.3 years.[8] There were no differences in sex distribution between the groups. The mean age at the incident event (64.1 years) was significantly lower in comparison to the mean age at the first (66.4 years) and second reinfarction (66.5 years), respectively.

Recurrent MIs differed from incident MIs in the frequency of comorbidities, laboratory values, ECG presentation, and therapy but not regarding 28-day mortality. The percentage of patients who were current smokers decreased after the incident MI and consequently the proportion of ex-smokers increased. The percentages of patients having typical chest pain symptoms were similar (ranging between 70% and 80% of all cases). Prehospital time was the highest for incident cases (median time: 157 min) and decreased for the second and third MI events (median: 134 min and 133.5 min) (Table 20.3). The percentage of patients living alone was higher with recurrent MIs than at the initial event. More patients were currently employed at the time of the first MI compared to at the time of reinfarction.[8]

Typical comorbidities and risk factors (diabetes, hypertension, hyperlipidemia, smoking, impaired renal function) were associated with an increased risk of hospitalized recurrent MI. Conversely, STEMI, being married, and having had CABG were predictors for a lower risk of hospitalized recurrent MI (Table 20.4).[8]

OUTCOMES WITH RECURRENT MYOCARDIAL INFARCTION

Outcomes with recurrent MI are related to the size of the infarction and the cumulative effect on left ventricular function. Other factors such as the severity of CAD, diabetes, modification of risk factors, and adherence to evidence-based therapies are important.

In ODYSSEY during 1.6 (0.8–2.4) and 1.3 (0.5–2.3) years of follow-up Type 1 and Type 2 MI respectively, mortality following the occurrence of type 2 MI (25.4%) was more than double that of patients with type 1 MI (11.9%).[6] In posthoc analyses, rates of death were 10.2% with alirocumab versus 13.4% with placebo (HR, 0.69; 95% CI, 0.48–1.00) following type 1 MI and 24.8% versus 25.9% (HR, 0.98; 95% CI, 0.62–1.56) following type 2 MI.

CAUSES AND PREDICTORS OF RECURRENT MYOCARDIAL INFARCTION

Causes of Recurrent Myocardial Infarction

There are a number of causes of recurrent MI related to features of the plaque,[14] features of the blood (thrombogenesis), and features of the patient (Table 20.5). Patients with severe coronary artery stenoses have an increased risk of MI not only because of the stenoses but also because the stenoses are markers for widespread atherosclerosis (Chapter X).

Several genetic mutations have been associated with an increased risk of MI.[15] At least 160 loci in genome-wide association studies (GWAS) have been associated with the risk of CAD.[15] In a recent study focusing on low-frequency and rare sequence variations in 55,736 individuals

TABLE 20.3 Characteristics of Incident Myocardial Infarction and First and Second Time Recurrent Myocardial Infarction.[8]

	INCIDENT MYOCARDIAL INFARCTION *N* = 11,871	FIRST RECURRENT MYOCARDIAL INFARCTION *N* = 1217	SECOND RECURRENT MYOCARDIAL INFARCTION *N* = 202	*P*-VALUE
Male	8469 (71.4)	887 (72.9)	148 (73.6)	.4299
Age (mean, SD)	64.1 (11.4)	66.4 (11)	66.5 (10.3)	<.0001
Comorbidities				
Hypertension	9052 (76.3)	1103 (90.7)	187 (93)	<.0001
Diabetes mellitus	3729 (31.4)	582 (47.9)	106 (52.7)	<.0001
Hyperlipidemia	6909 (58.3)	906 (74.5)	160 (79.6)	<.0001
Current smoker	3760 (31.7)	275 (22.6)	42 (20.9)	<.0001
Clinical Characteristics				
Typical chest pain symptoms	9239 (77.9)	950 (78.1)	146 (72.6)	.239
Prehospital time in minutes	157.0 (83–495)	134.0 (77–316.5)	133.5 (75–284.75)	.0043
Type of infarction				<.0001
STEMI	4275 (36)	252 (20.7)	35 (17.4)	
NSTEMI	6194 (52.2)	751 (61.8)	113 (56.2)	–
Bundle branch block	885 (7.5)	152 (12.5)	38 (18.9)	–
Ejection Fraction				<.0001
≤30%	665 (5.6)	92 (7.6)	11 (5.5)	
>30%	8536 (72)	774 (63.7)	113 (56.2)	
Renal Functions				
eGFR <30 mL/min/ 1.73 m^2	560 (4.7)	145 (11.9)	36 (17.9)	–
eGFR				<.0001
Days in intensive care				<.0001
mean (SD)	3.5 (5.5)	2.9 (4.9)	2.8 (3.9)	
Died within first 28 days	782 (6.6)	92 (7.6)	15 (7.5)	.3949
Laboratory Values				
Troponin I ng/mL	0.640 (0.13–4.07)	0.240 (0.06–1.12)	0.435 (0.12–2.2575)	<.0001
PCI	8040 (67.8)	810 (66.6)	132 (65.7)	.8666
Bypass	1703 (14.4)	107 (8.8)	12 (6)	0
Lysis	531 (4.5)	9 (0.7)	1 (0.5)	0
EBM at discharge	7853 (66.2)	825 (67.8)	127 (63.2)	.332
Family status				.0086
Married	7920 (66.8)	760 (62.5)	124 (61.7)	
Employment status				<.0001
Employed	2478 (20.9)	141 (11.6)	25 (12.4)	
Nationality German	10,792 (91)	1073 (88.2)	182 (90.5)	.0081

Categorical variables are presented as total numbers (percentages) and continuous variables are presented as median (25th and 75th quartile). *P*-values were calculated with Chi-Square tests for categorical variables and analysis of variance (ANOVA) for continuous variables.
CI, Confidence interval; *EBM*, evidence based medicine; *ECG*, electrocardiogram; *eGFR*, estimated glomerular filtration rate; *HR*, hazard ratio; *NSTEMI*, non-ST-elevation myocardial infarction; *PCI*, percutaneous coronary intervention; *STEMI*, ST-elevation myocardial infarction.
Adapted from Table 1 Schmitz T, Harmel E, Heier M, et al. Long-term predictors of hospitalized reinfarction after an incident acute myocardial infarction. *Life*. 2022;12(12):2090.

of European ancestry from nine cohorts for incident MI cases, ANGPTL4, a known locus to be associated with CAD, and a new locus LDLRAD1 was identified. No loci were significantly associated with all-cause mortality following a MI.[16]

Predictors of Recurrent Myocardial Infarction

In a national population-based cohort study in Sweden, 15,069 individuals who had an incident MI during 2008–2010 were investigated whether sociodemographic, labor market marginalization and medical characteristics were risk factors for recurrent MI within 1 year. The recurrent MI rate was very high at 35.5% (Table 20.1).[17] Higher risk of recurrent MI was associated with diabetes, renal insufficiency, previous stroke, cancer, somatic disorders, STEMI, and CABG. Also, lower education levels and living in small towns/villages were associated with a higher risk of recurrent MI. Being single without children at home was associated with a lower risk of recurrent MI. Unemployment was not associated with the risk of recurrent MI.

TABLE 20.4 Factors Shown to Be Associated with Recurrent Myocardial Infarction

- Increasing age
- Anterior MI
- Atrial fibrillation
- Cancer
- Chronic kidney disease
- Chronic obstructive pulmonary disease
- Coronary dissection
- Complex type C lesion:
  - Diffuse (>2 cm length)
  - Total occlusion >3 months old
  - Excessive tortuosity of proximal segment
  - Inability to protect major side branches
  - Extremely angulated segments >90°
  - Degenerated vein grafts with friable lesions
- Coronary embolism
- Diabetes
- Ejection fraction <50%
- Evidence of Restenosis
- Female sex
- Final coronary stenosis >30%
- Heart failure
- Higher levels of Lp(a)
- Hypertension
- Increased LDL-C
- Killip class >1
- Longer symptom onset-to-balloon time
- Longer stents
- Lower systolic blood pressure
- Mental illness, depression
- Multivessel disease
- No new Q waves
- Nonsmoking/smoking
- Not on β-blockers
- Obesity
- Percutaneous coronary intervention
- Presence of thrombus
- Previous CABG
- Previous MI
- Previous PCI
- Previous Stroke
- Regions and Race
- Shorter time to fibrinolysis
- Sociodemographic characteristics - being married, lower education
- Stroke
- Thrombocytosis
- Underutilization of guideline-directed medical therapy

CABG, Coronary artery bypass graft; *LDL-C,* low density lipoprotein-cholesterol; *Lp(a),* lipoprotein (a); *MI,* Myocardial infarction; *PCI,* percutaneous coronary intervention.

In a small study from Pakistan, 245 patients with incident MI were studied in 2018, and the recurrent MI in-hospital rate was 6.9% (Table 20.1).[18] Age, diabetes, and obesity (BMI >30 mg/kg^2) were associated with recurrent MI.

In a Taiwan Registry of 11,183 patients who had survived 1-year post-MI without recurrent MI or stroke, independent factors associated with a higher risk of recurrent MI or death included heart failure (HR, 1.19), hypertension (HR 1.16), age (65–75 vs. <65 years: HR, 1.29; 75–85 vs. <65 years: HR, 1.50; >85 vs. <65 years: HR, 1.70), diabetes (HR, 1.33), prior stroke (HR, 1.24), chronic kidney disease (HR, 1.4), atrial fibrillation (HR, 1.27), and underutilization of guideline-based medication (HR, 1.73).[6]

Factors that have been shown to be predictors of recurrent MI are shown in Table 20.4. Some have been contradictory in different studies (e.g., smoking). Independent predictors from ODYSSEY[7] are shown in Table 20.6 for type 1 MI and independent predictors for type 2 MI in Table 20.7.

TABLE 20.5 Causes of Recurrent Ischemia and Myocardial Infarction

- Ongoing thrombogenesis
- New plaque rupture, fissuring, or erosion
- Recurrent or new dissection
- Recurrent or new embolism
- Decreased supply and/or increased demand
- Periprocedural MI (associated with PCI or CABG)
- Stent thrombosis
- Restenosis
- Stopping antiplatelet therapy
- Genetic mutations

CABG, Coronary artery bypass grafting; *MI,* myocardial infarction; *PCI,* percutaneous coronary intervention.

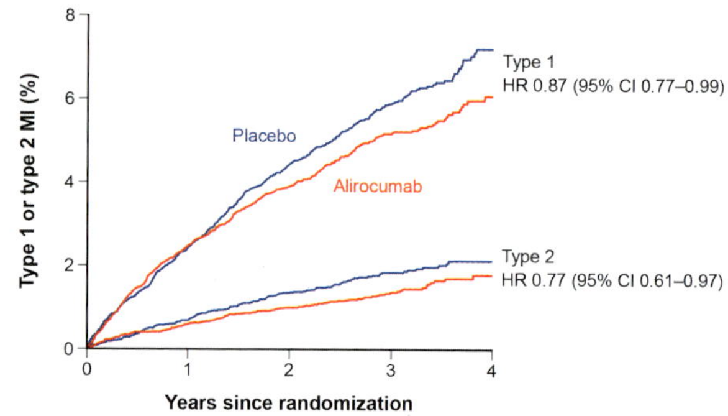

FIG. 20.4 Kaplan–Meier curves for the first occurrence of Type 1 and Type 2 myocardial infarctions and the effects of alirocumab over time.[7] *HR,* Hazard ratio; *MI,* myocardial infarction. (Reproduced from White HD, Steg PG, Szarek M, et al. Take home figure. Effects of Alirocumab on types of myocardial infarction: insights from the ODYSSEY trial. *Eur Heart J.* 2019;40(33):2801–2809.

PREVENTION OF RECURRENT MYOCARDIAL INFARCTION

Recurrent MI is most commonly the result of further plaque rupture or erosion with thrombus formation. Treatment has therefore been focused on the reduction of low-density lipoprotein cholesterol (LDL-C) and antithrombotic agents. Intensive LDL-C lowering with PCSK9 inhibitors may stabilize plaque and cause plaque regression.[19]

LDL-C reduction with statins and proprotein convertase subtilisin-kexin Type 9 (PCSK9) inhibitors reduces the risk of recurrent MI but less is known about the effects on types of MI.

ODYSSEY OUTCOMES (occurrence of cardiovascular events in patients who have recently experienced an acute coronary syndrome) compared the PCSK9 inhibitor alirocumab with placebo in 18,924 patients with recent ACS and elevated LDL-C (≥1.8 mmol/L) despite intensive statin therapy. In a prespecified analysis, the effects of alirocumab on types of MI were assessed. The median follow-up was 2.8 years. Alirocumab reduced MIs [HR, 0.85; 95% CI, 0.77–0.95; P = .003], with reductions in both Type 1 (HR 0.87, 95% CI, 0.77–0.99; P = .032) and Type 2 (0.77, 0.61–0.97; P = .025) (Fig. 20.4, Tables 20.6, 20.7, and 20.8). Achievement of LDL-C reduction with a PCSK-9 inhibitor below levels achievable with statins was shown to be an effective preventive strategy for both recurrent MI types.[7]

Antiplatelet drugs with ticagrelor and prasugrel, as above in ISAR-REACT 5, may reduce recurrent MI.[9] Anti-inflammatory drugs may stabilize coronary artery plaques

TABLE 20.6 Independent Predictors of Type 1 Myocardial Infarction Following Acute Coronary Syndrome in ODYSSEY[7]

BASELINE CHARACTERISTIC	HR (95% CI)	P-VALUE
Medical History		
Peripheral artery disease	1.61 (1.29–2.00)	<.0001
Percutaneous coronary intervention	1.51 (1.27–1.79)	<.0001
CABG	1.74 (1.45–2.09)	<.0001
Diabetes	1.57 (1.38–1.79)	<.0001
Current smoker	1.23 (1.06–1.42)	.006
Hypertension	1.54 (1.31–1.81)	<.0001
MI	1.46 (1.23–1.74)	<.0001
Heart failure	1.33 (1.12–1.57)	.001
Stroke	1.34 (1.02–1.75)	.034
Region		<.0001
Western Europe	Reference	
Eastern Europe	0.50 (0.41–0.61)	
North America	0.93 (0.77–1.13)	
South America	0.65 (0.51–0.84)	
Asia	2.03 (0.97–4.26)	
Rest of world	1.16 (0.92–1.46)	
LDL-C per 1-mmol/L increment	1.19 (1.11–1.27)	<.0001
GFR <60 mL/min/1.73 m²	1.37 (1.17–1.60)	.0001
Revascularization for index event	0.80 (0.70–0.91)	.0009
Race		.009
White	Reference	
Asian	0.38 (0.19–0.77)	
Black	1.37 (1.01–1.87)	
Other	0.97 (0.70–1.33)	
Alirocumab treatment	0.87 (0.77–0.99)	.029

CABG, Coronary artery bypass grafting; *CI,* confidence interval; *GFR,* glomerular filtration rate; *HR,* hazard ratio; *LDL-C,* low-density lipoprotein cholesterol; *MI,* myocardial infarction.
Reproduced from White HD, Steg PG, Szarek M, et al. Effects of Alirocumab on types of myocardial infarction: insights from the ODYSSEY trial. *Eur Heart J.* 2019;40(33):2801–2809, Table 2.

TABLE 20.7 Independent Predictors of Type 2 Myocardial Infarction Following Acute Coronary Syndrome in ODYSSEY[7]

BASELINE CHARACTERISTIC	HR (95% CI)	P-VALUE
GFR <60 mL/min/1.73 m²	2.05 (1.57–2.67)	<.0001
Medical History		
Peripheral artery disease	2.49 (1.83–3.39)	<.0001
Percutaneous coronary intervention	1.48 (1.09–2.01)	.012
COPD	2.26 (1.63–3.15)	<.0001
Heart failure	2.36 (1.80–3.09)	<.0001
Diabetes	1.76 (1.38–2.25)	<.0001
Hypertension	2.66 (1.79–3.97)	<.0001
MI	1.49 (1.11–2.01)	.009
Region		<.0001
Western Europe	Reference	
Eastern Europe	0.45 (0.30–0.65)	
North America	1.16 (0.83–1.64)	
South America	0.44 (0.25–0.76)	
Asia	1.23 (0.36–4.21)	
Rest of world	1.22 (0.77–1.94)	
Age category		<.0001
<65 years	Reference	
65–<75 years	1.46 (1.11–1.91)	
≥75 years	2.26 (1.58–3.23)	
Race		.021
White	Reference	
Asian	0.76 (0.24–2.36)	
Black	1.92 (1.22–3.02)	
Other	0.62 (0.27–1.45)	
HDL-C per 1-mg/dL increment	1.01 (1.00–1.02)	.017
Alirocumab treatment	0.77 (0.61–0.97)	.029

CI, Confidence interval; *COPD,* chronic obstructive pulmonary disease; *GFR,* glomerular filtration rate; *HDL-C,* high-density lipoprotein cholesterol; *HR,* hazard ratio; *MI,* myocardial infarction.
Reproduced from White HD, Steg PG, Szarek M, et al. Effects of Alirocumab on types of myocardial infarction: insights from the ODYSSEY Trial. *Eur Heart J.* 2019;40(33):2801–2809, Table 3.

and may decrease recurrent MI, see section 9 *The role of anti inflammatory drugs*.[20–23]

EFFECTS OF REVASCULARIZATION ON RECURRENT MYOCARDIAL INFARCTION

Revascularization has been shown to reduce recurrent MI after ACS and complete revascularization compared with incomplete revascularization has been shown to reduce rates of recurrent MI.[24]

Complete Revascularization Compared With Incomplete Revascularization

In the Complete versus Culprit-Only Revascularization Strategies to Treat Multivessel Disease after Early PCI for STEMI (COMPLETE) trial, 2016 patients with STEMI and successible culprit PCI were randomized to a strategy of either complete revascularization with PCI of angiographically significant nonculprit lesions or culprit-only revascularization.[24]

Follow-up was for a median of 3 years. The first co-primary outcome of cardiovascular death or MI occurred in 158 patients (7.8%) in the complete-revascularization group as compared with 213 patients (10.5%) in the culprit-lesion only PCI group (HR, 0.74; 95% CI, 0.60–0.91; $P = .004$)(Fig. 20.5). There was no difference in cardiovascular death; 2.9% complete-revascularization versus 3.2% culprit-only, MI was reduced with complete-revascularization 109 patients (5.4%) compared with 160 patients (7.9%) (HR, 0.68; 95% CI, 0.53–0.86) with culprit only revascularization. The following types of MI occurred less frequently in the complete-revascularization group than in the culprit-lesion-only PCI group: non-STEMI (3.3% vs. 5.2% events), STEMI (2.15 vs. 2.6%), and predominantly, MI type 1 (3.1% vs. 6.4%). The benefit of complete-revascularization emerged early (at around one month) with continued divergence of the cumulative event rates for several years (Fig. 20.5).[24] During the early period recurrent MI was mainly related to the culprit-lesion PCI. There was consistent benefit of complete revascularization regardless of whether nonculprit-lesion PCI was performed earlier, during the index hospitalization, or later, several weeks after discharge.

TABLE 20.8 Types of Myocardial Infarctions and Effects of Alirocumab[7]

	ALIROCUMAB		PLACEBO			
	PATIENTS WITH MI,[a] *N* (%)	TOTAL MIS	PATIENTS WITH MI,[a] *N* (%)	TOTAL MIS	TREATMENT HR (95% CI)[a]	*P*-VALUE[a]
Any MI	639 (6.8)	866	744 (7.9)	994	0.85 (0.77–0.95)	.003
Universal Classification						
Type 1	463 (4.9)	560	528 (5.6)	663	0.87 (0.77–0.99)	.032
Type 2	125 (1.3)	180	162 (1.7)	206	0.77 (0.61–0.97)	.025
Type 3	2 (<0.1)	2	0	0	–	–
Type 4a	22 (0.2)	23	28 (0.3)	29	0.94 (0.72–1.22)[f]	.62
Type 4b	50 (0.5)	55	46 (0.5)	49		
Type 4c	37 (0.4)	44	42 (0.4)	44		
Type 5	2 (<0.1)	2	3 (<0.1)	3	–	–
ECG Classification						
NSTEMI	437 (4.6)	576	529 (5.6)	692	0.82 (0.72–0.93)	.002
STEMI	92 (0.5)	96	109 (1.2)	116	0.84 (0.64–1.11)	.22
ECG not interpretable or not available	161 (1.7)	194	162 (1.7)	186	1.01 (0.81–1.25)	.96
Q-wave Classification						
Q Wave	52 (0.5)	52	71 (0.9)	73	0.73 (0.51–1.04)	.08
Non-Q Wave	483 (5.1)	634	560 (5.9)	725	0.86 (0.76–0.97)	.013
ECG not interpretable or available	146 (1.5)	180	165 (1.7)	196	0.88 (0.71–1.10)	.27

[a]Analysis of time to first type 1, type 2, or type 4a, 4b, 4c MI by Cox proportional hazards models, stratified by geographical region.
CI, Confidence interval; *ECG*, electrocardiogram; *HR*, hazard ratio; *MI*, myocardial infarction; *NSTEMI*, non-ST-elevation myocardial infarction; *STEMI*, ST-elevation myocardial infarction.
Reproduced from White HD, Steg PG, Szarek M, et al. Effects of Alirocumab on types of myocardial infarction: insights from the ODYSSEY trial. *Eur Heart J*. 2019;40(33):2801–2809, Table 2.

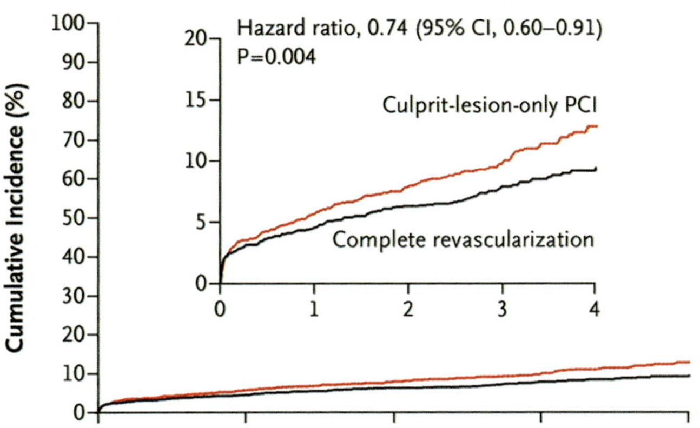

FIG. 20.5 Cumulative incidence of the first and second coprimary outcomes.[24] Panels A shows Kaplan–Meier estimates of the cumulative incidence of the first coprimary outcome (death from cardiovascular causes or new myocardial infarction). Insets show the same data on an enlarged y axis. *PCI*, Percutaneous coronary intervention. (Reproduced from Mehta SR, Wood DA, Storey RF, et al. Complete revascularization with multivessel PCI for myocardial infarction. *N Engl J Med*. 2019;381:1411–1421. Fig. 1 Page 1418.)

In the Direct Complete Versus Staged Complete Revascularization in Patients Presenting With Acute Coronary Syndromes and Multivessel Disease (BioVasc) trial, 764 patients with ACS and multivessel coronary disease were randomized to have revascularization of the culprit and other non-culprit lesions compared with staged complete-revascularization.[5] Immediate complete revascularization was noninferior for the one-year composite outcome of all-cause mortality, MI, any unplanned driven revascularization or cerebrovascular events (7.6% vs. 9.4%) (HR, 0.78; 95% CI, 0.55–1.11; *P* = .0011 (Fig. 20.6). At 1 year, MI as measured by the universal definition including type 1 and type 2 Mis, was lower in the complete revascularization group (1.9% vs. 4.5%) (HR, 0.41; 95 % CI, 0.22–0.76; *P* = .0045).[5]

Of patients with recurrent MI, 40% presented with STEMI and 60% with a non-ST-segment elevation MI. There was no heterogeneity in the study outcome based on ECG presentation.[5] The excess of MI in the staged strategy was mainly driven by early events that predominantly occurred in the time window between the index procedure and the planned date for the staged intervention. These events were not procedure-related events but type 1 MIs. An originally nonculprit lesion was identified by angiography as the cause for these events in almost all cases.

THE ROLE OF ANTIINFLAMMATORY DRUGS

Colchicine

Colchicine reduces inflammation by antagonizing the NOD-Like Receptor Protein 3 (NLRP3) inflammasome and cholesterol crystal-induced inflammation.[25] Treatment with colchicine may result in improvements in plaque morphology that may be driven by its anti-inflammatory properties (see Chapter 27).[26]

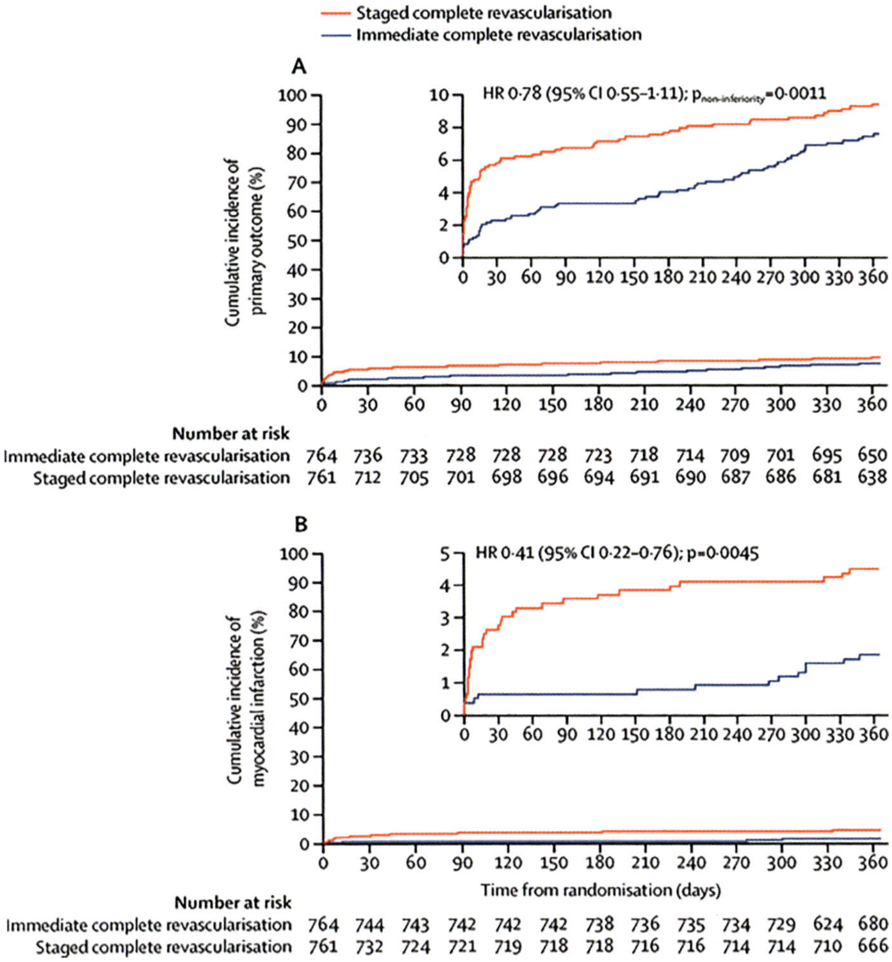

FIG. 20.6 Kaplan-Meier estimates of the primary outcome (A) and myocardial infarction (B) at 1 year.[5] The primary outcome was a composite of all-cause mortality, myocardial infarction, unplanned ischemia-driven revascularization, or cerebrovascular events at 1 year. Insets show a more detailed view of the same data on an enlarged y axis. *HR*, Hazard ratio. (Reproduced from Diletti R, den Dekker WK, Bennett J, et al. Immediate vs. staged complete revascularization in patients presenting with acute coronary syndrome and multivessel coronary disease (BIOVASC): a prospective, open-label, non-inferiority, randomized trial. Lancet. 2023;401:1172–1182. Fig. 2 Page 1179.)

In the Colchicine in Patient with acute coronary syndrome (COPS) study, 795 patients with ACS and evidence angiographically of CAD (≥30%) were randomized to receive colchicine 0.5 mg twice daily for one month or placebo,[20] and in the Colchicine Cardiovascular Outcomes trial, 4745 patients were randomized within 30 days of MI to receive colchicine 0.5 mg daily or placebo.[21] In a meta-analysis of these two RCTs with a pooled sample size of 5540 patients with 2778 (50.1%) receiving colchicine and 2762 (49.9%) placebo, patients receiving colchicine had a reduction in study-defined composite endpoint (5.5% vs. 7.6%) (OR, 0.67; 95% CI 0.46–0.98; $P = .04$) with a consistent trend in recurrent MI at longest available follow-up (OR, 0.89; 95% CI, 0.67–1.17; $P = .39$).[23] Further trials in ACS are underway (Chapter 27).

Canakinumab

In the Canakinumab Anti-inflammatory Thrombosis Outcomes study,[20] 10,061 patients with a history of MI and HS-CRP levels of ≥2 mg/L were randomly assigned to one of three doses of Canakinumab or to placebo.[19] HS-CRP levels were significantly reduced by Canakinumab without reducing LDL-C levels. The 150 mg dose reduced the composite of CV death, MI, and stroke at 3.7 years of follow-up. MI was reduced from 2.43 per 100 person-years with placebo to 2.06 per 100 person-years with Canakinumab, $P = .03$.

Association of Lipoprotein(a) and Recurrent Myocardial Infarction

Lp(a) has been shown to play a pathogenic role in atherothrombosis after ACS, but it is not clear whether Lp(a) is a predictor of recurrent events including recurrent MI. In a study from Switzerland, levels of Lp(a) were collected at the time of angiography from 1711 patients hospitalized for ACS. No association was found between elevated Lp(a) and MACE at 1 year nor was there an association with MI.[27]

In a prospective single-center registry in Korea of 12,064 patients between 2003 and 2013 with baseline Lp(a) measurements who underwent PCI, the primary outcome was a composite of cardiovascular death, spontaneous MI, and ischemic stroke.[28] From the registry, 3747 (31.1%) patients had high Lp(a) (>30 mg/dL), and 8317 (68.9%) patients had low Lp(a) (≤30 mg/dL). During a median follow-up of 7.4 years, the incidence rates of the primary outcomes were

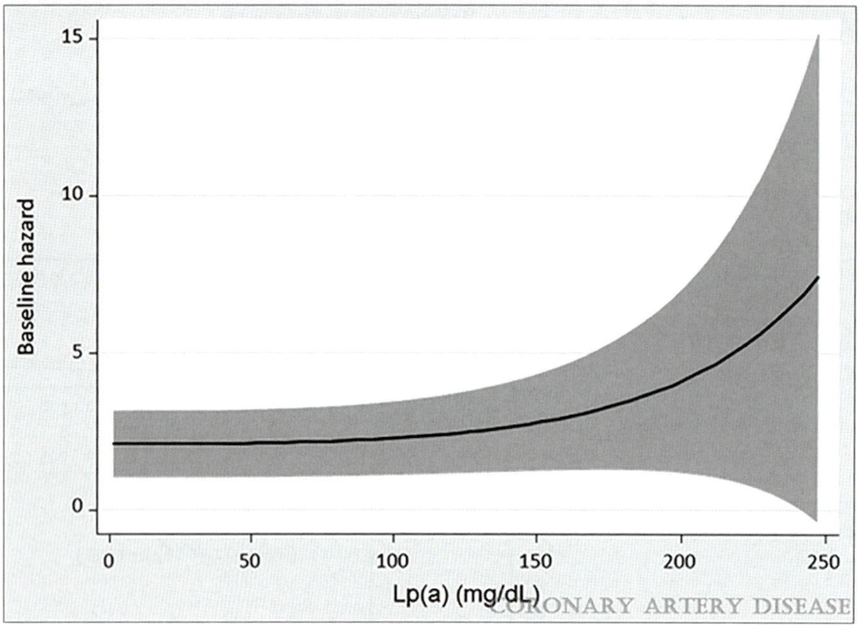

FIG. 20.7 Lipoprotein(a) and long-term recurrent infarction after an episode of ST-segment elevation myocardial infarction.[9] Lipoprotein Lp(a) and baseline hazard of reinfarction. *IRR*, Incidence rate ratio; (Reproduced from Miñana G, Gil-Cayuela C, Bodi V, et al. Lipoprotein(a) and long-term recurrent infarction after an episode of ST-segment elevation acute myocardial infarction. *Coron Artery Dis*. 2020;31(4):378–384. Fig. 2 page 381.)

2.0 per 100 person-years in the high-Lp(a) group and 1.6 per 100 person-years in the low-Lp(a) group (adjusted HR (aHR), 1.17; 95% CI, 1.05–1.30; *P* = .004). In addition, the risk of repeated revascularization was significantly higher in the high-Lp(a) group (aHR, 1.13; 95% CI, 1.02–1.25; *P* = .022). There was no relationship, per 100 person-years, to type 1 MIs, 0.6 low Lp(a) group versus 0.8 high Lp(a) group 1.16 (0.98–1.38), *P* = .08.

In a study that included 435 consecutive STEMI patients discharged from 2000 to 2003 in a single teaching center in Italy, after a median follow-up of 9.6years (4.1–15 years), 41.4% deaths and 30.6% MIs were recorded.[9] Higher values of Lp(a) in STEMI patients identified those at higher risk of recurrent MI (*P* = .020). Those with lipoprotein(a) values >95th percentile (≥135mg/dL) showed a higher risk of recurrent MI (incidence RR, 2.34; 95% CI, 1.37–4.02; *P* = .002). (Fig. 20.7) Levels of Lp(a) were not related to the risk of mortality (*P* = .245).[9]

In a study of 1711 patients from subgroups with ACS, levels of Lp(a) collected at the time of angiography were not predictive of cardiovascular outcomes including recurrent MI at one year; Lp(a) ≥ 30 mg/dL compared with <30 mg/dL 3.3% versus 3.5% adjusted HR, 1.02 (0.47–2.19).[27]

In the ODYSSEY trial, alirocumab reduced Lp(a) by an absolute change of 5.0 mg/dL ([IQR]: 0–13.5 mg/dL) and 23% ([IQR]: 47%–0%) relatively.[29] Lp(a) reductions with alirocumab were associated with reductions in MACE (composite of coronary heart disease, nonfatal MI, ischemic stroke or hospitalization for unstable angina). Reductions of Lp(a) (HR, 0.994; 95% CI, 0.990–999; *P* = .0090) and LDL-C (HR, 0.995; 95% CI, 0.993–0.997; *P* < .0001) independently contributed to the reduced risk of MACE. Among patients with high baseline Lp(a) levels (upper 2 quartile), alirocumab required treatment of 43 to 48 patients for a medium of 2.8 years to prevent 1 MACE. Trials are planned to assess the effects of siRNA and antisense oligonucleotides which reduce Lp(a) levels and effects on CV outcomes.

Plaque Morphology

In the Optical Coherence Tomography Morphologic and Fractional Flow Reserve Assessment in Diabetes Mellitus Patients (COMBINE OCT –FFR) trial optimal coherence tomography (OCT) detection of thin-cap fibroatheroma (TCFA) in diabetic patients with normal FFR, $n = 390$ patients, TCFA was detected in 98 patients (25%).[14] For the primary endpoint of MACE (cardiac mortality, target vessel MI, clinically driven target lesion revascularization or unstable angina requiring hospitalization) at 18 months was 13.3% in TCFA positive and 3.1% in TCFA negative patients (HR, 4.6; 95% CI, 1.99–10.89; *P* < .001) (Fig. 20.8).[14] TCFA was the strongest predictor of MACE (HR 5.12; 95% CI, 2.12–12.34; *P* < .001) And at 18 months follow-up the incidence of type 1 MI was 8.2% in patients with TCFA compared with 1.0% in patients without TCFA, HR, 8.26; (2.19–31.14), *P* = .002.[14]

ALGORITHM FOR THE DIAGNOSIS AND MANAGEMENT OF RECURRENT ISCHEMIA AND/OR RECURRENT MI

Fig. 20.9 shows an algorithm for the diagnosis and management of recurrent ischemia and/or recurrent MI depending on whether these occur.

Lifestyle modifications such as quitting smoking, body weight control, exercise, prevention of diabetes, and adherence to secondary evidence-based medications and rehabilitation are important to reduce the incidence of recurrent MI. Secondary prevention therapy is discussed in Chapter 29 and considerations regarding the use of

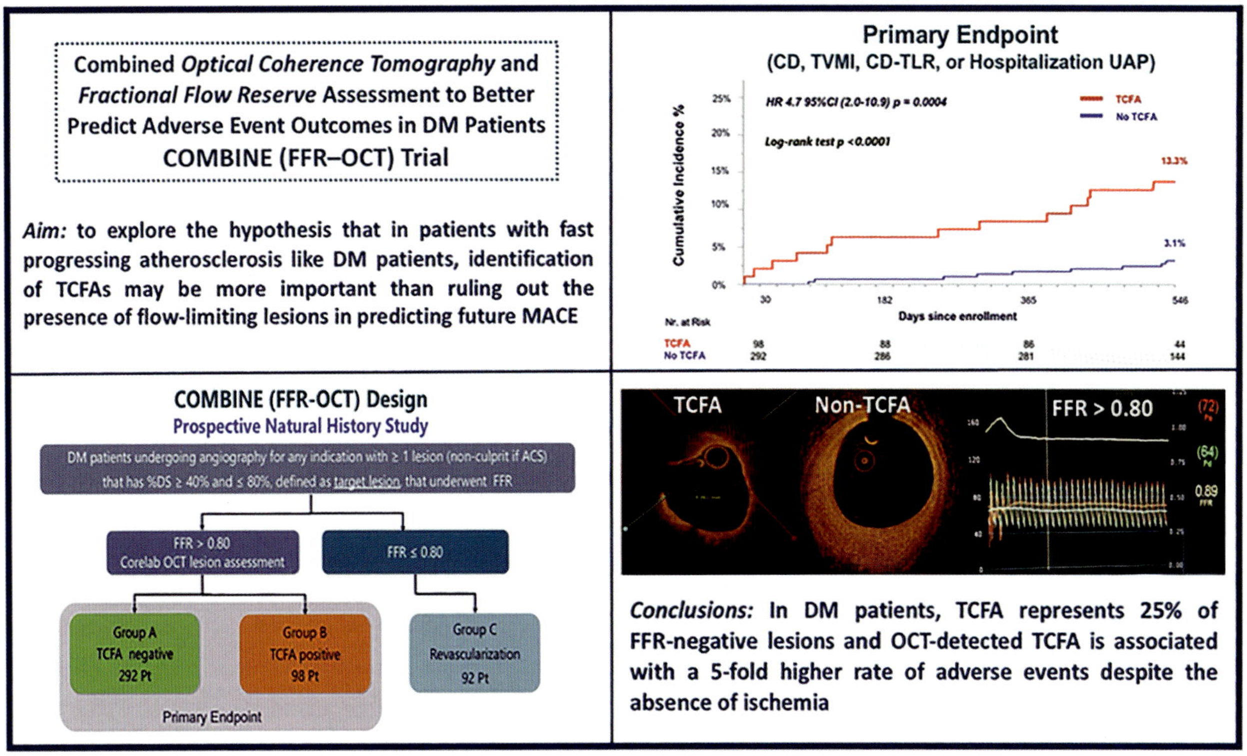

FIG. 20.8 Thin-cap fibroatheroma predicts clinical events in diabetic patients with normal fractional flow reserve: the COMBINE OCT–FFR trial – design and results.[14] *CD*, Clinically driven; *CD-TLR*, clinically driven target lesion revascularization; *DM*, diabetes mellitus; *FFR*, fractional flow reserve; *OCT*, Optical coherence tomography; *TCFA*, Thin-cap fibroatheroma; *TVMI*, target vessel myocardial infarction; *UAP*, unstable angina pectoris. (Reproduced from Kedhi E, Roleder T, Hermanides RS, et al. Thin-cap fibroatheroma predicts clinical events in diabetic patients with normal fractional flow reserve: the COMBINE OCT–FFR trial. *Eur Heart J.* 2021;42(45):4671–4679. Graphic abstract page 4672.)

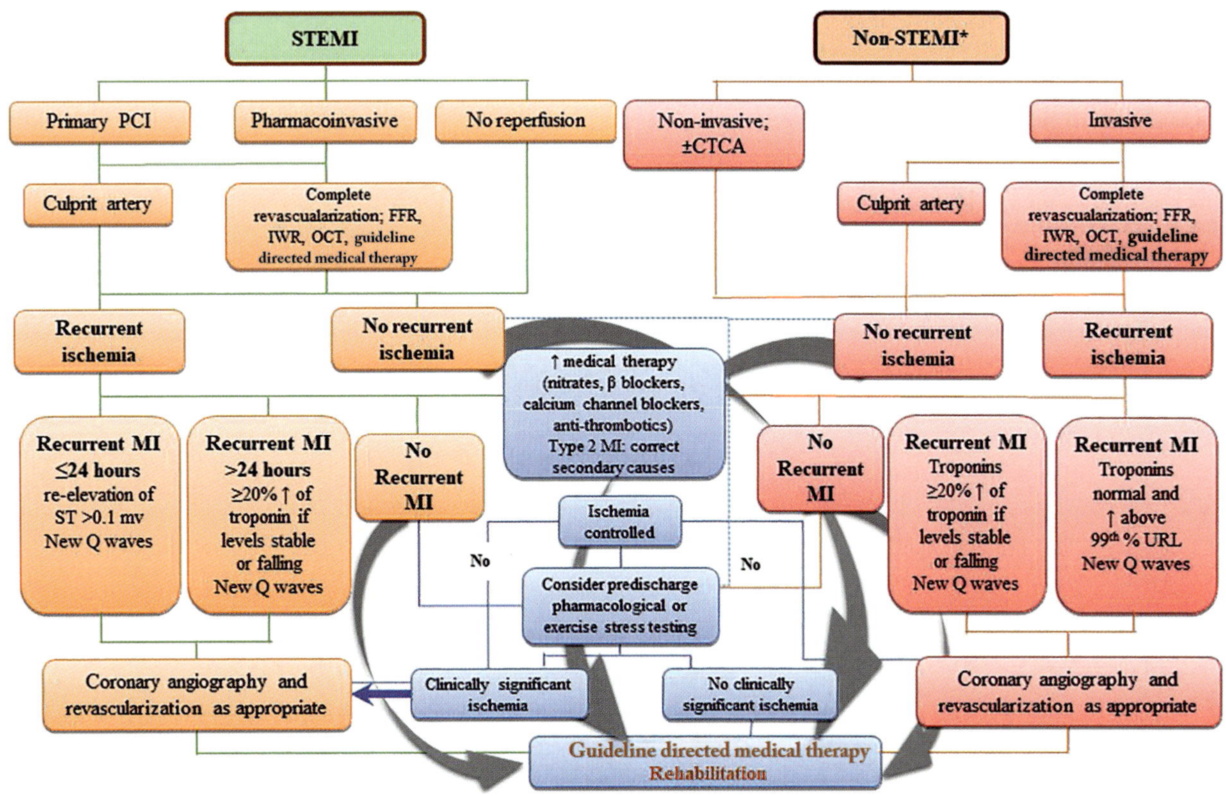

FIG. 20.9 Algorithm for the diagnosis and management of recurrent ischemia and/or recurrent myocardial infarction. *The management of type 2 MIs is to treat the cause of the supply/demand imbalance and to use preventative therapies if CAD is present. *CTCA*, Computerized tomographic coronary angiography;*FFR*, Fractional flow rate; *Ifr*, instantaneously wave-free rate; *OCT*, optimal coherence tomography; *URL*, uniform resource locator.

long-term antithrombotic therapies are reviewed in Chapters 25 and 26.

SUMMARY

Recurrent MI is associated with patient-focused adverse outcomes including increased hospital stay, complications, including heart failure, arrhythmias, increased rates of stroke, increased ischemia-driven revascularization, bleeding, and increased in-hospital and long-term mortality, all of which are associated with increased costs. Also, quality of life may be impaired.

As mortality from ACS has declined, the contribution of recurrent ischemic events to the composite of CV death and MI has increased, reflecting a change in competing risks with more patients being at risk of recurrent MI. There is a need for prolonged and close follow-up of patients after ACS, evaluating the presence of ischemia particularly in the first 90 days and in patients with risk factors for recurrent ischemia. Cardiac rehabilitation, prevention programs targeting traditional risk factors, and attention to prescribing and adherence to guideline directed medical therapy are important to reduce recurrent MI and to improve patient outcomes.

REFERENCES

1. Roth GA, Abate D, Abate KH, et al. Global, regional, and national age-sex-specific mortality for 282 causes of death in 195 countries and territories, 1980–2017: a systematic analysis for the global burden of disease study 2017. *Lancet.* 2018;392:1736–1788.
2. Thygesen K, Alpert JS, Jaffe AS, et al. Fourth universal definition of myocardial infarction (2018). *Circulation.* 2018;138:e618–e651. Erratum in: *Circulation.* 2018;138:e652.
3. Berwanger O, Santucci EV, de Barros e Silva PGM, et al. Effect of loading dose of atorvastatin prior to planned percutaneous coronary intervention on major adverse cardiovascular events in acute coronary syndrome. The SECURE-PCI randomized clinical trial. *JAMA.* 2018;319:1331–1340.
4. Nedkoff L, Briffa T, Murray K, et al. Risk of early recurrence and mortality in high-risk myocardial infarction patients: a population-based linked data study. *Int J Cardiovasc Risk Prev.* 2023;17:200185.
5. Diletti R, den Dekker WK, Bennett J, et al. Immediate versus staged complete revascularization in patients presenting with acute coronary syndrome and multivessel coronary disease (BIOVASC): a prospective, open-label, non-inferiority, randomised trial. *Lancet.* 2023;401:1172–1182.
6. Chen DY, Li CY, Hsieh MJ, et al. Predictors of subsequent myocardial infarction, stroke, and death in stable post-myocardial infarction patients: a nationwide cohort study. *Eur Heart J Acute Cardiovasc Care.* 2019;8:634–642.
7. White HD, Steg PG, Szarek M, et al. Effects of Alirocumab on types of myocardial infarction: insights from the ODYSSEY trial. *Eur Heart J.* 2019;40:2801–2809.
8. Schmitz T, Harmel E, Heier M, et al. Long-term predictors of hospitalized reinfarction after an incident acute myocardial infarction. *Life.* 2022;12:2090.
9. Miñana G, Gil-Cayuela C, Bodi V, et al. Lipoprotein(a) and long-term recurrent infarction after an episode of ST-segment elevation acute myocardial infarction. *Coron Artery Dis.* 2020;31:378–384.
10. Schüpke S, Neumann FJ, Menichelli M, et al. Ticagrelor or prasugrel in patients with acute coronary syndromes. *N Engl J Med.* 2019;381:1524–1534.
11. Sawano M, Lu Y, Caraballo C, et al. Sex difference in outcomes of acute myocardial infarction in young patients. *J Am Coll Cardiol.* 2023;81:1797–1806.
12. Furtado RHM, Nicolau JC, Magnani G, et al. Long-term ticagrelor for secondary prevention in patients with prior myocardial infarction and no history of coronary stenting: insights from PEGASUS-TIMI 54. *Eur Heart J.* 2020;41:1625–1632.
13. Chaitman BR, Alexander KP, Cyr D, et al. Myocardial infarction in the ISCHEMIA trial: impact of different definitions on incidence, prognosis, and treatment comparisons. *Circulation.* 2021;143:790–804.
14. Kedhi E, Berta B, Roleder T, et al. Thin-cap fibroatheroma predicts clinical events in diabetic patients with normal fractional flow reserve: the COMBINE OCT–FFR trial. *Eur Heart J.* 2021;42(45):4671–4679.
15. Hahn J, Fu YP, Brown MR, et al. Genetic loci associated with prevalent and incident myocardial infarction and coronary heart disease in the cohorts for heart and aging research in genomic epidemiology (CHARGE) consortium. *PLoS One.* 2020;15:e0230035.
16. Van der Harst P, Verweij N. Identification of 64 novel genetic loci provides an expanded view on the genetic architecture of coronary artery disease. *Circ Res.* 2018;122:433–443.
17. Wang M, Vaez M, Dorner TE, et al. Sociodemographic, labour market marginalisation and medical characteristics as risk factors for reinfarction and mortality within 1 year after a first acute myocardial infarction: a register-based cohort study of a working age population in Sweden. *BMJ Open.* 2019;9:e033616.
18. Mai K, Awan ID, Shaukat F. Evaluation of risk factors associated with reinfarction: a multicenter observational study. *Cureus.* 2019;11:e6063.
19. Nicholls SJ, Katoka Y, Nissen SE, et al. Effect of evolocumab on coronary plaque phenotype and burden in statin-treated patients following myocardial infarction. *JACC Cardiovasc Imaging.* 2022;15:1308–1321.
20. Ridker PM, Everett BM, Thuren T, et al. Antiinflammatory therapy with Canakinumab for atherosclerotic disease. *N Engl J Med.* 2019;377:1119–1131.
21. Tardif JC, Jiyz S, Water DD, et al. Efficacy and safety of low-dose colchicine after myocardial infarction. *N Engl J Med.* 2019;381:2497–2505.
22. Tong DC, Quinn S, Nasis A, et al. Colchicine in patients with acute coronary syndrome: the Australian cops randomized clinical trial. *Circulation.* 2020;142:1890–1900.
23. Nogic J, Mehta O, Tong D, et al. Colchicine in the management of acute coronary syndrome: a meta analysis. *Cardiol Ther.* 2023;12:171–181.
24. Mehta SR, Wood DA, Storey RF, et al. Complete revascularization with multivessel PCI for myocardial infarction. *N Engl J Med.* 2019;381:1411–1421.
25. Martinez GJ, Celermajer DS, Patel S. The NLRP3 inflammasome and the emerging role of colchicine to inhibit atherosclerosis-associated inflammation. *Atherosclerosis.* 2018;269:262–271.
26. Vaidya K, Arnott C, Martinez GJ, et al. Colchicine therapy and plaque stabilization in patients with acute coronary syndrome: a CT coronary angiography study. *JACC Cardiovasc Imaging.* 2018;11(2 Pt 2):305–316.
27. Gencer B, Rigamonti F, Nanchen D, et al. Prognostic value of elevated lipoprotein(a) in patients with acute coronary syndromes. *Eur J Clin Invest.* 2019;49:e13117.
28. Yoon YH, Ahn JM, Kang DY, et al. Association of lipoprotein(a) with recurrent ischemic events following percutaneous coronary intervention. *JACC Cardiovas Interv.* 2021;14:2059–2068.
29. Bittner VA, Szarek M, Aylward PE, et al. Effect of alirocumab on lipoprotein(a) and cardiovascular risk after acute coronary syndrome. *J Am Coll Cardiol.* 2020;75:133–144.
30. Galassa G, Angelis ED, Silverio A, et al. Predictors of recurrent ischemic events in patients with ST-segment elevation myocardial infarction. *Am J Cardiol.* 2021;159:44–51.

21 Heart Failure and Cardiogenic Shock in Acute Coronary Syndromes

ERIN A. BOHULA, DAVID. D. BERG, AND DAVID A. MORROW

INTRODUCTION

Acute coronary syndrome (ACS) is defined by acute myocardial ischemia, and, in the case of myocardial infarction (MI), resultant myocyte necrosis. If large in its territory or critical in its location, this injury can lead to loss of contractile function or other structural complications (Chapter 22) that result in insufficient cardiac output and consequent heart failure or cardiogenic shock. Despite significant advancements in the acute management of ACS, incident heart failure, including cardiogenic shock, still occurs in 10%–30% of patients during the initial hospitalization for ACS and is associated with at least a two-to-four-fold higher adjusted risk of in-hospital death compared to patients without heart failure.[1–4] Cardiogenic shock occurs in ~3%–10% of patients presenting with an acute MI and carries a staggering 30%–50% mortality rate.[1,2,5–8]

In this chapter, we will review the current understanding of the epidemiology, pathophysiology, evaluation, and management of heart failure and cardiogenic shock in ACS, in particular MI, henceforth referred to as ACS-HF and AMI-CS, respectively. The mechanical complications of MI are detailed in Chapter 22.

Defining and Classifying Heart Failure and Cardiogenic Shock

Heart failure in ACS is a clinical syndrome typically defined by evidence of pulmonary venous or central venous congestion. Irrespective of etiology, cardiogenic shock is characterized additionally by inadequate tissue or end-organ perfusion secondary to cardiac insufficiency.[9] This reduction in perfusion results in decreased oxygen and nutrient delivery to tissues, which if severe or protracted, can lead to multi-organ dysfunction and death. Generally accepted clinical criteria for shock include evidence of end-organ hypoperfusion, which may manifest as altered mental status, decreased urine output, acute kidney injury, cool or mottled extremities, acute liver injury, or lactic acidosis.[7,9,10] Historically, inclusion criteria for clinical trials of cardiogenic shock have also required frank or relative hypotension defined by a systolic blood pressure below 90 mm Hg for at least 30 minutes or a requirement for vasopressors to maintain adequate blood pressure; however, it should be noted that cardiogenic shock may be present without frank hypotension in the context of vasoconstriction, an entity referred to as normotensive cardiogenic shock.[7,9] Hemodynamic criteria suggestive of cardiogenic shock include an inadequate cardiac index, defined as <2.2 L/min/m^2 in the context of normal or elevated ventricular filling pressures.

Heart failure and cardiogenic shock can be categorized according to severity using one of several classification systems (Tables 21.1 and 21.2). The Killip classification system, which was derived specifically in patients with acute MI, is defined by physical exam findings consistent with heart failure, ranging from mild congestion to cardiogenic shock (Table 21.1). The Killip classification has a strong graded relationship with mortality following acute MI in which, compared to patients without any signs or symptoms of heart failure (Killip class I), patients with Killip class II-III heart failure have a fourfold higher risk of in-hospital mortality and those with cardiogenic shock, a 10-fold higher risk.[1,11] The New York Heart Association (NYHA) system describes a functional or symptomatic status, ranging from no symptomatic limitation of physical activity (NYHA class I) to symptoms with minimal exertion or symptoms at rest (NYHA class IV; Table 21.1). An indicator of heart failure severity, NYHA class is also associated with survival.[10,12] Investigators with the Interagency Registry of Mechanically Assisted Circulatory Support (INTERMACS) developed a classification system based on the combination of signs, symptoms, and level of therapeutic support, with the goal of refining the description of NYHA class III-IV and shock

TABLE 21.1 Heart Failure and Cardiogenic Shock Classification Systems

CLASSIFICATION	DEFINITION
Killip Classification	
Class I	No evidence of heart failure
Class II	Mild to moderate heart failure, including S3 gallop, rales less than one-half of the posterior lung fields, or jugular venous distension
Class III	Overt pulmonary edema
Class IV	Cardiogenic shock
NYHA Classification	
Class I	No limitation of physical activity
Class II	Slight limitation of physical activity. Comfortable at rest but ordinary physical activity results in symptoms of heart failure.
Class III	Marked limitation of physical activity. Comfortable at rest but less than ordinary activity causes symptoms of heart failure.
Class IV	Unable to carry on any physical activity without symptoms of heart failure or symptoms of heart failure at rest.
INTERMACS Classification	
Profile 1	Critical cardiogenic shock ("Crash and burn"); life-threatening hypotension despite rapidly escalating inotropic support
Profile 2	Progressive decline ("Sliding on inotropes"); declining function despite intravenous inotropic support
Profile 3	Stable but inotrope-dependent ("Dependent stability"); stable blood pressure, organ function, and symptoms on continuous intravenous inotropic support or temporary circulatory support or both with repeated failure to wean
Profile 4	Resting symptoms; stabilized close to normal volume status but experiences daily symptoms at rest or during activities of daily living (ADLs)
Profile 5	Exertion intolerant ("Housebound"); comfortable at rest or with ADLs, symptoms with any further activity
Profile 6	Exertion limited ("Walking wounded"); fatigues after first few minutes of anything beyond minor activity
Profile 7	Advanced NYHA III

NYHA, New York Heart Association; *INTERMACS*, Interagency Registry of Mechanically Assisted Circulatory Support.

patients in order to best define populations that would benefit from advanced therapies such as cardiac transplantation and mechanical circulatory support.[10,12] The INTERMACS profiles range from NYHA class III (INTERMACS 7), exertion limited (6), exertion intolerant (5), resting symptoms (4), stable but inotrope-dependent (3), progressive decline on inotropes (2) and critical cardiogenic shock (1) (Table 21.1). Finally, a shock classification scheme was developed by the Society for Cardiovascular Angiography and Interventions (SCAI) that defines five risk categories ranging from Stage A (at-risk) to Stage E (extremis) based on hemodynamic parameters, markers of tissue perfusion and response to interventions (Table 21.2).[13,14] The SCAI staging system has been shown to identify a strong gradient of risk for in-hospital mortality across a broad range of patients with cardiogenic shock (Fig. 21.1) including within subgroups defined by etiology (e.g., AMI-CS and CS without acute MI).[6,14,15]

In addition to classification systems that reflect illness severity, heart failure, and cardiogenic shock can be classified according to other characteristics, such as underlying etiology, heart failure chronicity, and hemodynamic phenotype. These distinctions reflect unique pathophysiologies, clinical trajectories, and outcomes and help to frame management. In terms of etiology, an important distinction is made according to whether the event was precipitated by an acute ischemic insult (Fig. 21.2).[9] Multiple registries have suggested that patients with acute myocardial infarction-related cardiogenic shock (AMI-CS) have worse outcomes compared with patients with HF-related cardiogenic shock (in the absence of ACS), possibly due to the acute nature of the insult which does not allow for chronic physiologic adaptation.[5,6,9,16]

Other classification schemes have used hemodynamic profiles (e.g., left, right, or biventricular congestion and/or pump dysfunction) or a combination of clinical, laboratory, and hemodynamic variables (e.g., noncongested, cardiometabolic, and cardiorenal) to further subclassify patients with shock.[6,17] Such strategies for refined phenotyping of patients are likely to have important implications for risk stratification, identification of homogenous study populations, and potentially for targeting specific therapeutic interventions to patients who will derive maximal benefit.[9]

EPIDEMIOLOGY AND OUTCOMES

Left or right ventricular failure is the predominant mechanism of cardiac insufficiency in ACS, accounting for approximately 75 percent of AMI-CS cases (Fig. 21.3). Mechanical causes of shock among patients with MI (Chapter 22), including ventricular septal rupture, severe mitral regurgitation, and free wall rupture with tamponade, accounted for 12% of shock cases in the Should We Emergently Revascularize Occluded Coronaries for Cardiogenic Shock (SHOCK) Trial Registry (Fig. 21.3); however, the global incidence of mechanical complications following acute MI has decreased over time due to the adoption of early reperfusion strategies.[18]

Incidence and Risk Factors

While estimates for the incidence of new-onset ACS-HF are variable due to differences in the study population, the heart failure definitions applied, and the observation period

TABLE 21.2 Society for Cardiovascular Angiography and Interventions (SCAI) Shock Stage Classification

STAGE	DESCRIPTION	PHYSICAL EXAM/BEDSIDE FINDING	BIOCHEMICAL MARKERS	HEMODYNAMICS
A At Risk	A patient who is not currently experiencing signs or symptoms of CS but is at risk for its development. These patients may include those with large acute myocardial infarction or prior infarction acute and/ or acute on chronic heart failure symptoms	Normal JVP Lungs sound clear Warm and well perfused • Strong distal pulses • Normal Mentation	Normal labs • Normal (at baseline) renal function • Normal lactic acid	Normotensive (SBP ≥100 or normal for patient) If hemodynamics done • Cardiac index ≥2.5 L/min/m² • CVP ≤ 10 mmHg • PCWP ≤ 15 mmHg • PA sat ≥65%
B Beginning CS	A patient who has clinical evidence of hemodynamic instability (including relative hypotension or tachycardia) without hypoperfusion.	Elevated JVP Warm and well perfused • Strong distal pulses • Normal mentation May include rales	Normal lactate Minimal renal function impairment Elevated BNP	SBP <90 mmHg *OR* MAP <60 mmHg *OR* >30 mmHg drop from baseline Pulse ≥ 100
C Classic CS	A patient who manifests with hypoperfusion that requires intervention (inotrope, pressor, or mechanical support, including ECMO) beyond volume resuscitation to restore perfusion. These patients typically present with relative hypotension.	*May include any of:* Looks unwell Panicked Ashen, mottled, dusky Volume overload Extensive rales Killip class 3 or 4 BiPAP or *mechanical* ventilation Cold, clammy Acute alteration in mental status Urine output <30 mL/h	*May include any of:* Lactate ≥2 mmol/L Creatinine 1.5x baseline *OR* >50% drop in eGFR Increased LFTs Elevated BNP	*May include any of:* SBP < 90 mmHg OR MAP < 60 mmHg OR > 30 mmHg drop from baseline *AND* drugs/ device used to maintain BP above these targets Hemodynamics • Cardiac index < 2.2 L/min/m² • PCWP > 15 mmHg
D Deteriorating/Doom	A patient that is similar to category C but is getting worse. Failure of initial support strategy to restore perfusion as evidenced by worsening hemodynamics or rising lactate.	*Any stage of C and worsening (or not improving) signs/ symptoms of hypoperfusion despite the initial therapy.*	*Any of Stage C AND:* lactate rising and persistently >2 mmol/L	*Any of Stage C AND:* Requiring multiple pressors *OR* Escalation pressor doses *OR* addition of MCS to maintain perfusion
E Extremis	Actual or impending circulatory collapse	Near pulselessness Cardiac collapse Mechanical ventilation Defibrillator used	CPR (A-modifier) pH ≤ 7.2 Lactate ≥ 8 mmol/L	Profound hypotension despite maximal hemodynamic support

BNP, B-type natriuretic protein; *CS*, cardiogenic shock; *CPR*, cardiopulmonary resuscitation; *CVP*, central venous pressure; *JVP*, jugular venous pressure; *LFTs*, liver function tests; *MCS*, mechanical circulatory support; *PA*, pulmonary artery; *PCWP*, pulmonary capillary wedge pressure; *SBP*, systolic blood pressure.

(i.e., at presentation, during hospitalization, or postdischarge), most studies have suggested that ACS-HF occurs in 10%–30% of patients with acute MI either at presentation or during hospitalization.[11] For patients without heart failure during the MI hospitalization, the risk of subsequent HF is highest in the first few months after discharge (~10%), then stabilizes at 1%–2% per year.[3] Several reports have suggested that the incidence of HF on admission has increased, possibly due to improvements in pre-hospital care that facilitate greater survival to admission.[3] In contrast, the incidence of HF development during hospitalization for acute MI has been decreasing. For example, the SWEDEHEART registry reported a decline in the incidence of in-hospital heart failure from 46% in 1996 to 28% in 2008. This trend is likely attributable to an increase in early, successful reperfusion as well as the increased sensitivity of troponin assays, which results in the diagnosis of acute MI in a population at lower risk for HF.[3] Risk factors for the development of heart failure after MI include older age, female sex, multivessel coronary disease, prior MI, prior HF or pre-existing LV systolic dysfunction, atrial fibrillation, diabetes, hypertension, chronic kidney disease, and elevated heart rate on presentation.[3,11]

Epidemiologic data are conflicting with respect to the trends in incidence in AMI-CS over time, variably reporting increasing, decreasing, and stable rates.[7] On balance, the data seem to support relative stability in the proportion of patients with AMI who develop CS, and the conflicting findings may reflect variation in research methodologies and reporting.[7] Importantly, however, the incidence of AMI, and particularly, STEMI, has been decreasing over time, such that the overall prevalence of AMI-CS is decreasing.[7,19] Concomitant with this epidemiologic trend, the global prevalence of heart failure is rising in the face of aging populations with a greater burden of obesity, diabetes, and other heart failure risk factors.[10,12] The confluence of these factors has led to an important finding: AMI-CS is no longer the dominant etiology underlying cardiogenic shock in contemporary registries.[5,6]

Risk factors for AMI-CS include STEMI, as compared to NSTEMI, with estimated rates of 6% to 10% and 2% to 4%, respectively.[1,2] Other risk factors for the development of AMI-CS, include older age, female sex, cardiac arrest on admission, anterior MI, left main coronary artery culprit lesion, and delayed or suboptimal revascularization.[7,20]

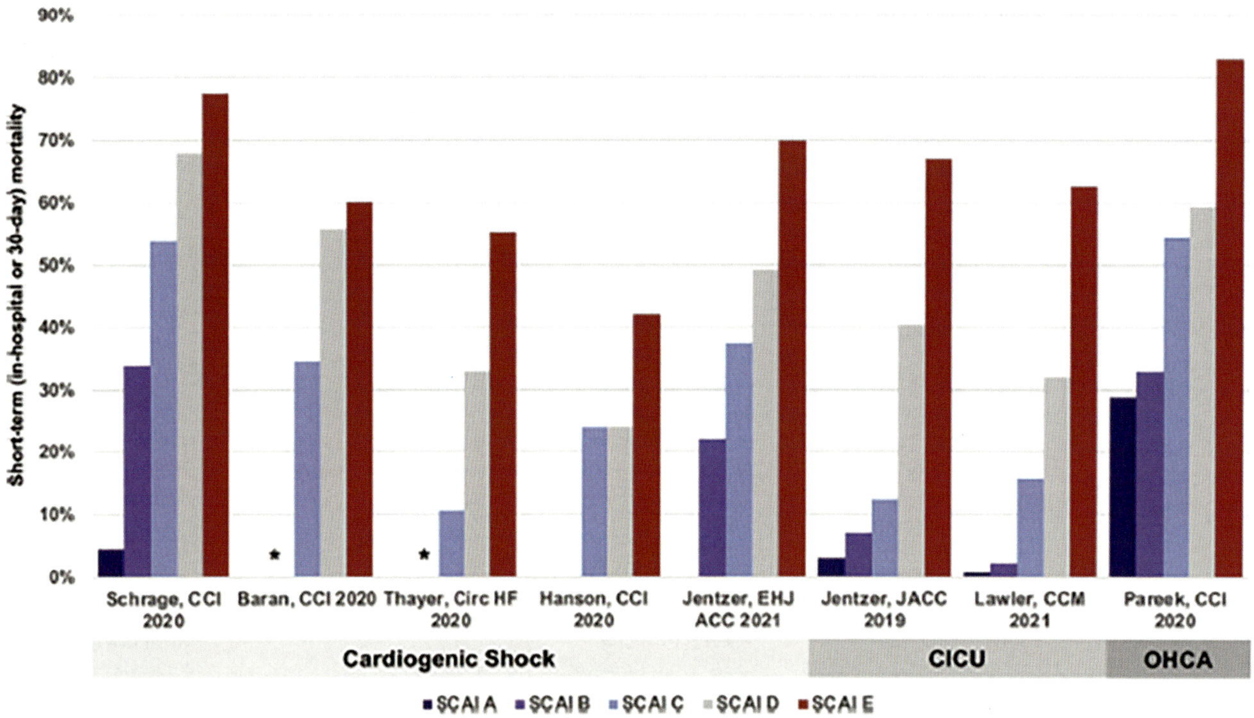

FIG. 21.1 Short-term mortality as a function of SCAI shock stages across multiple studies. *Indicates that no deaths were observed in SCAI Stage B patients. *CICU*, Cardiac intensive care unit; *OHCA*, out-of-hospital cardiac arrest; *SCAI*, Society for Cardiovascular Angiography and Interventions. (From Naidu et al. *JACC*. 2022;79(9):933–946.)

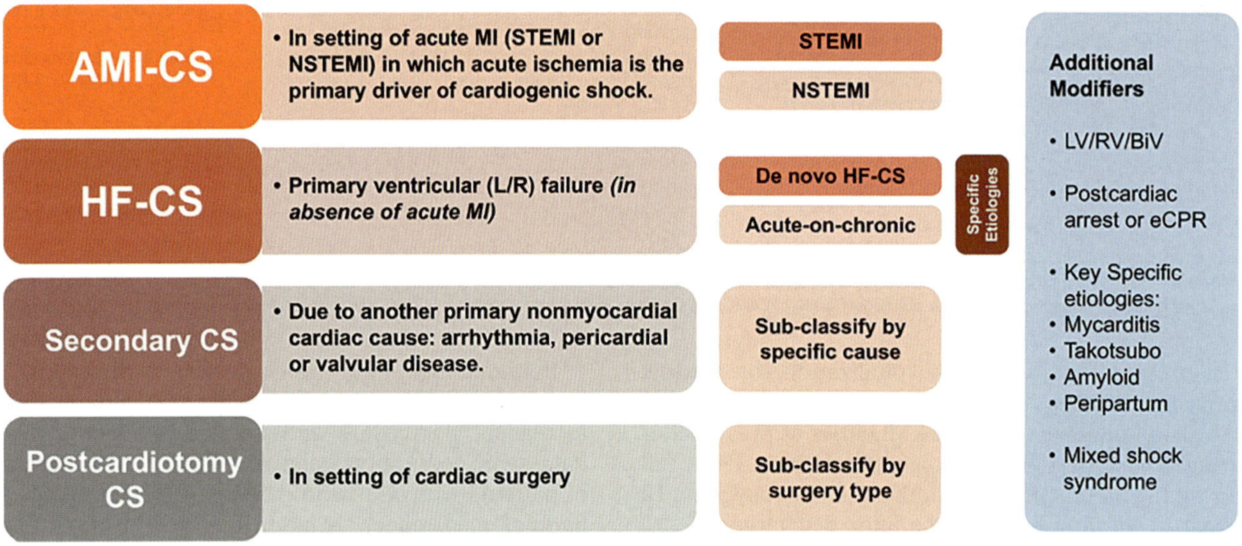

FIG. 21.2 Subcategories of cardiogenic shock. The Shock Academic Research Consortium (SHARC) outlined a framework for classifying cardiogenic shock into four main etiologic categories: AMI-CS, HF-CS, non-myocardial or secondary (e.g., arrhythmia, valvular, pericardial), and postcardiotomy cardiogenic shock. Further subclassifications are possibly by cause and/or chronicity. (From Waksman et al. *Circulation*. 2023;148:1113–11126.)

Outcomes with Heart Failure and Cardiogenic Shock

As described in the prior section, heart failure without cardiogenic shock continues to be a common complication of ACS and portends a worse prognosis. In the GRACE registry of 13,707 patients with ACS without shock or prior heart failure, presentation with heart failure or development of heart failure after admission identified patients with markedly higher in-hospital mortality compared to those without heart failure (12.0% vs. 17.8% vs. 2.8%, $P < .0001$), representing a greater than two-fold increased risk after adjustment for other predictors of mortality.[11] In addition to a higher risk of mortality, patients with ACS-HF are at a higher risk of recurrent MI, stroke, and recurrent hospitalization for heart failure.[11]

Although cardiogenic shock is a relatively infrequent complication of ACS, the mortality rate associated with the condition is staggeringly high. While the in-hospital mortality rates have decreased over the last 5 decades from 70% to 80% in the 1970s to around 30% to 50% currently, cardiogenic shock remains the major cause of death for patients hospitalized with acute MI (Fig. 21.4).[5–8,21] The improvement in mortality over time

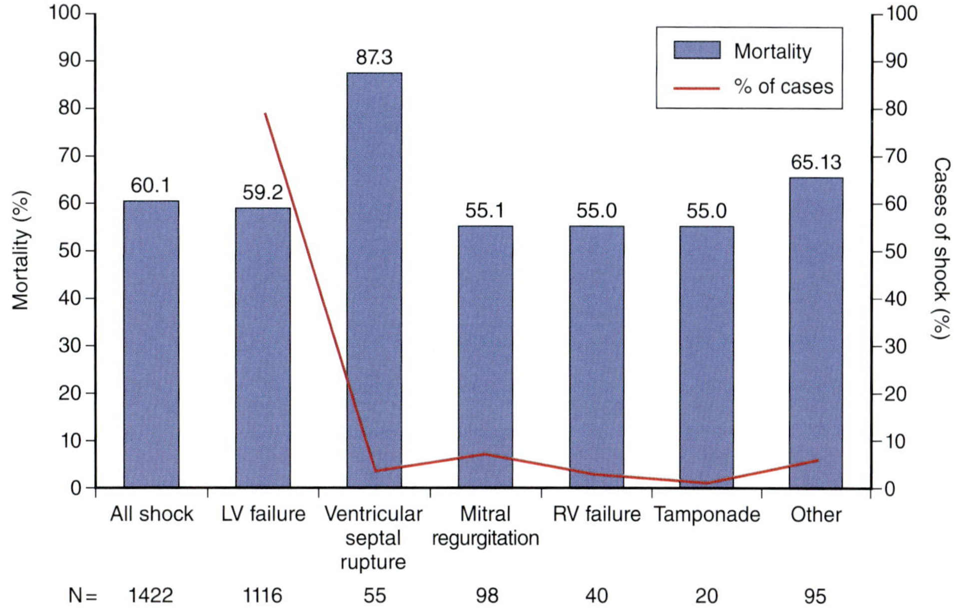

FIG. 21.3 **Mortality by etiology of cardiogenic shock following acute myocardial infarction.** In-hospital mortality rates are shown for the various primary etiologies of cardiogenic shock following AMI, including left ventricular failure (LVF), ventricular septal rupture (VSR), acute severe mitral regurgitation (MR), isolated right ventricular failure (RVF), cardiac tamponade/rupture (tamp) and other (includes prior severe valvular heart disease and excessive beta or calcium channel blockade). The proportion of patients in each category is shown. (Adapted from Hochman et al. *JACC.* 2000;36:1063–1070.)

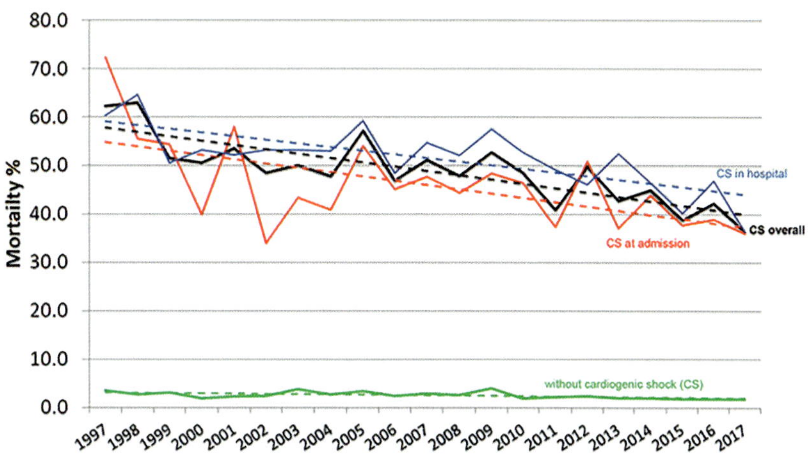

FIG. 21.4 **Trends in in-hospital mortality for AMI-CS.** The twenty-year trend in in-hospital mortality improved in the Acute Myocardial Infarction in Switzerland (AMIS) Plus Registry of 52,808 patients from 83 hospitals from 63% to 36% (*P*-trend <.001). PCI was the strongest independent predictor of survival in this dataset. (From Lukas et al. *Circulation: cardiovascular interventions.* 2019;12[4].)

is likely multi-factorial. For example, the options for and prioritization of reperfusion strategies for ACS have advanced significantly during this time period, as have processes of care for patients with cardiogenic shock.[22] In addition, multiple medical therapies that reduce the rate of recurrent cardiovascular events following ACS have been incorporated into standard practice, including high-intensity lipid-lowering therapies, potent antiplatelet agents, and neurohormonal antagonists, including beta blockers and inhibitors of the renin-angiotensin-aldosterone system (Chapter 29).[1,2,4,23,24]

Mortality Risk Prediction

As previously described in this chapter, the Killip and NYHA classification schemes, which are based on heart failure severity, are useful risk stratification tools with respect to mortality in the context of ACS.[10,12] Within the AMI-CS population, multiple other risk stratification tools have been shown to predict mortality, including the Sequential Organ Failure Assessment (SOFA) and IABP-SHOCK 2 scores; however, the previously described SCAI shock staging system has generally outperformed the other scores in terms of discrimination for mortality.[13–15] The SCAI shock staging system (Table 21.2) has been shown to identify a strong gradient of risk for in-hospital mortality across a broad population of patients with cardiogenic shock, including subpopulations defined by distinct etiologies, clinical settings, and hemodynamic profiles (Fig. 21.1).[6,14,15,25]

Hemodynamic variables and profiles have also proven useful in identifying high-risk AMI-CS patients. A depressed cardiac power output (CPO), that incorporates the product

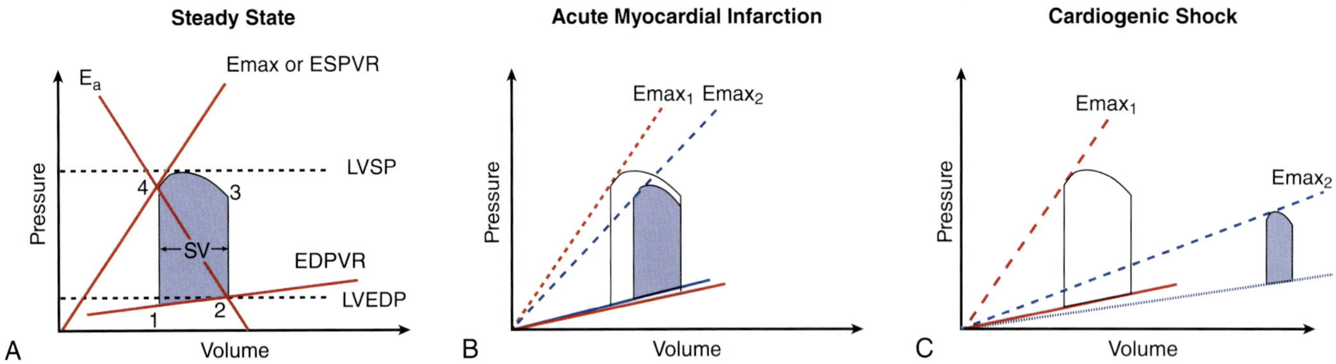

FIG. 21.5 Normal and pathologic pressure volume loops. Each pressure volume loop represents one cardiac cycle. (A) In the normal steady state, left ventricular filling occurs at the end of isovolumic relaxation (Phase 4 to 1) upon opening of the mitral valve (Point 1). The left ventricular end-diastolic pressure (LVEDP) is a function of the end-diastolic volume and myocardial compliance, represented by the end-diastolic pressure volume relationship (EDPVR). Once left ventricular volume is maximal at end-diastole (Point 2), isovolumic contraction begins (Phase 2–3). Systolic ejection occurs when left ventricular pressure exceeds aortic pressure, leading to aortic valve opening (Point 3), and continues until the point at which aortic pressure exceeds the left ventricular pressure, the end-systolic pressure-volume point (Point 4). The difference between the end-diastolic and end-systolic volume represents the stroke volume and area contained in the pressure-volume loop, the stroke work. (B) In the setting of an acute MI, left ventricular contractility is reduced, shifting the ESPV relationship down and reducing stroke volume. In addition, a decrease in myocardial compliance may lead to an increase in LVEDP. (C) In cardiogenic shock, LV contractility and stroke volume are severely reduced and LVEDP increased. (Adapted from Rihal CS, Naidu SS, Givertz MM, et al. 2015 SCAI/ACC/HFSA/STS clinical expert consensus statement on the use of percutaneous mechanical circulatory support devices in cardiovascular care: endorsed by the American Heart Assocation, the cardiological society of India, and Sociedad Latino Americana de Cardiologia Intervencion; Affirmation of Value by the Canadian Association of Interventional Cardiology-Association Canadienne de Cardiologie d'intervention. *J Am Coll Cardiol*. 2015;65(19):e7–e26.)

of mean arterial pressure and cardiac output, was found to be the strongest, independent hemodynamic predictor of in-hospital mortality in the SHOCK trial. In a more contemporary dataset from the Critical Care Cardiology Trials Network registry of 3603 cardiogenic shock patients with invasive hemodynamics, hemodynamic parameters reflecting decreased arterial tone (low mean arterial pressure, systolic blood pressure, and systemic vascular resistance) and right ventricular dysfunction (elevated right atrial pressure, right atrial pressure to pulmonary capillary wedge pressure ratio, and low pulmonary artery pulsatility index), but not CPO, were independently associated with worse outcomes.[26] Consistent with the notion that RV dysfunction portends worse outcomes, a separate study from the Cardiogenic Shock Working Group showed that right ventricular congestion was an independent predictor of mortality.[6]

Finally, there is much interest in applying sophisticated modeling approaches, such as machine learning techniques, to deeply phenotype cardiogenic shock patients to identify important sub-populations. One such effort from the Cardiogenic Shock Working Group and the Danish Retroshock Registry used clinical, hemodynamic, and laboratory data to identify three clusters of shock patients, broadly categorized as "non-congested," "cardiorenal," and "cardiometabolic," which were associated with mortality.[17] Novel biomarkers, such as markers of hemodynamic homeostasis (e.g., dipeptidyl amino-peptidase 3), have been shown to be associated with poor prognosis and mortality in cardiogenic shock patients; however, these biomarkers are not currently utilized for clinical risk stratification. Research is ongoing to employ "-omics" approaches (e.g., proteomic, transcriptomic, etc.) to phenotype cardiogenic shock patients in order to better understand pathophysiologic mechanisms, identify potential novel therapeutic targets, and improve prognostication.

PATHOPHYSIOLOGY

The pathophysiology of heart failure and cardiogenic shock is complex and dynamic, involving adaptive and maladaptive compensatory mechanisms coordinated by multiple organ systems.

Hemodynamic Considerations

The multiple myocardial and vascular parameters that determine stroke volume and work are represented in the left ventricular pressure-volume loops (Fig. 21.5A).[27] The left ventricular end-diastolic pressure is a function of the end-diastolic volume and myocardial compliance, represented by the end-diastolic pressure-volume relationship (EDPVR). The difference between the end-diastolic and end-systolic volume represents the stroke volume and area contained in the pressure-volume loop, the stroke work. The timing of the events in the cycle is determined by both myocardial and vascular characteristics. For example, the load-independent left ventricular contractility (E_{max}), described by the end-systolic pressure-volume relationship (ESPVR) across the range of loading conditions, and the effective arterial elastance (E_a) define the timing of aortic valve closure and therefore, of end-systole. E_a is a measure of arterial loading, approximated as the ratio of end-systolic pressure and stroke volume, and is influenced by peripheral resistance, vascular compliance and impedance, and systolic and diastolic time intervals. Stroke work or left ventricular pump efficiency is maximal when the ratio of effective arterial elastance and left ventricular contractility (E_a:E_{max}) approaches one.

In the setting of ACS, left ventricular contractility is reduced, thereby shifting the ESPVR down, and reducing stroke volume (Fig. 21.5B). In many cases, myocardial compliance decreases as well, shifting the EDPVR up and leading to an increase in left ventricular end-diastolic pressure for a given volume. If severe, these acute alterations

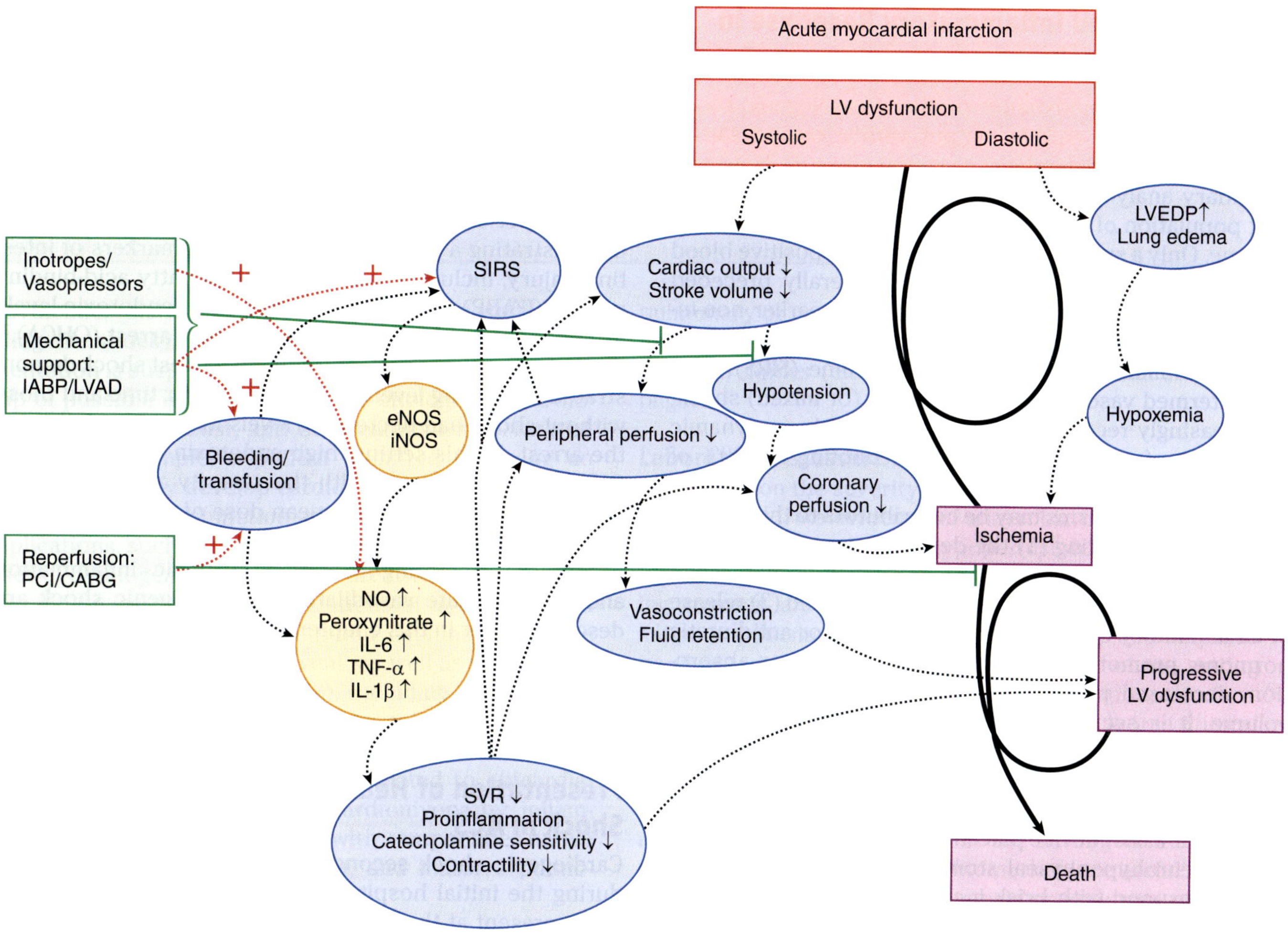

FIG. 21.6 **Pathophysiology of cardiogenic shock.** The classic shock spiral following acute myocardial infarction involves left ventricular dysfunction, leading to further ischemia, progressive ventricular dysfunction, and death. Systolic dysfunction results in insufficient cardiac output, hypotension, and peripheral and coronary hypoperfusion with subsequent ischemia. Diastolic dysfunction results in pulmonary congestion, hypoxemia, and additional ischemia. Finally, a systemic inflammatory response leads to inappropriate vasodilation with further hypotension, hypoperfusion, and ischemia as well as direct myocardial suppression, leading to worsened ventricular dysfunction. Several therapeutic strategies aim to abort this spiral through improvement in coronary perfusion (revascularization), myocardial contractility (inotropes), and peripheral perfusion (vasopressors and mechanical circulatory support). These therapeutic interventions may also contribute to bleeding, infection, and exacerbation of the systemic inflammatory response syndrome.
(Adapted from Reynolds & Hochman Circulation 2008;117(5):686–97 by Thiele et al. EHJ, 2015;36(20):1223–1230.)

in systolic and diastolic function can lead to decreased cardiac output, stroke work, and increased pulmonary congestion resulting in clinical heart failure.

In the extreme case of these perturbations (Fig. 21.5C), left ventricular contractile function is severely reduced, and left ventricular end-diastolic volume and pressures are significantly increased, culminating in cardiogenic shock. Unless interventions are made, cardiogenic shock begets worsened cardiogenic shock and death (Fig. 21.6). That is, the shock state, defined by inadequate cardiac output and congestion, results in a cascade of events that reinforce and exacerbate the underlying pathology of ischemia and progressive left ventricular dysfunction.

Impact of Altered Hemodynamics

The primary insult, myocardial ischemia across the spectrum of ACS and myocyte necrosis in the setting of an acute MI, results in reduced myocardial contractility and systolic dysfunction. The resultant reduction in cardiac output leads to hypotension and peripheral hypoperfusion. Hypotension can promote further ischemia and myocardial depression through decreased coronary perfusion, which can be exacerbated in the face of obstructive atherosclerotic lesions in non-culprit coronary vessels (Fig. 21.6). In an attempt to maintain perfusion to vital organs, the body releases endogenous catecholamines (e.g., norepinephrine) and other vasopressors (e.g., angiotensin II). These catecholamines and vasoconstrictors may mediate improved blood pressure through increased myocardial contractility and systemic vascular resistance (SVR); however, this increase in blood pressure may come at the cost of increased myocardial oxygen demand resulting from increased afterload and heart rate, promoting further ischemia. Hypoperfusion also activates the neurohormonal cascade resulting in sodium and fluid retention, thereby increasing perfusion through increased intravascular volume. However, in the setting of diastolic dysfunction, this can lead to a greater elevation of left ventricular end-diastolic pressures translating to more pulmonary edema and hypoxemia and further ischemia and progressive left ventricular dysfunction.

IN-HOSPITAL COMPLICATIONS

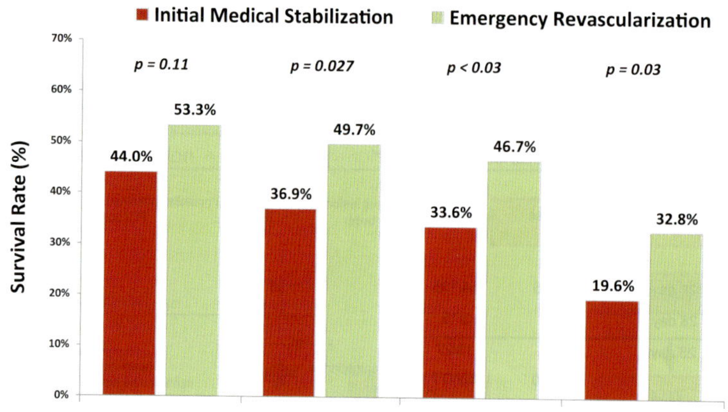

FIG. 21.10 Mortality benefit of early revascularization in patients with cardiogenic shock after acute myocardial infarction. The SHOCK Trial randomized 302 patients with STEMI and cardiogenic shock due to left ventricular failure to early revascularization within 6 h (ERV) or initial medical stabilization (IMS) with delayed revascularization more than 54 h after randomization, if appropriate. Survival rates in the ERV and IMS groups were 53.3% versus 44.0% (P = .11) at 30 days, 49.7% versus 36.9% (P = .027) at 6 months, 46.7% versus 33.6% (P < 0.03) at 1 year, and 32.8% versus 19.6% (P = .03) at 6 years, respectively. (Reproduced from Hochman et al. *JAMA*. 2006:295(21):2511.)

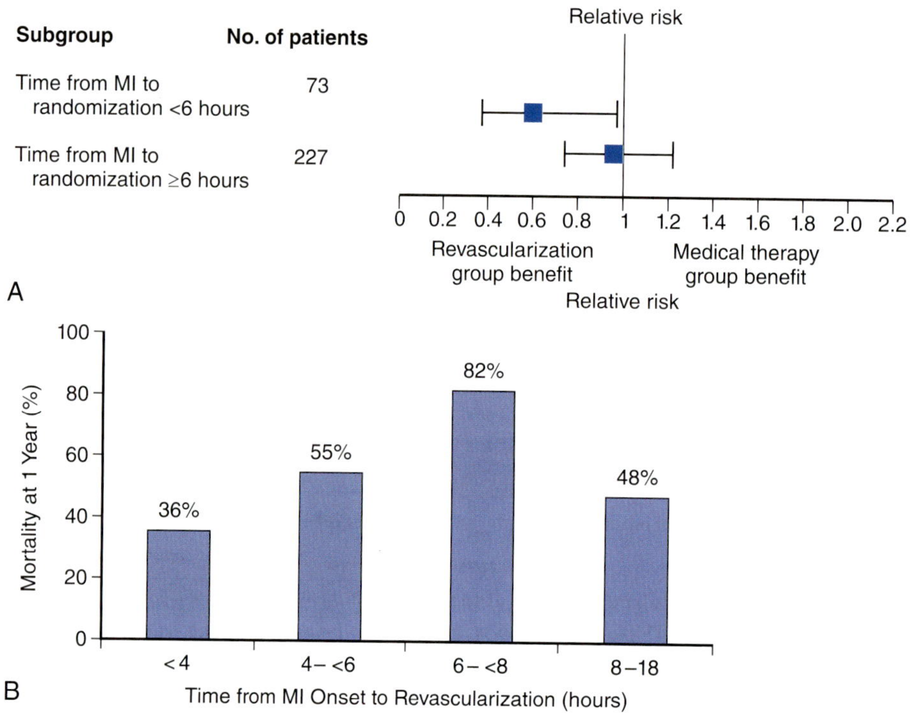

FIG. 21.11 Timing of revascularization in the SHOCK Trial. (A) Subgroup analysis for 30-day mortality comparing found no significant difference in benefit within the ERV by early (<6 h from MI onset) or later (≥6 h from MI onset) revascularization compared to IMS P-interaction = nonsignificant). (B) Within the ERV arm, mortality increased with increasing time from MI until after 8 h, which was thought to represent survivor bias. (From Hochman JS, Sleeper LA, Webb JG, et al. Early Revascularization in Acute Myocardial Infarction Complicated by Cardiogenic Shock. *N Engl J Med*. 1999;341:625–634.)

severe heart failure or shock is considered an indication for urgent angiography (Class I).

These recommendations are based on findings from the SHOCK Trial in which 49% (n = 152) of patients assigned to the early revascularization arm and 63% (n = 150) of those assigned to initial medical stabilization received fibrinolytic therapy for STEMI. Among patients randomized to initial medical therapy, administration of fibrinolytic therapy at the discretion of the treating physician was associated with a lower mortality rate at 1 year (unadjusted hazard ratio of 0.59, P = .01). However, among patients randomized to early revascularization, there was no association between administration of a fibrinolytic and subsequent mortality (unadjusted hazard ratio = 0.93, P = .76).

Although PCI is the preferred approach to revascularization when the coronary anatomy is suitable, favorable outcomes can also be achieved with early CABG. Of patients who underwent revascularization in the SHOCK trial, 63% had PCI and 37% had CABG. Despite higher rates of diabetes, three-vessel, and left main coronary disease in the CABG cohort, survival was similar at 1 year between patients who were revascularized with PCI compared with CABG (51.9% vs. 46.8%, P = .71). In patients with papillary muscle rupture, or acute severe mitral regurgitation related to MI, emergent surgical revascularization and valvular replacement may be preferable to a staged approach of percutaneous revascularization followed by surgical valve repair (Chapter 22).

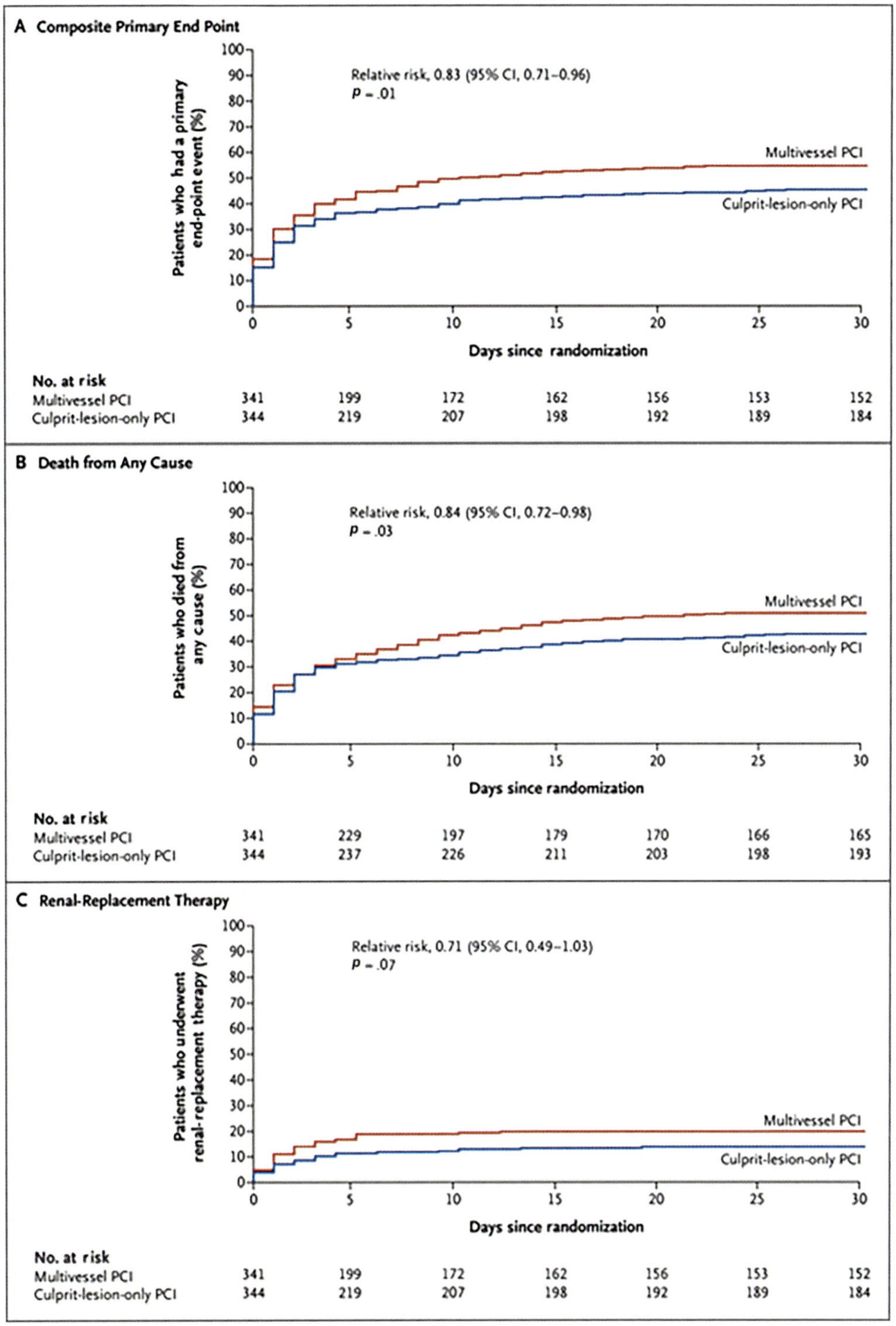

FIG. 21.12 Comparison of culprit-only versus immediate complete revascularization in AMI-CS in the CULPRIT-SHOCK trial. Results for the (A) primary composite endpoint of death from any cause or renal replacement therapy, (B) death from any cause, and (C) renal replacement in the CULPRIT-SHOCK trial comparing culprit-only versus immediate complete revascularization in patients with ACS (ST- and non-ST-elevation MI) and cardiogenic shock. (From Thiele et al. *N Engl J Med*. 2017;377:2419–2432.)

Non-Culprit Artery Revascularization in Shock

Multi-vessel disease is identified in 70%–90% of patients with cardiogenic shock and acute MI. In patients presenting with STEMI and multivessel disease *without shock*, multiple trials, including PRAMI (Preventive Angioplasty in Acute Myocardial Infarction, $n = 465$), DANAMI-3 PRIMULTI ($n = 627$), CvLPRIT (Complete Versus Lesion-Only Primary PCI trial, $n = 296$), and COMPLETE (Complete versus Culprit-Only Revascularization Strategies to Treat Multivessel Disease after Early PCI for STEMI, $n = 4041$), have demonstrated robust reductions in recurrent cardiovascular events with multi-vessel or complete revascularization compared to infarct-artery only revascularization in patients with STEMI.[41,42] In contrast, the CULPRIT-SHOCK (Culprit Lesion Only PCI versus Multivessel PCI in Cardiogenic Shock) trial, which randomized 706 patients with cardiogenic shock onset within 12 hours in the setting of acute MI (STEMI or NSTEMI) found that infarct-artery only revascularization was superior to immediate multi-vessel revascularization for the composite of death or renal replacement therapy at 30 days (45.9% vs. 55.4%, relative risk 0.83, 95% CI of 0.71–0.96, $P = .01$) as well as for death (relative risk 0.84, 95% CI 0.72–0.98, $P = .03$; Fig. 21.12). Notably, the benefit was consistent in patients with STEMI and NSTEMI. Additionally, approximately 18% of patients in the culprit-only arm went on to staged PCI for residual ischemic lesions, as evaluated by means of noninvasive testing or the use of fractional flow reserve, as outlined in the protocol. Based on the findings of the CULPRIT-SHOCK study, routine immediate revascularization of non-culprit lesions in patients with cardiogenic shock is not recommended; however, staged PCI of significant non-infarct related lesions may be considered.[2,4]

Pharmacotherapy

In general, the acute antithrombotic therapy and secondary preventive treatments for patients with acute MI and heart failure or shock should mirror that recommended for patients with an acute coronary event without heart failure or shock (Chapter 29). However, it is worthwhile to note that patients with hemodynamic instability were rarely included in the clinical trials supporting these guideline-based therapies. Furthermore, certain agents routinely utilized during treatment of an acute MI will exacerbate shock and are therefore contraindicated, including negative inotropic agents and antihypertensives. In addition, it is important to note that gastric and intestinal absorption of oral agents may be impaired in patients with shock. The roles of anticoagulant and antiplatelet agents are discussed in Chapter 12 and Chapter 13, respectively. Long-term secondary preventive therapies are discussed in Chapter 29. In this section, we focus our discussion on pharmacotherapy relevant to the acute management of heart failure and shock.

Agents with negative inotropic properties are contraindicated in cardiogenic shock. Specifically, these agents include beta blockers, non-dihydropyridine calcium channel blockers, such as verapamil and diltiazem, and specific classes of antiarrhythmics, notably class I sodium channel blockers (e.g., procainamide and quinidine) and certain class III agents (e.g., sotalol). If needed, amiodarone is the recommended antiarrhythmic of choice. Inhibitors of the renin-angiotensin system should not be administered in hypotensive patients with shock.

Vasoactive Medications

In addition to early coronary reperfusion, preservation of cardiac output, blood pressure and end-organ perfusion is paramount in patients with acute MI complicated by cardiogenic shock. These parameters can often be improved with a combination of pharmacologic and non-pharmacologic (e.g., advanced mechanical circulatory support) measures.

General Considerations

Inotropes and vasopressors may be administered with the goal of maintaining perfusion so as to preserve end-organ function. To achieve this goal, therapy is generally targeted at supporting the mean arterial pressure. Once the blood pressure is stabilized with resuscitation and/or vasopressor therapy, therapies can be tailored to address the underlying pathophysiology (e.g., addition of further inotropic support or vasodilator therapy).

In general, the dose of vasopressor and inotropic therapy should be maintained at the minimal dose and duration of therapy necessary to achieve these aims, as these agents can have adverse consequences. Catecholamines increase myocardial oxygen consumption and intracellular calcium, which can lead to arrhythmias or myocardial ischemia and cell death. Vasopressors can impair myocardial microcirculation promoting further ischemia. This concept is supported by the results of the SEPSISPAM trial of higher versus lower mean arterial pressure targets (80–85 mmHg vs. 65–70 mmHg) in septic shock showing no mortality benefit but higher rates of atrial fibrillation for the higher target.

Data to guide specific hemodynamic targets from PACs in patients with cardiogenic shock are very sparse. In the ESCAPE trial, treatment targets were a PCWP < 15 mmHg and a right atrial pressure of <8 mmHg. We generally titrate inotropic and vasodilator therapy to achieve a CI ≥2.2 L/min/m^2 and SVR 800–1000 dynes · sec/cm^5 with a PCWP < 15 mmHg. However, these goals are approximate, varying by the clinical setting and measures of end-organ function, such as urine output, as well as whether the patient is experiencing any adverse effects of therapy (e.g., tachyarrhythmia). Clinical signs of adequate end-organ perfusion should almost always take precedence over estimated hemodynamics from invasive monitoring.

The selection of specific inotropes or vasopressors should be guided by knowledge of their pharmacology and formulation of clear hemodynamic goals for the patient. The location and function of receptors targeted by these vasoactive medications are summarized in Table 21.4. Most vasoactive medications activate one or more of the adrenergic receptors. The alpha-1 adrenergic receptor is found in systemic vasculature and agonism results in arterial and venous smooth muscle contraction. Beta-1 receptors

TABLE 21.4 Vasoactive Medication Receptor Pharmacology

	LOCATION	RESPONSE TO RECEPTOR AGONISM
Adrenergic		
Alpha-1 (α-1)	Systemic vasculature	Arterial and venous smooth muscle contraction (vasoconstriction)
Beta-1 (β-1)	Myocardium	Increased contractility/inotropy Increased chronotropy
Beta-2 (β-2)	Splanchnic and skeletal muscle vasculature	Arterial smooth muscle relaxation (vasodilation)
Dopamine	Renal (D1, D2) and splanchnic vasculature (D2)	Renal arterial vasodilation Splanchnic vasodilation
Vasopressin	Systemic vasculature (V1) Renal collecting duct system (V2)	Arterial smooth muscle contraction (vasoconstriction) Water reabsorption via enhanced renal collecting duct permeability

are located in the myocardium where activation results in increased myocardial contractility and chronotropy. Activation of beta-2 receptors causes splanchnic and peripheral vasodilatation. Dopamine receptors (D1 and D2) are found on renal and splanchnic vasculature, resulting in vasodilatation in those beds. Finally, vasopressin receptor (V1 and V2) activation causes systemic vasoconstriction and water reabsorption in the kidneys, respectively.

Vasopressors

Dopamine

Dopamine is an endogenous catecholamine and precursor to epinephrine and norepinephrine. Dopamine has dose-dependent stimulation of dopamine, beta-1 and alpha-1 receptors (Table 21.5). At low doses, dopaminergic receptor stimulation predominates. Although "renal dosing" of dopamine was believed to improve urine output and renal protection in heart failure, this effect was not evident in a randomized control trial of patients with acute heart failure and renal dysfunction. At moderate doses, beta-1 activation results in augmentation of cardiac output and heart rate. At high doses, alpha-1 stimulation prevails, manifest as vasoconstriction.

While dopamine is an important option as a vasopressor, it may cause tachycardia and exacerbation of tachyarrhythmias. Compared with norepinephrine, treatment with dopamine at doses up to 20 μg/kg/min was associated with a higher rate of tachyarrhythmias (24.1% vs. 12.4%) among 1679 patients with shock in the Sepsis Occurrence in Acutely Ill Patients (SOAP)-II trial. Intriguingly, in a subgroup analysis among the patients with cardiogenic shock ($n = 280$, 17% of the total trial population) in SOAP II, dopamine was not only associated with more arrhythmic events but also with a trend toward increased 28-day mortality (approximately 50% vs. 40%, log-rank P value .03, P-interaction by shock type of septic, hypovolemic, and cardiogenic = 0.87).[28]

Norepinephrine

Norepinephrine is also an endogenous catecholamine that is a potent beta-1 and alpha-1 agonist (Table 21.5). The most prominent effect of norepinephrine is vasoconstriction secondary to alpha-1 stimulation. The effect of beta-1 stimulation on heart rate and cardiac output may be counterbalanced by reflex bradycardia and increased afterload that occurs as a result of increased SVR. In the SOAP II randomized trial, norepinephrine was similar to dopamine with respect to survival for the overall trial population with shock, including septic, hypovolemic, and cardiogenic but was associated with fewer complications.[28] The Surviving Sepsis Campaign recommends norepinephrine as the first vasoactive agent for sepsis with the possible addition of vasopressin to allow for norepinephrine dose reduction.[43] Norepinephrine is generally recommended over dopamine, except in cases of relative bradycardia or severe pulmonary hypertension.[28]

Epinephrine

Epinephrine, secreted from the adrenal medulla, is an activator of alpha and beta-adrenergic receptors, resulting in increased heart rate, cardiac output, and vascular tone (Tables 21.4 and 21.5). It is often reserved for refractory shock as a second- or third-line agent, anaphylaxis, or during cardiac arrest. Epinephrine use has been associated with a transient increase in lactate; the mechanism is believed to be due to exaggerated aerobic glycolysis through Na+/K+ ATPase stimulation within skeletal muscles, rather than to persistent tissue dysoxia. There are no data to suggest this transient increase in lactate worsens outcomes.

Epinephrine was compared to norepinephrine in OptimaCC (Study Comparing the Efficacy and Tolerability of Epinephrine and Norepinephrine in Cardiogenic Shock) in 57 patients with cardiogenic shock. Epinephrine was inferior to norepinephrine for the post-hoc composite outcome of refractory cardiogenic shock, defined as sustained hypotension, end-organ hypoperfusion, and hyperlactatemia, and high inotrope and vasopressor doses. Notably, this endpoint includes hyperlactatemia, which was observed in the OptimaCC trial and, as described above, may not be reflective of systemic hypoperfusion. While epinephrine is recommended during cardiac arrest according to the advanced cardiovascular life support algorithm, studies suggest that those who received epinephrine in the setting of out-of-hospital cardiac arrest had higher rates of return of spontaneous circulation, but equivalent or even worse survival and neurologic function.[44] Additional studies of epinephrine in cardiac arrest are needed to understand whether the adverse effects of epinephrine may outweigh the benefits.

Phenylephrine

Phenylephrine is a synthetic, selective alpha-1 agonist that results in systemic vasoconstriction and often, reflex bradycardia. Based on its potent vasoconstrictor properties, its use is primarily reserved for vasodilatory shock. As with other vasoconstrictors, phenylephrine can cause significant peripheral ischemia at high doses.

Vasopressin

Vasopressin: Vasopressin, or antidiuretic hormone (ADH), is a peptide hormone that is synthesized in the hypothalamus and secreted from the pituitary gland in response to decreased intravascular volume or plasma hyperosmolality. Its vasopressor activity is thought to result from arterial smooth muscle contraction mediated through V1 receptor agonism on the systemic vasculature (Table 21.5). Vasopressin is typically used for refractory vasodilatory shock, and particularly, septic shock. Vasopressin is often used as an adjunct in septic shock, allowing for lower doses of catecholamines, a strategy that was shown to have equivalent mortality to high dose norepinephrine in the Vasopressin and Septic Shock Trial (VASST).[43] We also occasionally use this 'adrenergic-sparing' approach in patients with severe heart failure, particularly in the setting of mixed cardiogenic and vasodilatory shock. This strategy is based on the hypothesis that endogenous vasopressin may fall over time due to the depletion of neurohypophyseal stores and norepinephrine-induced inhibition of vasopressin, and that vasopressin may counter the mechanisms underlying inflammatory vasodilation, including K_{ATP} channel activation and nitric oxide production.

Other Vasoconstrictors

Angiotensin II is a potent endogenous vasoconstrictor that has been approved for use in distributive shock.[45] This agent was shown to improve blood pressure in patients with catecholamine-resistant vasoplegic shock in the

TABLE 21.5 Inotropic and Vasopressor Dose Range, Receptor Binding, Indications, and Major Clinical Side Effects

DRUG	CLINICAL INDICATION(S)	DOSE RANGE	RECEPTOR BINDING α_1	β_1	β_2	DA	MAJOR SIDE EFFECTS
Catecholamines							
Dopamine	Shock (cardiogenic, vasodilatory) Symptomatic bradycardia unresponsive to atropine or pacing	2.0–20 μg/kg/min (max 50 μg/kg/min)	+++	++++	++	+++++	Severe hypertension (especially in patients taking nonselective beta-blocker) Ventricular arrhythmias Cardiac ischemia Tissue ischemia/gangrene (high doses or due to tissue extravasation)
Dobutamine	Low CO (decompensated HF, cardiogenic shock, sepsis-induced myocardial dysfunction) Symptomatic bradycardia unresponsive to atropine or pacing	2.0–10 μg/kg/min	+	+++++	+++	N/A	Tachycardia Increased ventricular response rate in patients with atrial fibrillation Ventricular arrhythmias Cardiac ischemia Hypotension
Norepinephrine	Shock (vasodilatory, cardiogenic)	0.01–3 μg/kg/min	++++	+++	+	N/A	Arrhythmias Bradycardia Peripheral (digital) ischemia Hypertension (especially in patients taking nonselective beta-blocker)
Epinephrine	Shock (cardiogenic, vasodilatory) Cardiac arrest Bronchospasm/anaphylaxis Symptomatic bradycardia or heart block unresponsive to atropine or pacing	*Infusion*: 0.01–0.10 μg/kg/min *Bolus*: 1 mg IV every 3–5 min (max. 0.2 mg/kg) *IM*: (1:1000): 0.1–0.5 mg (max 1 mg)	++++	++++	+++	N/A	Ventricular arrhythmias Severe hypertension Cardiac ischemia
Isoproterenol	Bradyarrhythmias (especially torsades de pointes) Brugada syndrome	2–10 μg/min	0	+++++	+++++	N/A	Ventricular arrhythmias Cardiac ischemia Hypertension, hypotension
Phenylephrine	Hypotension (vagally mediated, medication-induced) Increase MAP with AS and hypotension Decrease LVOT gradient in HCM	*Bolus*: 0.1–0.5 mg IV every 10–15 min *Infusion*: 0.4–9.1 μg/kg/min	+++++	0	0	N/A	Reflex bradycardia Hypertension (especially with nonselective beta-blockers) Severe peripheral and visceral vasoconstriction Tissue necrosis with extravasation
Other Agents							
Milrinone	Low CO (decompensated HF, after cardiotomy)	*Bolus*: 50 μg/kg bolus over 10–30 min *Infusion*: 0.375–0.75 μg/kg/min (dose adjustment necessary for renal impairment)	N/A				Ventricular arrhythmias Hypotension Cardiac ischemia Torsades de pointes
							Arrhythmias, enhanced AV conduction (increased ventricular response rate in atrial fibrillation)Hypotension Thrombocytopenia Hepatotoxicity
Vasopressin	Shock (vasodilatory, cardiogenic) Cardiac arrest	*Infusion*: 0.01–0.1 U/min (common fixed dose 0.04 U/min) *Bolus*: 40 U IV	V_1 receptors (vascular smooth muscle) V_2 receptors (renal collecting duct system)				Arrhythmias Hypertension Decreased CO (at doses >0.4 U/min) Cardiac ischemia Severe peripheral vasoconstriction causing ischemia (especially skin)Splanchnic vasoconstriction
Levosimendan	Decompensated HF	*Loading dose*: 12–24 μg/kg over 10 min *Infusion*: 0.05–0.2 μg/kg/min	N/A				Tachycardia, enhanced AV conduction Hypotension

α_1, α_1-adrenergic receptor; *AS*, aortic stenosis; *AV*, atrioventricular; β_1, β1-receptor; β_2, β_2-receptor; *CO*, cardiac output; *DA*, dopamine receptors; *HCM*, hypertrophic cardiomyopathy; *HF*, heart failure; *IM*, intramuscular; *IV*, intravenous; *LVOT*, left ventricular outflow tract; *MAP*, mean arterial pressure; *max.*, maximum; *N/A*, not applicable. *Receptor binding*: 0 = zero significant receptor affinity; + to +++++ = minimal to maximal relative receptor affinity.
Adapted from Overgaard CB, Dzavik V. *Circulation*. 2008;118(10):1047–1056.

Angiotensin II for the Treatment of High-Output Shock 3 (ATHOS-3) trial. Experience with this agent is limited in patients with cardiac insufficiency. Methylene blue is an inhibitor of guanylate cycle that decreases cGMP in vascular smooth muscle and results in vasoconstriction. Methylene blue increased mean arterial pressure and SVR as well as improved mortality in a small study of patients with vasoplegia following cardiopulmonary bypass ($n = 58$). Its use is contraindicated in cardiogenic shock with normal or high SVR due to a resultant decrease in cardiac output.

Inotropes

Inotropes augment cardiac output through an increase in contractility. Those agents used most for this effect (dobutamine and milrinone) also increase heart rate and reduce SVR (Table 21.5). Dobutamine is a synthetic sympathomimetic amine, and milrinone is a phosphodiesterase-3 enzyme (PDE) inhibitor; thereby, both agents result in increased intracellular cyclic AMP. Milrinone has a longer half-life than dobutamine (~2.5 h vs. 2 min with normal renal function) and also tends to be associated with greater pulmonary vasodilatation and fewer atrial tachyarrhythmic events. In the CAPITAL DOREMI study, a randomized trial of milrinone versus dobutamine in 192 subjects with cardiogenic shock, there were no significant differences in the primary composite of all-cause death, resuscitated cardiac arrest, heart transplant, mechanical circulatory support, myocardial infarction, transient ischemic attached, stroke or need for renal replacement therapy or the secondary endpoint of all-cause death between treatment arms.[46] It should be noted that in a randomized trial of acute heart failure without shock (Outcomes of a Prospective Trial of Intravenous Milrinone for Exacerbations of Chronic Heart Failure), milrinone did not improve mortality compared with placebo. As a result, inotropic therapy is typically restricted to those who cannot be managed with vasodilator and diuretic therapy alone. The CAPITAL DOREMI2 trial is currently underway to evaluate all-cause mortality in patients with cardiogenic shock randomized to a single-agent inotrope (dobutamine or milrinone) versus placebo.[47]

Levosimendan is a "calcium-sensitizer" that increases myofilament response to calcium at lower concentrations, thereby improving myocardial contractility without increasing oxygen demand or intracellular calcium overload. In addition, levosimendan has systemic and coronary vasodilatory effects through action on the K_{ATP} channels in vascular smooth muscle. Despite the theoretical benefits of increased contractility and vasodilatation in heart failure, a survival benefit has not been observed in larger-scale clinical trials.[48] While there appears to be a benefit in patients with cardiogenic shock, particularly when combined with catecholamines to maintain adequate perfusion pressures, the small number of patients studied with cardiogenic shock limits interpretation.[48]

Vasodilators

Nitrates are endothelium-independent vasodilators of the peripheral and coronary vasculature. Venodilation decreases cardiac preload and more modest, arterial dilation may result in decreased afterload. Additionally, nitrates can improve coronary flow, including via collaterals. Despite a lack of data showing a reduction in recurrent major adverse cardiovascular events, because of these favorable physiological effects viewed by expert consensus, intravenous nitroglycerin is recommended in patients with ACS and heart failure and/or persistent ischemia. Sodium nitroprusside is an intravenous vasodilator with a more balanced effect on venodilation and arteriodilation that is easily titrated and may be particularly useful in the setting of heart failure with hypertension or acute ischemic mitral regurgitation. Nitroprusside can produce significant hypotension and, in the setting of prolonged use or renal dysfunction, thiocyanate toxicity. Due to the arterial vasodilation and associated drop in blood pressure, neither agent should be used early in the setting of cardiogenic shock unless the hemodynamic profile reveals predominantly very high SVR with normal blood pressure (i.e., the normotensive shock phenotype). Vasodilators (particularly intravenous nitroglycerin) can be cautiously added in patients following stabilization of blood pressure to decrease preload and congestion.

Volume Management

Diuretics are the mainstay of therapy to reduce preload in patients with heart failure without shock. Intravenous loop diuretics are the recommended first line therapy, with bolus dosing and continuous infusions producing similar results in terms of symptoms, effective diuresis and outcomes.[10,12] Thiazide diuretics can be added to improve diuretic responsiveness. In patients hospitalized with acute heart failure, the addition of acetazolamide (versus placebo) to intravenous loop diuretics increased the rate of successful decongestion and reduced length of stay across the range of renal function and LVEF, at the cost of a greater rise in creatinine that was not sustained at 3 months.[49]

Ultrafiltration (UF) is generally reserved for patients with persistent congestion that is refractory to maximally-escalated medical therapy. This limited use is based on findings from Cardiorenal Rescue Study in Acute Decompensated Heart Failure (CARRESS-HF) where 188 patients with acute decompensated heart failure, progressive renal dysfunction and ongoing congestion were randomized to stepped medical therapy, including loop and thiazide diuretics and selective use of vasodilators and inotropes, or UF.[10] Ultrafiltration was inferior to medical therapy as assessed by worsening renal function in the UF arm compared to improved renal function in the medical therapy arm.

Additional Pharmacological Therapies for Heart Failure Without Shock

Renin-angiotensin-aldosterone system inhibition:
Inhibition of the renin-angiotensin-aldosterone system is recommended in post-MI patients with heart failure or left ventricular dysfunction based on improved survival. The rationale for inhibition of the renin-angiotensin-aldosterone system (RAAS) includes experimental and clinical evidence of a favorable impact on ventricular remodeling, improvement in hemodynamics, and reductions in heart failure.

Unequivocal evidence from randomized, placebo-controlled trials shows that ACE inhibitors reduce the rate of mortality in patients with reduced ejection fraction or clinical signs of heart failure after acute MI. In all but one trial in such patients, ACE inhibitor therapy was initiated between 3 and 16 days after MI and maintained for 1–4 years. In unselected patients with acute MI, ACE inhibitors administered for a short duration of therapy saves 5 lives per 1000 patients treated. In patients at higher risk of adverse remodeling, such as patients with anterior infarction, ACE inhibitors offer a greater benefit from early administration (11 lives saved per 1000). In patients with ventricular dysfunction or heart failure among whom ACE inhibitors were administered for longer duration (years), this benefit is greater with 42–76 lives saved per 1000 patients treated. In patients with acute MI at risk for heart failure, the mortality reduction with ACE inhibitors is accompanied by significant reductions in the development of heart failure, supporting the underlying pathophysiological rationale for administering this class of drugs in patients with acute MI. Patients with acute MI and anterior infarction, prior infarction, Killip Class II or greater, or evidence of depressed global ventricular function on an imaging study should receive life-long treatment with ACE inhibitors.

An alternative method of pharmacological inhibition of the RAAS is by administration of ARBs. The VALIANT trial compared the effects of the ARB valsartan versus captopril alone and in combination with captopril on mortality in patients with acute MI complicated by left ventricular systolic dysfunction and/or heart failure randomized within 10 days of MI.10 Rates of mortality were similar in the three treatment groups: 19.9 percent in the valsartan group, 19.3 percent in the valsartan plus captopril group, and 19.5 percent in the captopril alone group. The choice between ACE inhibition and an ARB following acute MI should be based on physician experience with the agents, patient tolerability, safety, convenience, and cost.

An angiotensin receptor/neprilysin inhibitor (ARNi) combines an ARB and an inhibitor of neprilysin, an enzyme that degrades natriuretic peptides, bradykinin, adrenomedullin, and other vasoactive peptides. The PARADISE-MI trial tested whether treatment with sacubitril-valsartan as compared with enalapril would also reduce cardiovascular death or HF hospitalization when initiated shortly after acute MI in patients with no previous HF but with reduced LVEF (≤40%) and/or pulmonary congestion. Although sacubitril-valsartan did not significantly reduce these outcomes relative to enalapril, the trend favored sacubitril-valsartan (HR 0.90, 95% CI 0.78–1.04), suggesting that the trial may have been underpowered. Moreover, given the superiority of sacubitril-valsartan in other HF settings, initiation of ARNi is also considered an appropriate first line alternative to ACE inhibitor or ARB therapy in patients with heart failure after acute MI.Aldosterone blockade is another pharmacological strategy for inhibition of the RAAS. The EPHESUS trial randomized 6642 patients with acute MI complicated by left ventricular dysfunction and heart failure to the selective aldosterone blocker eplerenone or placebo in conjunction with contemporary postinfarction pharmacotherapy.[10] During a mean follow-up period of 16 months, there was a 15% reduction in the relative risk of mortality favoring eplerenone. Cardiovascular mortality or hospitalization for cardiovascular events was also reduced by eplerenone. Serious hyperkalemia (serum potassium concentration >6 mmol/L) occurred in 5.5% of patients in the eplerenone group compared with 3.9% of patients in the placebo group ($P < .002$). We favor long-term administration of aldosterone blockade for high-risk patients following STEMI (ejection fraction <40%, clinical heart failure, diabetes mellitus) who are already receiving an ACE inhibitor and beta blocker and do not have contraindications. Given the small but definite increase in the risk of serious hyperkalemia when aldosterone blockade is prescribed, particularly when other measures for inhibition of the RAAS are used concurrently, periodic monitoring of the serum potassium level should be undertaken.

Beta-adrenergic blockers

Beta-adrenergic blockers: While beta blockade is recommended in the setting of uncomplicated acute MI (Class I), it is contraindicated with patients with shock and caution is recommended for patients at-risk for cardiogenic shock.[1,4] The recommendations for at-risk patients are based on findings from the Clopidogrel and Metoprolol in Myocardial Infarction Trial (COMMIT) in which 45,852 patients were randomized to early intravenous and subsequent high-dose oral metoprolol or placebo within 24 hours of MI, most of who presented with STEMI and were treated with fibrinolysis or medical therapy alone.[24] Lower rates of recurrent MI and ventricular fibrillation in those randomized to metoprolol were counterbalanced by higher rates of cardiogenic shock, particularly in those with older age (>70 years), lower systolic blood pressure (<120 mmHg), elevated heart rate (>110 beats per min) and late presentation. An observational study in the NCDR registry of 34,661 patients with NSTEMI or STEMI treated with more contemporary therapies, including PCI, found that in addition to older age, increased heart rate and lower blood pressure, a history of heart failure and left ventricular dysfunction (ejection fraction <40%) were risk factors for cardiogenic shock or death following beta blocker use.

In contrast, other studies have demonstrated improved long-term outcomes with sub-acute initiation of chronic beta blockade following MI in patients with left ventricular dysfunction or heart failure. For example, the Carvedilol Post-Infarct Survival Control in Left Ventricular Dysfunction (CAPRICORN) study, which randomized 1959 patients with reduced left ventricular systolic dysfunction following MI to carvedilol or placebo an average of 10 days post-MI, observed lower rates of death, recurrent MI and atrial and ventricular arrhythmias with beta blockade.[4,10] As a result, it recommended that beta blocker therapy be withheld in the first 24 hours for patients with heart failure or other risk factors for the development of shock. However, eligibility in-hospital for beta blocker therapy should be reassessed after 24 hours. Furthermore, patients with heart failure or left ventricular function should receive chronic beta blocker therapy for long-term secondary prevention.[1,4]Other Agents

Owing to the putative role of nitric oxide in causing inappropriately low systemic vascular resistance and myocardial depression in cardiogenic shock, tilarginine acetate, an inhibitor of nitric oxide synthase, was studied in patients with acute MI and cardiogenic shock (Fig. 21.9). The Tilarginine Acetate Injection in a Randomized International Study in Unstable MI Patients with Cardiogenic Shock (TRIUMPH) trial of 398 patients was stopped for futility with no difference in all-cause mortality at 30 days, despite an increase in blood pressure.[8]

Mechanical Circulatory Support

In severe cases of cardiogenic shock, pharmacologic therapy may not provide sufficient hemodynamic support. It is hypothesized that early and appropriate use of mechanical circulatory support (MCS) will interrupt the spiral of shock through improvement in cardiac output, blood pressure, and perfusion and therefore minimize ongoing ischemia, progressive ventricular dysfunction, development of multi-organ dysfunction, and death (Fig. 21.6). However, demonstration of an improvement in long-term survival in randomized trials is lacking with the exception of the use of microaxial flow-pump support (Impella CP) in patients with AMI-CS. The options and data for temporary MCS, including the intra-aortic balloon pump (IABP), Tandem Heart, Impella, and extracorporeal membrane oxygenation (ECMO) are discussed in this section.

Left Ventricular Support Devices

Intra-Aortic Balloon Pump (IABP)

The IABP was developed in the 1960s and remains the most employed left ventricular support device.[50] The IABP is a dual lumen device with an outer flexible balloon that is inflated with 20–50 cc of helium (Fig. 21.13). The device functions by counter-pulsation with inflation during diastole and deflation during systole (Fig. 21.14 and Table 21.6). Rapid deflation occurs at the start of systole during isovolumic contraction thereby reducing aortic end-diastolic pressure and left ventricular afterload, modestly augmenting cardiac output by ~0.5–1 L/min. Balloon inflation occurs at the beginning of diastole, just after the closure of the aortic valve, with a resultant increase in aortic diastolic pressure and coronary perfusion. The peak pressure of this diastolic augmentation is usually higher than peak systolic pressure and typically results in an increase in MAP despite providing afterload reduction.

The advantages of the IABP are ease of deployment, wide availability, and low cost. The most common arterial access site is the common femoral artery, although axillary and subclavian arterial access is also feasible (Table 21.6).

The IABP was studied in the largest, randomized trial of MCS devices in cardiogenic shock to date. The IABP SHOCK II trial demonstrated that treatment with an IABP as compared to usual care without an IABP did not significantly improve survival, renal function, or lactate clearance in AMI-CS patients undergoing PCI.[4] As a result, the routine use of an IABP in AMI-CS without mechanical complications is not recommended (class III).[40]

Impella Microaxial Flow Pumps

Impella support devices are non-pulsatile, microaxial flow pumps that use an Archimedes-screw design to propel blood from the inlet cannula situated in the left ventricle to the outlet area in the ascending aorta (Fig. 21.13 and Table 21.6). A performance (P) level is set, determining the rotational speed of the motor. The absolute flow, or device output, at any set performance level, is dependent on preload and afterload. A range of models exist that vary according to cannula size, maximum flows, and placement location. The Impella CP and 5.5 models can generate flows up to 3.5–4.0 and 5–5.5 L/min, respectively (Table 21.6). All models may be deployed through an axillary arterial approach; only the CP model may be placed percutaneously via the femoral artery.

Potential advantages of the Impella include direct unloading of the LV and relative ease of placement for Impella CP. While the Impella 5.5 requires surgical placement, it provides greater hemodynamic support and potentially lower rates of hemolysis than the CP. Limitations to the Impella devices include hemolysis, particularly at higher performance levels, inability to add an oxygenator, and challenges with device positioning and migration.

Until recently, adequately sized randomized trials comparing clinical outcomes of support with Impella versus no device in patients with cardiogenic shock had been lacking and comparisons of Impella versus alternate devices have demonstrated improved hemodynamics but had not been designed with sufficient statistical power to assess for potential mortality differences. However,[8] the DanGer shock trial evaluated Impella CP versus conventional guideline-driven treatment in patients with STEMI complicated by cardiogenic shock, excluding patients who remain comatose after cardiac arrest, and demonstrated a significant reduction with Impella support in the primary endpoint of all-cause mortality at 180 days[51,52] Death from any cause through 180 days occurred in 45.8% of the Impella group and 58.5% of the standard-care group (HR 0.74; (95% CI [0.55 to 0.99]; p=0.04). A composite safety endpoint of severe bleeding, limb ischemia, hemolysis, device failure, or worsening aortic regurgitation occurred in 24.0% of the Impella group and in 6.2% of the standard-care group (relative risk 4.74; 95% CI, 2.36 to 9.55). Moderate or severe bleeding and the need for renal replacement therapy were each increased ~2-fold and limb ischemia was increased ~5-fold in the Impella group.

TandemHeart

The TandemHeart percutaneous ventricular assist device is no longer commercially available. However, its history remains instructive regarding alternative frameworks for ventricular mechanical circulatory support. In its left-sided support configuration, the TandemHeart was used as a left atrial to aortic assist device (Fig. 21.13 and Table 21.6). The system consisted of a drainage catheter inserted into the left atrium via a trans-septal puncture approached from a femoral vein, a continuous flow external centrifugal pump and a return catheter that provided retrograde flow into a femoral artery. Flow, which ranged between 1–6 L/min, was dependent on the rotational speed of the pump, patient preload and afterload, and the diameter of the arterial cannula. An oxygenator could also be included in line to provide extracorporeal oxygenation, as needed.

A hemodynamic benefit of the TandemHeart system was that it directly unloaded the left atrium, reducing LV

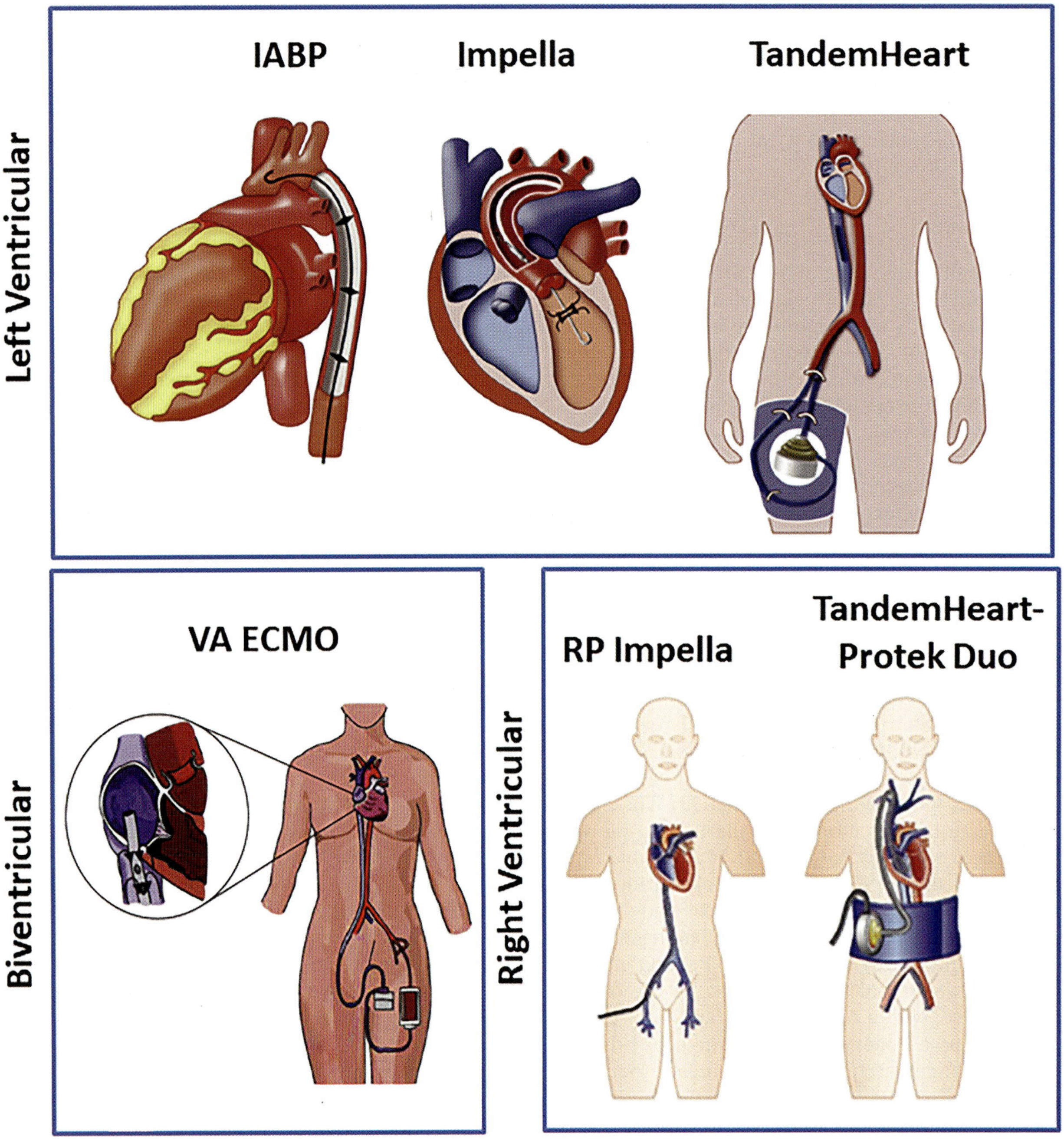

FIG. 21.13 Percutaneous temporary MCS devices. Left ventricular support devices include the intra-aortic balloon pump (IABP), Impella microaxial peripheral ventricular assist device, and the TandemHeart centrifugal pump. Impella 2.5, CP, and 5.0 may be placed via the femoral artery or via the axillary artery through a surgical graft. Right ventricular support devices include the RP Impella, TandemHeart pump with Protek Duo catheter, or VV-ECMO with the Protek Duo catheter (not shown). VA ECMO provides biventricular circulatory and ventilatory support. (Adapted from Thiele H, Ohman EM, de Waha-Thiele S, Zeymer U, Desch S. Management of cardiogenic shock complicating myocardial infarction: an update 2019. *Eur Heart J*. 2019;40(32):2671–2683.

end-diastolic pressure and pulmonary venous congestion (Table 21.6). This benefit had the potential to be counterbalanced by an increase in LV afterload due to the retrograde aortic flow. Disadvantages include the technical challenge of trans-septal catheter placement and large-bore femoral cannulation that is commensurate with cannula sizes for VA-ECMO.

As with other MCS devices, comparative data for TandemHeart with other devices were limited. TandemHeart was compared to IABP in a randomized trial of 42 patients presenting with cardiogenic shock. Patients randomized to TandemHeart had a higher cardiac index, higher MAP, and lower pulmonary capillary wedge pressure (PCWP) with no difference in clinical outcomes.[8]

Extra-Corporeal Membrane Oxygenation (ECMO)

VA-ECMO provides biventricular circulatory support as well as complete pulmonary support for oxygenation and ventilation. The basic peripheral VA-ECMO circuit includes a venous drainage cannula, an arterial/inflow cannula, an external centrifugal pump, and an oxygenator (Fig. 21.13 and Table 21.6). The venous/drainage cannula is placed into the right atrium or superior vena cava and serves as a conduit from which deoxygenated blood is transported via

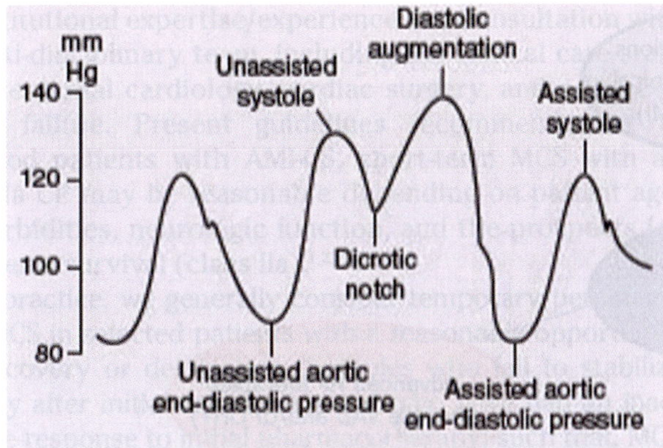

FIG. 21.14 Intra-aortic balloon pump pressure tracing. Aortic pressure tracing with an assist ratio of 1:2. As shown, balloon inflation occurs just prior to the dicrotic notch (aortic valve closure) and results in augmented diastolic pressure. Balloon deflation occurs near the end of diastole and results in an assisted end-diastolic pressure that is lower than the unassisted end-diastolic pressure, reflecting the lower afterload at the beginning of systole. The assisted systolic pressure is also lower than the unassisted pressure, again reflecting the reduction in afterload.

the pump through an oxygenator and is returned through an arterial/inflow cannula. The cannulas for VA-ECMO can be deployed peripherally or centrally (surgically). Like TandemHeart, the flow (range 1.5–6 L/min) is determined by the pump speed, patient preload and afterload, and inflow and outflow cannula sizes. Additionally, flow may be affected by high resistance across the oxygenator membrane, as can occur with pre- or post-membrane clot formation. In patients with severe renal insufficiency, a dialysis filter can be incorporated into the circuit.

The primary advantage of VA ECMO is that it provides full cardiopulmonary support, with biventricular circulatory and concomitant ventilatory support (Table 21.6). Additionally, VA ECMO may be deployed rapidly at the bedside, as is done during eCPR. The disadvantages are the requirement for large bore femoral cannulation in peripheral VA-ECMO, increased LV afterload due to retrograde return of flow via the femoral artery/distal aorta, and the significant risk of other complications, such as bleeding, limb ischemia, and North/South syndrome (upper body hypoxia). LV afterload induced by VA-ECMO can be minimized by limiting ECMO flows or counterbalanced by pharmacologically decreasing systemic vascular resistance or augmenting LV contractility. An alternative, commonly used approach to managing this increased afterload is via mechanical LV unloading or "venting" with concomitant use of an Impella or IABP. Additionally, atrial-septostomy or placement of a trans-septal LA cannula can be considered to allow for unloading via decompression of the left atrium.

Several trials of VA-ECMO in cardiogenic shock have recently been reported. The largest, ECLS-SHOCK, randomized 420 patients with AMI-CS within 12 hours of onset, a lactate of >3 mmol/L, and planned revascularization to early VA-ECMO or usual treatment, which allowed for use of other MCS devices in the setting of protocol-defined escalation.[52] There was no difference in the primary outcome of 30-day mortality (47.8% for VA-ECMO vs. 49.0% in usual care), with a 2.4- and 2.9-fold increased risk of moderate or severe bleeding and peripheral vascular complications requiring intervention, respectively. A meta-analysis of this and 3 other smaller trials similarly suggested no difference in mortality with a higher rate of complications with VA-ECMO.[53,54] Findings were consistent across several subgroups, including by magnitude of lactate elevation and preceding cardiac arrest. As such, it is unclear which, if any, populations might derive a mortality benefit from the routine use of VA-ECMO in AMI-CS; although it has been suggested that the selected phenotype enrolled in the DanGer trial might also benefit from VA-ECMO.

Right Ventricular Support Devices

Impella RP

The Impella RP, configured for right-sided support via femoral venous access, can generate a cardiac output of 4.0 L/

TABLE 21.6 Left-Sided Temporary Mechanical Circulatory Support Devices

FEATURE	IABP	IMPELLA (2.5, CP, 5.0, 5.5)	TANDEMHEART (TH)	VA ECMO (PERIPHERAL)
Max CO (L/min)	0.5	2.5, 4, 5, 5.5, respectively	5	6
Mechanism	Aortic counterpulsation	LV → Ao	LA → Ao	RA → Ao
SV	↑	↓	↓↓	↓↓
LV EDP	↓	↓↓	↓↓	↔/↑
LV Afterload	↓	-	↑	↑
Coronary Perfusion	↑	↑	↔/↑	↔/↑
RV support	No	No	No	Yes
Sheath (French)	7–8.5	12, 14, 23, and 23	A: 15–19 V: 21	A: 15–22 V: 21–25
Cannulation	Femoral, axillary, or subclavian	Femoral or axillary (surgical)	Femoral	Femoral or Central (surgical)
Resp Support	No	No	Yes (if oxygenator)	Yes
Relative Contraindication	Moderate/Severe AI or PAD; aortic dissection	Moderate/Severe AI or PAD; Critical aortic stenosis; LV thrombus; inability to anticoagulate	Moderate/Severe AI or PAD; left atrial thrombus; inability to anticoagulate	Moderate/Severe AI or PAD; inability to anticoagulate

Ao, Aorta; *AI*, aortic insufficiency; *CO*, cardia output; *EDP*, end-diastolic pressure; *IABP*, intraortic balloon pump; *LV*, left ventricle; *PAD*, peripheral artery disease; *RV*, right ventricular; *SV*, stroke volume.

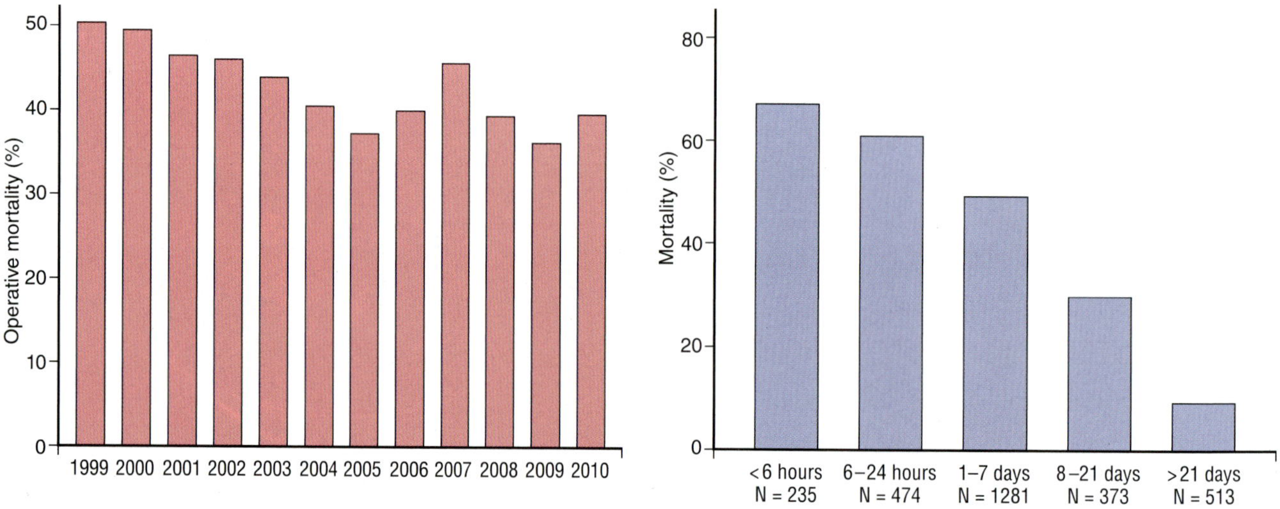

FIG. 22.14 Ventricular septal rupture surgical repair. Society of Thoracic Surgery National Database: ventricular septal defect repair in 2876 patients, 1999 to 2010. *(From Arnaoutakis GJ, et al: Surgical repair of ventricular septal defect after myocardial infarction: outcomes from the Society of Thoracic Surgeons National Database. Ann Thorac Surg 94:436, 2012.)*

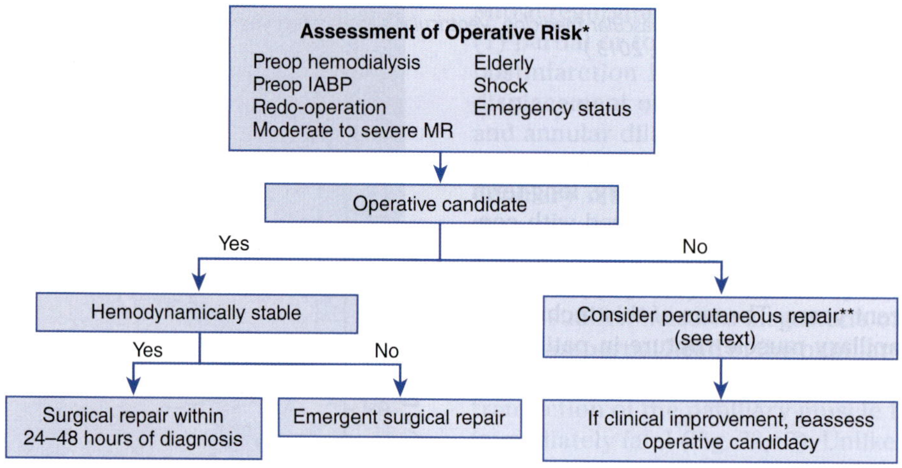

FIG. 22.15 Approach to ventricular septal rupture management. *Final risk assessment must be made in conjunction with the surgical team. **Should be considered if expertise is available. Should be followed by a definitive surgical repair if a satisfactory result is not achieved. *IABP*, Intra-aortic balloon pump; *MR*, mitral regurgitation.

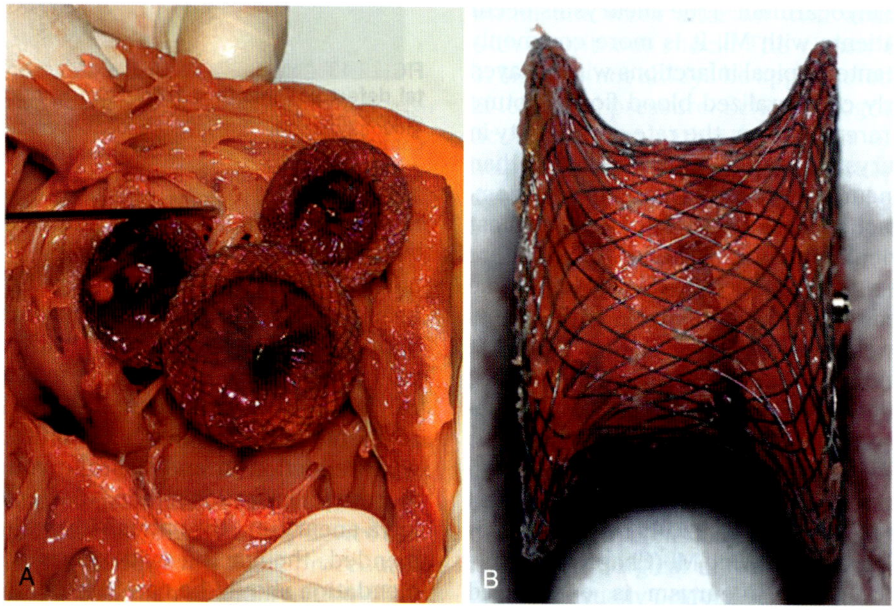

FIG. 22.16 Percutaneous closure of a ventricular septal defect (VSD). (**A**) Pathologic specimens of Amplatzer devices used to close a large post-infarction VSD. (**B**) Organized thrombus within the Amplatzer device. *(From Calvert P: Percutaneous Closure of Postinfarction Ventricular Septal Defect: In-Hospital Outcomes and Long-Term Follow-up of UK experience. Circulation 129:23, 2014.)*

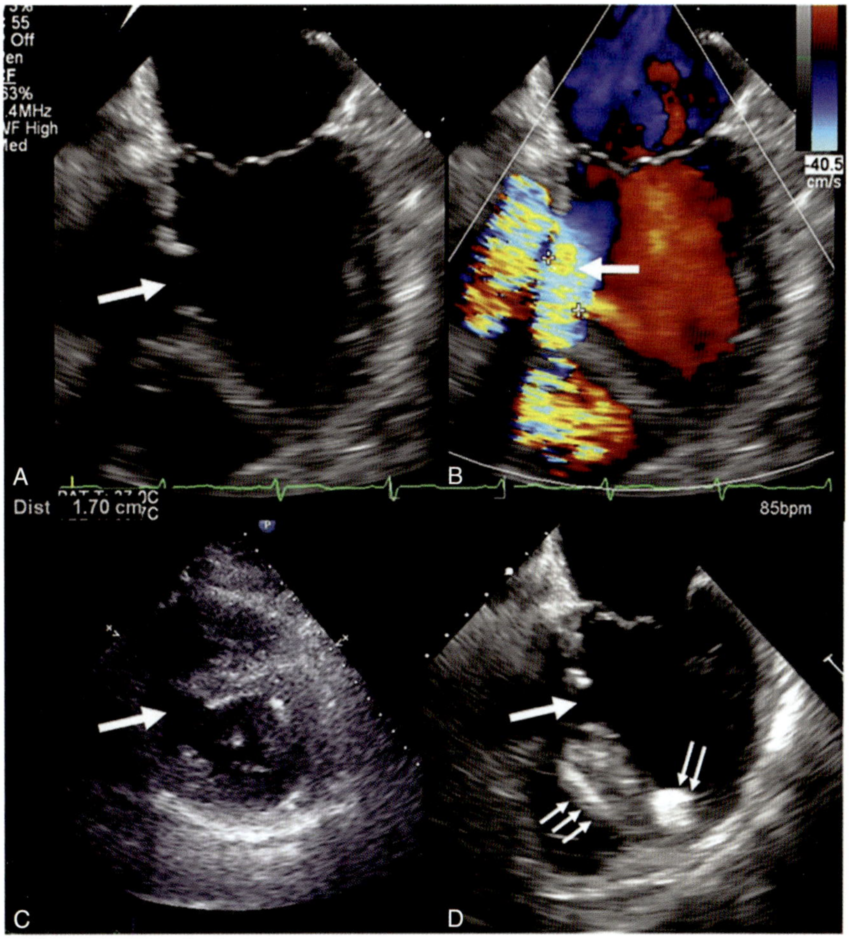

FIG. 22.17 Echocardiographic images of ventricular septal defects (VSDs) and percutaneous closure. (*All panels*) Ventricular septal defects (*single arrow*) on transesophageal echocardiogram. (**D**) Deployment of a 16-mm Amplatzer device (*double arrow*) still on the delivery cable (*triple arrow*). (From Amplatzer, Abbott are trademarks of Abbott or its related companies. Reproduced with permission of Abbott. © 2025 Abbott. All rights reserved.)

LEFT VENTRICULAR THROMBUS

During the acute phase of MI, endocardial inflammation, stasis of blood, and hypercoagulability can lead to mural thrombus formation and largely depend upon MI size and location (Fig. 22.18). Thrombus is most often seen in patients with large infarctions and associated aneurysms. The reported incidence of LV thrombus varies depending on the imaging modality used (e.g., echocardiography with or without contrast versus CMR) as well as the frequency and timing of cardiac imaging following MI (Figs. 22.19 and 22.e8). In the prereperfusion era, mural thrombus was associated with up to 60% of acute MI but is now likely less than 10%[13] due to the limitation of infarct size with rapid reperfusion. The predominant use of echocardiography as the diagnostic imaging modality may underestimate the true incidence. CMR has superior sensitivity and specificity in the detection of mural thrombus and is the current gold standard for its diagnosis.[13]

Clinical suspicion for LV thrombus should be considered for patients presenting with stroke or systemic embolism in the context of a recent (<3 months) MI, LV aneurysm, or decreased LV ejection fraction. The risk of thromboembolism due to mural thrombus has been reported to be as high as 16%, and increased risk is associated with thrombus mobility, its protrusion into the left ventricle, and time out of the anticoagulation therapeutic range.[13] Most thromboembolic events occur within the first 3 months of diagnosis.

There are no randomized trials evaluating the efficacy of extended duration of anticoagulation to prevent embolization in patients with LV thrombus after MI in the modern era. However, in studies of low molecular weight heparin during the initial hospitalization for acute MI, anticoagulation with the more effective anticoagulant also reduced the short-term risk of ischemic stroke. Current recommendations are based upon observational studies in patients with documented LV thrombus who had a reduced risk of embolization with anticoagulation and extrapolation from experiences when atrial fibrillation or heart failure complicate MI. Individual assessment regarding the risk of thromboembolization should be balanced against the risk of bleeding (Table 22.2). A recent scientific statement suggests that discontinuation of anticoagulation after 3 months should be considered if there is thrombus resolution and/or intercurrent major bleeding.[12]

Dual antiplatelet therapy (DAPT) does not appear to prevent mural thrombus formation in observational studies. It is reasonable to consider 3 months of

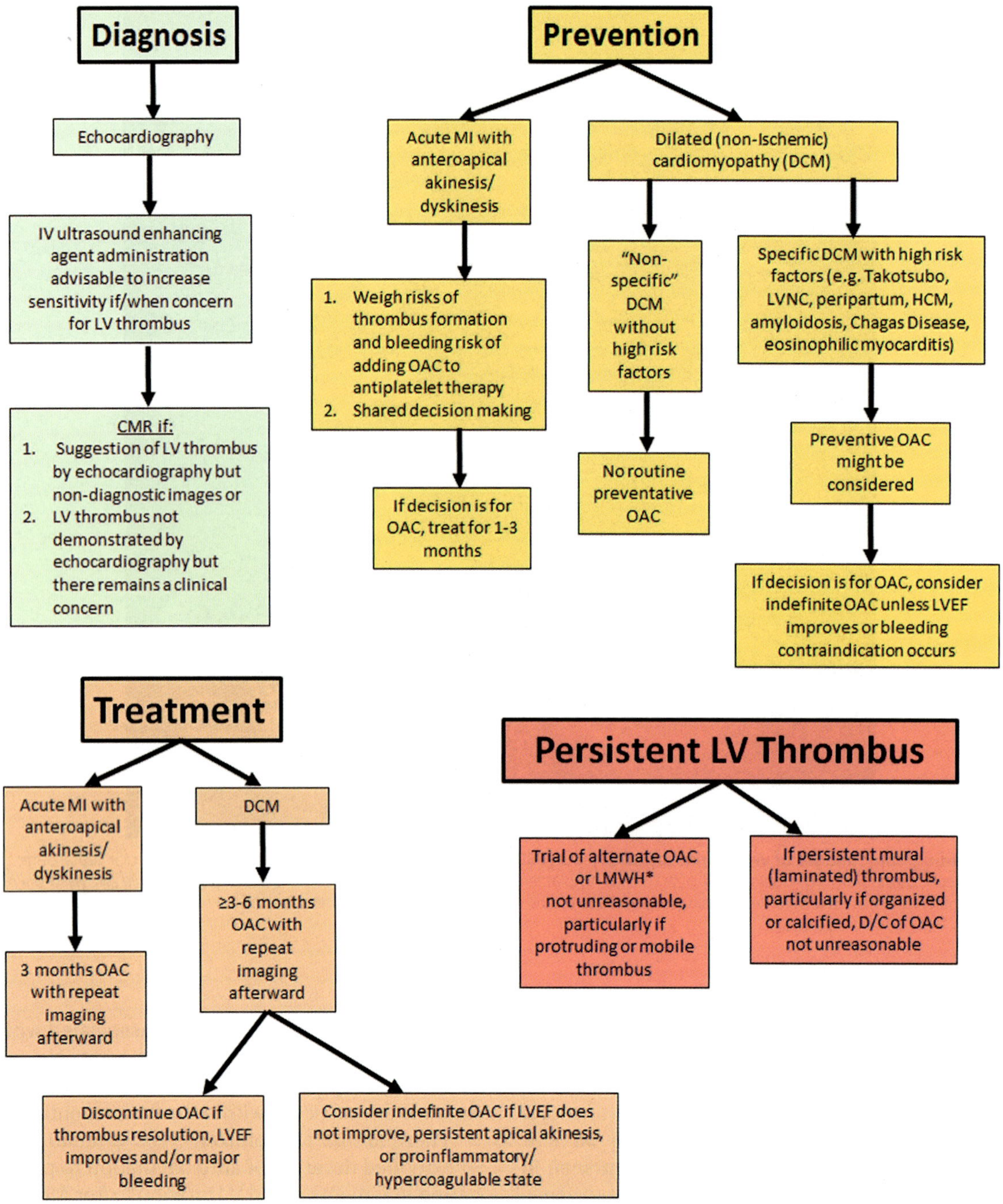

FIG. 22.18 Suggested strategies for the diagnosis, prevention and management of left ventricular thrombus. *CMR,* cardiac magnetic resonance; *D/C,* discontinuation; *DCM,* dilated cardiomyopathy; *HCM,* hypertrophic cardiomyopathy; *LMWH,* low-molecular-weight heparin; *LV,* left ventricular; *LVEF,* left ventricular ejection fraction; *LVNC,* left ventricular noncompaction; *MI,* myocardial infarction; *OAC,* oral anticoagulation; *VKA,* vitamin K antagonist. *Trial of *VKA* if persistent *LV* thrombus despite dual OAC; trial of dual OAC if persistent LV thrombus in the setting of consistent subtherapeutic international normalized ratio; and trial of LMWH if persistent LV thrombus in the setting of consistent therapeutic international normalized ratio. *(From: Levine G et al. Management of Patients at Risk for and With Left Ventricular Thrombus: A Scientific Statement From the American Heart Association. Circulation 146:15, 2022).*

anticoagulation in patients at high risk of thromboembolism, absent any data from prospective randomized data.[13] Direct oral anticoagulants (DOACs) are a reasonable alternative to vitamin K antagonists (VKA). In several meta-analyses of both randomized controlled trials and observational datasets, DOACs generally appear to be noninferior to VKA in relation to mortality, stroke, or LV thrombus resolution and are associated with less bleeding.[12] Surgical excision is rarely performed and generally limited to anecdotal reports when the thrombus is extremely large or performed during concomitant cardiac surgery (e.g., coronary bypass grafting).

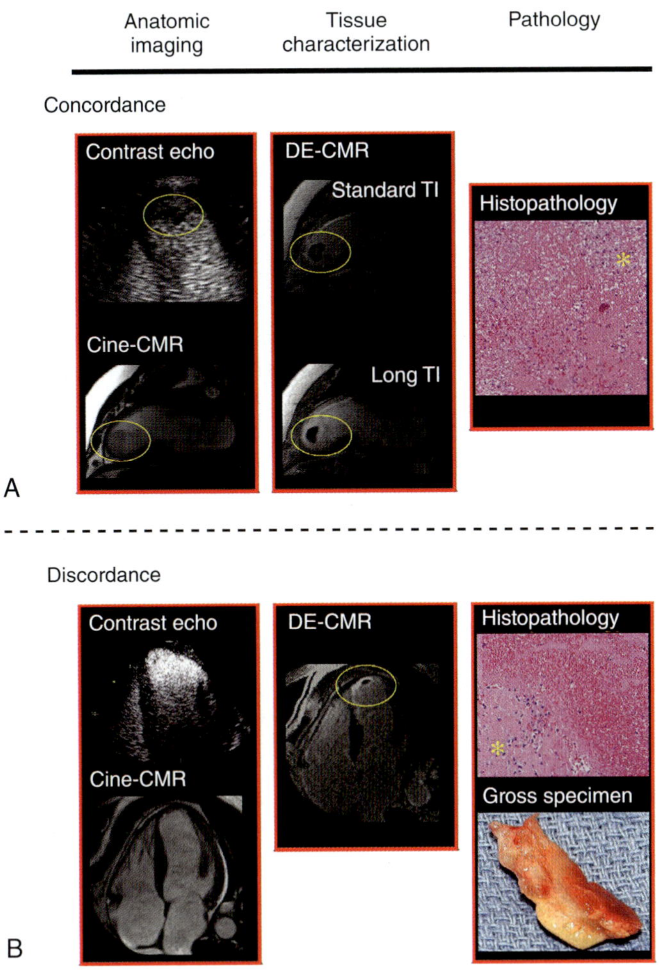

FIG. 22.19 Apical thrombus by anatomic and tissue characterization imaging. (**A**) Representative example of apical thrombus (*circle*) concordantly detected by anatomic imaging (*left,* contrast echocardiography four-chamber, cinecardiac magnetic resonance [CMR] two-chamber) and delayed enhancement (DE)- CMR (*center*). (**B**) Representative example of discordance between anatomic imaging and DE-CMR. DE-CMR identified a small mural thrombus (*circle*) within the apex. Cine-CMR and contrast echocardiography were interpreted as negative. For both examples, surgical resection enabled thrombus verification based on histopathology (*right,* hematoxylin and eosin stain, low power), which showed thrombus with associated fibroblasts (*asterisk*). *(From Weinsaft JW, et al: Contrast-enhanced anatomic imaging as compared to contrast-enhanced tissue characterization for detection of left ventricular thrombus. JACC Cardiovasc Imaging 2:972, 2009.)*

TABLE 22.2 Factors to Consider in Oral Anticoagulation Duration

Factors That Favor Continued OAC
Anteroapical MI with persistent akinesis
Protruding/mobile thrombus
Suspected or known cardioembolic event
Not high bleeding risk
Proinflammatory or hypercoagulable states
Recurrent LV thrombus
Factors That May or do not Favor Continued OAC
High bleeding risk
Concomitant antiplatelet therapy
Improvement in LVEF or focal akinesis
Persistent mural (laminated) thrombus, particularly if organized or calcified, despite therapeutic OAC

LV, Left ventricular; *LVEF*, left ventricular ejection fraction; *MI*, myocardial infarction; and *OAC*, oral anticoagulant.

REFERENCES

1. Tsao CW, Aday AW, Almarzooq ZI, et al. Heart disease and stroke statistics 2023 update, a report from the American Heart Association. *Circulation.* 2023;147:e93–e621.
2. Goldstein JA. Hemodynamic complications of right ventricular infarction. *JACC Case Rep.* 2021;3(9):1174–1176.
3. Femia G, French JK, Juergens C, et al. Right ventricular myocardial infarction: pathophysiology, clinical implications and management. *Rev Cardiovasc Med.* 2021;22(4):1229–1240.
4. Namana V, Gupta SS, Abbasi AA, Raheja H, Shani J, Hollander G. Right ventricular infarction. *Cardiovasc Revasc Med.* 2018;19:43–50.
5. Elbadawi A, Elgendy IY, Mahmoud K, et al. Temporal trends and outcomes of mechanical complications in patients with acute myocardial infarction. *JACC Cardiovasc Interv.* 2019;12(18):1825–1836.
6. Gong FF, Vaitenas I, Malaisrie SC, Maganti K. Mechanical complications of acute myocardial infarction: a review. *JAMA Cardiol.* 2021;6(3):341–349.
7. Matteucci M, Fina D, Jiritano F, et al. Treatment strategies for post-infarction left ventricular free-wall rupture. *Eur Heart J Acute Cardiovasc Care.* 2019;8(4):379–387.
8. Formica F, Mariani S, Singh G, et al. Postinfarction left ventricular free wall rupture: a 17-year single-centre experience. *Eur J Cardiothorac Surg.* 2018;53:150–156.
9. Damluji A, van Diepen S, Katz J, et al. Mechanical complications of acute myocardial infarction- a scientific statement from the American Heart Association. *Circulation.* 2021;144:e16–e35.
10. Giblett JP, Matetic A, Jenkins D, et al. Post-infarction ventricular septal defect: percutaneous or surgical management in the UK national registry. *Eur Heart J.* 2022;43:5020–5032.
11. Kilic A, Sultan I, Chu D, et al. Mitral valve surgery for papillary muscle rupture: outcomes in 1342 patients from The Society of Thoracic Surgeons Database. *Ann Thorac Surg.* 2020;110:1975–1982.
12. Levine GN, McEvoy JW, Fang JC, et al. Management of patients at risk for and with left ventricular thrombus: a scientific statement from the American Heart Association. *Circulation.* 2022;146:e205–e223.
13. Camaj A, Fuster V, Giustino G, et al. Left ventricular thrombus following acute myocardial infarction: JACC state-of-the-art review. *J Am Coll Cardiol.* 2022;7(10):1010–1022.

23 Arrhythmias and Sudden Cardiac Death After Myocardial Infarction

VARUN MALIK, JASON BRADFIELD, AND KALYANAM SHIVKUMAR

INTRODUCTION

Despite significant advances in the diagnosis and treatment of malignant cardiac arrhythmias, sudden cardiac death (SCD) constitutes 50% of all cardiovascular deaths, of which 25% to 50% represent the first symptomatic cardiac event.[1,2] In the last 2 to 3 decades, in the United States, approximately 230,000 to 350,000 deaths per year have been attributed to SCD.[1] It is widely acknowledged that most (approximately 80%) cases of SCD are due to coronary artery disease.[3] Therefore, there has been a great scientific push to advance our understanding of (1) the role of the burden of atherosclerosis and obstructive coronary disease in the outcome of SCD; (2) the electrophysiologic and structural remodeling effects of myocardial infarction (MI) upon the myocardium and, consequently, the propensity to develop lethal arrhythmias and (3) the effect of MI in producing ischemic cardiomyopathy. In conjunction with this inquiry at the "bench," there have been pivotal clinical studies at the "bedside" aimed at refining our stratification of SCD risk in patients with cardiovascular disease as well as guiding our approach to the management of high-risk patients such as those with ischemic cardiomyopathy. Despite these efforts, there are gaps in our knowledge in terms of the mechanisms and risk stratification of SCD. Since a significant number of patients die from out-of-hospital cardiac arrest with no cardiac monitoring at the time, the relationship between ischemia and presumed arrhythmia is difficult to ascertain. Although professional guidelines[1,2] suggest that patients at risk for SCD after MI often have an impaired left ventricular function (typically below 35%), SCD actually most commonly occurs in those with normal ejection fraction. Therefore, day-to-day clinical decision-making is complex, requiring significant clinical experience and judgment.

PATHOPHYSIOLOGY OF ARRHYTHMIAS IN MYOCARDIAL INFARCTION

Development of Preclinical Experimental Models

There is a need for preclinical (experimental models) to try to understand the mechanisms of SCD as well as ventricular arrhythmias (VA); particularly, ventricular fibrillation (VF) following MI. To this end, preparations have included: (1) in vitro models for cell-cell physiology; (2) ex vivo Langendorff perfusion models (both animal and human hearts); and (3) in vivo studies in both small and large animal models. In vitro models were developed because of the difficulty in obtaining microelectrode recordings from the beating heart. Various preparations can be used to examine transmembrane potentials or to detect changes in intracellular ion concentrations caused by ischemia. However, it is difficult to mimic the in vivo effects of ischemia, hypoxia, acidosis, and high potassium concentrations. The Langendorff perfusion model involves isolation of the heart and perfusion through the coronary arteries. The main disadvantage of this preparation is that the heart

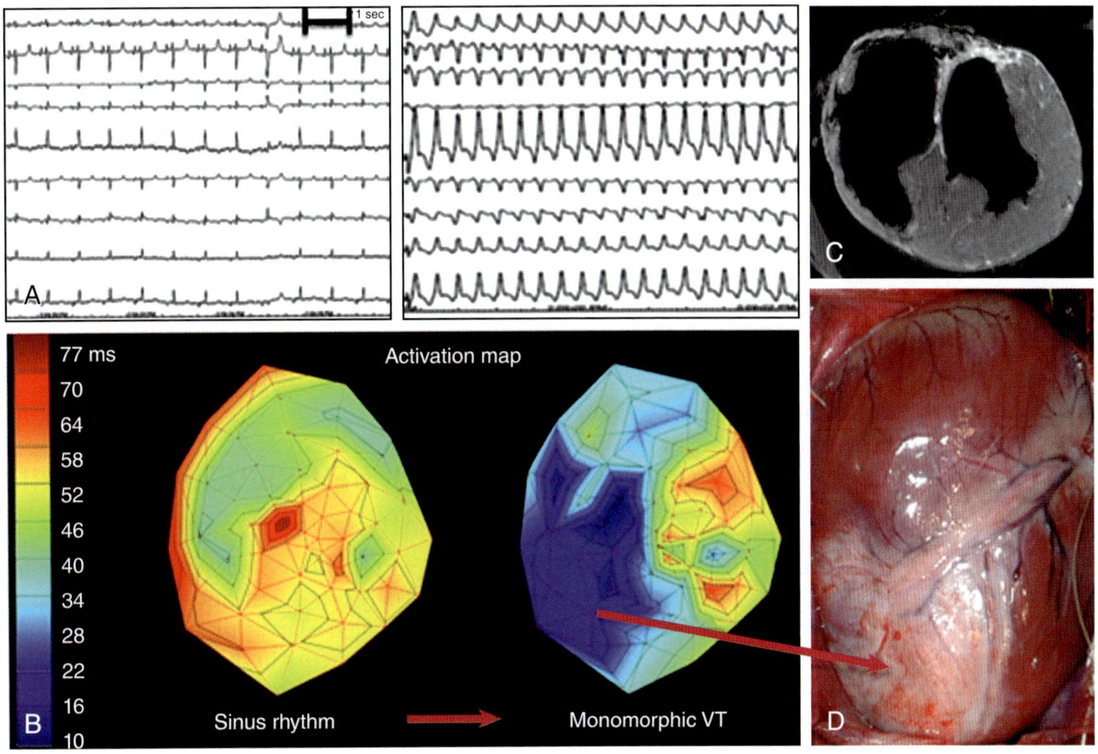

FIG. 23.1 Left anterior descending artery myocardial infarction in a porcine model with myocardial scar and ventricular tachycardia (VT). (A) A 12-lead electrocardiogram (ECG) shows sinus rhythm and subsequent VT in a porcine MI model (B) An example of a polar map of the activation time in sinus rhythm and VT, generated from a unipolar 56-electrode epicardial recording system, showing the earliest activation site in VT originating from the anterior wall of the left ventricle. A photo of the epicardial scar in vivo (D) in the same animal and cardiac magnetic resonance image (C) show the infarcted region.

is disconnected from the neural cardiac hierarchy (central nervous system, extrathoracic, and intrathoracic ganglia), which could alter arrhythmogenicity. Notably, this is similar to conditions following cardiac transplantation.

Many hurdles must be overcome in creating large animal models of MI and there are important limitations. The method of occlusion of the coronary artery varies. The coronary artery can either be ligated by means of a modified thoracotomy, embolized, or injected with ethanol (Fig. 23.e1). The duration of the ischemic period and the timing of reperfusion—early versus late versus nonreperfusion—both contribute to differing patterns of ischemia, scar, and border zones. Some investigators opt for a two-stage occlusion, with initial partial occlusion to create ischemic preconditioning and subsequent complete occlusion. In these studies, immediate lethal VA occur less frequently, probably owing to neural adaptation or memory to ischemia. Commonly, investigators will create a left anterior descending (LAD) infarct after the first diagonal (Fig. 23.e2) or a left circumflex artery infarct.

After 6 weeks, the substrate for subacute VA can be evaluated. However, arrhythmia induction in the terminal procedure is not guaranteed. Ventricular stimulation protocols, with up to three extra stimuli, at two different sites, epicardial and endocardial, are typically performed to assess for inducibility of ventricular tachyarrhythmia. On occasion, acute ischemia in a different territory can be induced in the setting of an already established chronic infarct to induce more electrical instability. Sympathetic stimulation with isoproterenol infusions or stellate ganglia stimulation is also employed to potentiate electrical instability. Despite these interventions, arrhythmia induction appears to occur in only 30% to 60% of canines and slightly more frequently in porcine models. Cardiac 3-dimensional electroanatomic substrate mapping and cardiac imaging modalities such as magnetic resonance imaging (MRI) or echocardiography often are combined to provide additional information on the relationship of scar to VA inducibility (Fig. 23.1).

Differences exist in coronary vascular anatomy among species. Porcine models have limited or no coronary collaterals, so in such preparations, at the time of infarction, VF due to accelerated cell death is common. Canine coronary artery occlusion results in a predominantly subendocardial infarction, versus transmural infarction seen in the porcine model. Differences in collateral development and patterns of infarction can alter the experimental model and its relation to clinical findings. Thus, experimental models, upon which our current understanding of cardiac arrhythmias after MI or SCD is based, are imperfect at mimicking the human condition.

Cellular Electrophysiologic Effects of Myocardial Ischemia

Myocardial ischemia affects the resting membrane potential and inward and outward currents, altering conduction, refractoriness, and automaticity. During ischemia, an initial increase in extracellular K^+ results in a reduction in resting membrane potential.[4] Within the first 15 minutes of ischemia, these changes in resting membrane potential are rapidly reversible and can return to normal. The changes in extracellular K^+ occur in two phases: After the first 15 minutes, a plateau or slight decrease is seen in extracellular K^+, which then starts to rise again in the second phase, corresponding with irreversible cell death. It is thought that the plateau phase may be related to the release of catecholamines, which pushes K^+ intracellularly owing to enhanced activation of the Na^+-K^+ pump. This pump, which is responsible for K^+ influx into the cell, is energy consuming. A reduction in available energy in the first 10 to 15 minutes may result in depression of the Na^+-K^+ pump. Efflux of K^+ is due to a complex set of changes that are a result of net inward currents and accumulation of ischemic metabolites. Other elements that contribute to membrane potential alterations, such as Ca^{2+} and magnesium, potentially have some effect on depolarization as a consequence of intracellular accumulation. Additionally, accumulation of the metabolites of phospholipids in the ischemic myocardium may affect the membrane potential.

Myocardial Scar Development Secondary to Ischemia

After 15 to 20 minutes of complete coronary occlusion in a canine model, signs of cell death are evident. The exact timing of cell death with occlusion in humans is not clear. MI can result in transmural necrotic myocardial tissue, but more commonly seen are patchy areas of surviving myocytes. During ischemia, the cells die gradually, and the infarct can increase in size, initially being localized to the subendocardial layer and then spreading to the endocardium and mid- and subepicardium. This pattern evolves because under normal conditions, the coronary blood supply is greatest in the mid- and subepicardial layers, and collaterals are more numerous in the subepicardium. After ischemic injury, necrotic myocardium is replaced by fibrotic tissue that surrounds the surviving myocytes. Ischemia results in abnormal refractoriness, abnormal conduction velocities, altered excitability, and automaticity, which can facilitate ventricular arrhythmias.[4] Importantly, surrounding the infarcted tissue, a "border zone" separates normal myocytes from the scar. Several recent studies highlight the arrhythmogenicity of this area, which is independent of left ventricular ejection fraction (LVEF).[5–8] Scar characterization with magnetic resonance imaging (MRI) using late gadolinium enhancement has provided key observations. Areas of scar border zones, and the presence of channels (which correlate with VA substrate identified by voltage mapping during ablation) were much more likely in those with VA post-ST-elevation MI (STEMI) than in matched controls who presented with STEMI and without VA during follow-up.[5] The MRI in this nested, retrospective case-control substudy of the Danish Acute Myocardial Infarction-3 multicenter trial and the Danegaptide phase II proof-of-concept clinical trial was taken 3 months after presentation with STEMI and acute percutaneous coronary intervention (PCI).[5] In an animal study, the border zone of anterior-septal infarcts (studied 4 weeks following coronary occlusion) was associated with the origin of ventricular ectopic beats, delayed after depolarizations and spontaneous action potentials corresponding with ventricular ectopic beats (in vitro) as well as VA at elevated heart rates. This area was susceptible to heightened sympathetic efferent (autonomic) tone.[6]

LVEF remains suboptimal in the characterization of the risk of VA and SCD following acute MI. The assessment of substrate for VA (channels within scar), border zone area, and perhaps alterations within the border zone in terms of arrhythmogenicity and autonomic function represent research priorities.

A border zone region can contain essential regions of slow conduction (channels) for reentrant substrates or function as a site of focal impulse origin (Fig. 23.2).

TIMING OF VENTRICULAR ARRHYTHMIAS

Early Ventricular Arrhythmias

Early VA (within 30 min of ischemia) occur in two phases according to (both small and large) animal models.[4] The first phase, called Harris phase *1a* (made up of so-called immediate VA), occurs in the first 2 to 10 minutes after coronary occlusion, with the highest incidence of arrhythmias at approximately 5 to 6 minutes. The second phase, called *1b*, usually occurs from 12 to 30 minutes after coronary occlusion, with a peak at 15 to 20 minutes. It is unclear if humans have the same 2-phase response with early arrhythmias.

The underlying mechanism appears to be different for each phase. *Phase 1a arrhythmias* appear to demonstrate conduction slowing and delayed activation of the subepicardial electrograms. The electrograms in these arrhythmias are markedly heterogeneous, with the sharp action potential becoming slurred and biphasic and even spanning diastole (diastolic bridging). Other features include an increase in the refractory period and marked conduction delay. It is thought that phase 1a arrhythmias are caused by reentrant arrhythmias with an appropriately timed trigger, such as a premature ventricular contraction (PVC). Heterogeneous electrical activation between the epicardium and the endocardium, and a delay after depolarization, facilitates reentry.

Phase 1b arrhythmias are thought to be a result of endogenous catecholamine release, which could occur in the 12- to 30-minute period after MI. Information is lacking about whether arrhythmias occur in the same pattern in humans during the first 30 minutes of ischemia. After 3–6 hours, arrhythmias are very infrequent and after 8 to 24 hours, PVCs gradually increase in frequency.

Delayed Ventricular Arrhythmias

Delayed VA occur 24 to 72 hours after MI, with PVCs, accelerated idioventricular rhythms, and ventricular tachycardia (VT)/VF seen on the electrocardiogram (ECG). The autonomic component of the peripheral nervous system appears to play a critical role in the emergence of delayed VA. In fact, autonomic modulation with therapies such as thoracic epidural anesthesia or sympathetic denervation is recognized to reduce the incidence of VA related to MI.[9]

Several mechanisms may underlie delayed VA. Long cycle lengths with a long coupling interval PVC, late in

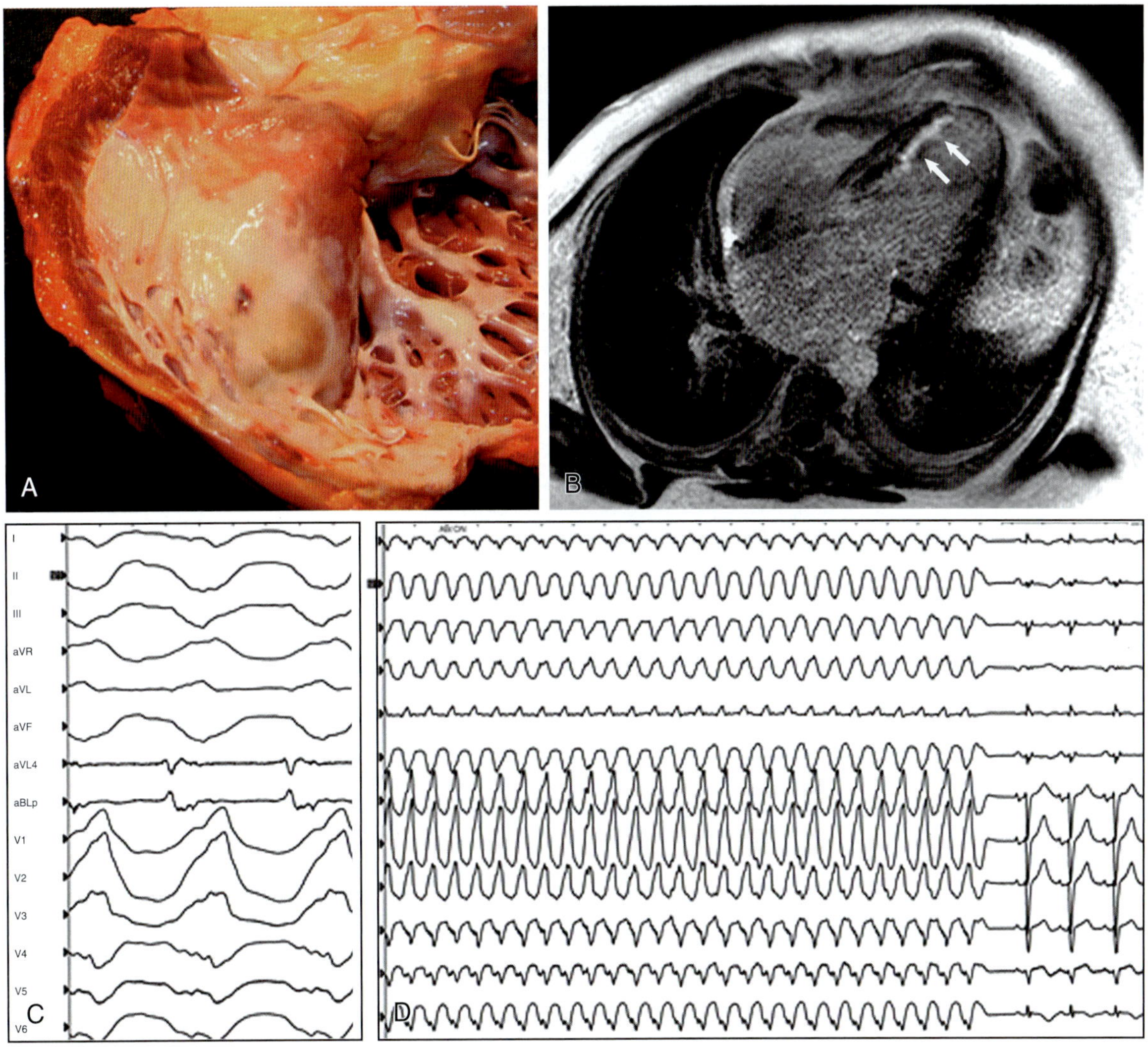

FIG. 23.2 Ventricular tachycardia originating from a myocardial scar. (A) Histopathologic transverse section through the left ventricle. (B) Cardiac magnetic resonance image of a septal hypodense region (*arrows*) indicative of scar. (C and D) These 12-lead electrocardiogram traces show ventricular tachycardia originating from the left ventricular substrate. (A) (From Wallace A. *McAlpine Collection*. UCLA Cardiac Arrhythmia Center.)

diastole, may result in abnormal impulse initiation. Normally, sinus rhythm prevents activation of ectopic pacemakers by overdrive suppression, but once the sinus rate slows or has pauses, ectopic pacemaker tissue can become active, generating ectopic ventricular rhythms, through an automatic mechanism. Triggered activity due to early afterdepolarizations can result in reentrant arrhythmias.

As a consequence of the lack of clinical studies, the relevance of comparisons of acute phase arrhythmias between animal models and humans is uncertain. In relation to the delayed VA, more data are available to help correlate findings in experimental models and in clinical practice.

Reperfusion Arrhythmias

Experimental models suggest that at least 3 minutes of ischemia is required for the development of reperfusion arrhythmias. In the era of primary PCI for MI, reperfusion arrhythmias are commonly seen, ranging from isolated PVCs, accelerated idioventricular rhythms, and VT and VF. In experimental models, phases of arrhythmias related to reperfusion are evident, with none occurring after less than 3 minutes of ischemia. Arrhythmias are more frequent when the ischemic period is increased from 5 minutes to 20 to 30 minutes. Reperfusion arrhythmias are less frequent after 30 to 60 minutes. These arrhythmias are a result of washout of ions such as lactate and potassium and of toxic metabolites from the ischemic zone and also oxidative stress, all of which alter autonomic function.

In humans, the most common rhythm with reperfusion is accelerated idioventricular rhythm, with rates ranging from 70 to 100 beats/min. The absence of reperfusion arrhythmias is thought to be a negative prognostic indicator in that it is suggestive of a longer ischemic period than had been potentially realized. In experimental models, when reperfusion is performed early, a sudden and almost immediate restoration of action potentials to the ischemic area occurs. In the early stages of reperfusion, the action potentials are abnormal, with alternating low to high amplitude. Within the myocardium, marked heterogeneity of action potentials, along with the addition of a trigger, can act as a substrate for arrhythmias. This heterogeneity tends to decrease after the first 30 seconds of reperfusion.

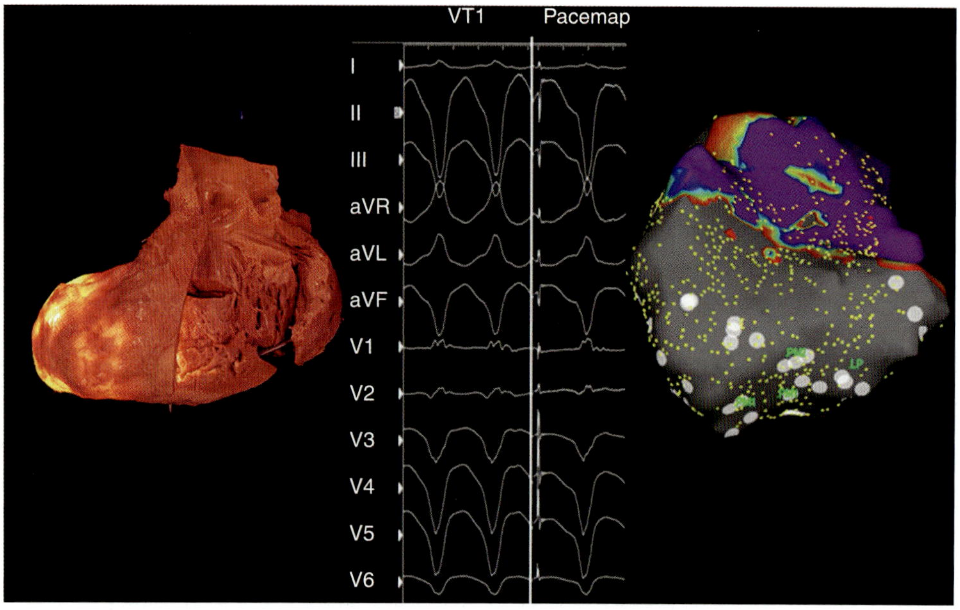

FIG. 23.3 Anterior myocardial infarction resulting in aneurysmal anteroapical left ventricular (LV) wall. In the example shown, consequent apical thinning is evident on transillumination through the LV apex with a 12-lead electrocardiogram of the ventricular tachycardia (VT) originating from around the scar. A pace map from the critical isthmus shows a pattern identical to the ventricular tachycardia, and an electroanatomic map demonstrates a large anteroapical region of myocardial scar surrounded by a border zone. (From Wallace A. *McAlpine Collection*. UCLA Cardiac Arrhythmia Center.)

Late or Chronic Ventricular Arrhythmias

Late VA occur approximately 1 to 3 weeks after MI, as the infarct evolves and starts to heal. After the early-phase arrhythmias, fewer VAs are typically seen from 72 hours to 5 days, and then frequent PVCs predominate. The burden of early arrhythmias unfortunately does not predict the frequency of late arrhythmias. The absence of in-hospital or early arrhythmias does not predict the absence of late arrhythmias.

Risk factors predictive of late arrhythmias are the size of the scar, presence of aneurysms, multivessel disease, and anterior location of the MI (Fig. 23.3). Before discharge, in the setting of these risk factors, treadmill exercise testing may be helpful in risk stratification (see Chapter 14). The development of arrhythmias during exercise testing is predictive of an increased risk for SCD. Electrophysiology testing for induction of ventricular arrhythmias by programmed stimulation is predominantly helpful for late or chronic ventricular arrhythmias (at least greater than 3 weeks following infarct). This utility is because chronic ventricular arrhythmias tend to be reentrant in nature as described in the next section.

MECHANISM OF VENTRICULAR ARRHYTHMIAS

Reentrant Arrhythmias

Reentrant (ventricular) tachycardias require a zone of slow conduction and unidirectional block that occurs due to the development of scar tissue following MI with heterogeneous substrate defined by patches of the electrically inactive scar; channels through the scar, (areas of slow conduction); and border zones of abnormal, electrically active tissue surrounding scar regions. The longer it takes for the impulse to traverse the area of slow conduction, the more time is required for the impulse to emerge from the zone of reentry, and the longer the coupling interval before the onset of tachycardia. Either a single loop or multiple loops may be present within a reentrant circuit (Fig. 23.4). Such loops often take a 3-dimensional course involving the endocardium, mid-myocardium, and the epicardial surfaces. The inscription of the QRS morphology (exit of the reentrant ventricular tachycardia circuit) may be remote from the sites of the critical isthmus.[10] Reentrant tachycardias can be terminated by a critically timed premature stimulus that collides with the reentrant circuit, rendering it refractory. Capture of the ventricular electrical activity with pacing that does not affect the tachycardia (presence of an excitable gap) also is indicative of a reentrant arrhythmia, and progressive fusion with entrainment is a diagnostic feature of reentry. Resetting of the reentrant arrhythmia to abort the tachycardia also may occur if pacing delivers a premature stimulus within the circuit. In other words, when resetting occurs, the QRS of the tachycardia occurs earlier than expected (advances) as a result of the paced stimulus.

Triggered Arrhythmias

Triggered activity is dependent on afterdepolarizations, either early or late, with at least one action potential preceding it. Triggered activity displays features of both automaticity and reentry. If afterdepolarizations are of sufficient magnitude, they can generate another action potential. The action potential can result from either spontaneous leakage of positive ions intracellularly or a premature ventricular beat (Fig. 23.5). Two distinct types of triggered activity exist: pause-dependent arrhythmias and catecholamine-dependent arrhythmias. During a pause, if the afterdepolarization reaches the cellular threshold, another action potential can be generated. This circumstance can allow for impulse initiation from the trigger and subsequent sinus node suppression. With catecholamine-dependent triggers, delayed afterdepolarizations lead to the generation of another action potential secondary to an increase in sympathetic activity.

Various groups of investigators have studied the benefits of opting for permanent pacing immediately over inserting a temporary pacing system. This approach may provide a short-term survival benefit in hospital, but it appears that the mortality rate on discharge is similar. If the AV block is a result of increased parasympathetic tone, adenosine release, or potassium fluxes, then the AV block could be transient, such as in the case of a right coronary artery occlusion. It is more likely to be permanent with an LAD occlusion. The presence of a stable escape rhythm eliminates the need to intervene immediately, and telemetry monitoring can be adequate, allowing time for the AV block to potentially resolve. Treating high-degree AV block with inotropic agents or atropine can be problematic because increasing the heart rate may potentially worsen the AV conduction, resulting in a more profound bradycardia.

Bundle Branch Block

Further defining bundle branch block (BBB) associated with MI may be helpful in relation to prognostic significance, such as left versus right, duration, and time of appearance. BBB can be transiently associated with MI or persistent. BBB post MI is associated with increasing age and comorbid conditions such as diabetes and heart failure during hospitalization. Compared with those with right BBB (RBBB), patients with left BBB (LBBB) exhibit a higher prevalence of comorbid conditions. Also, new LBBB is associated with higher mortality as well as structural abnormalities such as cardiomyopathy due to the larger area of myocardial damage required to elicit LBBB following MI. The time of appearance and duration of the bundle branch block have different prognostic significances, and the presence of BBB may help with risk stratification.

SUMMARY

SCD secondary to MI continues to be a major public health problem. Despite substantial advances in the treatment of myocardial ischemia, in a meaningful proportion of patients, MI may be complicated by conduction system disease, ventricular arrhythmias, or may precipitate SCD, often as the only clinical event. Therefore, it is imperative to understand the pathophysiology of SCD and VA, and then identify risk factors and optimize risk stratification techniques.

CLASSIC REFERENCES

1. Harris AS, Bisteni A, Russell RA, et al. Excitatory factors in ventricular tachycardia resulting from myocardial ischemia; potassium a major excitant. *Science*. 1954;119:200–203.
2. Janse MJ, Wit AL. Electrophysiological mechanisms of ventricular arrhythmias resulting from myocardial ischemia and infarction. *Physiol Rev*. 1989;69:1049–1169.

REFERENCES

1. Al-Khatib SM, Stevenson WG, Ackerman MJ, et al. 2017 AHA/ACC/HRS guideline for management of patients with ventricular arrhythmias and the prevention of sudden cardiac death: a report of the American College of Cardiology/American Heart Association task force on clinical practice guidelines and the heart rhythm society. *Heart Rhythm*. 2018;15:e73–e189. https://doi.org/10.1016/j.hrthm.2017.10.036.
2. Zeppenfeld K, Tfelt-Hansen J, de Riva M, et al. 2022 ESC guidelines for the management of patients with ventricular arrhythmias and the prevention of sudden cardiac death. *Eur Heart J*. 2022;43:3997–4126. https://doi.org/10.1093/eurheartj/ehac262.
3. Wong CX, Brown A, Lau DH, et al. Epidemiology of sudden cardiac death: global and regional perspectives. *Heart Lung Circ*. 2019;28:6–14. https://doi.org/10.1016/j.hlc.2018.08.026.
4. Ferrero JM, Gonzalez-Ascaso A, Matas JFR. The mechanisms of potassium loss in acute myocardial ischemia: new insights from computational simulations. *Front Physiol*. 2023;14:1074160. https://doi.org/10.3389/fphys.2023.1074160.
5. Thomsen AF, Bertelsen L, Jons C, et al. Scar border zone mass and presence of border zone channels assessed with cardiac magnetic resonance imaging are associated with ventricular arrhythmia in patients with ST-segment elevation myocardial infarction. *Europace*. 2023;25:978–988. https://doi.org/10.1093/europace/euac256.
6. Amoni M, Claus P, Dries E, et al. Discrete sites of frequent premature ventricular complexes cluster within the infarct border zone and coincide with high frequency of delayed afterdepolarizations under adrenergic stimulation. *Heart Rhythm*. 2021;18:1976–1987. https://doi.org/10.1016/j.hrthm.2021.07.067.
7. Zegard A, Okafor O, de Bono J, et al. Myocardial fibrosis as a predictor of sudden death in patients with coronary artery disease. *J Am Coll Cardiol*. 2021;77:29–41. https://doi.org/10.1016/j.jacc.2020.10.046.
8. Zegard A, Okafor O, de Bono J, et al. Greyzone myocardial fibrosis and ventricular arrhythmias in patients with a left ventricular ejection fraction >35. *Europace*. 2022;24:31–39. https://doi.org/10.1093/europace/euab167.
9. Bradfield JS, Ajijola OA, Vaseghi M, Shivkumar K. Mechanisms and management of refractory ventricular arrhythmias in the age of autonomic modulation. *Heart Rhythm*. 2018;15:1252–1260. https://doi.org/10.1016/j.hrthm.2018.02.015.
10. Tung R, Raiman M, Liao H, et al. Simultaneous endocardial and epicardial delineation of 3D reentrant ventricular tachycardia. *J Am Coll Cardiol*. 2020;75:884–897. https://doi.org/10.1016/j.jacc.2019.12.044.
11. Dusi V, Zhu C, Ajijola OA. Neuromodulation approaches for cardiac arrhythmias: recent advances. *Curr Cardiol Rep*. 2019;21:32. https://doi.org/10.1007/s11886-019-1120-1.
12. Podolecki T, Lenarczyk R, Kowalczyk J, et al. Prognostic significance of complex ventricular arrhythmias complicating st-segment elevation myocardial infarction. *Am J Cardiol*. 2018;121:805–809. https://doi.org/10.1016/j.amjcard.2017.12.036.
13. Behnes M, Mashayekhi K, Weiss C, et al. Prognostic impact of acute myocardial infarction in patients presenting with ventricular tachyarrhythmias and aborted cardiac arrest. *J Am Heart Assoc*. 2018;7:e010004. https://doi.org/10.1161/JAHA.118.010004.
14. Venkateswaran RV, Moorthy MV, Chatterjee NA, et al. Diabetes and risk of sudden death in coronary artery disease patients without severe systolic dysfunction. *JACC Clin Electrophysiol*. 2021;7:1604–1614. https://doi.org/10.1016/j.jacep.2021.05.014.
15. Frederiksen TC, Dahm CC, Preis SR, et al. The bidirectional association between atrial fibrillation and myocardial infarction. *Nat Rev Cardiol*. 2023;20:631–644. https://doi.org/10.1038/s41569-023-00857-3.
16. Sandhu RK, Dron JS, Liu Y, et al. Polygenic risk score predicts sudden death in patients with coronary disease and preserved systolic function. *J Am Coll Cardiol*. 2022;80:873–883. https://doi.org/10.1016/j.jacc.2022.05.049.
17. Sramko M, Abdel-Kafi S, Wijnmaalen AP, et al. Head-to-head comparison of t1 mapping and electroanatomical voltage mapping in patients with ventricular arrhythmias. *JACC Clin Electrophysiol*. 2023;9:740–748. https://doi.org/10.1016/j.jacep.2022.10.035.
18. van der Bijl P, Delgado V, Bax JJ. Imaging for sudden cardiac death risk stratification: current perspective and future directions. *Prog Cardiovasc Dis*. 2019;62:205–211. https://doi.org/10.1016/j.pcad.2019.04.005.
19. Gomez-Mesa JE, Marquez-Murillo M, Figueiredo M, et al. Inter-American Society of Cardiology (CIFACAH-ELECTROSIAC) and latin-American Heart Rhythm Society (LAHRS): multidisciplinary review on the appropriate use of implantable cardiodefibrillator in heart failure with reduced ejection fraction. *J Interv Card Electrophysiol*. 2023;66:1211–1229. https://doi.org/10.1007/s10840-022-01425-4.
20. Kovoor JG, Deshmukh T, von Huben A, et al. Optimizing electrophysiology studies to prevent sudden cardiac death after myocardial infarction. *Europace*. 2023;25:euad219. https://doi.org/10.1093/europace/euad219.
21. de Groot JR. Implantable cardioverter-defibrillators in non-ischaemic cardiomyopathy: a need or not? *Neth Heart J*. 2023;31:87–88. https://doi.org/10.1007/s12471-023-01765-4.
22. Chung MK, Patton KK, Lau CP, et al. 2023 HRS/APHRS/LAHRS guideline on cardiac physiologic pacing for the avoidance and mitigation of heart failure. *Heart Rhythm*. 2023;20(9):e17–e91. https://doi.org/10.1016/j.hrthm.2023.03.1538.
23. Tian Y, Wittwer ED, Kapa S, et al. Effective use of percutaneous stellate ganglion blockade in patients with electrical storm. *Circ Arrhythm Electrophysiol*. 2019;12:e007118. https://doi.org/10.1161/CIRCEP.118.007118.
24. Sanghai S, Abbott NJ, Dewland TA, et al. Stellate ganglion blockade with continuous infusion versus single injection for treatment of ventricular arrhythmia storm. *JACC Clin Electrophysiol*. 2021;7:452–460. https://doi.org/10.1016/j.jacep.2020.09.032.
25. Fudim M, Qadri YJ, Waldron NH, et al. Stellate ganglion blockade for the treatment of refractory ventricular arrhythmias. *JACC Clin Electrophysiol*. 2020;6:562–571. https://doi.org/10.1016/j.jacep.2019.12.017.
26. Nonoguchi NM, Adachi M, Nogami A, et al. Stellate ganglion phototherapy using low-level laser: a novel rescue therapy for patients with refractory ventricular arrhythmias. *JACC Clin Electrophysiol*. 2021;7(10):1297–1308. https://doi.org/10.1016/j.jacep.2021.04.015.
27. Markman TM, Hamilton RH, Marchlinski FE, Nazarian S. Case series of transcutaneous magnetic stimulation for ventricular tachycardia storm. *JAMA*. 2020;323:2200–2202. https://doi.org/10.1001/jama.2020.3833.
28. Natale A, Zeppenfeld K, Della Bella P, et al. Twenty-five years of catheter ablation of ventricular tachycardia: a look back and a look forward. *Europace*. 2023;25:euad225. https://doi.org/10.1093/europace/euad225.

24 Epidemiology and Management of Bleeding in Acute Coronary Syndromes

SUNIL V. RAO AND LOUAI RAZZOUK

INTRODUCTION

Clinical outcomes after acute coronary syndrome (ACS) have significantly improved over time. A significant proportion of the reduction in mortality has been the result of development and adoption of potent anticoagulant and antiplatelet therapies coupled with invasive risk stratification in high-risk patients (see Chapters 12 and 13, Chapters 25, and 26). In addition, the use of secondary prevention strategies to control risk factors has further improved long-term outcomes (see Chapter 29). Although antithrombotic medications reduce the risk of recurrent ischemic events, they increase the risk of bleeding and the need for blood transfusion. Paradoxically, bleeding events are associated with a subsequent higher risk for myocardial infarction (MI), stroke, stent thrombosis, and death. Randomized trials of "bleeding avoidance strategies" (BAS) in patients with ACS have demonstrated a reduction in adverse events, including mortality.[1] Because of the availability of BAS, the use of management strategies that reduce ischemia while minimizing bleeding has the potential to further improve outcomes. This chapter summarizes the epidemiology and management of bleeding events in ACS.

EPIDEMIOLOGY OF BLEEDING

Reported Incidence of Bleeding: Influence of Definitions

The reported incidence of major bleeding events among patients with ACS varies greatly depending on the definition used, the fidelity with which the events are identified, the types of antithrombotic therapies used, and whether invasive risk stratification with revascularization is pursued. Before discussing the incidence of bleeding in ACS, it is important to review how bleeding is defined. Several schemas exist, but a few have been consistently used to identify bleeding events across randomized trials or registries that include ACS patients. Bleeding events as defined by several of these classification systems have also been correlated with other adverse events such as recurrent MI, stroke, stent thrombosis, and death (see section on Bleeding and Outcomes).

Most bleeding definitions are made up of specific data elements that broadly fall into three categories: changes in hemoglobin or hematocrit; clinical events (e.g., gastrointestinal bleeding or intracranial hemorrhage); and consequences (e.g., blood transfusion or fatal bleeding). The extremes of bleeding definitions could focus solely on either changes in hemoglobin or on clinical events, and either could "cast the net" too widely—that is, identify events that would not be considered bleeding events by most clinicians or too narrowly by identifying only the most severe bleeding events and missing other less severe but clinically important, events. Most definitions include combinations of all three categories. Table 24.1 displays commonly used bleeding definitions across randomized trials and registries.

Established Definitions

Thrombolysis in Myocardial Infarction and Global Use of Strategies to Open Occluded Arteries Definitions

Historically, the most commonly used definitions were the thrombolysis in myocardial infarction (TIMI) and global use of strategies to open occluded (GUSTO) arteries bleeding scales. The TIMI definition was developed in the context of fibrinolytic therapy for ST-elevation MI (STEMI) and was generally based on decreases in hemoglobin. The categorization for TIMI bleeding originally consisted of minimal, minor, and major bleeding, defined according to the degree of hemoglobin change. Because intracranial hemorrhage is the most feared complication of fibrinolytic therapy, it was included as part of the TIMI major bleeding definition. Since its original development, the TIMI bleeding definition has evolved to include a qualifier that bases the required decrease in hemoglobin on whether a clinically overt bleeding event has occurred (Table 24.1). The GUSTO definition was also developed in the context

TABLE 24.1 Sample Bleeding Definitions in ACS Clinical Trials and Registries

TRIAL/DEFINITION	PATIENT POPULATION	INTERVENTION	BLEEDING DEFINITION

Thrombolysis in Myocardial Infarction (TIMI)	ACS, PCI	N/A	Major
			• Any intracranial bleeding (excluding microhemorrhages <10 mm evident only on gradient-echo MRI)
			• Clinically overt signs of hemorrhage associated with a drop in hemoglobin of ≥5 g/dL
			• Fatal bleeding (bleeding that directly results in death within 7 days)
			Minor
			• Clinically overt (including imaging), resulting in hemoglobin drop of 3 to <5 g/dL
			Requiring medical attention
			  • Any overt sign of hemorrhage that meets one of the following criteria and does not meet criteria for a major or minor bleeding event, as defined above
			    • Requiring intervention (medical practitioner-guided medical or surgical treatment to stop or treat bleeding, including temporarily or permanently discontinuing or changing the dose of a medication or study drug)
			    • Leading to or prolonging hospitalization
			    • Prompting evaluation (leading to an unscheduled visit to a healthcare professional and diagnostic testing, either laboratory or imaging)
			Minimal
			• Any overt bleeding event that does not meet the criteria above
			
			Bleeding in the setting of CABG
			• Fatal bleeding (bleeding that directly results in death)
			• Perioperative intracranial bleeding
			• Reoperation after closure of the sternotomy incision for the purpose of controlling bleeding
			• Transfusion of ≥5 U PRBCs or whole blood within a 48-h period; cell saver transfusion will not be counted in calculations of blood products.
			• Chest tube output >2 L within a 24-h period

Global Use of Strategies to Open Occluded arteries (GUSTO)	ACS, PCI	N/A	Severe or life-threatening • Intracerebral hemorrhage • Resulting in substantial hemodynamic compromise requiring treatment Moderate • Requiring blood transfusion but not resulting in hemodynamic compromise Mild • Bleeding that does not meet above criteria
SYNERGY	NSTE-ACS	Enoxaparin vs. heparin	TIMI & GUSTO
PURSUIT	NSTE-ACS	Eptifibatide/heparin vs. heparin	TIMI & GUSTO

CURE	NSTE-ACS	Aspirin vs. aspirin + clopidogrel	Major bleeding
			• Life-threatening
			  • Fatal
			  • Intracranial
			  • Requiring surgical intervention
			  • Results in hypotension
			  • Decrease in Hgb ≥5 g/dL
			  • Requires ≥4 units of blood
			• Other major
			  • Requires transfusion of 2 or 3 units
			  • Intraocular

GUSTO IIb	NSTE-ACS	Hirudin vs. heparin	GUSTO
CURRENT-OASIS 7`	NSTE-ACS	High-dose aspirin vs. low-dose aspirin; high-dose clopidogrel vs. standard dose clopidogrel	Severe bleeding • Fatal • Requiring transfusion ≥4 U of PRBCs or equivalent whole blood • Resulting in hemoglobin drop ≥5 g/dL • Leading to hypotension that requires inotropes • Requiring surgery • Symptomatic intracranial hemorrhage Other major bleeding • Requiring transfusion of 2–3 U of PRBCs or whole blood • Significantly disabling, intraocular bleeding leading to significant loss of vision
OASIS-5	NSTE-ACS	Fondaparinux vs. enoxaparin	Major bleeding • Fatal, intracranial, retroperitoneal, intraocular leading to vision loss • Decrease in Hgb ≥3 g/dl adjusted for transfusion • Transfusion of 2 units of red blood cells

TABLE 24.1 Sample Bleeding Definitions in ACS Clinical Trials and Registries—cont'd

TRIAL/DEFINITION	PATIENT POPULATION	INTERVENTION	BLEEDING DEFINITION
ACUITY & HORIZONS-MI	NSTE-ACS	Bivalirudin alone vs. heparin or enoxaparin + GP IIb/IIIa vs. bivalirudin + GP IIb/IIIa	Major bleeding • Intracranial or intraocular bleeding • Hemorrhage at the access site requiring intervention • Hematoma with a diameter of at least 5 cm • Reduction in hemoglobin levels of at least 4 g/dL without an overt bleeding source or at least 3 g/dL with such a source • Reoperation for bleeding • Transfusion of a blood product.
ACTION-GWTG	ACS	n/a	• Absolute Hgb decrease of ≥4 g/dL (baseline to nadir) • Intracranial hemorrhage • Documented or suspected retroperitoneal bleed • Any red cell blood transfusion with baseline Hgb ≥9 g/dL or any red cell transfusion with Hgb <9 g/dL and a suspected bleeding event.
CRUSADE	NSTE-ACS	n/a	Major bleeding • Absolute decrease in hematocrit concentration by 12% from baseline • Intracranial hemorrhage • Retroperitoneal bleeding • Red blood cell transfusion due to bleeding.
GRACE	NSTE-ACS		• Life-threatening bleeding requiring a transfusion of >2 U PRBCs • Resulting in a decrease in hematocrit of >10% • Occurring intracerebrally • Resulting in stroke or death
TRITON TIMI 38	NSTE-ACS		TIMI
PLATO	NSTE-ACS		Major life-threatening • Fatal • Intracranial • Intrapericardial with cardiac tamponade • Resulting in hypovolemic shock or severe hypotension that requires pressors or surgery • Clinically overt or apparent bleeding associated with decrease in hemoglobin >5 g/dL • Requiring transfusion of ≥4 units whole blood or PRBCs Other major • Significantly disabling (e.g., intraocular with permanent vision loss) • Associated drop in hemoglobin of 3–5 g/dL • Requiring transfusion of 2–3 U whole blood or PRBCs Any major • Any one of the above criteria

of fibrinolytic therapy for STEMI and was based solely on clinical events. GUSTO bleeding is categorized as mild, moderate, or severe, and again, intracranial hemorrhage is considered severe according to the GUSTO definition.

Capture of Bleeding Events

Another factor that may affect the incidence of bleeding is the method for detecting events. Clinical trials often use independent clinical events committees that review source documents (medical charts) to detect adverse events. This approach minimizes the risk of bias at the site level. In contrast, registries generally do not use adjudication and rely on site-identified events. This aspect is particularly true of registries in which the primary purpose is quality improvement rather than comparing the effectiveness of one treatment with another. As such, the rates of bleeding are often higher in clinical trials than in registries, despite the inclusion of higher-risk patients in the latter.

Bleeding Academic Research Consortium Definition

To overcome some of the challenges posed by different bleeding definitions, several groups have attempted to develop a standardized approach to classifying and reporting bleeding events. Rather than developing a new definition, the Academic Research Consortium (ARC) proposed a list of standardized data elements that should be recorded in the case report form for a clinical trial of antithrombotic therapy (or the data collection form of a registry of ACS). These data elements can then either be reported separately or combined to reconstruct other bleeding definitions. The ARC, which originally consisted of members from four academic research organizations that designed and executed pivotal trials of drug-eluting stents, developed a set of standardized definitions for endpoints used in coronary stent trials. Periprocedural bleeding was not considered in their initial deliberations; however, subsequent iterations of ARC have developed definitions for bleeding endpoints for ACS trials, transcatheter valve trials, and peripheral arterial disease trials. The Bleeding Academic Research Consortium (BARC) definition of bleeding for use in ACS trials is shown in Table 24.2.

Bleeding Incidence

In-hospital Bleeding

The rate of in-hospital bleeding in patients presenting with ACS encompasses peri-procedural bleeding and remains an important determinant of outcomes. The presence of numerous clinical trial and registry databases has created a deep knowledge base regarding risk factors and risk indicators associated with hemorrhagic complications in ACS. A major

TABLE 24.2 Bleeding Academic Research Consortium Definition of Bleeding

Type 0: no bleeding

Type 1: bleeding that is not actionable and does not cause the patient to seek unscheduled performance of studies, hospitalization, or treatment by a health care professional; may include episodes leading to self-discontinuation of medical therapy by the patient without consulting a health care professional

Type 2: any overt, actionable sign of hemorrhage (e.g., more bleeding than would be expected for a clinical circumstance, including bleeding found by imaging alone) that does not fit the criteria for type 3, 4, or 5 but does meet at least one of the following criteria: (1) requiring nonsurgical, medical intervention by a health care professional, (2) leading to hospitalization or increased level of care, or (3) prompting evaluation

Type 3

- Type 3a
  - Overt bleeding plus hemoglobin drop of 3 to <5 g/dL (provided hemoglobin drop is related to bleed), corrected for transfusion
  - Any transfusion with overt bleeding
- Type 3b
  - Overt bleeding plus hemoglobin drop ≥5 g/dL (provided hemoglobin drop is related to bleed), corrected for transfusion
  - Cardiac tamponade
  - Bleeding requiring surgical intervention for control (excluding dental/nasal/skin/hemorrhoid)
  - Bleeding requiring intravenous vasoactive agents
- Type 3c
  - Intracranial hemorrhage (does not include microbleeds or hemorrhagic transformation, does include intraspinal)
  - Subcategories confirmed by autopsy or imaging or lumbar puncture
  - Intraocular bleed compromising vision

Type 4: CABG-related bleeding

- Perioperative intracranial bleeding within 48 h
- Reoperation after closure of sternotomy for the purpose of controlling bleeding
- Transfusion of ≥5 U whole blood or packed red blood cells within a 48-h period
- Chest tube output ≥2 L within a 24-h period

Type 5: fatal bleeding

- Type 5a
  - Probable fatal bleeding; no autopsy or imaging confirmation but clinically suspicious
- Type 5b
  - Definite fatal bleeding; overt bleeding or autopsy or imaging confirmation

risk for bleeding is the use of invasive procedures, such as cardiac catheterization, percutaneous coronary intervention, and coronary artery bypass grafting (CABG), which compounds the risk for bleeding in patients treated with potent antithrombotic medications. The widespread adoption of these procedures has led to the broad categorization of bleeding into either "access-site related bleeding" or "nonaccess-site related bleeding." This categorization also facilitates the grouping of BAS, which can be directed at the vascular access site or systemically (see the section on Bleeding Avoidance Strategies). The proportion of bleeding related to the vascular access site appears to vary with the patient's clinical presentation. In the context of ACS, patients with non-ST-elevation (NSTE)-ACS have a higher proportion of nonaccess-site bleeding. This observation is borne out in registry data and in randomized clinical trials. For example, in the National Cardiovascular Data Registry's Cath-PCI registry of the bleeding events that occurred in NSTE-ACS patients who underwent PCI, two-thirds of the bleeds were not related to the access site. Similarly, in the RIVAL trial, which compared radial with femoral access in 7021 patients with ACS (>70% of whom had NSTE-ACS), two-thirds of major bleeding was unrelated to the vascular access site. In contrast, patients with STEMI not only have a higher rate of bleeding, but a larger proportion of these patients (approximately 50%) have bleeding related to the vascular access site.[2] These differences are likely related to the much higher use of PCI and its attendant intense antithrombotic therapy among patients with STEMI.

Another common etiology of in-hospital bleeding in ACS is drug-induced thrombocytopenia and bleeding due to antithrombotic treatment. Heparin is the most commonly used antithrombotic medication associated with thrombocytopenia, but so are glycoprotein IIb/IIIa inhibitors (GPI) and potent oral antiplatelet agents. The management of antiplatelet therapy in ACS patients with thrombocytopenia is particularly challenging as these patients are prone to more bleeding and thrombotic events. The use of GPI has decreased over the last two decades with the advent of novel stent platforms with lower thrombotic risks and potent oral antiplatelet agents with rapid platelet inhibition (see Chapter 13). Cangrelor is a nucleotide-mimetic intravenous $P2Y_{12}$ receptor antagonist that reduces bleeding complications in the peri-procedure setting as compared to clopidogrel and is not associated with acquired thrombocytopenia. Given its potency and pharmacokinetics with rapid onset and offset, it has utility in potentially reducing bleeding in ACS patients with thrombocytopenia or at risk thereof.[3]

Post Acute Coronary Syndrome Discharge Bleeding

Patients undergoing revascularization percutaneously or surgically are often discharged on dual antiplatelet therapy (DAPT),[4] which increases the risks of nonaccess-site bleeding. The most common serious bleeding complication related to DAPT is gastrointestinal in etiology, and it is even more challenging given its insidious clinical presentation. Aspirin, which directly inhibits cyclooxygenase-1 reduces the protective effects of prostaglandins on the endothelium, is a common culprit in upper gastrointestinal bleeding etiology. Furthermore, ticagrelor and prasugrel have both been associated with higher risk of GI bleeding as compared to clopidogrel. Intracranial bleeding (ICB) is another important source of bleeding, often with serious consequences. Patients with concomitant oral anticoagulant or with prior history of ICB are at a significantly higher risk, and management remains a challenge due to the scarce number of events in randomized controlled trials. Risk stratification of patients prior to initiation of antiplatelet and antithrombotic therapies is therefore crucial to prevent the bleeding events.

Risk Scores for Bleeding

In addition to clinical presentation, published risk models for bleeding have identified a variety of demographic and clinical features that are associated with a higher risk for bleeding complications. Because most bleeding events in ACS occur early, either during the index hospitalization or within 30 days, most of these models have used in-hospital or 30-day bleeding as the primary outcome. A commonly used bleeding prediction model is one derived from the ACUITY and HORIZONS-MI clinical trials, which examined a bivalirudin strategy in patients with NSTE-ACS or STEMI, respectively, who underwent primary PCI.[5] Both trials used the same definition of bleeding, and the combined trials consisted of 17,421 patients. The overall rate of non-CABG–related major bleeding was 7.4%. Baseline covariates independently associated with bleeding included age, female sex, elevated serum creatinine, elevated white blood cell count, preexisting anemia, NSTEMI, and STEMI. One treatment covariate—the use of heparin plus a glycoprotein IIb/IIIa inhibitor—was also a significant predictor. The model has reasonable discrimination, with a c-index of 0.74. The goodness-of-fit was evaluated by comparing predicted with observed bleeding. Finally, an integer risk score was developed for use at the bedside (Fig. 24.1).

Another model was derived from the CRUSADE registry, which is used for risk adjustment in an ACS quality

								Add to score
Gender	Male 0			Female +8				
Age (years)	<50 0	50–59 +3	60–69 +6	70–79 +9	≥80 +12			
Serum creatinine (mg/dL)	<1.0 0	1.0– +2	1.2– +3	1.4– +5	1.6– +6	1.8– +8	≥2.0 +10	
White blood cell count (×10^9)	<10 0	10– +2	12– +3	14– +5	16– +6	18– +8	≥20 +10	
Anemia	No 0			Yes +6				
Presentation	STEMI +6	NSTEMI - Raised biomarkers +2		NSTE-ACS - Normal biomarkers 0				
Antithrombotic medications	Heparin plus a GPI 0			Bivalirudin monotherapy −5				
	Total score*							

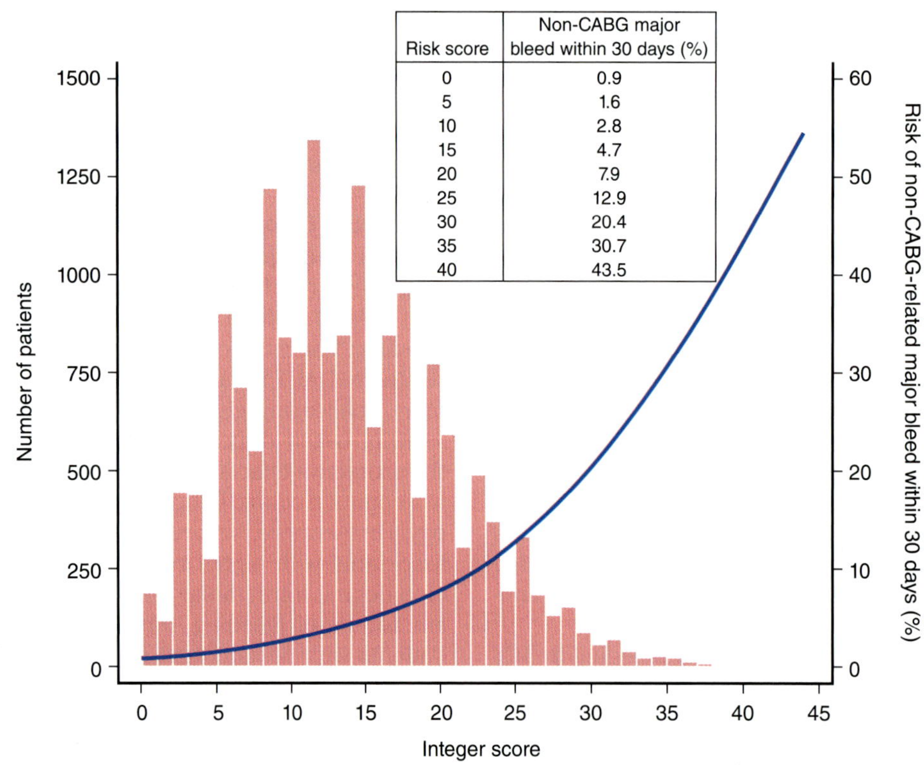

Risk score	Non-CABG major bleed within 30 days (%)
0	0.9
5	1.6
10	2.8
15	4.7
20	7.9
25	12.9
30	20.4
35	30.7
40	43.5

FIG. 24.1 An integer risk score for non-CABG-related major bleeding within 30 days of patient presentation with acute coronary syndrome and distribution of the risk score with subsequent probability of non-CABG-related major bleeding.

TABLE 24.3 Predictors of Bleeding from Selected Bleeding Prediction Risk Scores

DATA SOURCE	NCDR CATHPCI REGISTRY	ACTION-GWTG REGISTRY	ACUITY + HORIZONS MI CLINICAL TRIAL DATA	BLUE CROSS-BLUE SHIELD CONSORTIUM REGISTRY[a]
Population	PCI	ACS	ACS undergoing PCI	PCI
Risk Factors				
Age	X	X	X	
Sex	X	X	X	
Weight/BMI	BMI	Weight	–	Height and Weight
Renal	Chronic kidney disease	Baseline creatinine	Baseline creatinine	Baseline creatinine
Preexisting anemia	Baseline hemoglobin	Baseline hemoglobin	Anemia	–
Presentation	• STEMI • Shock • Cardiac arrest within 24 h of PCI	• Systolic blood pressure • Admission heart rate • Heart failure/shock on admission • ECG changes	NSTEMI or STEMI	• CAD presentation • Anginal classification • Heart failure within prior 2 weeks • Cardiogenic shock in 24 h prior to PCI • Preprocedure cardiac markers (CKMB, Troponin I/T)
History	Prior PCI	• Diabetes mellitus • Peripheral artery disease	–	• Diabetes mellitus • Chronic lung disease
Interventions	Urgent or emergent/ salvage PCI	–	–	–
Medications	–	Warfarin use	Unfractionated heparin + glycoprotein IIb/IIIa inhibitor	–
Other	–	–	White blood cell count	–

[a]Outcome is in-hospital blood transfusion.

improvement registry. This model included only NSTE-ACS patients and did not include treatment variables so that site-level bleeding outcomes could be benchmarked and allow for process changes to reduce bleeding risk at centers with high bleeding rates. Using 71,277 patients as the development data set and 17,857 patients as the validation data set, the investigators identified eight independent predictors of major bleeding (defined according to the registry; see Table 24.1). These risk indicators included baseline hematocrit, baseline creatinine clearance, baseline heart rate, female sex, heart failure at presentation, baseline systolic blood pressure, previous vascular disease, and diabetes mellitus. The c-indices in the development and validation cohorts were 0.72 and 0.71, respectively. Similar to the ACUITY bedside risk score, the investigators developed the "CRUSADE" bleeding risk score, which showed an increase in the predicted probability as the score increased.[6]

These published models share certain predictors of bleeding, namely, chronic kidney disease, anemia, and female sex (Table 24.3). Chronic kidney disease likely predisposes to bleeding through reduced clearance of antithrombin agents (especially those that are predominantly renally cleared) and platelet dysfunction. Anemia is likely a marker of occult bleeding that may be exacerbated in the setting of aggressive antithrombotic therapy. In addition, baseline anemia may increase the likelihood of blood transfusion, which is an element of the bleeding definition in many studies. The mechanism underlying the association between female sex and higher bleeding risk has yet to be elucidated. Women presenting with ACS are more likely to be older, to have lower body mass, and to have impaired renal function. As such, overdosing of antithrombotic medications may be responsible for some degree of the increased risk (see the section on Preventive Strategies); however, such overdosing does not appear to fully explain the apparent independent association. Further research is needed to understand if there are reversible causes of bleeding in women with ACS.

While not specific to patients presenting with ACS, the Academic Research Consortium for High Bleeding Risk (ARC-HBR) established a list of major and minor clinical criteria to identify patients at HBR who are undergoing PCI.[7] HBR was defined as a BARC 3 or 5 bleeding risk ≥4% at 1 year or a risk of an intracranial hemorrhage of ≥1% at 1 year. Patients are defined as HBR if they met at least 1 major or 2 minor ARC-HBR criteria (Table 24.4). This risk score was evaluated in a large cohort of patients undergoing PCI, and the risk score successfully identified patients at increased risk for bleeding: bleeding events at 1 year were 9.1% in the HBR group versus 3.2% in the non-HBR population.[8] The study also demonstrated an increase in bleeding risk in patients who met the HBR definition multiple times. Patients who met ARC-HBR criteria were also at increased risk of thrombotic events and all-cause mortality, which limits the utility of this definition as a stand-alone risk stratification tool.

BLEEDING COMPLICATIONS AND OUTCOMES

Associated Clinical and Nonclinical Outcomes

Clinical Outcomes

Not all bleeding events in ACS patients have equally adverse outcomes. The severity of bleeding, the timing of the medical intervention, and the patient's overall underlying health status all play important roles in determining the impact of bleeding on clinical outcomes. Several studies describe an

TABLE 24.4 Major and Minor Criteria for Academic Research Consortium HBR at the Time of PCI

MAJOR	MINOR
Anticipated use of long-term oral anticoagulation	Age ≥ 75 years
Severe or end-stage CKD (eGFR < 30 ml/min)	Moderate CKD (eGFR 30-59 mL/min)
Hemoglobin < 11 g/dL	Hemoglobin 11–12.9 g/dL for men Hemoglobin 11–11.9 g/dL for women
Spontaneous bleeding requiring hospitalization or transfusion in past 6 months, or any time if recurrent	Spontaneous bleeding requiring hospitalization or transfusion within the past 12 months not meeting the major criterion
Moderate or severe baseline thrombocytopenia (platelet count < 100 x 10^9/L)	Long-term use of oral NSAIDs or steroids
Previous spontaneous ICH (at any time) Previous traumatic ICH within past 12 months Presence of brain AVM Moderate or severe ischemic stroke within past 6 months	Any ischemic stroke at any time not meeting the major criterion
Liver cirrhosis with portal hypertension	
Active malignancy (excluding non-melanoma skin cancer) within past 12 months	
Non-deferrable major surgery on DAPT	
Recent major surgery or major trauma within 30 days before PCI	

HBR, High bleeding risk; *PCI*, percutaneous coronary intervention; *CKD*, chronic kidney disease; *eGFR*, estimated glomerular filtration rate; *NSAID*, nonsteroidal anti-inflammatory drugs; *ICH*, intracerebral hemorrhage; *AVM*, arteriovenous malformation; *DAPT*, dual antiplatelet therapy.

association between bleeding (regardless of definition) in the ACS population and adverse outcomes, including death, MI, stroke, unplanned revascularization, and stent thrombosis. One of the earliest studies in ACS was published by Moscucci and colleagues, who examined the GRACE registry.[9] Of 24,045 patients with ACS (including unstable angina, NSTEMI, and STEMI), 3.9% had a bleeding event (4.8% in STEMI, 4.7% in NSTEMI, and 2.3% in unstable angina). Similar to previous studies, older age, female sex, renal insufficiency, and history of bleeding were associated with an increased risk of bleeding. After adjustment for potential confounders, major bleeding as defined by the GRACE registry was associated with higher in-hospital mortality. Intermediate-term outcomes have been examined in a variety of studies using different bleeding definitions. In an analysis by Rao and colleagues that examined 26,452 ACS patients enrolled in the PURSUIT, PARAGON B, and GUSTO IIb trials, there was a stepwise increase in risk between GUSTO bleeding severity and 30-day and 6-month death.[10] Other studies by Eikelboom and colleagues, Manoukian and colleagues, and Segev and colleagues describe a significant association between the OASIS, ACUITY, and the Canadian ACS definitions of major bleeding in ACS patients and adverse short- and long-term outcomes, including stroke and stent thrombosis.[9] With respect to a "standardized" definition, Ndrepepa and colleagues examined the association between BARC-defined bleeding and 1-year mortality and found that BARC type 2 or greater bleeding was associated with significantly higher 1-year mortality compared with type 0 (no bleeding), with an adjusted hazard ratio of 2.72.

Because of the slight differences in bleeding definitions across studies, it is tempting to compare the prognostic impact of various scales. Rao and colleagues examined 15,898 patients from two ACS clinical trials that used both the GUSTO and TIMI definitions of bleeding to categorize bleeding severity. When applied separately, each scale identified patients as having had bleeding events that were missed by the other scale. In addition, both GUSTO and TIMI bleeding were associated with an increased risk for 30-day death or MI when examined separately. When both definitions were included in the same model, increasing GUSTO bleeding severity was associated with a stepwise increase in the adjusted hazard of death or MI, whereas TIMI bleeding was no longer correlated with outcomes. These data suggest that data elements reflecting clinical events may have more prognostic value than laboratory-based measures; however, this study, as well as others, demonstrated that clinically overt bleeding that results in a decrease in hemoglobin is also associated with adverse outcomes.

Cost of Care

In the setting of ACS, bleeding complications are also associated with increased costs of care. Bleeding events in ACS may involve various medical interventions, such as blood transfusions, diagnostic testing, and in some cases repeat cardiovascular procedures, which extend the hospital length of stay and contribute to an increased cost of care. Rao and colleagues examined data from the economic substudy of the GUSTO IIb trial, which included 1235 patients from the United States, and found that hospital length of stay and costs increased as bleeding severity increased.[11] After adjustment for baseline differences among patients, each bleeding event was associated with a $3770 increase in costs, and each transfusion event was associated with a $2080 increase. Interestingly, when recurrent MI and bleeding were considered separately, patients who experienced a bleeding event incurred more costs than those who incurred a recurrent MI. Those who experienced both had the highest costs.

Potential Mechanisms of Bleeding and Increased Mortality

It is important to note that the associations between bleeding and outcomes come from posthoc observational analyses of clinical trial data or registry data. As such, assigning causality is problematic. Certainly, intracranial hemorrhage

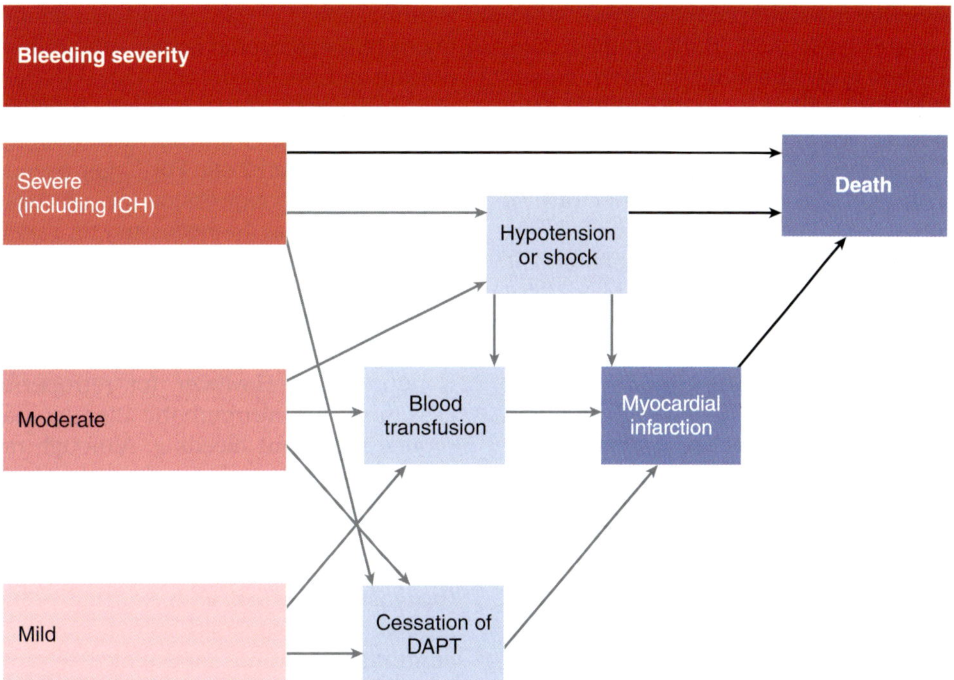

FIG. 24.2 Potential mechanisms underlying the relationship between bleeding complications and mortality. (From Rao SV. The conundrum of reducing ischemic and bleeding events after PCI. *JACC* 2015;65(14):1421–1423).

or frank exsanguination can lead directly to death, but such severe bleeding events are exceedingly rare in the contemporary era of ACS management. More commonly, in-hospital bleeding consists of procedure-related bleeding (e.g., access site hematomas), or on occasion, gastrointestinal bleeding. Bruising or ecchymoses generally characterize bleeding during long-term outpatient therapy with dual antiplatelet therapy. It is difficult to ascribe a direct causal link between these types of bleeding events and subsequent mortality. Therefore, other mechanisms must be involved. Fig. 24.2 shows the potential mechanism underlying the association between bleeding and adverse outcomes. First, confounding must be considered; patients in these data sets who develop bleeding complications are fundamentally different from those who do not in both measured and unmeasured ways. Even the most robust statistical adjustment is unlikely to account for these confounders. Second, bleeding complications likely lead to discontinuation of secondary prevention therapies. Third, there may be an independent role of blood transfusion on outcomes that is distinct from bleeding. Finally, chronic blood loss during the posthospitalization period can result in anemia, which may compromise oxygen delivery to the myocardium, resulting in an increased risk for recurrent MI.

Discontinuation of Antithrombotic Therapies

ACS patients who experience bleeding complications are more likely to have secondary prevention therapies discontinued. In an analysis of the GRACE registry, Spencer and colleagues found that patients who developed in-hospital major bleeding were less likely to have received aspirin (ASA), thienopyridines, and parenteral antithrombin therapy.[10] This difference in the use of guideline-directed medical therapies was estimated to account for a significant proportion of the increased risk for in-hospital mortality. Similarly, an analysis of ACS patients enrolled in the PREMIER registry demonstrated an association between in-hospital bleeding and lower use of ASA and thienopyridine at discharge. These patients were less likely to be restarted on therapy up to 1 year after hospitalization, which may account for the correlation between in-hospital bleeding and subsequent stent thrombosis.

Anemia and Transfusions

As described previously, many bleeding definitions include the data element of red blood cell transfusion. The advantage of incorporating transfusions into a definition is that it represents a discrete event that can be recorded with a date and time. The disadvantage is that clinical practice may dictate the use of transfusion even in the absence of clinically overt bleeding. Moreover, there may be an independent association beyond bleeding between transfusion and adverse outcomes among patients with ischemic heart disease. Several observational studies have shown this association, and adequately powered prospective randomized trials of transfusion thresholds in the ACS population are lacking. Mechanistically, transfusion may affect myocardial oxygenation by limiting oxygen delivery to already ischemic myocardial tissue. In the setting of hypoxia, oxygen delivery is maintained through compensatory vasodilation. This vasodilatory response may be attenuated in coronary vessels that have significant stenosis, and in response, the heart rate increases as a further compensatory response. Increased heart rate in the setting of ACS increases oxygen demand, and although transfusion may seem to increase oxygen delivery, preclinical studies indicate that stored red blood cells are devoid of nitric oxide and 2,3 diphosphoglycerate, further augment vasoconstriction, and do not increase tissue oxygenation.

Two small prospective randomized pilot trials compared transfusion strategies in ACS. Both studies compared a threshold of 8 g/dL (hematocrit 24%) versus 10 g/dL (hematocrit of 30%) and came to different conclusions. The CRIT-Pilot trial randomized 65 patients with ACS and found that a liberal transfusion strategy (i.e., transfusion for a hematocrit ≤30%) resulted in a higher rate of in-hospital death, recurrent MI, or new or worsening heart failure compared with a conservative strategy (liberal 38% vs. restrictive 13%; $P = .046$). In contrast, in the MINT Pilot trial, which randomized 110 patients with ACS and a hemoglobin of less than 10 g/dL, a liberal transfusion strategy resulted in a lower rate of 30-day death, MI, or unplanned revascularization (10.9% vs. 25.5%; $P = .054$). In addition, the rate of 30-day death was lower in those assigned to the liberal strategy (1.8% vs. 17%; $P = .032$).[12] The subsequent full Myocardial Ischemia and Transfusion (MINT) trial was a randomized clinical trial that investigated the optimal blood transfusion strategy among 3500 patients with acute myocardial infarction and comorbid anemia.[12a] The trial demonstrated that a liberal transfusion goal (Hgb ≥10 g/dL) was not superior to a restrictive strategy (Hgb 7 to 8 g/dL) with respect to 30-day all-cause mortality or recurrent myocardial infarction (MI); however the endpoint of cardiac death, which was not independently adjudicated, was significant higher among patients assigned to a restrictive strategy. A prespecified subgroup analysis revealed that participants with type I MI and anemia had higher rates of death or MI at 30 days in the restrictive strategy when compared with those assigned to the liberal strategy (RR, 1.32; 95% CI, 1.04 to 1.67).[12b] This trend towards benefit did not occur in participants with type II MI (risk ratio, 1.05; 95% CI, 0.85 to 1.29). Further research is needed to investigate the impact of different transfusion strategies on long-term outcomes in patients with type I MI.

Approximately 15% to 40% of hospitalizations in ACS patients are complicated by anemia. Anemia, which is defined by the World Health Organization as a hemoglobin less than 13 g/dL, is an independent predictor of major adverse cardiovascular events (MACEs) and mortality in patients across the spectrum of ACS. The pathophysiology underlying poor outcomes in anemic ACS patients may be explained by the combination of reduced oxygen delivery to the already hypoxic myocardium and the high myocardial oxygen demand secondary to the compensatory increases in heart rate and stroke volume. These compensatory mechanisms can result in a deleterious disparity between myocardial oxygen supply and demand.

MANAGEMENT OF BLEEDING COMPLICATIONS

Once a bleeding complication develops, management depends on its severity and location. Mild bleeding events like bruising or ecchymoses can be managed conservatively without stopping antithrombotic therapy. For patients who have undergone invasive evaluation or primary PCI for STEMI, vascular access site bleeding complications can range from superficial hematomas to arteriovenous fistulae and arterial pseudoaneurysms to more severe complications like retroperitoneal hematomas. Superficial access site hematomas can be managed with local compression. Most arteriovenous fistulae formed as a complication of percutaneous femoral arterial access are not hemodynamically significant and close spontaneously. Arterial pseudoaneurysms can occur with either femoral, brachial, or radial artery access, and most will resolve without specific treatment if they are less than 2 cm. For larger pseudoaneurysms, ultrasound-guided compression or ultrasound-guided thrombin injection may be necessary. In rare cases of extremely large pseudoaneurysms, surgical ligation is needed. Radial artery pseudoaneurysms almost always resolve with prolonged compression using a radial hemostatic band. In all of these situations, continuation of dual antiplatelet therapy is appropriate. However, for retroperitoneal hematomas, cessation of antithrombotic therapy may be necessary to reduce persistent bleeding. Although rare, retroperitoneal hematomas are associated with a higher mortality rate because of the large volume of blood that can accumulate in the retroperitoneal space in an occult fashion.

Nonaccess-site bleeding most commonly occurs from the gastrointestinal tract. For bleeding events that are mild or not associated with hemodynamic compromise, continuation of dual antiplatelet therapy may be appropriate while the source of bleeding is investigated. However, for hemodynamically significant gastrointestinal bleeding, cessation of antithrombotic therapy is reasonable until the bleeding source is identified and definitively treated. Intravenous proton pump inhibitors are useful to minimize bleeding and prevent recurrences. Antithrombotic therapy, especially dual antiplatelet therapy, should be restarted as soon as possible after the bleeding event has resolved.

Bleeding events that occur during ACS hospitalization or during PCI (e.g., coronary artery perforation) when antithrombin agents are being administered may require reversal of the anticoagulant effect. For indirect thrombin inhibitors like unfractionated heparin and enoxaparin, protamine sulfate is useful to reverse the anticoagulation. Protamine fully reverses unfractionated heparin and reverses 60% to 80% of the effect of enoxaparin.

PREVENTIVE STRATEGIES

Because options for management are limited and rooted in discontinuation of antithrombotic therapy, prevention of bleeding complications is essential to achieving the best outcomes in ACS. Preventive strategies fall broadly into three categories: appropriate dosing and use of antithrombotic therapies; use of targeted anticoagulants; and vascular access strategies (Table 24.5). In many patients, a combination of these approaches may result in the lowest bleeding risk.

Dosing and Selection of Antithrombotic Therapies

In the hospital setting, inappropriate administration and dosing of antithrombotic, antiplatelet, and glycoprotein IIb/IIIa inhibitor therapy have been implicated as a preventable cause of bleeding among ACS patients. An analysis from the CRUSADE registry of ACS patients reported that 42% of patients received at least one excess dose of antithrombotic agent during their hospitalization. Excess

TABLE 24.5 Strategies to Minimize Bleeding Risk

Pharmacological	Appropriate dosing of antithrombotic medications • Dosing adjusted for renal function if medication is renally cleared • Dosing of unfractionated heparin to maintain aPTT 50–70 sec • Caution with potent antiplatelet agents (prasugrel contraindicated) in patients age ≥75 yrs, body weight <60 kg, previous stroke or TIA • Use of low-dose (≤100 mg) aspirin during long-term therapy with dual antiplatelet therapy Targeted anticoagulants • Fondaparinux • Bivalirudin
Vascular access	Radial approach Appropriate positioning of femoral arteriotomy

[a]*PTT*, Activated partial thrombin time; *TIA*, transient ischemic attack.

dosing of an antithrombotic agent was directly associated with increased rates of bleeding and prolonged length of hospital stay. Risk factors for receiving excessive doses of unfractionated heparin, low–molecular-weight heparin, or glycoprotein IIb/IIIA inhibitors included advanced age, female sex, low body weight, diabetes mellitus, and heart failure. The authors reported that 15% of major bleeding events in ACS patients were preventable with proper bleeding risk assessment and proper administration of anticoagulants. In women, excess dosing may account for up to 25% of the bleeding risk.[13] In this context, it is important to carefully adjust the doses of renally cleared agents, such as eptifibatide and low–molecular-weight heparins, in patients with renal insufficiency; dosing of intravenous unfractionated heparin should be weight-based and aPTT values should be maintained in the range of 50 to 70 seconds.

In the long-term treatment phase of ACS management, reduction of bleeding risk depends on using low-dose ASA and avoiding more potent $P2Y_{12}$ inhibitors in patients with contraindications. In a posthoc analysis of 12,562 ACS patients enrolled in the CURE trial, Peters and colleagues described an increased incidence of major bleeding directly associated with ASA dose (ASA alone: dose 100 mg; 1.9%, 101–199 mg; 2.8%, 200 mg; 3.7%; $P = .0001$; ASA + clopidogrel: dose 100 mg; 3.0%, 101–199 mg; 3.4%, 200 mg; 4.9%; $P = .0009$). There was no significant effect of the ASA dose on efficacy. The only randomized trial of ASA dosing in ACS is the CURRENT-OASIS 7 trial. This trial compared high-dose (600 mg followed by 150 mg/d for 7 days) with standard dose (300 mg followed by 75 mg/d) clopidogrel and high- versus low-dose ASA (300–325 mg/day vs. 75–100 mg/d). At 30 days, there was no difference in efficacy or safety between the high- and low-dose ASA strategies. The effect of ASA dose on safety after 30 days was not assessed in the CURRENT trial, and until further data are available, it seems reasonable to lower doses of ASA 30 days after an ACS event to minimize the bleeding risk.

Antiplatelet Agents and Urgent Coronary Artery Bypass Grafting

A major bleeding risk with clopidogrel use is the risk associated with coronary artery bypass surgery. Because clopidogrel provides irreversible inhibition of the $P2Y_{12}$ receptor, its antiplatelet effect is reversed only when new platelets are generated. Therefore, studies have indicated an increased risk of surgical bleeding if CABG is undertaken within 5 days of clopidogrel therapy. To minimize this risk, it is reasonable to wait 5 to 7 days after clopidogrel discontinuation before proceeding with bypass surgery; importantly, there does not appear to be a risk of increased ischemic events during this waiting period. A strategy of platelet reactivity testing for the timing of CABG after patients were treated with DAPT was shown to be noninferior to the standard of care in ACS patients and significantly shortened the waiting time for CABG by 24 hours, thus reducing hospital expenses.[14]

More potent $P2Y_{12}$ inhibitors are available for use in ACS patients and lead to greater platelet inhibition than clopidogrel, and consequently, have higher bleeding risk. Prasugrel, a thienopyridine that provides greater inhibition of platelet aggregation compared with clopidogrel, was associated with an increased risk of CABG-related bleeding in the TRITON-TIMI 38 trial (see Chapter 13).[5] Ticagrelor, a $P2Y_{12}$ inhibitor that reversibly binds to the receptor, also provides greater platelet inhibition than clopidogrel. In the PLATO trial, ticagrelor plus ASA was also more efficacious than clopidogrel plus ASA in patients with ACS, with a reported significant reduction in CABG-related bleeding.[5] The pattern of CABG-related bleeding may be caused by the reversible nature of the $P2Y_{12}$ inhibition of ticagrelor, but it is more likely that it is caused by differences in the applied definition of CABG-related bleeding and trial protocol. The PLATO trial mandated discontinuation of the study drug several days before planned CABG, thus minimizing the risk for CABG-related bleeding. Prasugrel requires discontinuation at least 7 days and ticagrelor at least 5 days before CABG to minimize surgical bleeding risk.

Duration of DAPT and De-escalation

Societal guidelines have a class I recommendation for a DAPT duration of therapy of 12 months in patients undergoing PCI for ACS, but this duration can be reduced or extended based on the patient's bleeding and thrombotic risks.[15] Discontinuation of the $P2Y_{12}$ inhibitor and continuation of aspirin monotherapy was the traditional single antiplatelet regimen; however, recent data suggest that discontinuation of aspirin and continuation of the $P2Y_{12}$ inhibitor may be more advantageous, and there has been a paradigm shift with respect to single antiplatelet regimens (SAPT). A trial of Ticagrelor monotherapy after 3 months in patients treated with Sirolimus-eluting stents for ACS demonstrated superiority for NACE over DAPT.[16] Therefore, for patients at high risk of bleeding, the European guidelines have a recommendation to consider discontinuation of $P2Y_{12}$ inhibitor after 3 months (Class IIa) or discontinuation of aspirin at 3 to 6 months (Class IIa). Similar to the European guidelines, ACC/AHA/SCAI recommend the discontinuation of aspirin at 1 to 3 months in all patients (class IIa) or the discontinuation of the $P2Y_{12}$ inhibitor at 6 months for select patients at high bleeding risk or overt bleeding on DAPT (class IIb).

De-escalation from a potent $P2Y_{12}$ inhibitor to clopidogrel after a brief period post ACS, when the ischemic risk is highest, is another approach to reduce bleeding risk without impacting thrombotic outcomes (Fig. 24.3). A CYP2C19 genotype-guided strategy to select the oral

guidelines in North America recommend interruption of OAC with the exception of emergency PCI.[7–9] The 2020 ACC expert consensus decision pathway provide practical recommendations for patients requiring an invasive approach.[8] For patients requiring emergent interventions, VKA or DOAC therapy is held, and percutaneous coronary intervention performed without delay. If possible, a radial approach is preferred because of the lower risk of bleeding. For nonemergent PCI, OAC is held, and the procedure could be performed when the INR < 2.0 for VKAs or when DOAC are withheld for at least 2 half-lives for radial PCI; and for at least 4 half-lives for transfemoral approaches. OAC is usually resumed 24 hours post-PCI unless there are bleeding complications.

PATIENTS WITH ACS WITHOUT A SEPARATE INDICATION FOR OAC

Patients with ACS are at risk of recurrent atherothrombosis despite treatment with antiplatelet therapy. These events are thought to be mediated in part by a persistent acquired hypercoagulable state, as evidenced by elevated blood levels of coagulation biomarkers (such as d-dimer, prothrombin fragments, and thrombin-antithrombin complexes) after the index event. By suppressing persistent hypercoagulability, the addition of OAC to antiplatelet therapy has the potential to prevent recurrent events, but has the downside of an increased risk of bleeding. Strategies that have been evaluated to mitigate bleeding risk in patients treated with the combination include a shift from VKA to DOACs, the use of lower dose of DOACs, and shortening the duration of dual antiplatelet therapy. Novel factor XI inhibitors that are hypothesized to prevent thrombosis with little impact on hemostasis are presently undergoing evaluation in randomized trials.

Initial Anticoagulation

In the immediate period after ACS, the goal of adding anticoagulant to DAPT is to prevent thrombus progression or new thrombus formation at the site of plaque disruption, facilitate clot lysis, and prevent thrombus formation on guidewires and coronary stents during percutaneous coronary interventions. Three classes of parenteral anticoagulants are approved for the acute treatment of patients with ACS: heparins, which include unfractionated heparin (UFH) and low-molecular-weight heparin (LMWH), a direct thrombin inhibitor, bivalirudin, and a synthetic pentasaccharide, fondaparinux. These anticoagulants have different pharmacological profiles (e.g., half-life, renal clearance, reversibility), and fondaparinux is less effective than unfractionated heparin in preventing catheter thrombosis, but all have been shown to be effective in preventing recurrent ischemic events in patients with ACS (see Chapter 12).

In the early trials of LMWH, treatment with a parenteral anticoagulant was evaluated for durations of up to 60 days but the main benefits appeared to be confined to the first 14 days. With the routine adoption of early invasive management strategies and rapid hospital discharge, the duration of parenteral anticoagulation has been shortened, largely for pragmatic reasons and potentially at the cost of reduced efficacy. To address this issue, the H-REPLACE trial examined whether oral treatment with rivaroxaban, a factor Xa inhibitor, could replace enoxaparin in the initial management of patients with STEMI. In H-REPLACE, 2055 participants with ACS who missed the primary reperfusion window for STEMI or did not undergo an early invasive strategy for management of NSTE-ACS were randomized 1:1:1 to oral rivaroxaban 2.5 mg or 5 mg or 1 mg/kg subcutaneous enoxaparin twice daily in addition to dual antiplatelet therapy for a mean duration of 3.7 days.[10] The primary safety outcome was a composite of major bleeding, clinically relevant nonmajor bleeding, and minor bleeding according to the International Society of Thrombosis and Hemostasis (ISTH) definitions and the primary efficacy outcome was major adverse cardiovascular event (MACE), a composite of death from cardiac causes, MI, stroke, or revascularization during a 6-month follow-up period. The noninferiority margins for the primary safety and efficacy outcomes were 1.24 and 1.185, respectively. When compared with enoxaparin, both rivaroxaban 2.5 mg (hazard ratio, HR: 0.68; 95% CI, 0.43–1.07) and 5 mg (HR: 0.88; 95% CI, 0.70–1.09) were noninferior in terms of bleeding. For MACE, noninferiority was reached for rivaroxaban 5 mg (HR: 0.60; 95% CI, 0.31–1.16) but not for rivaroxaban 2.5 mg (HR: 0.68; 95% CI, 0.36–1.30). Based on these results, rivaroxaban appears to be an attractive oral alternative to parenteral anticoagulation for the initial management of ACS but is not currently approved for this indication.[11]

Long-Term Oral Anticoagulation for Acute Coronary Syndrome

Table 25.1 summarizes the pharmacology of oral anticoagulants that have been approved for long-term management of patients after acute coronary syndrome.

Vitamin K Antagonists

In a meta-analysis of 14 trials involving 25,307 patients with recent ACS, the combination of moderate intensity warfarin (INR 2–3) and aspirin compared with aspirin alone reduced the risk of MI, ischemic stroke or death by about 25% (9.4% vs. 12.3%) but increases the risk of major bleeding by more than two-fold (2.6% vs. 1.1%), and there was no mortality benefit.[12] Most of these trials were performed prior to the introduction of DAPT which was subsequently demonstrated in randomized trials to reduce MACE with a more acceptable bleeding risk than warfarin, and in the case of the combination of ticagrelor and aspirin reduced mortality compared with aspirin alone. With the added inconvenience of VKA management, warfarin has had only limited uptake for long-term secondary prevention following MI. However, the results provided proof of principle for the use of dual pathway inhibition (combination of anticoagulant and antiplatelet therapy) and prompted reevaluation of combination therapy when the direct oral thrombin or factor Xa inhibitors were introduced as alternatives to VKAs.

Direct Oral Anticoagulants

Unlike VKAs, DOACs are administered in fixed doses without laboratory monitoring and have a lower potential for food and drug interactions. Large, randomized trials for VTE prevention and treatment and for stroke prevention in AF demonstrated that DOACs were at least as effective as conventional anticoagulants and associated with a lower risk of life-threatening bleeding.[13]

TABLE 25.1 Pharmacology of Oral Anticoagulants for Secondary Prevention in Acute Coronary Syndrome

	WARFARIN	RIVAROXABAN
Target	VKORC1	Factor Xa
Dosing and frequency	Variable	Fixed, 2.5 mg twice daily
Routine monitoring	Yes, dose adjusted to an INR target of 2.0–3.0	No
Half-life	20–60 h	9–13 h
Hepatic metabolism	100%	57%
Renal clearance	<1%	66%[a]
Antidote	Vitamin K and PCC	Andexanet alfa, PCC
Approval for ACS management	Yes	2.5 mg twice daily approved in Europe but not in the United States

INR, International normalized ratio; *PCC*, prothrombin complex concentrates; *VKORC1*, vitamin K epoxide reductase complex subunit 1
[a]1/3 of active drug is cleared as unchanged drug, and another 1/3 of active drug, which is metabolized to inactive metabolites, is also cleared by the kidneys.

Phase 2 trials evaluated direct oral thrombin inhibitors (ximelagatran and dabigatran) as well as factor Xa inhibitors (rivaroxaban, apixaban, darexaban, and TAK 442) in patients with ACS. Only rivaroxaban and apixaban were further evaluated in phase 3 trials for this indication. Ximelagatran was withdrawn from the market because of hepatotoxicity, and the results with the other agents were not sufficiently promising to progress to evaluation in phase 3 trials.

Apixaban

In the Apixaban for Prevention of Acute Ischemic Events 1 (APPRAISE-1) trial, the direct FXa inhibitor, apixaban (5 mg–20 mg) was compared to placebo in 1751 patients within 7 days of presentation with ACS, who were treated with standard antiplatelet therapy (aspirin or DAPT). The two highest-dose apixaban arms (10 mg twice daily, 20 mg daily) were discontinued on the recommendation of the data monitoring committee because of excess total bleeding. Compared with placebo, apixaban resulted in a dose-dependent increase in major or clinically relevant nonmajor bleeding. Apixaban 2.5 mg twice daily and 10 mg once daily resulted in lower rates of ischemic events compared with placebo with the balance of risk-benefit favoring the 10-mg once daily dose. Patients treated with the combination of clopidogrel and aspirin appeared to have an attenuated benefit of apixaban, and a higher risk of bleeding compared with those treated with aspirin alone. Based on the results indicating favorable risk-benefit of 10 mg once daily, a 5 mg twice daily dose was selected for testing in the phase 3 APPRAISE-2 trial. In APPRAISE-2, apixaban 5 mg twice daily (a therapeutic anticoagulant dose) was compared to placebo in 7392 patients with recent ACS who received standard medical therapy (aspirin and/or clopidogrel). Because of a substantial (2.5-fold) increase in major bleeding with no signal of benefit, the trial was terminated early.[14]

Rivaroxaban

In the phase II Anti-Xa Therapy to Lower Cardiovascular Events in Addition to Standard Therapy in Subjects with Acute Coronary Syndrome–Thrombolysis in Myocardial Infarction 46 (ATLAS ACS-TIMI 46) trial, the direct FXa inhibitor, rivaroxaban (5–20 mg dose) was compared to placebo in 3491 patients within 7 days of presentation with ACS and who were treated with standard antiplatelet therapy (aspirin or DAPT). Rivaroxaban was associated with a dose-dependent increase in clinically significant bleeding events, with a trend towards a reduction in the primary efficacy endpoint of death, MI, stroke, or severe recurrent ischemia requiring revascularisation. Two rivaroxaban dosing regimens, namely 2.5 mg and 5 mg twice daily were selected for testing in the phase 3 ATLAS ACS 2-TIMI 51 trial.

In the phase III ATLAS-ACS-2 TIMI 51, rivaroxaban (2.5 mg and 5 mg twice daily) was compared with placebo in 15,526 patients who were treated with standard antiplatelet therapy (aspirin or DAPT) within 7 days of presentation with ACS. The primary efficacy outcome was a composite of death from cardiovascular causes, MI, or stroke; and primary safety outcome was TIMI major bleeding not related to coronary-artery bypass grafting. Participants received study drugs for a mean of 13 months and up to 31 months. Both regimens significantly reduced the primary efficacy outcome and increased the risk of major bleeding, but the lower dose of rivaroxaban resulted in less bleeding than the higher dose. The 2.5 mg twice daily dose also significantly reduced cardiovascular death and overall mortality.[14] Based on this favorable risk-benefit profile, the 2.5 mg twice daily dose was approved by the European Medicine Agency for the prevention of atherothrombotic events in adult patients after ACS with elevated cardiac biomarkers, but it has not been approved by the US FDA.

Factor XI Inhibitors

The Study to Gather Information About the Proper Dosing and Safety of the Oral FXIa Inhibitor BAY 2433334 in Patients Following an Acute Heart Attack (PACIFIC-AMI) is the first phase II trial to examine the addition of an oral FXIa inhibitor to DAPT in patients presenting within 5 days of a MI.[15] In this trial, 1601 patients with recent acute MI receiving DAPT (80% received ticagrelor or prasugrel) were randomized to oral asundexian (10, 20, or 50 mg daily) or placebo. The main safety outcome was bleeding defined as Bleeding Academic Research Consortium type 2, 3, or 5 bleeding, and the efficacy outcome was a composite of cardiovascular death, MI, stroke, or stent thrombosis. Asundexian produced near complete inhibition of FXIa activity without increasing bleeding, but there was no evidence of an efficacy signal even with the higher doses (pooled asundexian 20–50 mg vs. placebo: HR, 1.05 [90% CI, 0.69–1.61]). These results suggest that inhibition of FXIa may be a safer approach to anticoagulation in patients with a recent ACS who are receiving DAPT, but it remains to be seen if this approach is effective.

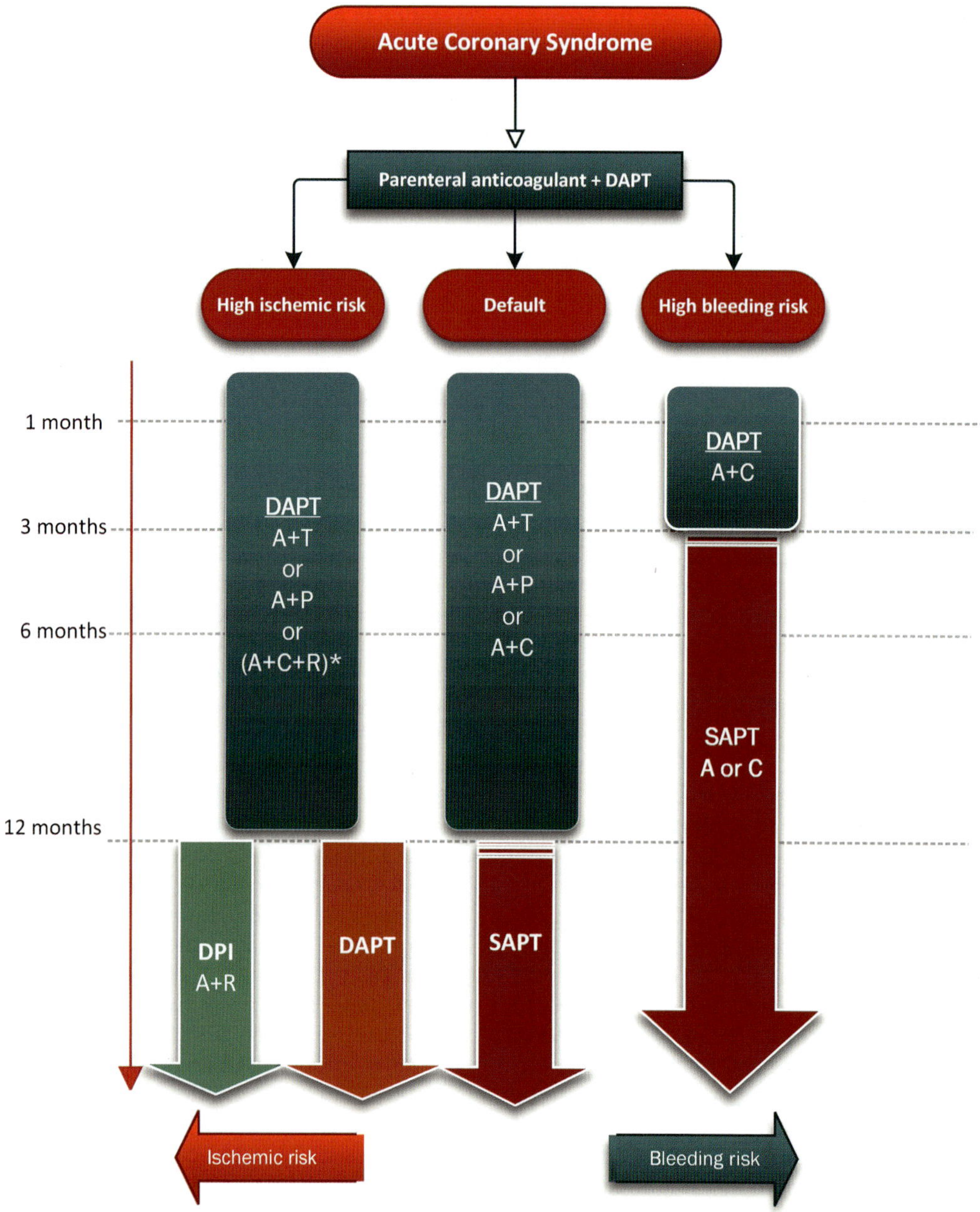

FIG. 25.1 Suggested antithrombotic therapy after acute coronary syndrome. Following an acute coronary syndrome, guidelines recommend dual antiplatelet therapy (DAPT) with aspirin and a newer generation $P2Y_{12}$ inhibitor in preference to clopidogrel for at least 12 months, after which patients could be switched to single antiplatelet agent such clopidogrel or a newer generation $P2Y_{12}$ inhibitor like ticagrelor or to dual pathway inhibition (DPI) with the combination of very low dose rivaroxaban (2.5 mg twice daily) and aspirin. In patients at high thrombotic and ischemic risk, antithrombotic therapy can be intensified by prolonging the duration of DAPT beyond 12 months or switching to DPI after 12 months. Oral anticoagulation has limited role in the first 12 months post ACS. *In some countries (but not US), very low-dose rivaroxaban could be added to clopidogrel based DAPT for 12 months post ACS. In patients at high risk of bleeding or with recent bleeding, a shorter duration of clopidogrel-based DAPT is recommended before switching to single antiplatelet agent. High bleeding risk is defined according to the Academic Research Consortium High Bleeding Risk (ARC-HBR) criteria,[27] and high thrombotic or ischemic risk is defined according to the ACC/AHA DAPT guideline. *A*, Aspirin; *C*, clopidogrel; *DAPT*, dual antiplatelet therapy; *DPI*, dual pathway inhibition; *P*, prasugrel; *R*, rivaroxaban 2.5 mg twice daily; *SAPT*, single platelet therapy; *T*, ticagrelor. (From Collet J-P, Thiele H, Barbato E, et al. 2020 ESC guidelines for the management of acute coronary syndromes in patients presenting without persistent ST-segment elevation: the task force for the management of acute coronary syndromes in patients presenting without persistent ST-segment elevation of the European Society of Cardiology (ESC). *Eur Heart J*. 2020;42:1289–1367, and Byrne RA, Rossello X, Coughlan JJ, et al. 2023 ESC guidelines for the management of acute coronary syndromes: developed by the task force on the management of acute coronary syndromes of the European Society of Cardiology (ESC). *Eur Heart J*. 2023;44:3720–3826.)

Approach to Oral Antithrombotic Therapy After Acute Coronary Syndrome

In the initial management of ACS, parenteral anticoagulation in addition to dual antiplatelet therapy is the standard of care and guidelines do not recommend OAC at this time (Fig. 25.1). In patients invasively managed and without bleeding contraindications, the American College of Cardiology/American Heart Association (ACC/AHA) and European Society of Cardiology (ESC) guidelines recommend DAPT for at least 12 months with ticagrelor or prasugrel in preference to clopidogrel, and in patients who are medically managed, ticagrelor is the preferred P2Y12 inhibitor.[6,16,17] In patients with high risk of bleeding or recent bleeding, the duration of DAPT could be shortened (≤3 months) before switching to single antiplatelet therapy.

Following the acute phase, it remains unclear whether patients should be treated with oral anticoagulant in addition to contemporary DAPT with potent P2Y12 inhibitors (ticagrelor or prasugrel). Although the addition of rivaroxaban 2.5 mg twice daily to DAPT reduced ischemic events and cardiovascular mortality in ATLAS-TIMI ACS 51, most patients were treated with aspirin and clopidogrel in this trial, and the risk-benefit of this approach for patients receiving potent P2Y12 inhibitors, such as ticagrelor or prasugrel, is unclear. The ESC guidelines provide a Class IIb recommendation (level of evidence B) for the addition of rivaroxaban 2.5 mg twice daily to clopidogrel-based DAPT in select patients with ACS who are at high ischemic risk and who have no history of stroke or transient ischemic events and no bleeding contraindications.[4]

After 12 months of treatment, stable patients can stop DAPT and continue single antiplatelet agents (Fig. 25.1), but patients at high thrombotic or ischemic risk could continue DAPT or consider a switch to the combination of rivaroxaban 2.5 mg twice daily and aspirin (dual pathway inhibition) based on the findings of the COMPASS trial,[4] which demonstrated that the combination reduced MACE as well as overall mortality.

PATIENTS WITH ACUTE CORONARY SYNDROME WHO ARE STARTING OR RESUMING ORAL ANTICOAGULATION FOR A SEPARATE INDICATION

Patients presenting with ACS often have or develop comorbid conditions that require long-term anticoagulation. About 1 in 10 patients with ACS have atrial fibrillation (AF), and about 1 in 15 develop left ventricular thrombus following a STEMI. Other patients may require anticoagulation for the management of venous thromboembolism, for mechanical valve replacement, or for antiphospholipid antibody syndrome. For these indications, anticoagulation is more effective than DAPT, but DAPT is the standard of care for patients with ACS. Such quandary prompted the use of triple therapy (combination of DAPT and therapeutic anticoagulation) with the intent of preventing both coronary ischemic and other thromboembolic events, but the benefit-risk profile of triple therapy is suboptimal because the risk of major bleeding with triple therapy is unacceptably high, at least 10% per year.[18] Randomized trials in patients with AF undergoing percutaneous coronary interventions (PCI) for coronary artery disease have demonstrated that dual pathway compared with triple therapy reduces bleeding without compromising efficacy, and guidelines are now recommending dual over triple therapy for most patients with AF and ACS.[5,7,8,19,20] The same approach is commonly followed for patients with indications for OAC other than AF.

Atrial Fibrillation in Patients With Acute Coronary Syndrome

To reduce bleeding in patients requiring both anticoagulant and antiplatelet therapy, two approaches have been evaluated: the early transition from DAPT to single antiplatelet therapy with clopidogrel, and the shift from VKA to DOAC-based therapy. These approaches have been tested mostly in patients with AF undergoing PCI for coronary artery disease, of whom some had ACS. In a meta-analysis of four randomized trials that included 10,026 AF patients undergoing PCI, the combination of these two approaches, that is, the switch from VKA to DOAC and the use of single antiplatelet therapy rather than DAPT reduced major bleeding and intracranial hemorrhage (ICH) by 51% and 74%, respectively.[21] More specifically, the shift to SAPT and the shift from VKA to DOAC-based therapy resulted in a 42% and 30% reduction in major bleeding, respectively.[21] The rates of major adverse cardiovascular events (OR, 1.02; 95% CI, 0.71–1.97) were similar but the CI for the estimate was wide. Similarly, the estimates for recurrent MI (OR, 1.18; 95% CI, 0.81–1.72) and for stent thrombosis (OR, 1.41; 95% CI, 0.71–2.76) did not show significant difference but the wide CI could not exclude the potential of an excess of these events and argues for a short duration of triple therapy in patients at very high ischemic risk. These results have prompted revisions of clinical practice guidelines, which now recommend dual antithrombotic therapy over triple therapy in most patients but allow for the option of extending triple therapy in patients at high risk of stent thrombosis or recurrent ACS (Fig. 25.2).[5,7,8,19,20]

Managing Oral Anticoagulant and Antiplatelet Therapy in Patients with Acute Coronary Syndrome and Atrial Fibrillation (Without Mechanical Valve Replacement or Moderate-Severe Rheumatic Mitral Valve Stenosis)

The AHA/ACC/Heart Rhythm Society guidelines recommend that clinicians assess stroke risk in patients with ACS and AF using the CHA2DS2-VASc score and prescribe anticoagulation if the CHA2DS2-VASc score is ≥2 for males and ≥3 for females.[8,19] Patients with lower scores could be offered DAPT, but oral anticoagulant therapy could still be considered in patients with additional risk factors (left atrial enlargement, cardiomyopathy, or rheumatic valvular disease), and in those who prefer anticoagulation therapy and do not have an unacceptable risk of bleeding. Modifiable risk factors for bleeding can be identified using validated risk prediction tools (HAS-BLED, HEMORR2HAGES, or ATRIA).[8]

Guidelines recommend a DOAC over VKA because of the lower risk of bleeding and an early transition to single antiplatelet therapy with clopidogrel (within 1 week for most patients) and continued for up to 12 months after ACS or coronary stent implantation, after which time antiplatelet therapy could be stopped if the patient is stable (Fig. 25.2).[5,6,8,19,20] Clopidogrel is the preferred antiplatelet agent because of the lack of safety data with more potent P2Y12 inhibitors. Select patients at high risk of stent thrombosis or recurrent ACS can continue DAPT for up to 1 month following a recent ACS if there is no bleeding contraindication (Fig. 25.2). Table 25.2 details the dosing for DOACs in AF.

Venous Thromboembolism in Patients With Acute Coronary Syndrome

The standard therapy for acute venous thromboembolism is therapeutic anticoagulation and the 2020 ACC expert consensus decision pathway gives preference to DOACs over

and management of atrial fibrillation of the European Society of Cardiology (ESC) developed with the special contribution of the European Heart Rhythm Association (EHRA) of the ESC. *Eur Heart J.* 2021;42:373–498.
6. Byrne RA, Rossello X, Coughlan JJ, et al. 2023 ESC guidelines for the management of acute coronary syndromes: developed by the task force on the management of acute coronary syndromes of the European Society of Cardiology (ESC). *Eur Heart J.* 2023;44:3720–3826.
7. Angiolillo DJ, Bhatt DL, Cannon CP, et al. Antithrombotic therapy in patients with atrial fibrillation treated with oral anticoagulation undergoing percutaneous coronary intervention: a North American perspective: 2021 update. *Circulation.* 2021;143:583–596.
8. Kumbhani DJ, Cannon CP, Beavers CJ, et al. 2020 ACC expert consensus decision pathway for anticoagulant and antiplatelet therapy in patients with atrial fibrillation or venous thromboembolism undergoing percutaneous coronary intervention or with atherosclerotic cardiovascular disease. *J Am Coll Cardiol.* 2021;77:629–658.
9. Andrade JG, Aguilar M, Atzema C, et al. The 2020 Canadian Cardiovascular Society/Canadian Heart Rhythm Society comprehensive guidelines for the management of atrial fibrillation. *Can J Cardiol.* 2020;36:1847–1948.
10. Zhou S, Xiao Y, Zhou C, et al. Effect of rivaroxaban vs. enoxaparin on major cardiac adverse events and bleeding risk in the acute phase of acute coronary syndrome: the H-REPLACE randomized equivalence and noninferiority trial. *JAMA Netw Open.* 2023;6:e2255709.
11. Berwanger O. Rivaroxaban for patients with acute coronary syndromes—where do we stand? *JAMA Netw Open.* 2023;6:e2255724.
12. Capodanno D, Bhatt DL, Eikelboom JW, et al. Dual-pathway inhibition for secondary and tertiary antithrombotic prevention in cardiovascular disease. *Nat Rev Cardiol.* 2020;17:242–257.
13. Carnicelli AP, Hong H, Connolly SJ, et al. Direct oral anticoagulants versus warfarin in patients with atrial fibrillation: patient-level network meta-analyses of randomized clinical trials with interaction testing by age and sex. *Circulation.* 2022;145:242–255.
14. Chan NC, Weitz JI. Antithrombotic agents. *Circ Res.* 2019;124:426–436.
15. Rao SV, Kirsch B, Bhatt DL, et al. A multicenter, phase 2, randomized, placebo-controlled, double-blind, parallel-group, dose-finding trial of the oral factor XIa inhibitor asundexian to prevent adverse cardiovascular outcomes after acute myocardial infarction. *Circulation.* 2022;146:1196–1206.
16. Capodanno D, Alfonso F, Levine GN, et al. ACC/AHA versus ESC guidelines on Dual antiplatelet therapy: JACC guideline comparison. *J Am Coll Cardiol.* 2018;72:2915–2931.
17. Lawton JS, Tamis-Holland JE, Bangalore S, et al. 2021 ACC/AHA/SCAI guideline for coronary artery revascularization: a report of the American College of Cardiology/American Heart Association joint committee on clinical practice guidelines. *J Am Coll Cardiol.* 2022;79:e21–e129.
18. Rein NV, Heide-Jørgensen U, Lijfering WM, et al. Major bleeding rates in atrial fibrillation patients on single, dual, or triple antithrombotic therapy. *Circulation.* 2019;139:775–786.
19. January CT, Wann LS, Calkins H, et al. 2019 AHA/ACC/HRS focused update of the 2014 AHA/ACC/HRS guideline for the management of patients with atrial fibrillation: a report of the American College of Cardiology/American Heart Association task force on clinical practice guidelines and the Heart Rhythm Society in collaboration with the society of thoracic surgeons. *Circulation.* 2019;140:e125–e151.
20. Steffel J, Collins R, Antz M, et al. 2021 European Heart Rhythm Association practical guide on the use of non-Vitamin K antagonist oral anticoagulants in patients with atrial fibrillation. *Europace.* 2021;23:1612–1676.
21. Lopes RD, Hong H, Harskamp RE, et al. Safety and Efficacy of antithrombotic strategies in patients with atrial fibrillation undergoing percutaneous coronary intervention: a network meta-analysis of randomized controlled trials. *JAMA Cardiol.* 2019;4:747–755.
22. Levine GN, McEvoy JW, Fang JC, et al. Management of patients at risk for and with left ventricular thrombus: a scientific statement from the American Heart Association. *Circulation.* 2022;146:e205–e223.
23. Kwok CS, Bennett S, Borovac JA, et al. An evidence-based evaluation of left ventricular thrombus treatment, outcomes, and resolution: a systematic review, pooled analysis and meta-analysis. *Coron Artery Dis.* 2023;34:260–273.
24. Wang TY, Svensson LG, Wen J, et al. Apixaban or warfarin in patients with an On-X mechanical aortic valve. *NEJM Evid.* 2023;2:EVIDoa2300067.
25. Connolly SJ, Karthikeyan G, Ntsekhe M, et al. Rivaroxaban in rheumatic heart disease–associated atrial fibrillation. *N Engl J Med.* 2022;387:978–988.
26. Khairani CD, Bejjani A, Piazza G, et al. Direct oral anticoagulants vs. Vitamin K antagonists in patients with antiphospholipid syndromes. *J Am Coll Cardiol.* 2023;81:16–30.
27. Urban P, Mehran R, Colleran R, et al. Defining high bleeding risk in patients undergoing percutaneous coronary intervention. *Circulation.* 2019;140:240–261.

26 Antiplatelet Therapy After Acute Coronary Syndrome

SIDDHARTH M. PATEL, MICHELLE L. O'DONOGHUE, AND MARC S. SABATINE

INTRODUCTION

Myocardial infarction (MI) is classically caused by atherothrombosis (see Chapters 1 and 32), with platelets playing a pivotal role in clot formation following plaque rupture or erosion. As such, antiplatelet therapy is an important cornerstone in the management of atherothrombosis (see Chapter 13). Moreover, patients with prior MI have a heightened risk of recurrent atherothrombotic events, thereby increasing the anticipated benefit from longer duration or more potent antiplatelet therapy (Figs. 26.1 and 26.2).

However, existing antiplatelet therapies also increase bleeding risk. Accordingly, the type, intensity, and duration of antiplatelet therapy after MI should be tailored in accordance with the patient's risk of subsequent ischemic events and of bleeding. This chapter considers the rationale for antiplatelet therapy for long-term secondary prevention in patients with MI, reviews trials of specific agents and strategies, and describes the application of clinical trial evidence in clinical practice.

EPIDEMIOLOGY OF RECURRENT ATHEROTHROMBOSIS

Myocardial Infarction as a Marker of Long-Term Atherothrombotic Risk

Several modern observational data sets have characterized long-term ischemic risk in patients with previous atherothrombosis. An analysis of data for 64,977 stable outpatients enrolled in the REduction of Atherothrombosis for Continued Health (REACH) Registry evaluated the risk of cardiovascular death, MI, and stroke over a 4-year period based on a clinical history of either cardiovascular risk factors only, known atherosclerosis but no previous ischemic event, or a previous ischemic event (Fig. 26.3). Those with a prior ischemic event had the highest risk of cardiovascular death, MI, or stroke at 4 years when compared with patients with stable atherosclerosis or risk factors alone. Although this risk was higher for those within 1 year of their event, it remained heightened for those patients who had survived more than a year from their most recent event.

Types of Atherothrombotic Events in Stable Patients With Previous Myocardial Infarction

In patients presenting with acute MI, the risk of early ischemic complications is typically a combination of issues related to the culprit coronary lesion or associated coronary interventions, as well as vulnerable/significant nonculprit lesions throughout the coronary vasculature. More potent antiplatelet strategies reduce the risk of periprocedural MI (type 4a MI) occurring in the setting of percutaneous coronary intervention (PCI; see Chapter 11) and stent thrombosis (type 4b MI), as well as recurrent spontaneous MI (type 1 MI).[1,2] After discharge, however, the risk of stent-related complications decreases, whereas the risk of recurrent spontaneous events persists (see Fig. 26.2). In studies of cardiovascular events occurring after successful PCI in patients with acute coronary syndrome (ACS), rates of recurrent events related to the culprit lesion and to nonculprit lesions were similar (Fig. 26.4). In addition, nonculprit lesions leading to recurrent atherothrombosis frequently were angiographically mild at initial angiography but were associated with markers of instability, including lipid-rich thin-cap fibroatheromas (see Chapter 10).

Collectively, these data indicate that as patients stabilize after an acute MI, the type of recurrent coronary event for which they are at risk may evolve from those related to both culprit and nonculprit lesions and coronary intervention, to those primarily occurring in the setting of de novo plaque rupture elsewhere in the coronary tree (see Fig. 26.2).

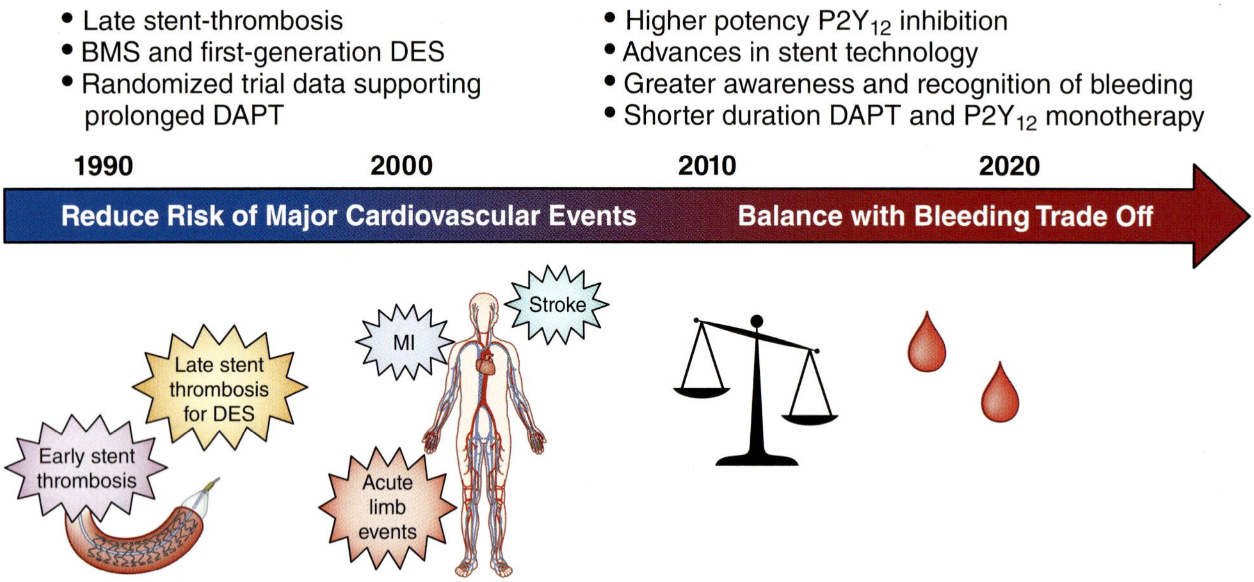

FIG. 26.1 Evolution in the role of $P2Y_{12}$ inhibition and dual antiplatelet therapy in patients with previous myocardial infarction. *BMS*, Bare metal stent; *DAPT*, dual antiplatelet therapy; *DES*, drug-eluting stent.

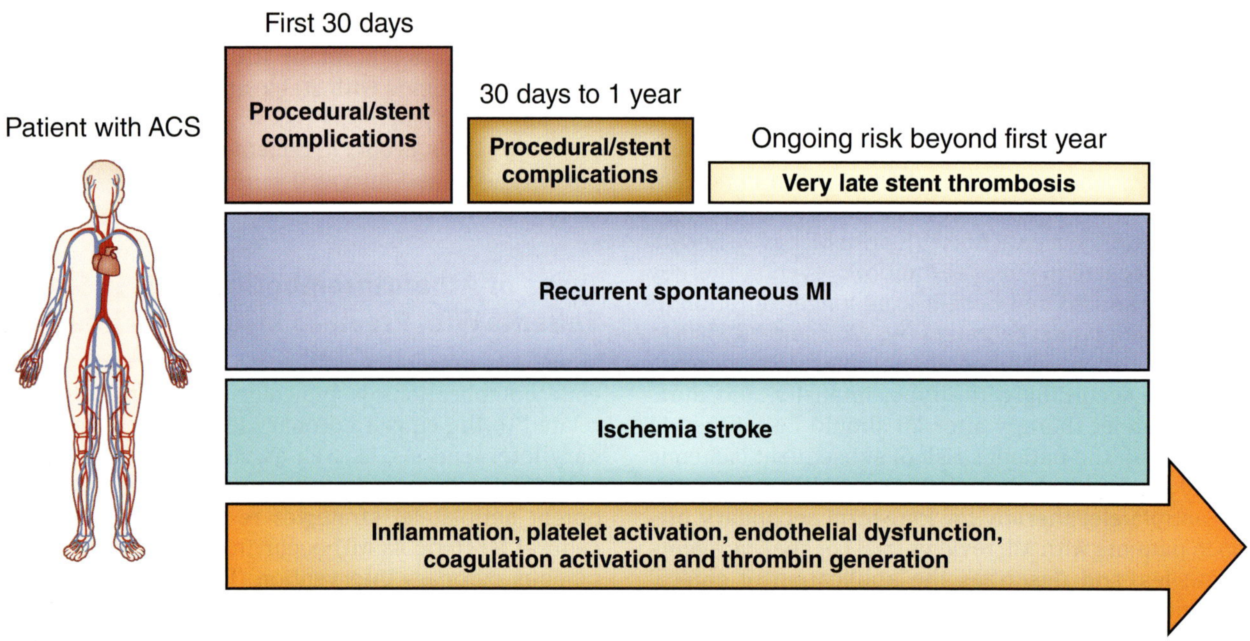

FIG. 26.2 Risk of ischemic events over time in patients presenting with spontaneous myocardial infarction (MI). The risk for recurrent spontaneous MI and ischemic stroke, in the context of a pro-thrombotic milieu persists in the longer term in patients with a prior ACS, whereas the risk of procedural and stent-related complications is highest in the period immediately following PCI or the ACS presentation. *ACS*, acute coronary syndrome; *PCI*, percutaneous coronary intervention.

Rationale for Antiplatelet Therapy for Long-Term Secondary Prevention

Given the heightened long-term risk for recurrent atherothrombotic events among patients with prior MI, both oral antiplatelet and anticoagulant strategies have been intensely studied for long-term secondary prevention. In particular, several antiplatelet agents targeting differing pathways of platelet activation that can be used alone or in combination are currently employed early after an MI and may further offer clinical benefit in more stable patients with chronic coronary disease. The use of low-dose anticoagulants as adjunctive therapy is covered in Chapter 25.

CLINICAL TRIALS OF ANTIPLATELET THERAPY FOR SECONDARY PREVENTION AFTER MYOCARDIAL INFARCTION

Aspirin

Aspirin has been studied for ischemic risk reduction in multiple randomized trials and analyzed in a meta-analysis conducted by the Antithrombotic Trialists' Collaborative. In early iterations of the meta-analysis, a total of 287 randomized, controlled studies involving 135,000 patients in trials of a variety of antiplatelet agents were combined and showed a reduction in 36 serious vascular events

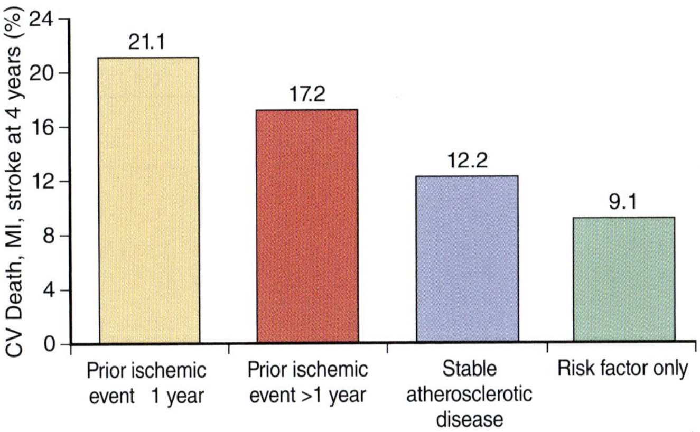

FIG. 26.3 Rate of cardiovascular (CV) death, myocardial infarction (MI), or stroke at 4 years by history of previous ischemic event, stable atherosclerotic disease, or risk factors only. (Adapted from Bhatt DL, Eagle KA, Ohman EM, et al. Comparative determinants of 4-year cardiovascular event rates in stable outpatients at risk of or with atherothrombosis. *JAMA*. 2010;304:1350–1357.)

prevented per 1000 patients with previous MI treated for 2 years (Fig. 26.5A).[3] A subsequent analysis that focused specifically on the efficacy and safety of aspirin for primary and secondary prevention included 6 trials in patients with previous MI and 10 trials in patients with previous stroke or transient ischemic attack (TIA). In the secondary prevention population, aspirin reduced the risk of any serious vascular event by 19% (hazard ratio [HR], 0.81; 95% confidence interval [CI], 0.75–0.87), with an absolute risk reduction of 1.49% per year versus placebo.[3] There were consistent relative risk reductions in coronary mortality, myocardial infarction, and ischemic stroke.

In a study considering the safety of antiplatelet therapy, aspirin increased the risk of major extracranial bleeding, primarily gastrointestinal bleeding (absolute risk increase of 0.4% per year) and hemorrhagic stroke (absolute risk increase of 0.01% per year).[3] Overall, a net benefit was achieved with aspirin for secondary prevention due to the ischemic risk in that population. The CURRENT-OASIS 7 trial evaluated whether high-dose (300–325 mg daily) aspirin is superior to low-dose aspirin (75–100 mg daily) for 30 days in patients presenting with ACS (Fig. 26.5B).[4] In this acute setting, in which potent platelet inhibition might be expected to be most beneficial, there was no difference in the composite of cardiovascular death, MI, or stroke with high- versus low-dose aspirin (HR, 0.97; 95% CI, 0.86–1.09; $P = .61$); however, the rates of major gastrointestinal bleeding ($P = .04$) and minor bleeding ($P = .04$) were higher. The pragmatic open-label ADAPTABLE study evaluated low-dose (81 mg) versus high-dose (325 mg) aspirin in 15,076 stable patients with established atherosclerotic cardiovascular disease, among which 5305 patients (35.2%) had prior MI.[5] There was no difference in the composite of all-cause mortality, hospitalization for MI or stroke between dosing arms (HR, 1.02; 95% CI, 0.91–1.14; $P = .75$), or hospitalization for major bleeding requiring transfusion (HR, 1.18; 95% CI, 0.79–1.77; $P = .41$). Notably, however, there was a high cross-over rate from high-dose to the low-dose arm (41.6%). Collectively, these data indicate that the ischemic benefit from aspirin is likely achieved at a low dose (≤100 mg daily) and that higher doses may result in more bleeding.

Beyond differences in dosing, the formulation of aspirin may also play a role in its antiplatelet effect, with concerns raised regarding the oral bioavailability of enteric-coated aspirin. In a study of 400 healthy volunteers, those receiving non-coated aspirin were more likely to have suppression of platelet aggregation compared to those receiving enteric-coated aspirin, with subsequent suppression of platelet aggregation in the enteric-coated group achieved after receiving ex vivo aspirin. However, a secondary analysis of the ADAPTABLE trial showed no differences in ischemic or bleeding events for coated versus noncoated aspirin, albeit the use of aspirin with enteric coating was not randomly allocated.[6] The implications of different aspirin formulations with respect to cardiovascular outcomes,

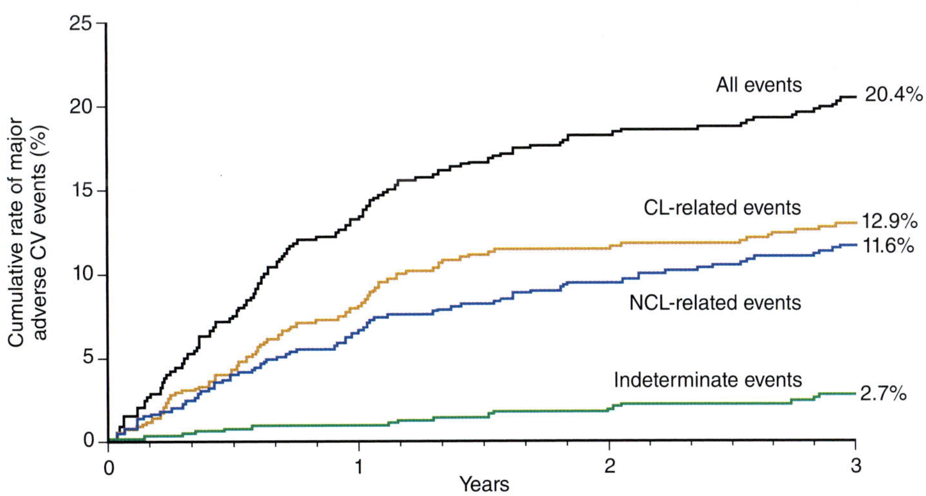

FIG. 26.4 Rates of cardiovascular (CV) death, cardiac arrest, myocardial infarction, or rehospitalization for unstable or progressive angina (major adverse CV events) related to culprit lesions (CL), nonculprit lesions (NCL), and events of indeterminate origin. CL-related events were those adjudicated to be recurrent diseases at the sites of originally treated culprit lesions; NCL-related events were adjudicated to be at sites of nonculprit lesions. Some patients had both CL-related and NCL-related events, and some patients had multiple CL-related events, multiple NCL-related events, or both at different times (in which case the first event is represented in the time-to-event curve). (Adapted from Stone GW, Maehara A, Lansky AJ, et al. A prospective natural-history study of coronary atherosclerosis. *N Engl J Med*. 2011;364:226–235.)

Category of Trial	No. of Trials with Data	No. (%) of Vascular Events: Allocated Antiplatelet	No. (%) of Vascular Events: Adjusted Controls	Observed-Expected	Variance	Odds Reduction (SE) (%)
Previous MI	12	1345/9984 (13.5)	1708/10,022 (17.0)	–159.8	567.6	25 (4)
Acute MI	15	1007/9568 (10.4)	1370/9644 (14.2)	–181.5	519.2	30 (4)
Previous stroke/ transient ischemic attack	21	2045/11,493 (17.8)	2464/11,527 (21.4)	–152.1	625.8	22 (4)
Acute stroke	7	1670/20,418 (8.2)	1858/20,403 (9.1)	–94.6	795.3	11 (3)
Other high risk	140	1638/20,359 (8.0)	2102/20,543 (10.2)	–222.3	737.0	26 (3)
Subtotal: all except acute stroke	188	6035/51,494 (11.7)	7644/51,736 (14.8)	–715.7	2449.6	25 (2)
All trials	**195**	**7705/71,912 (10.7)**	**9502/72,139 (13.2)**	**–810.3**	**3244.9**	**22 (2)**

Heterogeneity of odds reductions between:
5 categories of trial: ^{2} = 21.4, df = 4; P = .0003
Acute stroke vs other: ^{2} = 18.0, df = 1; P = .00002

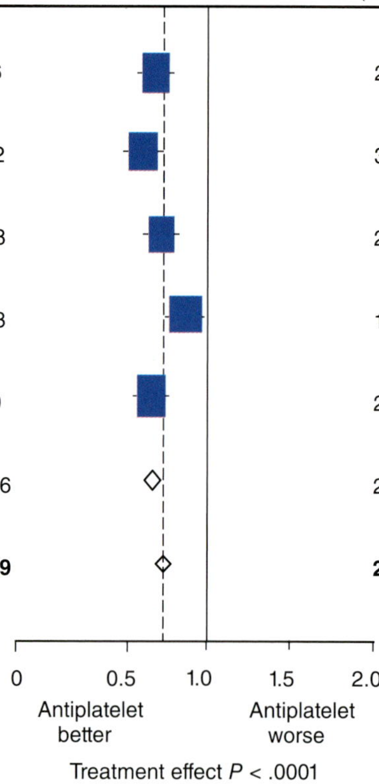

A

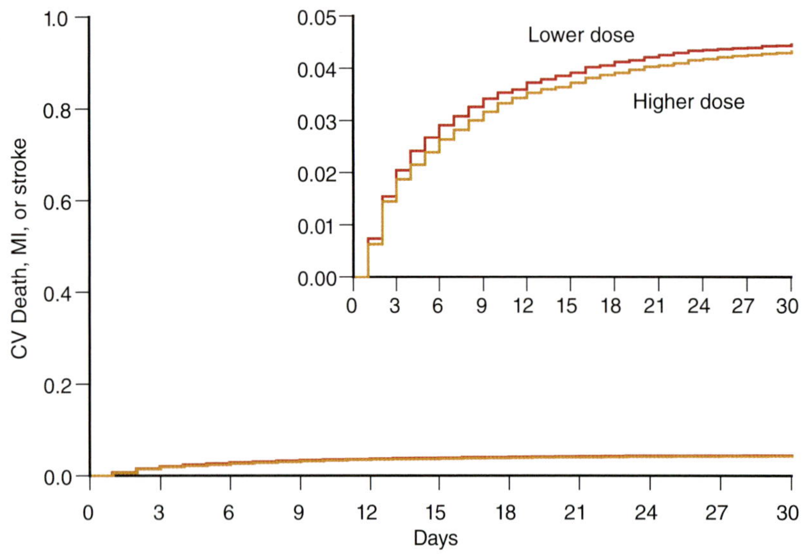

B

FIG. 26.5 (A) The proportional effects of antiplatelet therapy on the composite of cardiovascular (CV) death, myocardial infarction (MI), or stroke by risk category. (B) CV death, MI, or stroke at 30 days for patients presenting with acute coronary syndrome and randomly assigned to receive high-dose (*yellow*) or low-dose (*red*) aspirin. ([A] From Antithrombotic Trialists' Collaboration. Collaborative meta-analysis of randomised trials of antiplatelet therapy for prevention of death, myocardial infarction, and stroke in high-risk patients. *BMJ*. 2002;324:71–86. [B] Adapted from CURRENT-OASIS 7 Investigators, Mehta SR, Bassand JP, et al. Dose comparisons of clopidogrel and aspirin in acute coronary syndromes. *N Engl J Med*. 2010;363:930–942.)

specifically among patients with a prior ACS, have not been examined.

P2Y$_{12}$ Inhibitors and Dual Antiplatelet Therapy

Inhibition of platelet activation through blockade of the P2Y$_{12}$ adenosine diphosphate (ADP) receptor has been demonstrated to be effective in reducing the risk of CV events. Each of the available oral agents (clopidogrel, prasugrel, and ticagrelor) is described in greater detail in Chapter 13 (see Fig. 13.2 and Table 13.1).

A strategy of dual antiplatelet therapy (DAPT) with the second-generation thienopyridine, clopidogrel, added to aspirin versus aspirin alone, was studied in the CURE trial which enrolled patients presenting with non-ST-elevation ACS, with slightly less than half undergoing angiography.[1,2] In CURE, a DAPT regimen with clopidogrel reduced the recurrence of cardiovascular

(CV) death, MI, or stroke by approximately 20% in both the first 30 days (RR, 0.75; 95% CI 0.69 to –0.92) and in landmark analyses from 30 days through 12 months (RR, 0.82; 95% CI 0.70–0.95) versus aspirin alone, albeit at the expense of increased major and minor bleeding (see Chapter 13).

Following the results of CURE, the TRITON-TIMI 38 trial demonstrated a reduction in CV death, MI, or stroke with prasugrel, a higher potency $P2Y_{12}$ inhibitor, compared with clopidogrel, on a background of aspirin therapy in patients presenting with ACS with planned PCI (see Chapter 13).[1,2] Subsequent landmark analyses demonstrated persistent benefit over time with prasugrel versus clopidogrel (31% reduction in MI and 55% reduction in stent thrombosis from 3 days through end of study). Although there was an increased risk of non-CABG-related major bleeding (HR, 1.39; 95% CI, 1.02–1.89; $P = .036$), the net clinical benefit continued to favor prasugrel during the late phase of the study (HR, 0.87; 95% CI 0.77–0.95; $P = .028$). In contrast, in TRILOGY ACS, which examined a similar strategy of DAPT with prasugrel versus clopidogrel in 9326 patients with ACS but without planned revascularization, no greater benefit was seen for ischemic events with prasugrel compared with clopidogrel (HR for composite of CV death, MI and stroke: 0.96; 95% CI 0.86–1.07; $P = .45$) at a median follow-up of 17 months.[1,2] Accordingly, the benefit of higher potency DAPT may be more likely to be realized among those undergoing revascularization for ACS compared to those with medically managed ACS.

Paralleling the findings from TRITON-TIMI 38, the PLATO trial also demonstrated greater longer-term efficacy with use of the higher potency $P2Y_{12}$ inhibitor, ticagrelor, compared with clopidogrel for DAPT among patients presenting with ACS (see Chapter 19), with the majority (61%) undergoing PCI.[1,2] Beyond 30 days, ticagrelor reduced the risk of CV death, MI, and stroke by 20% (HR 0.80; 95% CI 0.70–0.91; $P < .001$) but with a significant increase in non-CABG-related major bleeding (HR 1.34, 95% CI 1.05–1.71; $P = .02$) compared with clopidogrel in this population.

Taken together, these data support DAPT for 1 year after ACS to reduce the risk of major vascular events, with higher potency regimens further reducing ischemic risk but increasing bleeding risk. The only large, head-to-head comparison of prasugrel versus ticagrelor was the open-label ISAR-REACT 5 trial, which enrolled 4018 patients presenting with ACS (41% STEMI, 46% NSTEMI, 13% unstable angina).[7] In ISAR-REACT 5, ticagrelor increased the risk of the primary endpoint composite of death, myocardial infarction, and stroke at 1 year compared with prasugrel (9.3% vs. 6.9%; HR, 1.36; 95% CI, 1.09–1.70; $P = .006$) without any difference in BARC type 3–5 bleeding (5.4% vs. 4.8%; HR, 1.12; 95% CI, 0.83–1.51; $P = .46$). These findings were unexpected given the similar pharmacodynamic properties of prasugrel and ticagrelor and difficult to reconcile given the similar magnitude of relative risk reduction observed for both prasugrel and ticagrelor over clopidogrel in TRITON-TIMI 38 and PLATO, respectively. Thus, further validation of this observation in additional studies would be helpful.

Longer Duration of Dual Antiplatelet Therapy

CHARISMA

Landmark analyses of CURE, TRITON-TIMI 38, and PLATO demonstrating the sustained benefit of DAPT in patients out to approximately 1 year after ACS raised the possibility that prolonged DAPT even beyond 1 year might yield additional benefit. This hypothesis was first tested broadly in the Clopidogrel and Aspirin versus Aspirin Alone for the Prevention of Atherothrombotic Events (CHARISMA) trial.[8] A total of 15,603 patients were randomly assigned to receive clopidogrel 75 mg daily or matching placebo, with all receiving aspirin (75–162 mg daily), over a median period of 28 months. Overall, there was no significant benefit of adding clopidogrel to aspirin for reducing cardiovascular death, MI, or stroke (risk ratio [RR], 0.93; $P = .22$), and there was an increase in GUSTO moderate or severe bleeding (HR, 1.48; 95% CI, 1.24–1.78; $P < .001$), driven primarily by increased moderate bleeds.

However, when stratified by the presence or absence of established cardiovascular disease, a marginally significant interaction (*P*-interaction = 0.045) for efficacy was observed, with those having established symptomatic disease deriving benefit reducing in MACE (HR, 0.88; 95% CI, 0.77–0.998), whereas those who had only atherothrombotic risk factors (i.e., primary prevention cohort) did not. A subsequent post-hoc analysis of the data explored the efficacy and safety of aspirin and clopidogrel for secondary prevention in more detail. In the subset of 3846 patients with previous MI, a significant reduction in cardiovascular death, MI, or stroke was observed (HR, 0.77; 95% CI, 0.61–0.98; $P = .031$) (Fig. 26.6).

DAPT Trial

In the Dual Antiplatelet Therapy after Drug Eluting (DAPT) trial, patients with prior PCI who tolerated DAPT (with either clopidogrel or prasugrel) for 12 months, without experiencing a major adverse cardiovascular or cerebrovascular event, repeat revascularization, or moderate or severe bleeding, were subsequently randomized to have their $P2Y_{12}$ inhibitor withdrawn or to continue for an additional 18

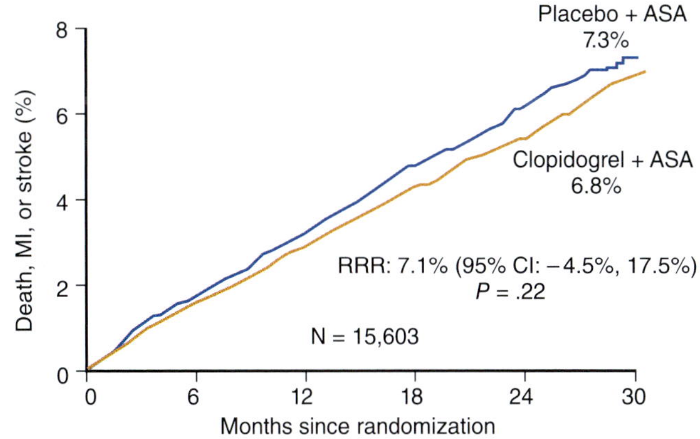

FIG. 26.6 Cardiovascular (CV) death, myocardial infarction (MI), or stroke at 30 months with clopidogrel and aspirin (*orange*) vs. aspirin alone (*blue*) in patients with previous MI. *ASA*, Acetylsalicylic acid; *HR*, hazard ratio. (Adapted from Bhatt DL, Flather MD, Hacke W, et al. Patients with prior myocardial infarction, stroke, or symptomatic peripheral arterial disease in the CHARISMA trial. *J Am Coll Cardiol*. 2007;49:1982–1988.)

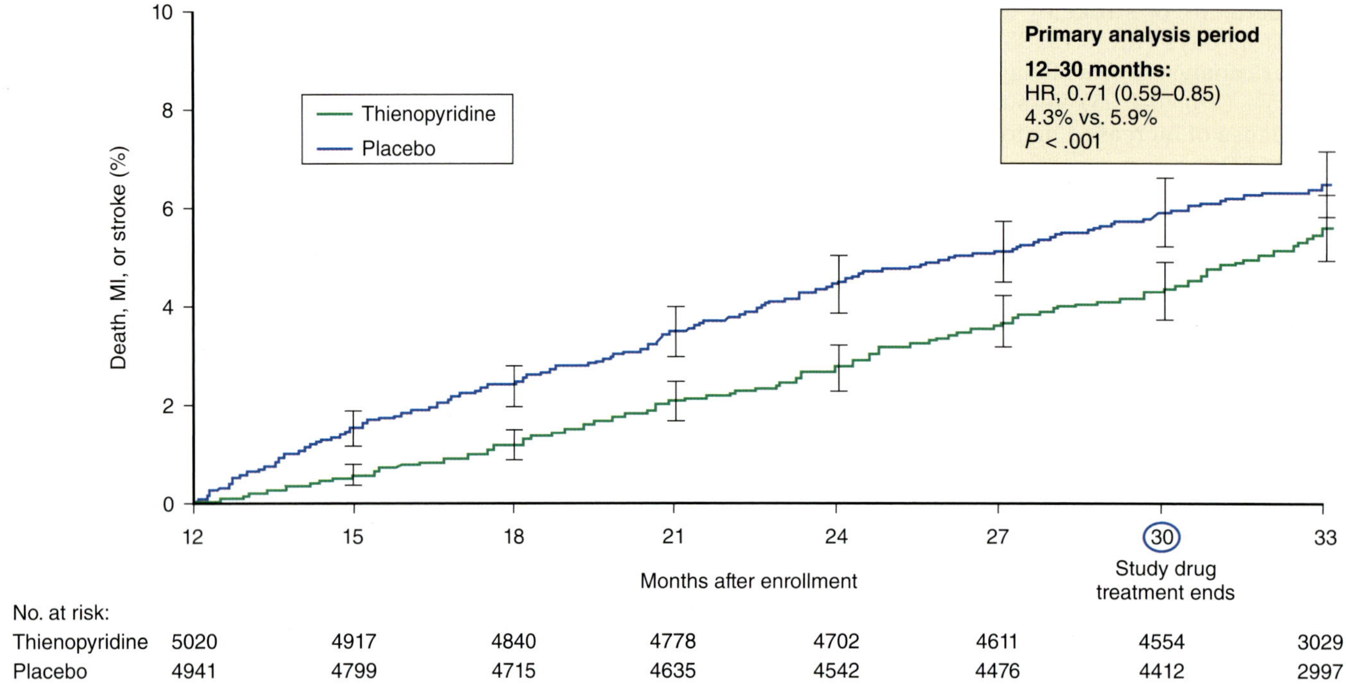

FIG. 26.7 Death, myocardial infarction (MI), or stroke at 33 months from coronary intervention. Patients who were event-free and tolerating therapy were randomly selected at 12 months to continue $P2Y_{12}$ inhibition and aspirin (*blue*) or to stop $P2Y_{12}$ inhibition (*green*). At month 30, patients randomly selected to continue at 12 months (*blue*) also stopped $P2Y_{12}$ inhibition. (Adapted from Mauri L, Kereiakes DJ, Yeh RW, et al. Twelve or 30 months of dual antiplatelet therapy after drug-eluting stents. *N Engl J Med*. 2014;371:2155–2166.)

months.[2,8] Because the primary criterion for enrollment was a coronary procedure, the population was heterogeneous, including patients undergoing PCI for ACS (42%) in addition to stable angina (38%) or other reasons (20%). Overall, the trial showed a significant reduction in both coprimary endpoints of stent thrombosis (0.4% vs. 1.4%; HR, 0.29; 95% CI, 0.17–0.48; $P < .001$) and the MACE composite of death, MI, or stroke (4.3% vs. 5.9%; HR, 0.71; 95% CI, 0.59–0.85; $P < .001$) (Fig. 26.7). Bleeding was increased with more prolonged DAPT (GUSTO-defined moderate or severe bleeding rate: 0.66% per year; 2.5% vs. 1.6% at 18 months; HR, 1.61; 95% CI, 1.21–2.16; $P = .001$), a difference driven primarily by moderate bleeding (ARI of 0.7% at 18 months; $P = .004$).

A subsequent subgroup analysis evaluated the efficacy and safety of continued DAPT versus $P2Y_{12}$ inhibitor withdrawal in the 3576 subjects presenting with acute MI.[2] There was a significantly greater magnitude of benefit with prolonged DAPT (*P*-interaction = 0.03) in the acute MI subset (3.9% vs. 6.8%; HR, 0.56; 95% CI, 0.42–0.76; $P < .001$) at the cost of increased GUSTO moderate or severe bleeding (1.9% vs. 0.8%; HR, 2.38; 95% CI, 1.27–4.43; $P = .005$).

PEGASUS-TIMI 54 Trial

The Prevention of Cardiovascular Events in Patients with Prior Heart Attack Using Ticagrelor Compared to Placebo on a Background of Aspirin–Thrombolysis in Myocardial Infarction 54 (PEGASUS-TIMI 54) trial was designed to address the hypothesis that the more potent $P2Y_{12}$ inhibitor ticagrelor offers additional benefit to aspirin alone in patients who are 1–3 years post MI.[2,8] Patient selection was enriched for ischemic risk factors and those with a history of ischemic stroke, intracranial bleeding or gastrointestinal bleeding within the previous 6 months were excluded. Patients were randomly assigned to receive one of two doses of the ticagrelor (90 mg or 60 mg twice daily) or a matching placebo, with all patients receiving low-dose aspirin. At a median of 33 months, both doses of ticagrelor significantly reduced the composite of cardiovascular death, MI, or stroke (60-mg dose: HR, 0.84; 95% CI, 0.74–0.95; $P = .004$; 90-mg dose: HR, 0.85; 95% CI, 0.75–0.96; $P = .008$) (Fig. 26.8). The efficacy of ticagrelor was directionally consistent for all components of the primary endpoint including cardiovascular death. Both doses significantly increased TIMI major bleeding (60-mg dose: HR, 2.32; $P < .001$; 90-mg dose: HR, 2.69; $P < .001$), with no significant excess of fatal or intracranial bleeds. Based on the data from this trial, for every 10,000 patients who began treatment with ticagrelor 60 mg bid, 42 primary endpoint events would be prevented whereas 31 TIMI major bleeds would be caused.

Pooled Analysis of Prolonged DAPT Trials

The results of the CHARISMA previous-MI subgroup, the DAPT previous-MI subgroup, and PEGASUS-TIMI 54 were pooled together with those for the MI subgroups in several other trials in a meta-analysis evaluating prolonged DAPT ($N = 20{,}203$) with a $P2Y_{12}$ inhibitor plus aspirin versus aspirin alone ($N = 13{,}232$) for secondary prevention.[9] Consistent with the individual trials, the pooled analysis showed a significant reduction in the composite of cardiovascular death, MI, or stroke with prolonged DAPT (Fig. 26.9). In this pooled analysis with greater statistical power, the addition of a $P2Y_{12}$ inhibitor to aspirin also significantly reduced the risk of CV death ($P = .03$) (Fig. 26.e1). There was no statistically significant difference in the rate of intracranial hemorrhage or fatal bleeding (Fig. 26.10).

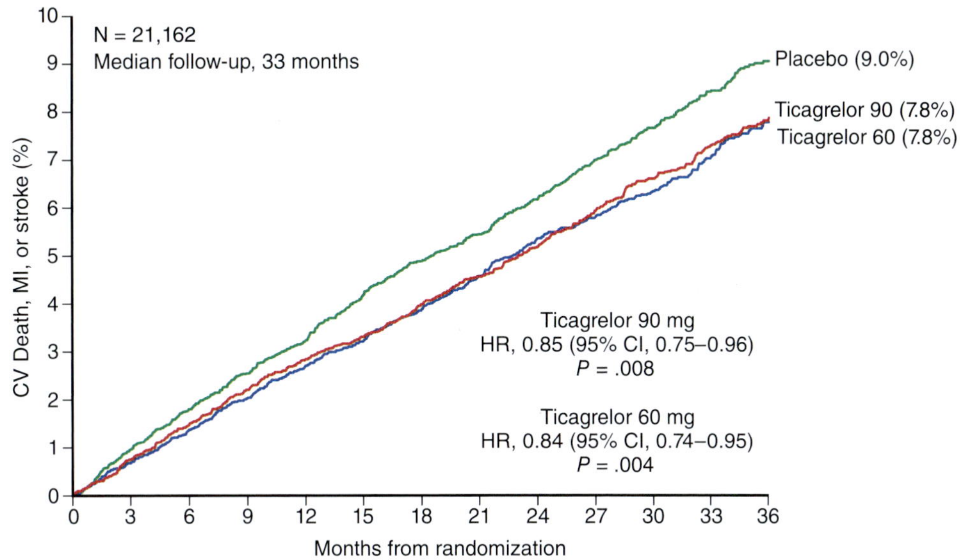

FIG. 26.8 Cardiovascular (CV) death, myocardial infarction (MI), or stroke at 2 years in patients with a history of MI (1–3 years previously) randomly assigned to a regimen of ticagrelor 60 mg twice daily (*blue*), ticagrelor 90 mg twice daily (*red*), or placebo (*green*). All patients received low-dose aspirin. (Adapted from Bonaca MP, Bhatt DL, Cohen M, et al. Long-term use of ticagrelor in patients with prior myocardial infarction. *N Engl J Med*. 2015;372:1791–1800.)

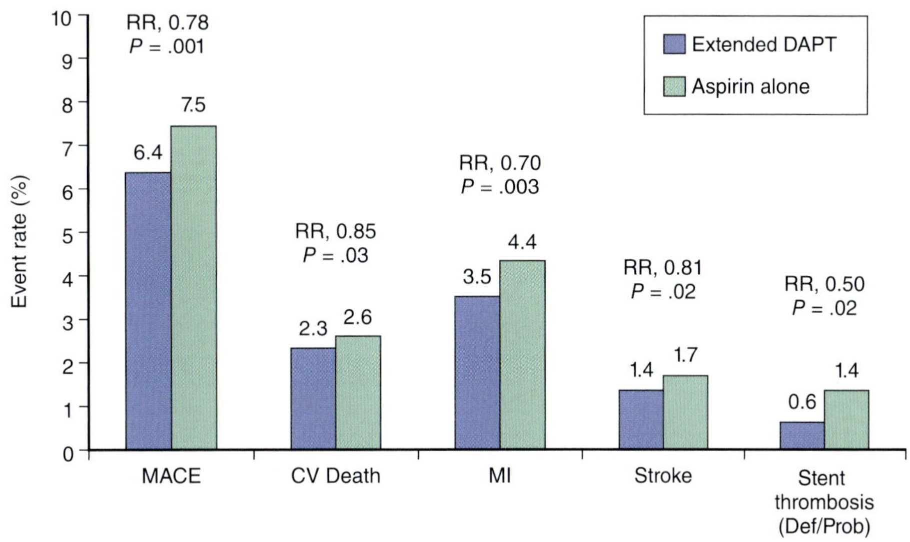

FIG. 26.9 Rates of ischemic outcomes with extended dual-antiplatelet therapy with aspirin and a P2Y12 inhibitor (*blue*) vs. aspirin alone (*green*) for long-term secondary prevention after myocardial infarction. *CV*, Cardiovascular; *MACE*, major adverse cardiac event; *RR*, risk ratio.

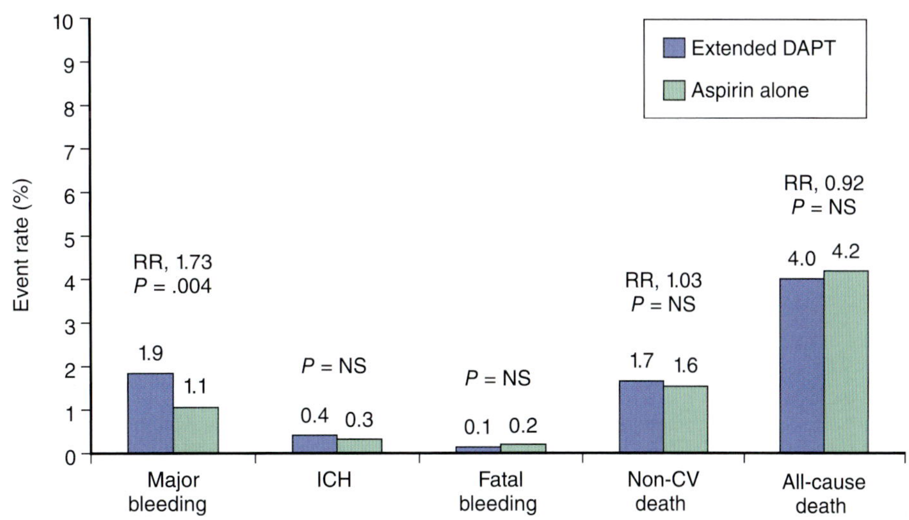

FIG. 26.10 Rates of safety outcomes with extended dual-antiplatelet therapy with aspirin and a $P2Y_{12}$ inhibitor (*blue*) vs. aspirin alone (*green*) for long-term secondary prevention after myocardial infarction. *CV*, Cardiovascular; *ICH*, intracranial hemorrhage; *NS*, not significant; *RR*, risk ratio.

Dual Versus Triple Antithrombotic Therapy With Oral Anticoagulation

Studies suggest that up to 10% of patients undergoing PCI have an indication for long-term oral anticoagulation, typically in the context of atrial fibrillation (AF), and up to 30% of patients with AF undergo PCI.[2,8] In the WOEST trial conducted in the era of vitamin K antagonist-based anticoagulation, 573 patients undergoing PCI were randomized to receive either clopidogrel or aspirin and clopidogrel, with both arms receiving warfarin titrated to a therapeutic INR (i.e., dual antithrombotic therapy [DAT] versus triple antithrombotic therapy [TAT]).[2,8] AF was the indication for anticoagulation in most patients (69%). DAT with clopidogrel and warfarin reduced the primary safety endpoint of any bleeding at 1 year (19.4% vs. 44.4%; HR, 0.36; 95% CI, 0.26–0.50; $P < .0001$), without an increase in ischemic events (death, MI, stroke, target-vessel revascularization, or stent thrombosis: 11.1% vs. 17.6%; HR, 0.60; 95% CI, 0.38–0.94; $P = .025$), compared to TAT.

Several pivotal trials have subsequently examined contemporary direct oral anticoagulants (DOAC) in a DAT versus TAT strategy in patients with AF undergoing PCI, with a subset also comparing DOAC versus warfarin as the OAC strategy.[2,8] Notably, each of these studies taken individually lacks sufficient power to reliably detect differences in ischemic events. However, a subsequent meta-analysis of four pivotal trials ($N = 10{,}234$) examined DAT versus TAT using DOAC.[10] The proportion of patients presenting with ACS and the time from PCI (or ACS) to randomization varied considerably across the included trials (ACS: 17%–52%; enrollment beginning 4 hours following PCI up to 14 days after presentation). As well, one of the included trials (PIONEER AF-PCI) used a reduced-dose DOAC for the DAT strategy, compared with warfarin for the TAT strategy. In that context, the meta-analysis demonstrated a consistent benefit of DAT versus TAT across all bleeding endpoints including intracranial hemorrhage, but with a trade-off in ischemic events, specifically stent thrombosis (see Fig. 26.11).[10]

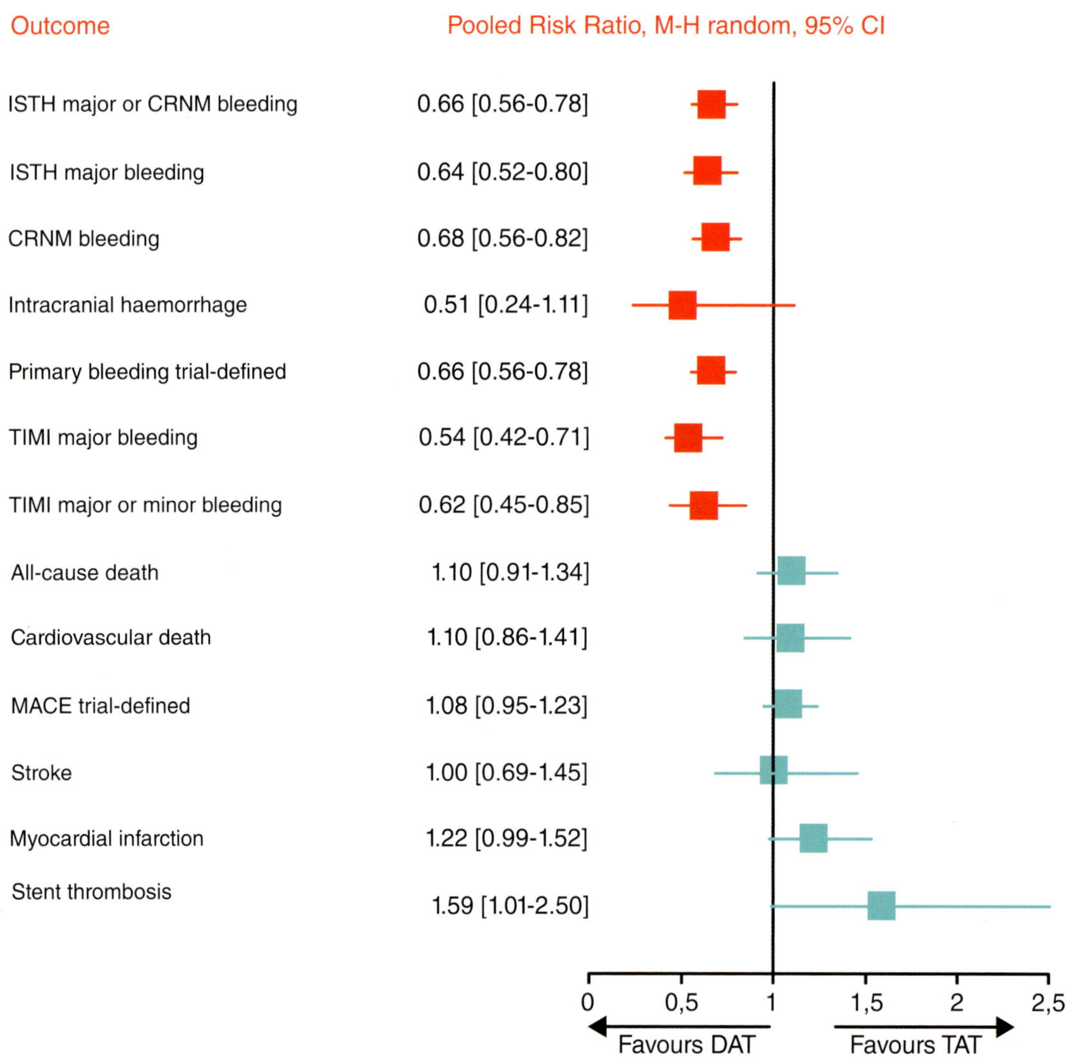

FIG. 26.11 Meta-analytic summary of dual antithrombotic vs. triple antithrombotic therapy on bleeding and ischemic events. *CRNM*, clinically relevant non-major; *DAT*, double antithrombotic therapy; *ISTH*, International Society on Thrombosis and Haemostasis; *MACE*, major adverse cardiovascular events; *TAT*, triple antithrombotic therapy; *TIMI*, thrombolysis in myocardial infarction. (Adapted from Gargiulo G, Goette A, Tijssen J, et al. Safety and efficacy outcomes of double vs. triple antithrombotic therapy in patients with atrial fibrillation following percutaneous coronary intervention: a systematic review and meta-analysis of non-vitamin K antagonist oral anticoagulant-based randomized clinical trials. *Eur Heart J*. 2019;40:3757–3767.)

However, the risk of stent thrombosis in this population is likely highest immediately following PCI as described previously. In a secondary analysis of the AUGUSTUS trial, which randomized patients using a 2 × 2 factorial design, first to a strategy of apixaban-based versus warfarin-based OAC with $P2Y_{12}$ inhibitor therapy, followed by randomization to either aspirin or matching placebo, the majority of stent thrombosis events occurred within the first 30 days after randomization, with numerically higher rates in the nonaspirin group irrespective of randomized OAC (aspirin vs. nonaspirin: 0.6% vs. 1.1%, HR: 0.58; 95% CI, 0.28–1.22).[11] These data indicate that a strategy of upfront TAT may be beneficial in reducing ischemic events in the highest risk period immediately following PCI, shortly after which transition to a DAT strategy may be more preferable (within the first month) owing to the substantially greater risk of bleeding with TAT. Moreover, as clopidogrel was used for $P2Y_{12}$ inhibition in approximately 90% of patients enrolled across these trials, limited data exist examining ticagrelor or prasugrel in a DAT strategy with OAC.

Furthermore, data regarding longer-term antiplatelet therapy beyond 1 year in patients receiving OAC remains limited. The AFIRE trial randomized 2236 patients with AF undergoing coronary revascularization (with PCI or CABG) at least 1 year prior or otherwise with angiographically confirmed CAD to rivaroxaban or combination therapy with rivaroxaban and a physician-selected antiplatelet agent (70% aspirin, 27% $P2Y_{12}$ inhibitor, 2% other).[12] The trial was terminated prematurely on recommendation from the data and safety monitoring committee. Rivaroxaban monotherapy reduced the primary endpoint (stroke, systemic embolism, MI, unstable angina requiring revascularization, all-cause death) compared with combination therapy (4.1% vs. 5.8%; HR, 0.72; 95% CI, 0.55–0.95; $P < .001$), a finding which was driven primarily by all-cause death (1.9% vs. 3.4%; HR 0.55; 95% CI, 0.38–0.81) with a limited number of other ischemic events.[12] Major bleeding was also reduced with rivaroxaban monotherapy versus combination therapy (1.6% vs. 2.8%; HR, 0.59; 95% CI, 0.39–0.89; $P = .01$).[12] Larger randomized trials with longer duration of follow-up are necessary to further elucidate whether there exists a benefit of more prolonged antiplatelet therapy in patients receiving OAC.

Protease Activated Receptor Antagonism

Protease-activated receptor 1 (PAR-1), the primary receptor for thrombin on human platelets, has also been identified as a potential therapeutic target in secondary prevention. Vorapaxar, an oral competitive antagonist of PAR-1, has been studied both in the ACS setting and for longer-term secondary prevention. The Thrombin Receptor Antagonist in Secondary Prevention of Atherothrombotic Ischemic Events (TRA2°P)–Thrombolysis in Myocardial Infarction (TIMI) 50 trial randomly assigned a broad population of patients with atherosclerotic vascular disease (previous MI, symptomatic peripheral arterial disease, or ischemic stroke) to receive vorapaxar or matching placebo, with background therapy permitted at the discretion of the treating physician (94% aspirin, with 78% also on thienopyridine in the subset with previous MI).[4]

In TRA2°P-TIMI 50, vorapaxar significantly reduced the primary endpoint of cardiovascular death, MI, or stroke (HR, 0.87; 95% CI, 0.80–0.94; $P < .001$) at 3 years, but with an increase in GUSTO-defined moderate or severe bleeding (ARI 1.7%; HR, 1.66; 95% CI, 1.43–1.93; $P < .001$) as well as in intracranial hemorrhage (HR, 1.94; 95% CI, 1.39–2.70; $P < .001$). Notably, however, there was marked heterogeneity in the absolute risk for intracranial hemorrhage, with a greater absolute risk in those with a history of stroke (2.4% with vorapaxar vs. 0.9% with placebo; $P < .001$) compared to those without (0.6% with vorapaxar group vs. 0.4% with placebo; $P = .049$). Accordingly, vorapaxar is approved for clinical use based on its overall efficacy in a secondary prevention population but is contraindicated in patients with prior stroke or TIA owing to the risk of intracranial hemorrhage.

Individualizing Antiplatelet Therapy Based on Patient Factors

Collectively, these data indicate that there exists a fundamental trade-off with respect to ischemic and bleeding risk, such that decision making around longer or higher potency regimens of antiplatelet therapy necessitates individualization for patient-specific risk factors of recurrent ischemia and bleeding. As such, comprehensive patient-specific risk assessment inclusive of clinical risk factors, platelet function testing, and genetics may inform clinical decision making regarding the duration and intensity of antiplatelet therapy.

Clinical Risk Scores to Help Determine Duration of DAPT

The DAPT score was developed to assess the net benefit of prolonged DAPT beyond 1 year after coronary stenting using data from the DAPT trial.[13] Several patient and angiographic characteristics were independently associated with the benefit of prolonged DAPT and assigned an integer weight. Patients with a low score had a smaller ARR in MI or stent thrombosis at 18 months (ARR, 0.52%) relative to patients with a high score (ARR, 1.90%) (Fig. 26.12). Moreover, patients with a low DAPT score had more bleeding with DAPT (ARI, 1.44%) at 18 months relative to those who had a high score (ARI, 0.38%) (see Fig. 26.12).

Following the DAPT score, the PRECISE-DAPT score was developed to assess the bleeding risk of DAPT at the very outset following PCI and guide the duration of therapy.[13] Five clinical and laboratory variables were independently associated with the risk of bleeding, and thresholds were developed for the assignment of various integer weights in the risk score. Patients with low scores had a reduction in MI, definite stent thrombosis, stroke, or target-vessel revascularization (ARD, −4.13% [−6.09% to −2.15%]) with longer (12–24 months) versus shorter (3–6 months) DAPT duration, without a significant difference observed for TIMI major or minor bleeding (ARD, +0.14% [−0.22% to +0.49%]) at 1 year (see Fig. 26.13). In contrast, those with high scores had no difference in the ischemic composite (ARD, +1.54% [−3.27% to +6.32%]) at 1 year with longer compared to shorter DAPT duration but did experience greater bleeding (ARD, +2.61 [+0.19% to +4.99%]).

In a subsequent analysis of PEGASUS-TIMI 54, a stepwise patient selection algorithm was developed (Fig. 26.14).[14] Patients with either low hemoglobin or prior hospitalization

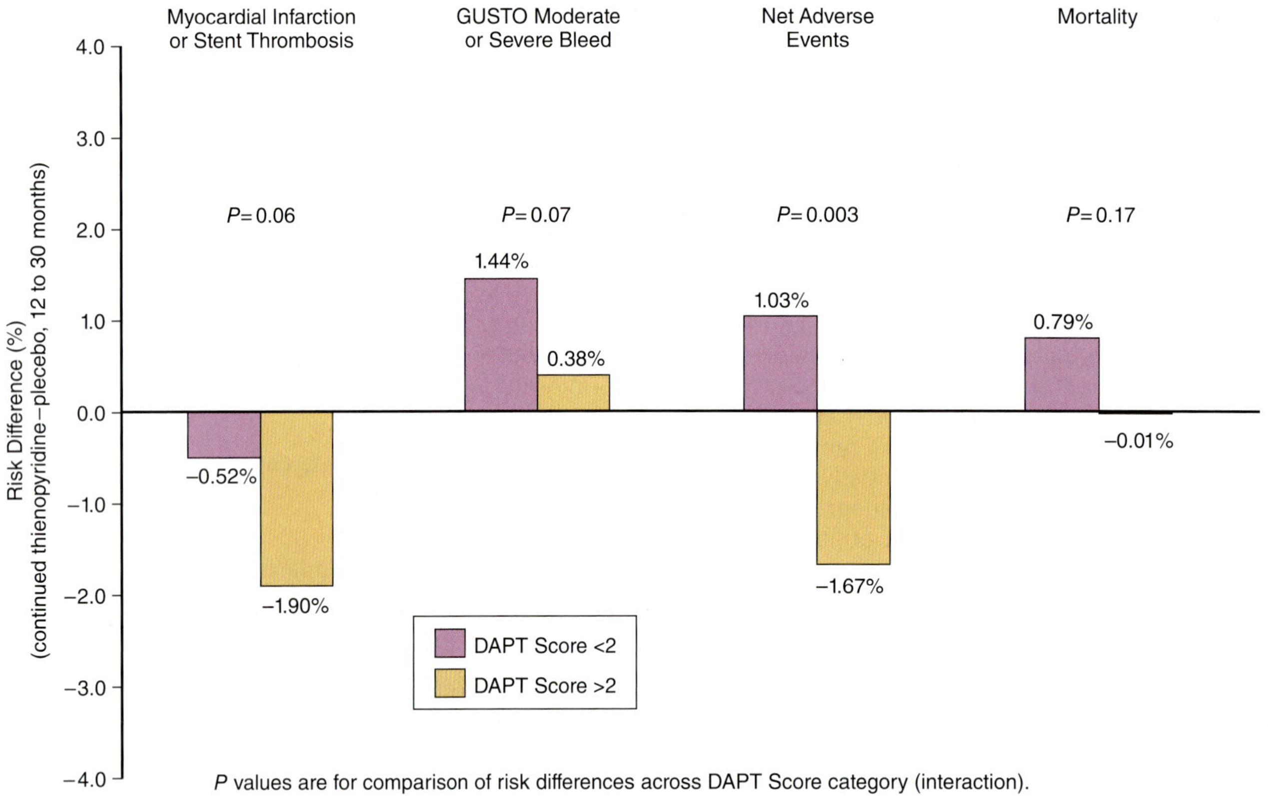

FIG. 26.12 The absolute risk difference in efficacy and safety events with extended-duration clopidogrel vs. placebo on a background of aspirin, stratified by DAPT risk score (<2 in *purple*, >2 in *yellow*). (Data from Yeh RW, Secemsky E, Kereiakes DJ, et al. LBCT 03: individualizing treatment duration of dual antiplatelet therapy after percutaneous coronary intervention: an analysis from the DAPT study. *JAMA*. 2016;315:1735–1749.)

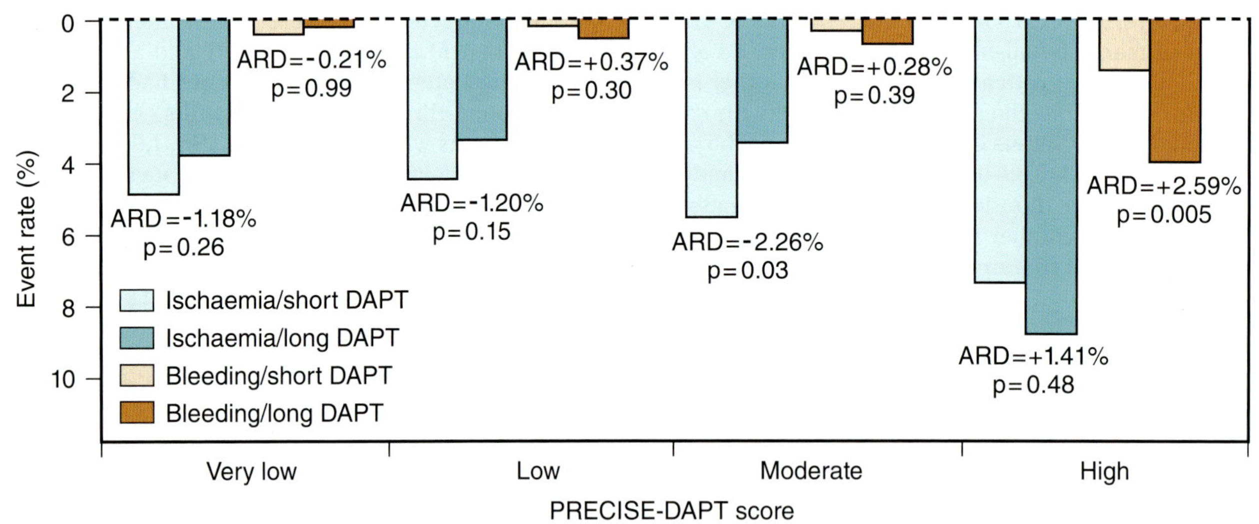

FIG. 26.13 Absolute risk difference for prolonged (12–24 months) vs. short (3–6 month) duration of DAPT for ischemia (MI, definite stent thrombosis, stroke, or target-vessel revascularization) and bleeding (TIMI major and minor) by quartile of PRECISE-DAPT score. *ARD*, Absolute risk difference; *MI*, myocardial infarction; *TIMI*, thrombolysis in myocardial infarction. (Adapted from Costa F, van Klaveren D, James S, et al. Derivation and validation of the predicting bleeding complications in patients undergoing stent implantation and subsequent dual antiplatelet therapy (PRECISE-DAPT) score: a pooled analysis of individual-patient datasets from clinical trials. *Lancet*. 2017;389:1025–1034.)

for bleeding were designated as being high bleeding risk. Among the remainder of patients without either of these risk factors designated as low bleeding risk, ischemic risk was then assessed based on six clinical variables. In patients at high bleeding risk, prolonged DAPT with ticagrelor increased TIMI major bleeding at 3 years compared with placebo (ARD, +2.3% [+0.6%–3.9%]]), without a difference observed for CV death, MI, or stroke (ARD +0.08% [-2.4% to +2.4%]) (Fig. 26.14).[14] In contrast, among patients at low bleeding risk, a stepwise increase in the ARR for ischemic

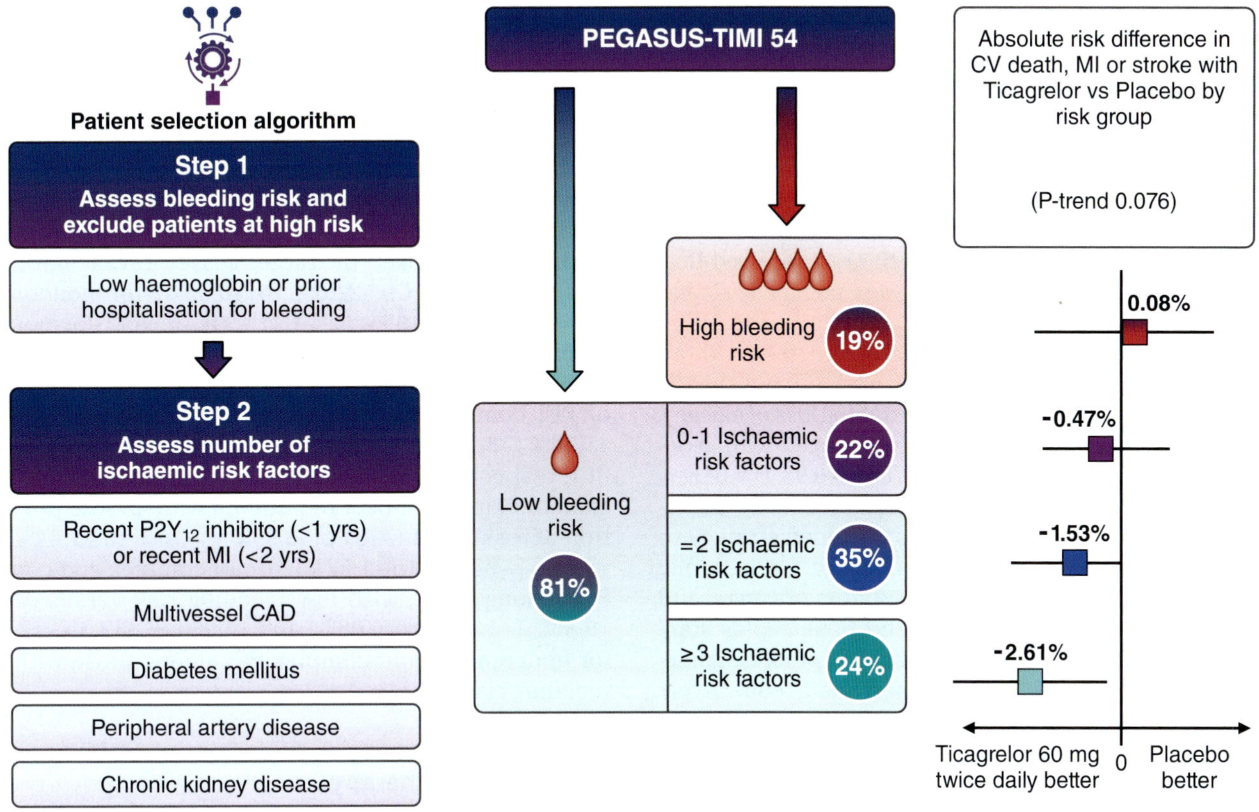

FIG. 26.14 Patient selection algorithm based on bleeding and ischemic risk for prolonged DAPT from PEGASUS-TIMI 54. In patients at high bleeding risk, prolonged DAPT with ticagrelor 60 mg increased TIMI major bleeding at 3 years without a difference in ischemic outcomes compared with aspirin only. However, among patients at low bleeding risk, there was a stepwise increase in the absolute benefit with prolonged DAPT for reduction in ischemic events with an increasing number of ischemic risk factors. *CAD*, Coronary artery disease; *MI*, myocardial infarction. (Adapted from Bonaca MP, Im K, Magnani G, et al. Patient selection for long-term secondary prevention with ticagrelor: insights from PEGASUS-TIMI 54. *Eur Heart J.* 2022;43:5037–5044.)

events was observed with increasing number of ischemic risk factors (≤1, 2, 3: ARD of -0.5%, −1.5%, and −2.6% at 3 years, respectively; *P*-trend = .03), with a similar incidence of TIMI major bleeding across ischemic risk groups (*P*-trend for ARD = 0.96).[14] Consistent with greater ARR for ischemic events, there was also a stepwise increase in the ARR for CV death (≤1, 2, 3 ischemic risk factors: ARD of -0.2%, −0.9%, and −1.6% at 3 years, respectively; *P*-trend = 0.018) and all-cause mortality (ARD of −0.3%, −0.5%, and −2.0%; *P*-trend = 0.03).

While application of such risk scores for patient selection should ideally be evaluated with prospective randomization, they represent a potential mechanism for individualizing the ischemic risk of a post-ACS patient and evaluating their benefit and risk with more long-term potent secondary prevention with antiplatelet therapy.

Platelet Function and Genetic Testing

Among the $P2Y_{12}$ inhibitors, clopidogrel has been demonstrated to have significant interindividual variability, with implications for recurrent ischemic events, particularly stent thrombosis, as well as for bleeding.[13] Genetic polymorphisms in CYP2C19, the cytochrome P450 enzyme responsible for converting clopidogrel to its active metabolite, have been identified to contribute, at least in part, to the marked variability observed in response to clopidogrel.[15] As well, results of platelet function testing (PFT) have been demonstrated to predict both atherothrombotic and bleeding events for patients on clopidogrel in observational studies.

The TROPICAL-ACS trial evaluated a strategy of PFT-guided early de-escalation among patients with ACS treated with PCI.[4] Patients in the guided de-escalation group underwent PFT at day 14, following 7 days of initial prasugrel therapy and a subsequent 7 days of clopidogrel therapy on a background of aspirin. Those with high platelet reactivity (HPR) on PFT were transitioned to prasugrel to complete the 12-month duration of treatment, whereas those without HPR were maintained on clopidogrel. This guided de-escalation strategy was compared with uniform antiplatelet therapy with prasugrel for a 12-month duration in the control arm. The guided de-escalation strategy was noninferior to standard treatment with prasugrel for the primary outcome of CV death, MI, stroke, or BARC type 2–5 bleeding at 1 year (HR, 0.81; 95% CI 0.61–1.06; *P* for noninferiority = .0004), with no differences observed when separately considering only ischemic events (CV death, MI, stroke: HR, 0.77; 95% CI 0.48–1.21; *P* for noninferiority = 0.01). Bleeding was numerically lower with the guided de-escalation strategy but did not reach statistical significance (any BARC bleeding: HR, 0.83; 95% CI 0.65–1.06; *P* = .14).

With respect to genotyping, the TAILOR-PCI trial enrolled 5302 patients undergoing PCI for either ACS (82%) or stable CAD (18%), with randomization to either clopidogrel for all, versus a genotype-guided strategy with ticagrelor (or prasugrel) among those identified as carrying a CYP2C19 loss-of-function variant, with clopidogrel for the rest. There was a nonsignificant but numerically lower rate of CV death, MI, stroke, severe recurrent ischemia, or stent thrombosis at 1 year with the genotype-guided escalation strategy (4.0% vs. 5.9%; HR, 0.66; 95% CI 0.43–1.02; P = .06).[16] The Popular Genetics trial approached this issue from a different perspective. Patients presenting with STEMI undergoing primary PCI were randomized to a standard of care of ticagrelor or prasugrel for all versus a genotype-guided arm in which noncarriers were de-escalated to clopidogrel and the rest received ticagrelor or prasugrel.[17] Ischemic events were nominally similar with the use of a genotype-guided strategy for de-escalation to clopidogrel compared with prasugrel or ticagrelor without genotype guidance (HR, 0.83; 95% CI 0.53–1.31), but the CIs were wide and could not exclude a substantial loss of efficacy. PLATO major and minor bleeding were reduced with genotype-guided treatment (HR, 0.78; 95% CI 0.61–0.98; P = .04).

Notably, each of these individual trials are likely underpowered to compare a guided versus unguided strategy to guide $P2Y_{12}$ inhibitor selection, particularly for ischemic events. While higher potency $P2Y_{12}$ inhibitors prasugrel and ticagrelor are now widely available and preferred as standard of care over clopidogrel across clinical practice guidelines immediately following ACS, these data collectively highlight the potential role for PFT and genetic testing to guide decision making regarding longer term antiplatelet therapy, where bleeding risk remains a concern. Such data may be helpful to guide de-escalation of antiplatelet therapy.

De-escalation of Antiplatelet Therapy

As described earlier, while longer duration and higher potency DAPT has been demonstrated to reduce recurrent atherothrombotic events among patients with prior ACS, bleeding during chronic treatment remains an issue. Moreover, subsequent advances in medical therapy and stent technology from the initial clinical trials that demonstrated the benefit of higher potency and longer duration of DAPT may have shifted the relative balance of ischemic and bleeding risk in a contemporary post-ACS patient population. Importantly, there is also an increasing prevalence of older, fragile, and multi-comorbid patients undergoing PCI for ACS, a subset which was typically excluded from clinical trials and may represent a particularly high bleeding risk group. In view of this shifting epidemiology, there is increasing interest in de-escalation of antiplatelet therapy following the early phase of ACS to minimize longer-term bleeding without a significant trade-off in recurrent ischemic events. Such de-escalation may be unguided and based solely on clinical judgment or may be guided by PFT and genetic testing as noted earlier.

Shorter DAPT Strategies With Continued Aspirin Monotherapy

Several trials have examined a shorter DAPT duration of 3–6 months compared to the standard 12-month duration, followed by aspirin monotherapy, with mixed results. Notably, each trial taken in isolation has been underpowered to assess risk for ischemic events following an abbreviated duration of DAPT, with many often including directionally opposing ischemic and bleeding endpoints in the primary composite outcome.

An individual patient-level meta-analysis pooled eight clinical trials (N = 14,963) to compare a DAPT duration of 3–6 months to ≥12 months followed by aspirin monotherapy, with further stratification by both bleeding risk (using the PRECISE-DAPT score) and PCI complexity.[18] In those at lower bleeding risk, there was evidence of greater benefit with prolonged DAPT for ischemic events (ARD at 24 months for composite of MI, definite stent thrombosis, stroke, or target-vessel revascularization of −1.14% [95% CI −2.26% to −0.02%] for noncomplex PCI and −3.86% [95% CI −7.71% to +0.06%] for complex PCI). However, those at high bleeding risk did not appear to benefit from the longer DAPT duration irrespective of PCI complexity (ARD of +1.45% [−1.84%+4.72%] and +1.30% [−6.99% to +9.57%] for noncomplex and complex PCI, respectively). These findings were consistent when examined in the subset of patients with an ACS presentation across trials (ARD of -3.39% [−5.37% to −1.44%] and −8.08% [−14.86% to −1.52%] for noncomplex and complex PCI among those with low bleeding risk versus ARD of +0.86% [−4.34% to +6.08%] and +4.96 [−6.86% to +17.22%] for noncomplex and complex PCI among those with high bleeding risk).

Shorter DAPT Strategies With Continued $P2Y_{12}$ Inhibitor Monotherapy

While aspirin has traditionally remained the backbone of antiplatelet regimens since the very early days of PCI, accumulating data indicates that $P2Y_{12}$ inhibitor monotherapy may offer a reduction in ischemic events without a significant trade-off in bleeding risk when compared with aspirin monotherapy. Clopidogrel was first studied head-to-head against aspirin as monotherapy for secondary prevention in the Clopidogrel versus Aspirin in Patients at Risk of Ischemic Events (CAPRIE) trial.[8] A total of 19,185 patients with stable atherosclerotic vascular disease (6302 in the recent MI subgroup and 8446 with previous MI) were randomly assigned to receive either clopidogrel 75 mg daily or aspirin 325 mg daily, with follow-up periods ranging from 1 to 3 years. At a mean of 1.91 years of follow-up, clopidogrel was superior to aspirin for reducing the composite of cardiovascular death, MI, or stroke (relative risk reduction, 8.7%; P = .043), with a modest absolute risk reduction (ARR) of 0.51%. Notably, bleeding was similar for clopidogrel versus aspirin monotherapy, with less frequent gastrointestinal bleeding observed for those randomized to clopidogrel.

The more recent HOST-EXAM trial examined a long-term monotherapy strategy of clopidogrel versus aspirin in stable patients with prior PCI from South Korea.[19] A total of 5530 patients who remained event free at a median of 1 year following PCI underwent open-label randomization to either clopidogrel 75 mg or aspirin 100 mg daily and followed for 24 months. For the primary composite outcome of all-cause mortality, MI, stroke, readmission for ACS, or major bleeding, clopidogrel monotherapy was superior to aspirin monotherapy as a long-term maintenance strategy (5.7% vs. 7.7%; HR, 0.73; 95% CI, 0.59–0.90; P = .003). Additionally, there was a reduction in the thrombotic composite of cardiovascular death, MI, stroke, ACS readmission, and stent thrombosis (3.7% vs. 5.5%; P = .003) and BARC type 2–5 bleeding (2.3% vs. 3.3%; $P = .036$), without any effect modification when stratified by setting of index PCI (acute MI = 1987 patients and ACS = 3921 patients). In a subsequent extension study of the subset of patients ($N = 4717$) who remained on randomized therapy for a median follow-up of 5.8 years from randomization, the benefit of clopidogrel over aspirin was sustained with lower BARC type 2–5 bleeding (4.5% vs. 6.1%; $P = .016$) and lower occurrence of the thrombotic composite (8.1% vs. 11.9%; $P < .001$).[20]

In the setting of data supporting the potential better efficacy and safety profile of long-term clopidogrel monotherapy over aspirin monotherapy, trials have examined a strategy of early de-escalation to $P2Y_{12}$ inhibitor monotherapy compared with a conventional 1-year DAPT regimen. The TWILIGHT trial randomized 7119 patients undergoing PCI with high-risk features for ischemia or bleeding after an initial 3-month period of DAPT with aspirin and ticagrelor to either ticagrelor monotherapy or continued DAPT for 1 year.[21] Importantly, patients were required to be free of a recurrent ischemic event or major bleeding in the first 3 months to be eligible. Ticagrelor monotherapy after 3 months reduced the primary endpoint of BARC type 2, 3 or 5 bleeding (HR, 0.56; 95% CI 0.46–0.65; $P < .001$), without an increased risk of CV death, MI, or stroke (HR, 0.99; 95% CI, 0.78–1.25; P for noninferiority < .001) compared with DAPT for 1 year. These results were directionally consistent among subgroups of patients presenting with non-ST-elevation ACS (64.8%) as well as those with prior MI (29.7%),[22] though notably patients presenting with ST-elevation MI were excluded. The TICO trial examined a similar strategy across the spectrum of ACS ($N = 3056$; 36% STEMI, 34% NSTEMI, 30% unstable angina), without the requirement for a 3-month event-free period prior to enrollment.[23] In a pooled analysis of TWILIGHT and TICO, no differences were observed for the secondary ischemic endpoint of CV death, MI, or ischemic stroke with ticagrelor monotherapy for months 3–12 versus DAPT (HR, 0.89; 95% CI 0.66–1.20; $P = .22$) with a significant reduction in BARC 3 or 5 bleeding (HR, 0.37; 95% CI 0.24–0.56; $P < .001$).[24]

However, optimal selection of any one $P2Y_{12}$ inhibitor for monotherapy remains uncertain, with trials to date yielding mixed results particularly for clopidogrel. Specifically, while trials have demonstrated a consistent reduction in bleeding with discontinuation of aspirin, results for ischemic events with clopidogrel monotherapy have been mixed. In the SMART-CHOICE and STOPDAPT-2 trials, which evaluated a strategy of clopidogrel monotherapy beginning at 1–3 months compared with continued DAPT for 1 year among patients undergoing PCI, there was no clear excess in ischemic events, albeit in the context of wide confidence intervals which could not exclude clinically important risk (SMART-CHOICE: HR, 1.19; 95% CI, 0.76–1.85; STOPDAPT-2: HR, 0.79; 95% CI 0.49–1.29). These results were consistent in the limited subset of patients presenting with ACS in each trial (58% in SMART-CHOICE and 38% in STOPDAPT-2). However, in the STOPDAPT-2 ACS trial, which examined a strategy of clopidogrel monotherapy at 1–2 months after PCI compared with DAPT for 1 year in patients presenting with ACS ($N = 4169$), the rate of the primary endpoint was greater in the clopidogrel monotherapy group (3.2% vs. 2.8%; HR, 1.14; 95% CI, 0.80–1.62; $P = .06$ for noninferiority), which was driven by an excess in ischemic events (CV death, MI, definite stent thrombosis or stroke; 2.8% vs. 1.9%; HR, 1.50; 95% CI, 0.99–2.26).[25]

While the bulk of trials examining $P2Y_{12}$ monotherapy have required DAPT for an initial 1–3 prior to de-escalation, recent trials have now examined a strategy of even earlier de-escalation. The STOPDAPT-3 trial randomized 5966 patients in Japan presenting with either ACS (75%, with 43% having STEMI) and/or with high bleeding risk to a strategy of either low-dose prasugrel monotherapy (without aspirin) or DAPT with aspirin and low-dose prasugrel immediately following PCI.[26] In the prasugrel monotherapy arm, there was a greater rate of ischemic events (HR for CV death, MI, definite stent thrombosis, or ischemic stroke, 1.12; 95% CI, 0.87–1.45; $P = .01$ for noninferiority) at one month without a reduction in BARC type 3 or 5 bleeding (HR, 0.95; 95% CI 0.75–1.20. $P = .66$ for superiority). These results suggest immediate de-escalation to monotherapy following PCI, particularly with a lower dose prasugrel regimen, may still be associated with higher ischemic risk. However, other trials employing more conventional dosing of $P2Y_{12}$ inhibitor monotherapy for earlier de-escalation have demonstrated no difference in ischemic outcomes. The T-PASS trial randomized 2850 patients in South Korea presenting with ACS (40% STEMI, 35% NSTEMI, 25% unstable angina) to a strategy of ticagrelor monotherapy after <1 month of DAPT (with aspirin discontinuation at a median of 16 days [IQR 12–25 days] after ACS) versus continued DAPT with ticagrelor for 1 year.[27] No differences were observed for ischemic events (composite of CV death, MI, stent thrombosis, or ischemia-driven revascularization: 1.5% vs. 2.2%; HR, 0.68; 95% CI, 0.39–1.18; $P = .17$) when aspirin was discontinued early, with a reduction in BARC type 3c/5 bleeding with ticagrelor monotherapy (1.2% vs. 3.4%; HR, 0.35; 95% CI, 0.20–0.61; $P < .001$).

Notably, each of the individual trials examining de-escalation to $P2Y_{12}$ monotherapy is likely underpowered to assess for differences in ischemic events. In a meta-analysis of 5 clinical trials examining a strategy of $P2Y_{12}$ monotherapy after 1–3 months of DAPT ($N = 32,145$), in the subset of patients presenting with ACS (56%), there was a marked reduction in bleeding without excess in ischemic events with de-escalation to $P2Y_{12}$ monotherapy compared with DAPT (Fig. 26.15).[28]

Collectively, these data suggest that de-escalation to $P2Y_{12}$ monotherapy after 1–3 months of DAPT may be beneficial in reducing bleeding risk without a significant tradeoff in risk for ischemic events, with very limited data for even earlier de-escalation. However, the optimal choice of $P2Y_{12}$ inhibitor for monotherapy remains uncertain. Moreover, considering the marked interindividual variability observed with clopidogrel, whether selection should be personalized on the basis of PFT or genetic testing remains unclear. As well, uncertainties remain regarding the optimal timing of transition to monotherapy following ACS, and whether such a strategy should be continued indefinitely beyond 12 months.

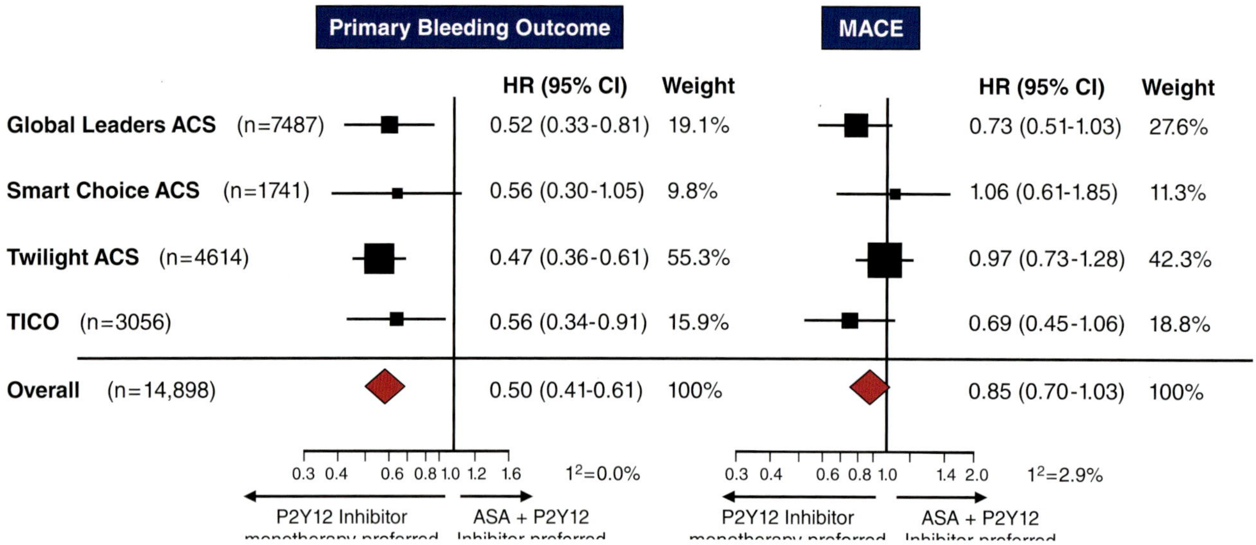

FIG. 26.15 **Relative hazard of bleeding and major adverse cardiovascular events among patients treated with $P2Y_{12}$ monotherapy vs. DAPT 1–3 months after an ACS.** In the subset of patients presenting with an ACS included in the meta-analysis, $P2Y_{12}$ monotherapy 1–3 months after ACS presentation reduced bleeding without increasing the risk for ischemic events compared with conventional DAPT. (Adapted from O'Donoghue ML, Murphy SA, Sabatine MS. The safety and efficacy of aspirin discontinuation on a background of a P2Y(12) inhibitor in patients after percutaneous coronary intervention: a systematic review and meta-analysis. *Circulation*. 2020;142:538–545.)

PRACTICAL APPROACH TO ANTIPLATELET THERAPY AFTER MYOCARDIAL INFARCTION

Although the evidence from large randomized, controlled trials supports the efficacy of antiplatelet therapy for long-term secondary prevention of adverse events after MI, the multiple options for selection of individual agents and their combinations as well as the need to balance bleeding risk have complicated application of these findings in clinical practice. This section outlines potential strategies for treatment with antiplatelet agents for secondary prevention after MI.

Given the differences in trial designs and possible heterogeneity of benefits related to the stability and time from the ACS presentation, an important consideration for decision making is whether the patient is within 1 year of the most recent ACS. Accordingly, considerations for clinical decision making with respect to antiplatelet regimens entail both the time from most recent ACS as well as the patient's specific bleeding and ischemic risk profile.

Patients Within 1 Year From the Most Recent Myocardial Infarction

The risk of recurrent atherothrombosis is highest during the first year after an MI, and net clinical outcomes are clearly improved by adding another antiplatelet agent to aspirin during this period, except for subgroups of patients with contraindications to antithrombotic therapy or at particularly high risk for serious bleeding. In patients without high bleeding risk, we suggest adherence to current professional society guidelines many of which continue to recommend a third-generation $P2Y_{12}$ inhibitor (ticagrelor or prasugrel) with aspirin for 12 months after ACS (Fig. 26.1).

For patients at higher bleeding risk, de-escalation to $P2Y_{12}$ inhibitor monotherapy after 1–3 months of dual antiplatelet therapy appears to be reasonable to minimize bleeding risk (Fig. 26.16), though this should be weighed against risk factors for recurrent ischemia. The choice of the optimal $P2Y_{12}$ inhibitor for monotherapy remains uncertain; however, owing to prior data regarding the variability in response to clopidogrel and the totality of data examining ticagrelor monotherapy, ticagrelor may be preferred when opting for $P2Y_{12}$ inhibitor monotherapy. Moreover, for patients who require concomitant oral anticoagulation (e.g., those with atrial fibrillation), aspirin should be discontinued in favor of dual antithrombotic therapy (i.e., $P2Y_{12}$ inhibitor and anticoagulant) until 12 months post ACS.

Patients at or Beyond 1 Year From Myocardial Infarction

For patients who tolerate DAPT through the first 12 months following ACS without any bleeding complications, consideration should be given to the appropriateness of a long-term antiplatelet regimen, weighing ischemic and bleeding risk. In those at high ischemic risk, consideration may be given to a prolonged DAPT strategy (Fig. 26.16). Alternatively, patients may be de-escalated to monotherapy; while classically this has been with discontinuation of $P2Y_{12}$ inhibitor in support of ongoing aspirin monotherapy, long-term $P2Y_{12}$ monotherapy may be at least equally as efficacious and perhaps offer lower bleeding risk though data to date for long-term secondary prevention are lacking. The role of long-term antiplatelet therapy for patients receiving oral anticoagulant therapy remains incompletely studied as previously described.

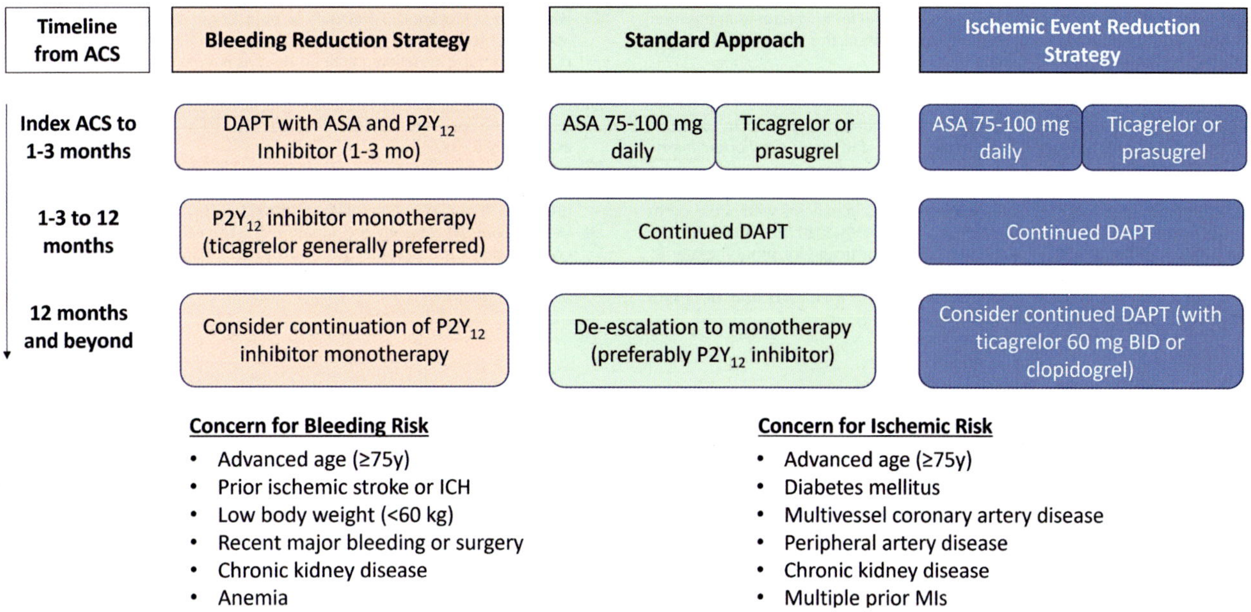

FIG. 26.16 A schema for considering antiplatelet therapies as secondary prevention after acute coronary syndrome. *ASA*, Acetylsalicylic acid (aspirin); *ICH*, intracranial hemorrhage.

SUMMARY

In addition to its near-term complications, MI reflects an underlying diffuse and chronic condition with a natural history marked by a "stuttering" clinical course and by a substantial risk of recurrent atherothrombosis that extends for years beyond the initial acute event, albeit with the most significant risk being in the early phase following MI. This disease state is characterized by a risk not only of recurrent MI but also of future events across vascular beds (e.g., stroke and peripheral vascular events) which lead to permanent disability and shorten lifespan. The history of MI, therefore, is an indication to the clinician of an underlying condition that warrants chronic treatment.

Antiplatelet therapy not only is effective in managing the acute event but also mitigates the long-term risk of recurrence. The reduction in ischemic events must be balanced against an increased risk of bleeding. In the coming years, more sophisticated strategies for assessing this risk-benefit balance, including applications of machine learning to refine risk stratification are likely to become available to facilitate such therapeutic risk stratification with increasing greater precision.

A number of open questions remain regarding the optimal type and duration of antiplatelet therapy after MI, particularly the optimal duration and choice of aspirin versus $P2Y_{12}$ inhibitor for monotherapy in the long term. This remains a complex and rapidly evolving landscape with the continued evolution of optimal treatment strategies expected over the next few years.

REFERENCES

1. Lawton JS, Tamis-Holland JE, Bangalore S, et al. 2021 ACC/AHA/SCAI guideline for coronary artery revascularization: executive summary: a report of the American College of Cardiology/American Heart Association joint committee on clinical practice guidelines. *Circulation*. 2022;145:e4–e17.
2. Byrne RA, Rossello X, Coughlan JJ, et al. 2023 ESC guidelines for the management of acute coronary syndromes. *Eur Heart J*. 2023;44:3720–3826.
3. Jacobsen AP, Raber I, McCarthy CP, et al. Lifelong aspirin for all in the secondary prevention of chronic coronary syndrome: still sacrosanct or is reappraisal warranted? *Circulation*. 2020;142:1579–1590.
4. Gawaz M, Geisler T, Borst O. Current concepts and novel targets for antiplatelet therapy. *Nat Rev Cardiol*. 2023;20:583–599.
5. Jones WS, Mulder H, Wruck LM, et al. Comparative effectiveness of aspirin dosing in cardiovascular disease. *N Engl J Med*. 2021;384:1981–1990.
6. Sleem A, Effron MB, Stebbins A, et al. Effectiveness and safety of enteric-coated vs uncoated aspirin in patients with cardiovascular disease: a secondary analysis of the ADAPTABLE randomized clinical trial. *JAMA Cardiol*. 2023;8:1061–1069.
7. Schupke S, Neumann FJ, Menichelli M, et al. Ticagrelor or prasugrel in patients with acute coronary syndromes. *N Engl J Med*. 2019;381:1524–1534.
8. Knuuti J, Wijns W, Saraste A, et al. 2019 ESC guidelines for the diagnosis and management of chronic coronary syndromes. *Eur Heart J*. 2020;41:407–477.
9. Howard CE, Nambi V, Jneid H, Khalid U. Extended duration of dual-antiplatelet therapy after percutaneous coronary intervention: how long is too long? *J Am Heart Assoc*. 2019;8:e012639.
10. Gargiulo G, Goette A, Tijssen J, et al. Safety and efficacy outcomes of double vs. triple antithrombotic therapy in patients with atrial fibrillation following percutaneous coronary intervention: a systematic review and meta-analysis of non-vitamin K antagonist oral anticoagulant-based randomized clinical trials. *Eur Heart J*. 2019;40:3757–3767.
11. Lopes RD, Leonardi S, Wojdyla DM, et al. Stent thrombosis in patients with atrial fibrillation undergoing coronary stenting in the AUGUSTUS trial. *Circulation*. 2020;141:781–783.
12. Yasuda S, Kaikita K, Akao M, et al. Antithrombotic therapy for atrial fibrillation with stable coronary disease. *N Engl J Med*. 2019;381:1103–1113.
13. Gorog DA, Ferreiro JL, Ahrens I, et al. De-escalation or abbreviation of dual antiplatelet therapy in acute coronary syndromes and percutaneous coronary intervention: a consensus statement from an international expert panel on coronary thrombosis. *Nat Rev Cardiol*. 2023;20:830–844.
14. Bonaca MP, Im K, Magnani G, et al. Patient selection for long-term secondary prevention with ticagrelor: insights from PEGASUS-TIMI 54. *Eur Heart J*. 2022;43:5037–5044.
15. Bergmark BA, Mathenge N, Merlini PA, et al. Acute coronary syndromes. *Lancet*. 2022;399:1347–1358.
16. Pereira NL, Farkouh ME, So D, et al. Effect of genotype-guided oral P2Y12 inhibitor selection vs conventional clopidogrel therapy on ischemic outcomes after percutaneous coronary intervention: the TAILOR-PCI randomized clinical trial. *JAMA*. 2020;324:761–771.
17. Claassens DMF, Vos GJA, Bergmeijer TO, et al. A genotype-guided strategy for oral P2Y(12) inhibitors in primary PCI. *N Engl J Med*. 2019;381:1621–1631.
18. Costa F, Van Klaveren D, Feres F, et al. Dual antiplatelet therapy duration based on ischemic and bleeding risks after coronary stenting. *J Am Coll Cardiol*. 2019;73:741–754.
19. Koo BK, Kang J, Park KW, et al. Aspirin versus clopidogrel for chronic maintenance monotherapy after percutaneous coronary intervention (HOST-EXAM): an investigator-initiated, prospective, randomised, open-label, multicentre trial. *Lancet*. 2021;397:2487–2496.

20. Kang J, Park KW, Lee H, et al. Aspirin versus clopidogrel for long-term maintenance monotherapy after percutaneous coronary intervention: the HOST-EXAM extended study. *Circulation*. 2023;147:108–117.
21. Mehran R, Baber U, Sharma SK, et al. Ticagrelor with or without aspirin in high-risk patients after PCI. *N Engl J Med*. 2019;381:2032–2042.
22. Chiarito M, Baber U, Cao D, et al. Ticagrelor monotherapy after PCI in high-risk patients with prior MI: a prespecified TWILIGHT substudy. *JACC Cardiovasc Interv*. 2022;15:282–293.
23. Kim BK, Hong SJ, Cho YH, et al. Effect of ticagrelor monotherapy vs ticagrelor with aspirin on major bleeding and cardiovascular events in patients with acute coronary syndrome: the TICO randomized clinical trial. *JAMA*. 2020;323:2407–2416.
24. Baber U, Jang Y, Oliva A, et al. Safety and efficacy of ticagrelor monotherapy in patients with acute coronary syndromes undergoing percutaneous coronary intervention: an individual patient data meta-analysis of TWILIGHT and TICO randomized trials. *Circulation*. 2024;149:574–584.
25. Watanabe H, Morimoto T, Natsuaki M, et al. Comparison of clopidogrel monotherapy after 1 to 2 months of dual antiplatelet therapy with 12 months of dual antiplatelet therapy in patients with acute coronary syndrome: the STOPDAPT-2 ACS randomized clinical trial. *JAMA Cardiol*. 2022;7:407–417.
26. Natsuaki M, Watanabe H, Morimoto T, et al. An Aspirin-Free Versus Dual Antiplatelet Strategy for Coronary Stenting: STOPDAPT-3 Randomized Trial. *Circulation*. 2024;149:585–600.
27. Hong SJ, Lee SJ, Suh Y, et al. Stopping aspirin within 1 month after stenting for ticagrelor monotherapy in acute coronary syndrome: the T-PASS randomized noninferiority trial. *Circulation*. 2024;149(8):562–573.
28. O'Donoghue ML, Murphy SA, Sabatine MS. The safety and efficacy of aspirin discontinuation on a background of a P2Y(12) inhibitor in patients after percutaneous coronary intervention: a systematic review and meta-analysis. *Circulation*. 2020;142:538–545.

27 Anti-inflammatory Therapy After Acute Coronary Syndrome

JEAN-CLAUDE TARDIF

INTRODUCTION

Atherosclerotic cardiovascular disease is the leading cause of mortality and disability worldwide. Atherosclerosis is a complex process involving multiple inflammatory signaling pathways, through its different stages of initiation, progression, and destabilization.[1] An acute exacerbation of cardiovascular inflammation has been demonstrated in acute coronary syndromes (ACS), in addition to the chronic atherosclerosis-related inflammatory process. Despite existing guideline-based secondary prevention strategies focused on lipids and thrombosis, the residual risk of subsequent vascular events remains high, emphasizing the need to identify additional therapeutic targets in order to further improve patient outcomes.

The question regarding the magnitude of residual risks of cardiovascular events attributed to elevated cholesterol and inflammation has recently been addressed in a contemporary clinical setting of statin-treated patients.[2] This meta-analysis of three recent randomized trials having included 31,245 patients aimed at comparing the strength of the association between residual inflammatory risk (reflected by the plasma concentration of high-sensitivity C-reactive protein) and cardiovascular events and mortality with the association between residual cholesterol risk (reflected by the plasma concentration of LDL-cholesterol) and cardiovascular events and mortality. Among patients intensively treated with statins, the strength of the association of residual inflammatory risk with cardiovascular events and mortality appeared to be higher than that of residual cholesterol risk. More precisely, individuals with higher levels of high-sensitivity C-reactive protein (top vs. bottom quartile) had large and statistically significantly increased hazard ratios (HRs) for major adverse cardiovascular events (1.31), cardiovascular mortality (2.68), and all-cause mortality (2.42). In contrast, individuals with higher levels of LDL-cholesterol (top vs. bottom quartile) had modestly increased HRs for major adverse cardiovascular events (1.08, P =.10), cardiovascular mortality (1.27), and total mortality (1.16). These results support the potential of inflammation reduction therapy for the prevention of cardiovascular events in patients with ACS.

Colchicine is a medication that has been used for years for the treatment of inflammatory disorders such as gout, pericarditis, and familial Mediterranean fever.[3–5] It is a derivative from the plant *Colchicum automnale*, used as an Old Egyptian remedy for joint inflammation, and was isolated by two French scientists (Pelletier and Caventou) in the 18th century. Colchicine is a lipid-soluble drug characterized by a bioavailability of 44%, a low-affinity binding with albumin of 32%, cytochrome P450 3A4-related metabolism, and predominant liver excretion.[6] Colchicine is contraindicated in patients with severe renal dysfunction and has a relatively narrow therapeutic index, with effective plasma concentrations ranging from 0.5 to 3 ng/mL.[6] It concentrates preferentially in white blood cells, which results in anti-inflammatory effects even at low doses.[7] Colchicine is characterized by broad antiinflammatory actions as it inhibits leukocyte tubulin polymerization and the NOD-like receptor protein 3 (NLRP3) inflammasome, which are involved in the activation of the interleukin1ß/6 signaling pathway. Its specific actions and effects include (among others) alteration of neutrophil deformability and motility, antimitotic properties in leukocytes, inhibition of cholesterol crystal-induced coronary atherogenesis, and reduction of the expression of cellular adhesion molecules.[8–11] Colchicine also reduces the production of inflammatory biomarkers,[6,12,13] and stabilizes coronary plaques among patients with a recent ACS.[14] In patients undergoing percutaneous coronary intervention, colchicine attenuates the increase of circulating interleukin-6 and high-sensitivity C-reactive protein levels at 24 hours[12] and attenuates neutrophil extracellular trap formation.[15] In patients with stable coronary artery disease, colchicine at a dose of 0.5 mg once daily for 30 days is associated with significant reductions of inflammatory biomarkers related to the NLRP3 inflammasome pathway (IL-6 and IL-18), of circulating high-sensitivity C-reactive protein, and of proteins involved in neutrophil degranulation.[16]

In this chapter, the evidence is summarized to support the use of colchicine in secondary prevention of atherosclerotic cardiovascular disease, including after ACS.

INFLAMMATION REDUCTION IN ACS

Colchicine has been tested in patients with a recent myocardial infarction. The COLchicine Cardiovascular Outcomes Trial (COLCOT) recruited 4745 patients within the first 30 days following a myocardial infarction who were randomized to receive either low-dose colchicine (0.5 mg per os daily) or matched placebo.[17] Exclusion criteria were the presence of severe heart failure, left ventricular ejection fraction lower than 35%, stroke within the previous 3 months, type 2 index myocardial infarction, coronary-bypass surgery either within the previous 3 years or planned, a history of noncutaneous cancer within the previous 3 years, inflammatory bowel disease or chronic diarrhea, neuromuscular disease, nontransient creatine kinase level greater than three times the upper limit of the normal range (unless due to infarction), clinically significant nontransient hematologic abnormalities, severe renal disease with a serum creatinine level that was greater than two times the upper limit of the normal range, severe hepatic disease, drug or alcohol abuse, systemic glucocorticoid use, or clinically significant sensitivity to colchicine. Patients were enrolled a mean of 13.5 days after myocardial infarction and followed for a median of 22.6 months. Aspirin, a second antiplatelet agent, and a statin were used in 99%, 98%, and 99% of patients, and percutaneous coronary intervention was performed in 93% of patients for their index myocardial infarction.

After a median follow-up of 22.6 months, the primary efficacy endpoint, a composite of death from cardiovascular causes, resuscitated cardiac arrest, myocardial infarction, stroke, or urgent hospitalization for angina leading to coronary revascularization, occurred in 5.5% of participants randomized to colchicine and in 7.1% of participants randomized to placebo (HR: 0.77; 95% confidence interval (CI): 0.61–0.96). Therefore, colchicine led in COLCOT to a significant reduction of 23% in the occurrence of the primary endpoint.[17] The effect of colchicine on all of the components contributed to the benefit on the primary endpoint, although the efficacy was more pronounced on strokes (HR: 0.26; 95% CI: 0.10–0.70) and urgent hospitalizations for angina leading to revascularization (HR: 0.50; 95% CI: 0.31–0.81). Colchicine was also associated with a relative risk reduction of 34% in the total number of primary endpoint events (first and recurrent) compared to placebo (rate ratio 0.66, 95% CI 0.51–0.86).[17]

A post-hoc analysis from COLCOT demonstrated that early initiation of colchicine (within the first 3 days post-myocardial infarction) was associated with an even greater reduction (48%) in the risk of the composite primary endpoint compared to placebo (HR 0.52, 95% CI 0.32–0.84).[18] This subgroup analysis lends support to the hypothesis that early initiation of colchicine following ACS may offer incremental value with inhibition of the acute-phase inflammation response. In addition, a cost-effectiveness analysis in COLCOT demonstrated that the addition of colchicine to the standard of care in patients after a myocardial infarction was economically dominant, meaning that it led to cost savings, based on both in-trial (24 months) and lifetime (20 years) incremental cost-effectiveness ratios.[19]

The Australian Colchicine in Patients with Acute Coronary Syndrome (COPS) trial was a smaller study conducted in patients having presented with an ACS.[20] COPS was a multicenter, randomized, double-blind, placebo-controlled trial that enrolled 795 patients with acute coronary syndrome and angiographic evidence of coronary artery disease.[20] Patients were managed with either percutaneous coronary intervention or medical therapy and were assigned to receive either colchicine (0.5 mg twice daily for the first month, then 0.5 mg daily for 11 months) or placebo. The primary outcome was a composite of all-cause mortality, ACS, unplanned ischemia-driven urgent revascularization, and noncardioembolic ischemic stroke. At 365 days of follow-up, colchicine was associated with a non-significant reduction in the risk of the primary composite endpoint when compared to placebo (HR 0.65, 95% CI 0.38–1.09).[20] The smaller than anticipated sample size, short duration of follow-up, incomplete rate of follow-up, and lack of power (a total of 62 primary endpoint events were reported throughout the trial) most likely accounted for the numerically lower but non-statistically significant difference observed for the primary endpoint.[20] In a post-hoc analysis evaluating a composite endpoint similar to the COLCOT trial primary endpoint, the event risk among patients receiving colchicine was half that seen in the placebo group (5.0% with colchicine vs. 9.5% with placebo; HR: 0.51; 95% CI: 0.29–0.89; $P = .019$).

The recently completed Colchicine and Spironolactone in Patients With MI/SYNERGY Stent Registry trial (CLEAR-SYNERGY) randomized 7062 participants (from 104 centers in 14 countries (including approximately 2500 patients in 4 sites in Macedonia and 500 patients in Serbia)) with myocardial infarction treated with percutaneous coronary intervention to colchicine versus placebo. The vast majority of patients were enrolled after a ST elevation myocardial infarction (95%). The protocol of that study was amended, following the results of the COLCOT and LoDoCo2 trials, to lower the dosage of colchicine from 0.5 mg twice daily to once daily). The median duration of follow-up was 3 years. The primary composite endpoint of cardiovascular death, myocardial infarction, stroke, or ischemia-driven revascularization occurred in 9.1% of patients allocated to colchicine and 9.3% allocated to placebo (hazard ratio (HR) 0.99, 95% confidence interval [CI] 0.85-1.16), $p = .93$). There was a reduction of 22% in the incidence of a primary endpoint event with colchicine versus placebo before the pandemic, which was lost during the pandemic, with an interaction between the COVID-19 phase and the treatment effect ($p < .10$). The inverted relationship between the incidence of non-fatal myocardial infarction and all-cause deaths in CLEAR-SYNERGY is consistent with the published impact of COVID-19 on cardiovascular clinical care and major under-reporting of non-fatal events (Tardif JC, Kouz S. Efficacy and safety of colchicine and spironolactone after myocardial infarction: the CLEAR-SYNERGY trial in perspective. Eur Heart J Acute Cardiovasc Care 2024;13:843-844). Furthermore, inflammation was not controlled in the colchicine arm of CLEAR-SYNERGY with a least-squares mean hs-CRP of 3.0 mg/L (95% CI 2.6-3.5), in contrast to the on-treatment median values of 1.12 mg/L (IQR: 0.77-2.10) in COLCOT and 0.94 mg/L (IQR: 0.53-1.93) in LoDoCo2. These data are important, given that CANTOS has previously shown that inflammation reduction therapy lowers the incidence of cardiovascular events only in those with an on-treatment hs-CRP <2.0 mg/L (as in COLCOT and LoDoCo2), but not in those with hs-CRP ≥ 2.0 mg/L (as in CLEAR-SYNERGY) (Ridker PM, MacFayden JG, Everett BM, et al. Relationship of C-reactive protein reduction to cardiovascular event reduction following treatment with canakinumab: a secondary analysis from the CANTOS randomised controlled trial. Lancet 2018;391:319-328). This might also explain at least in part the strange lack of benefit of colchicine, and even a trend for worsening, on the occurrence of pericarditis (HR 1.53, 95% CI 0.88-2.65) in CLEAR-SYNERGY. These important issues makes the results of CLEAR-SYNERGY uncertain and uninterpretable.

INFLAMMATION REDUCTION IN CHRONIC CORONARY DISEASE

A discussion of the benefits of colchicine in chronic coronary artery disease is relevant in this chapter on inflammation reduction, because the ACS setting eventually gives way to the more chronic stage of atherosclerotic cardiovascular disease.

The impact of colchicine on cardiovascular event reduction was first studied in the Low-Dose Colchicine (LoDoCo) randomized trial, in which 532 patients with angiographically-proven stable coronary artery disease were randomized to receive colchicine 0.5 mg daily or no colchicine.[21] Among the participants randomized to colchicine, 32 stopped the study drug early due to adverse effects, and the protocol allowed to replace them with additional participants. All patients, whether or not they stopped the study drug due to adverse effects, were included in the intention-to-treat analysis. The majority of study participants were treated with at least one antiplatelet agent and high-dose statin as part of their secondary prevention treatment, and 55%–60% were also treated with an angiotensin-converting enzyme inhibitor. The primary efficacy endpoint, a composite of ACS, fatal and non-fatal out-of-hospital cardiac arrest, and non-cardioembolic ischemic stroke, occurred in 5.3% of the participants in the colchicine group and in 16.0% of participants in the control group (HR: 0.33; 95% CI: 0.18–0.59), after a median follow-up of 36 months. This was largely driven by an excess of non-stent-related ACS in the control group compared with colchicine. Despite the large magnitude of the absolute and relative risk reductions, the results of the LoDoCo trial were nevertheless viewed as hypothesis-generating given the small sample size, lack of a placebo-control or participant blinding, and limited verification of adherence in participants randomized to colchicine.

The results of the subsequent placebo-controlled, double-blind, randomized Low-Dose Colchicine-2 (LoDoCo2) trial were consistent with the findings of the original LoDoCo trial.[22] In this study, 6528 patients with evidence of coronary disease on invasive coronary angiography, computed tomography angiography, or a coronary-artery calcium score of at least 400 Agatston units, and considered stable for at least 6 months were included. Key exclusion criteria were the presence of at least moderate renal impairment, severe heart failure, and at least moderate valvular disease requiring intervention. All participants entered a 1-month run-in period in which they were treated with open-label colchicine 0.5 mg once daily to ascertain tolerance. Following the run-in period, 5522 patients (84.6%) were randomized to either colchicine 0.5 mg daily or placebo; 1006 patients (15.4%) were not randomized, mainly due to perceived adverse effects. The primary endpoint, a composite of cardiovascular death, spontaneous myocardial infarction, ischemic stroke, or ischemia-driven coronary revascularization, occurred in 6.8% of participants in the colchicine group and in 9.6% of the participants in the placebo group (HR: 0.69; 95% CI: 0.57–0.83; $P < .001$) after a median follow-up of 28.6 months. Individual endpoints of myocardial infarction and ischemia-driven coronary revascularization were significantly reduced with colchicine, but not ischemic strokes. Death from any cause occurred in 2.6% and in 2.2% of participants randomized to colchicine and placebo, respectively (HR: 1.12; 95% CI: 0.86–1.71). Results were consistent across multiple prespecified subgroups, including in male and female participants.

The consistency of the results of the LoDoCo and LoDoCo2 trials in patients with stable coronary artery disease along with those of COLCOT in patients having suffered a myocardial infarction, in addition to the established safety profile of colchicine, position this inexpensive medication as an important addition in the secondary prevention of cardiovascular events in patients with coronary disease. In LoDoCo2, the number-needed-to-treat over a mean follow-up duration of 28.6 months was 35, which is consistent with the benefits of aspirin, statin, and antihypertensive therapy in secondary prevention.[23] Notably, this benefit was obtained despite the fact that almost all patients received these other guideline-recommended therapies during the trial.

Several meta-analyses of randomized controlled trials have confirmed that colchicine decreases the risk of major cardiovascular events, myocardial infarction, stroke, and coronary revascularization, but not of cardiovascular death, in secondary prevention of coronary artery disease.[24–26] Our own meta-analysis, which included the results of COLCOT, LoDoCo, COPS, and LoDoCo2 and a total of 11,594 patients, demonstrated that colchicine was associated with a reduction of 32% in the incidence of the composite of cardiovascular mortality, myocardial infarction, ischemic stroke, and urgent coronary revascularization in comparison with placebo (Fig. 27.1).[24] Colchicine also significantly reduced the incidence of myocardial infarction by 38%, stroke by 62%, and urgent coronary revascularization by 44% compared to placebo.[24]

Reassuringly, these benefits were observed without an increase in gastrointestinal safety concerns.[24–27] With regards to the safety of colchicine, pooled risk ratios from LoDoCo2 and COLCOT demonstrated no statistically significant difference in the incidence of infections, hospitalizations for gastrointestinal events, and diagnoses of cancer between

TABLE 27.1 Approval of Colchicine by the US Food and Drug Administration in June 2023

- "Colchicine 0.5 mg once daily is indicated to reduce the risk of myocardial infarction, stroke, coronary revascularization, and cardiovascular death in adult patients with established atherosclerotic disease or with multiple risk factors for cardiovascular disease."
- "Concurrent use of strong cytochrome P450 3A4 inhibitors or P-glycoprotein inhibitors with colchicine is contraindicated, including in patients with hepatic or renal impairment."
- "Colchicine is contraindicated in patients with preexisting blood dyscrasias, renal failure, and severe hepatic impairment."

coronary artery disease (as was the case in COLCOT and LoDoCo2 that have included more than 10,000 patients followed for more than 2 years), atrial fibrillation, and heart failure. In the absence of severe renal disease, colchicine is often used in patients with heart failure who develop gout triggered by the use of a loop diuretic.

Colchicine causes relatively few adverse effects, which tend to be mild and tolerable. The most frequent are gastrointestinal symptoms, such as flatulence, nausea, abdominal pain, and diarrhea. However, at the low dose of 0.5 mg once daily used in COLCOT, the incidence of total gastrointestinal adverse events was not significantly higher with colchicine than with placebo.[17] In COLCOT, nausea (1.8% and 1.0%, respectively; $P = .02$) and flatulence (0.6% and 0.2%, respectively; $P = .02$), were more frequent with colchicine than placebo. Blood dyscrasias such as agranulocytosis and aplastic anemia have been reported very rarely with colchicine. Therefore, a complete blood count should be considered annually, although such abnormalities were not reported more frequently with colchicine than with placebo in the COLCOT and LoDoCo2 trials.[17,20,22] In COLCOT, a small increase in the risk of pneumonias was observed (21 with colchicine [0.9%] vs. 9 with placebo [0.4%]; $P = .03$), but no such trend was observed in LoDoCo2 where hospitalization for pneumonia was observed in 1.7% and 2.0% of participants, respectively (HR: 0.84; 95% CI: 0.56–1.24). A recent meta-analysis has not shown a significant increase in the risk of pneumonias with colchicine compared to placebo in patients with coronary artery disease.[24] Therefore, in light of both the good safety and tolerability of colchicine, the risk-benefit profile favors the use of colchicine in most eligible patients in secondary prevention of athrosclerotic cardiovascular disease.

REGULATORY APPROVAL, GUIDELINE RECOMMANDATIONS

The United States Food and Drug Administration has approved colchicine in 2023 (Table 27.1), with the following label: "Colchicine 0.5 mg once daily is indicated to reduce the risk of myocardial infarction, stroke, coronary revascularization, and cardiovascular death in adult patients with established atherosclerotic disease or with multiple risk factors for cardiovascular disease. Concurrent use of strong cytochrome P450 3A4 inhibitors or P-glycoprotein inhibitors with colchicine is contraindicated, including in patients with hepatic or renal impairment. Colchicine is contraindicated in patients with preexisting blood dyscrasias, renal failure, and severe hepatic impairment." Health Canada had previously approved low-dose colchicine in 2021 for the indication of "the reduction of atherothrombotic events in adult patients with existing coronary artery disease, in addition to standard therapies, including LDL-cholesterol lowering and antithrombotic drug treatment."

The 2023 AHA/ACC/ACCP/ASPC/NLA/PCNA guidelines for the management of patients with chronic coronary disease, the European guidelines both for the management of acute coronary syndromes and for cardiovascular prevention, as well as the South American guidelines have all given a positive class 2b recommendation for colchicine 0.5 mg once daily for the secondary prevention of atherosclerotic cardiovascular events.[33,34] More recently, the European guidelines were updated and assigned a class 2a recommendation for colchicine in secondary cardiovascular prevention (Vrints C, Andreotti F, Koskinas KC, et al. 2024 ESC Guidelines for the management of chronic coronary syndromes. Eur Heart J 2024;45:3415-3537).

PRACTICAL INTEGRATION OF LOW-DOSE COLCHICINE IN CLINICAL PRACTICE

Along with other guideline-recommended secondary prevention strategies and lifestyle modifications, colchicine at a dose of 0.5 mg once daily should be considered in patients with a recent ACS or with established stable coronary artery disease to improve cardiovascular outcomes.

The issue of polypharmacy is sometimes mentioned by physicians as the reason for having to choose between further lipid-lowering treatment or inflammation-reducing therapy in statin-treated patients. It is time to reconsider our answer to this apparent problem considering the worldwide burden of atherosclerotic cardiovascular disease and the cost-effectiveness of colchicine.[19,28] Serious consideration should be given to applying the successful model of four treatment pillars in heart failure to the multifaceted prevention of atherothrombotic events in patients with coronary disease. Physicians should no longer consider intensive lipid lowering and inflammation reduction as mutually exclusive but rather as complementary approaches in statin-treated patients with atherosclerotic cardiovascular disease.

Because colchicine is metabolized by cytochrome P450 3A4 and is a substrate for P-glycoprotein, it should not be used with strong P-glycoprotein inhibitors such as clarithromycin (the use of azithromycin is acceptable), and the concomitant use of strong and moderate cytochrome P450 3A4 inhibitors (including grapefruit juice) should be avoided particularly in patients with hepatic or renal impairment. Strong cytochrome P450 3A4 inhibitors include, but are not limited to, ritonavir, itraconazole, ketoconazole, and clarithromycin. The dosage of colchicine should also be reduced in patients receiving moderate to high doses of diltiazem or verapamil. Concomitant use of colchicine with high-intensity statin therapy has been well tolerated in COLCOT. Colchicine should not be used in patients with an estimated glomerular filtration rate <30 mL/min/1.73 m^2. A pharmacokinetic study has shown that the dosage of 0.5 mg once daily of colchicine will very rarely cause accumulation in patients with moderate kidney dysfunction, in contrast to the dosage of 0.6 mg once daily with which higher plasma levels can occasionally occur in that setting.[35] Fortunately, the dosage of 0.5 mg once daily of colchicine is now available in several countries including the United States.

A recent meta-analysis found that colchicine use throughout pregnancy was not associated with an increased incidence of miscarriage or major fetal malformations.[36] Indeed, the incidence of miscarriage was significantly lower in women who took colchicine compared with those who did not.

CONCLUSION

Low-dose (0.5 mg once daily) colchicine reduces the risk of ischemic cardiovascular events on a background of excellent standard care, irrespective of whether the patient has suffered a myocardial infarction or presents with stable coronary artery disease. In light of the positive results from COLCOT, LoDoCo2, and meta-analyses, its good safety and tolerability profile, and cost-effectiveness, inflammation reduction with low-dose colchicine should always be considered to treat patients with ACS in the absence of severe renal dysfunction.

SUMMARY

Acute coronary syndromes encompass a group of clinical conditions caused most often by the rupture or the erosion of an atherosclerotic plaque. Inflammation is central to the initiation and progression of atherosclerosis and to the destabilization of plaque leading to an ACS. Inflammation reduction therapy has been shown in large clinical trials to reduce the risk of ischemic cardiovascular events, both in patients with a recent ACS and in those with chronic coronary disease. Low-dose colchicine has been approved by the US Food and Drug Administration and has entered the American and European guidelines for the prevention of atherothrombotic events.

REFERENCES

1. Libby P, Loscalzo J, Ridker PM, et al. Inflammation, immunity, and infection in atherothrombosis: JACC review topic of the week. *J Am Coll Cardiol*. 2018;72:2071–2081.
2. Ridker PM, Bhatt DL, Pradhan AD, Glynn RJ, MacFadyen JG, Nissen SE. Inflammation and cholesterol as predictors of cardiovascular events among patients receiving statin therapy: a collaborative analysis of three randomised trials. *Lancet*. 2023;401:1293–1301.
3. FitzGerald JD, Dalbeth N, Mikuls T, et al. 2020 American College of Rheumatology guideline for the management of gout. *Arthritis Care Res (Hoboken)*. 2020;72:744–760.
4. Bouabdallaoui N, Tardif JC. Repurposing colchicine for heart disease. *Annu Rev Pharmacol Toxicol*. 2022;62:121–129.
5. Imazio M, Nidorf M. Colchicine and the heart. *Eur Heart J*. 2021;42:2745–2760.
6. Marquis-Gravel G, Goodman SG, Anderson TJ, et al. Colchicine for prevention of atherothrombotic events in patients with coronary artery disease: review and practical approach for clinicians. *Can J Cardiol*. 2021;37:1837–1845.
7. Deftereos SG, Beerkens FJ, Shah B, et al. Colchicine in cardiovascular disease: in-depth review. *Circulation*. 2022;145:61–78.
8. Martínez GJ, Celermajer DS, Patel S. The NLRP3 inflammasome and the emerging role of colchicine to inhibit atherosclerosis-associated inflammation. *Atherosclerosis*. 2018;269:262–271.
9. Roubille F, Merlet N, Busseuil D, et al. Colchicine reduces atherosclerotic plaque vulnerability in rabbits. *Atheroscler Plus*. 2021;45:1–9.
10. Fiolet ATL, Nidorf SM, Mosterd A, Cornel JH. Colchicine in stable coronary artery disease. *Clin Ther*. 2019;41:30–40.
11. Slobodnick A, Shah B, Krasnokutsky S, et al. Update on colchicine, 2017. *Rheumatology (Oxford)*. 2018;57(suppl 1):i4–i11.
12. Shah B, Pillinger M, Zhong H, et al. Effects of acute colchicine administration prior to percutaneous coronary intervention. *Circ Cardiovasc Interv*. 2020;13:e008717.
13. Sun M, Dubé MP, Hennessy T, Rhainds D, Hillis GS, Tardif JC. Low-dose colchicine and high-sensitivity C-reactive protein after myocardial infarction: a combined analysis using individual patient data from the COLCOT and LoDoCo-MI studies. *Int J Cardiol*. 2022;363:20–22.
14. Vaidya K, Arnott C, Martínez GJ, et al. Colchicine therapy and plaque stabilization in patients with acute coronary syndrome: a CT coronary angiography study. *JACC Cardiovasc Imaging*. 2018;11:305–316.
15. Vaidya K, Tucker B, Kurup R, et al. Colchicine inhibits neutrophil extracellular trap formation in patients with acute coronary syndrome after percutaneous coronary intervention. *J Am Heart Assoc*. 2021;10:e018993.
16. Opstal Tjerk SJ, Hoogeveen Renate M, Fiolet Aernoud TL, et al. Colchicine attenuates inflammation beyond the inflammasome in chronic coronary artery disease. *Circulation*. 2020;142:1996–1998.
17. Tardif JC, Kouz S, Waters DD, et al. Efficacy and safety of low-dose colchicine after myocardial infarction. *N Engl J Med*. 2019;381:2497–2505.
18. Bouabdallaoui N, Tardif JC, Waters DD, et al. Time-to-treatment initiation of colchicine and cardiovascular outcomes after myocardial infarction in the colchicine cardiovascular outcomes trial (COLCOT). *Eur Heart J*. 2020;41:4092–4099.
19. Samuel M, Tardif JC, Khairy P, et al. Cost-effectiveness of low-dose colchicine after myocardial infarction in the colchicine cardiovascular outcomes trial (COLCOT). *Eur Heart J Qual Care Clin Outcomes*. 2021;7:486–495.
20. Tong DC, Quinn S, Nasis A, et al. Colchicine in patients with acute coronary syndrome: the Australian COPS randomized clinical trial. *Circulation*. 2020;142:1890–1900.
21. Nidorf SM, Eikelboom JW, Budgeon CA, Thompson PL. Low-dose colchicine for secondary prevention of cardiovascular disease. *J Am Coll Cardiol*. 2013;61:404–410.
22. Nidorf SM, Fiolet ATL, Mosterd A, et al. Colchicine in patients with chronic coronary disease. *N Engl J Med*. 2020;383:1838–1847.
23. Nelson K, Fuster V, Ridker PM. Low-dose colchicine for secondary prevention of coronary artery disease: JACC review topic of the week. *J Am Coll Cardiol*. 2023;82:648–660.
24. Samuel M, Tardif JC, Bouabdallaoui N, et al. Colchicine for secondary prevention of cardiovascular disease: a systematic review and meta-analysis of randomized controlled trials. *Can J Cardiol*. 2021;37:776–785.
25. Fiolet ATL, Opstal TSJ, Mosterd A, et al. Efficacy and safety of low-dose colchicine in patients with coronary disease: a systematic review and meta-analysis of randomized trials. *Eur Heart J*. 2021;42:2765–2775.
26. Xia M, Yang X, Qian C. Meta-analysis evaluating the utility of colchicine in secondary prevention of coronary artery disease. *Am J Cardiol*. 2021;140:33–38.
27. Stewart S, Yang KCK, Atkins K, Dalbeth N, Robinson PC. Adverse events during oral colchicine use: a systematic review and meta-analysis of randomised controlled trials. *Arthritis Res Ther*. 2020;22:28.
28. Tardif JC, Samuel M. Inflammation contributes to cardiovascular risk in patients receiving statin therapy. *Lancet*. 2023;401:1245–1247.
29. Deftereos S, Giannopoulos G, Raisakis K, et al. Colchicine treatment for the prevention of bare-metal stent restenosis in diabetic patients. *J Am Coll Cardiol*. 2013;61:1679–1685.
30. Deftereos S, Giannopoulos G, Angelidis C, et al. Anti-inflammatory treatment with colchicine in acute myocardial infarction: a pilot study. *Circulation*. 2015;132:1395–1403.
31. Ridker PM, Everett BM, Thuren T, et al. Antiinflammatory therapy with canakinumab for atherosclerotic disease. *N Engl J Med*. 2017;377:1119–1131.
32. Roubille F, Tardif JC. Colchicine for secondary cardiovascular prevention in coronary disease. *Circulation*. 2020;142:1901–1904.
33. Virani SS, Newby LK, Arnold SV, et al. 2023 AHA/ACC/ACCP/ASPC/NLA/PCNA guideline for the management of patients with chronic coronary disease. *J Am Coll Cardiol*. 2023;82:833–955.
34. Byrne RA, Rossello X, Coughlan JJ, et al. 2023 ESC guidelines for the management of acute coronary syndromes. *Eur Heart J*. 2023;44(38):3720–3826. Erratum in: *Eur Heart J*. 2024;45(13):1145.
35. Robinson PC, Terkeltaub R, Pillinger MH, et al. Consensus statement regarding the efficacy and safety of long-term low-dose colchicine in gout and cardiovascular disease. *Am J Med*. 2022;135:32–38.
36. Indraratna PL, Virk S, Gurram D, Day RO. Use of colchicine in pregnancy: a systematic review and meta-analysis. *Rheumatology*. 2018;57:382–387.

28 Management of the Patient With ACS in the Absence of Obstructive Coronary Artery Disease (MINOCA, SCAD, Coronary Artery Spasm)

HARMONY R. REYNOLDS AND NATHANIEL R. SMILOWITZ

INTRODUCTION

The most common cause of acute coronary syndrome (ACS) is atherosclerotic coronary artery disease with thrombosis present in 85%–95% of cases. This chapter will address the remaining causes, namely, spontaneous coronary artery dissection (SCAD), myocardial infarction with nonobstructive coronary arteries (MINOCA), and coronary artery spasm (Fig. 28.1). Female patients are more likely than males to have one of these diagnoses when presenting with a clinical syndrome suggesting myocardial infarction (MI).

Before delving into each of these entities, it should be noted that MINOCA is a working diagnosis that encompasses several different underlying causes. The term "suspected MINOCA" or a provisional diagnosis of MINOCA is often used until an underlying cause is identified, because diagnostic testing directed at finding the underlying cause may reveal a MINOCA mimic, that is, an alternate, nonischemic cause such as myocarditis or cardiomyopathy (Fig. 28.2). Once an alternate cause is found, MINOCA is no longer the diagnosis.

Coronary artery spasm is an underlying cause of MINOCA, but it may also cause ischemia at rest without evidence of myocardial injury, that is, unstable angina. The term "nonobstructive coronary arteries" in cases of coronary spasm refers to the appearance of the arteries after administration of nitroglycerin; that is, it refers to the fixed component of obstruction, not dynamic obstruction due to spasm.

SCAD typically causes angiographically evident obstruction of the arterial lumen, though it may not be identified on initial review because of the long, smooth nature of these stenoses in many cases. SCAD occasionally causes mild-to-moderate narrowing of the lumen, with an appearance that can resemble normal tapering of the artery or a focal mild atherosclerotic plaque. When SCAD is not apparent by invasive coronary angiography, the diagnosis can be made using intracoronary imaging such as intravascular ultrasound (IVUS) or optical coherence tomography (OCT). Nonobstructive SCAD appears to be a rare cause of MINOCA, occurring in 1%–4% of cases.[1]

SPONTANEOUS CORONARY ARTERY DISSECTION

SCAD is a cause of ACS that is mechanistically distinct from atherothrombotic disease, affecting patients with different demographics than typical acute MI. Treatment differs from typical acute MI, both in terms of the approach to coronary revascularization and medical therapy. Though both SCAD and atherothrombotic disease led to acute MI and its sequelae, such as ventricular arrhythmia, heart failure, shock, and sudden cardiac death, the similarities end there. SCAD is a common cause of ACS in young women and may be even more common than recognized, given the barriers to making an accurate diagnosis. Thus, all cardiovascular medicine providers need to be familiar with the approach to the diagnosis of SCAD and the evidence for management.

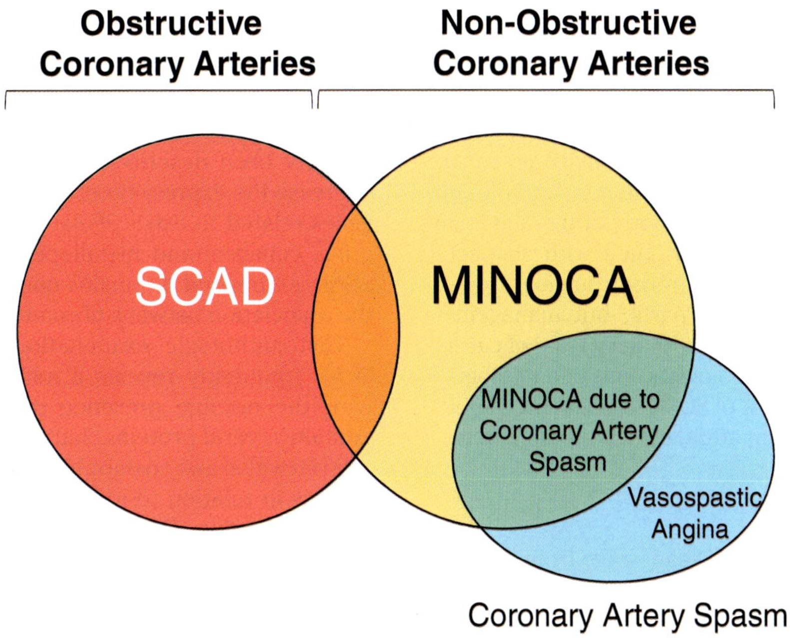

FIG. 28.1 **Relationship between MINOCA, SCAD, and coronary spasm.** The figure depicts the relationship between the diagnoses addressed in this chapter. SCAD is an angiographic diagnosis that causes luminal narrowing and rarely meets the criteria for MINOCA *(overlap in orange represents 1%–3% of MINOCA cases)*. Coronary artery spasm is a cause of MINOCA *(green)* but may also cause unstable angina *(blue)*. MINOCA is a working diagnosis with several underlying causes.

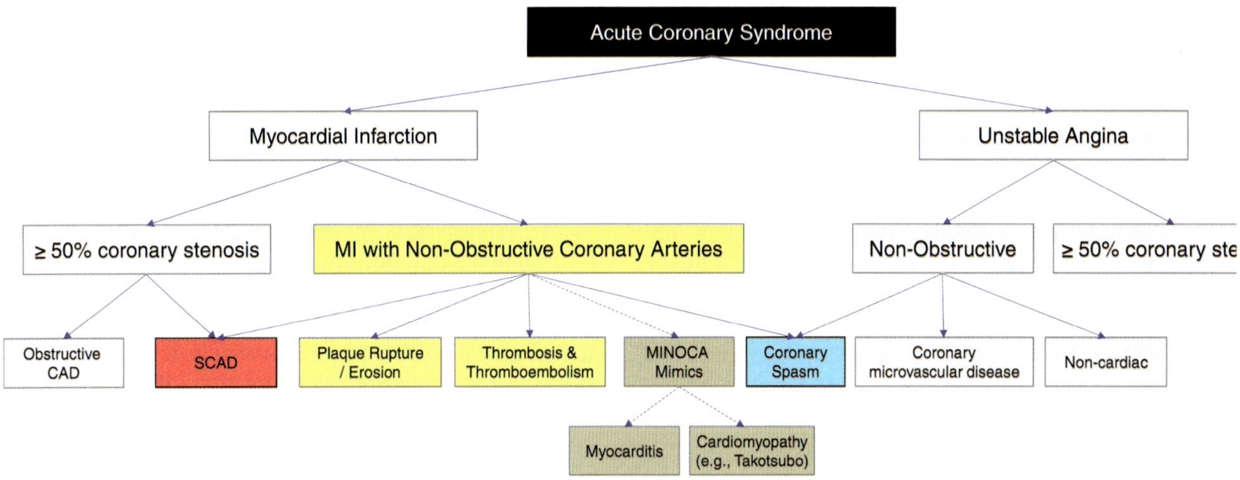

FIG. 28.2 **Diagnoses associated with obstructive and nonobstructive coronary arteries in acute coronary syndromes.** Acute coronary syndrome encompasses myocardial infarction (MI), in which there is biomarker evidence of myocardial necrosis, and unstable angina, in which there is not. MI can occur with angiographic stenosis of ≥50%, due either to atherosclerotic coronary artery disease (CAD) or spontaneous coronary artery dissection (SCAD). MI cases without 50% or greater stenosis on angiography are termed MI with nonobstructive coronary arteries *(MINOCA, yellow)*. There is a variety of underlying causes of MINOCA, including plaque disruption (rupture or erosion), thrombosis, thromboembolism, and coronary artery spasm. Some patients with a provisional diagnosis of MINOCA are found to have a mimic syndrome rather than MI during evaluation, such as myocarditis, takotsubo syndrome, or hypertrophic or nonischemic cardiomyopathy. Unstable angina is most frequently caused by atherosclerotic CAD, as is the case for MI. When a nonobstructive angiographic appearance is observed, the differential diagnosis includes coronary artery spasm, coronary microvascular disease, or a mimic syndrome of noncardiac chest pain. This chapter focuses on MINOCA, SCAD, and coronary artery spasm.

Epidemiology

The true prevalence of SCAD remains unknown because there is wide variability in physician knowledge about the disorder and its angiographic features. About 90% of affected patients are female, and the average age at presentation is 45–55 across studies.[2] Patients of both sexes can be affected at any age, however. Overall, approximately 1%–4% of MI cases are believed to be due to SCAD, but prevalence varies widely with patient demographics.[2] It is estimated that 25%–35% of women presenting with MI under the age of 50–60 have SCAD. Some cases (<5%–10%) occur in patients with inherited arteriopathies or inflammatory diseases including vasculitis. Precipitating physical or emotional stress is reported in at least half of patients. Physical stressors that can trigger SCAD include heavy lifting/isometric exercise, intense aerobic exercise, a strong Valsalva maneuver (e.g., vomiting), and hormone fluctuations associated with the pregnancy/postpartum state and use of exogenous hormones. SCAD is strongly associated with fibromuscular dysplasia in other vascular beds.[3] Occasionally, a patient with ACS may report a history of carotid dissection or FMD, and suspicion for SCAD should be very high. More commonly, FMD is identified in other vascular beds based on evaluation prompted by a new SCAD diagnosis.

SCAD is the most common cause of MI among pregnant or recently postpartum women (43% of such cases), particularly in the third trimester or the early postpartum period.[2,4] SCAD in pregnancy may be associated with more severe presentation, such as multivessel involvement or heart failure; affected patients require counseling about future risks in any additional pregnancies.[5] Pregnant women with suspected SCAD should undergo invasive coronary angiography as would their nonpregnant counterparts, but management decisions should involve a multidisciplinary team of cardiologists, obstetricians, anesthesiologists, and neonatologists. Once diagnosed, management of SCAD in pregnancy should be similar to the nonpregnant adult, as described herein.

Clinical Presentation

The clinical presentation of SCAD can range from acute MI to ventricular arrhythmias and sudden cardiac death. ST elevation is common, present in one-quarter to two-thirds of cases. Approximately 2%–5% of patients have cardiogenic shock, and up to 10% may have ventricular arrhythmia.

Mechanisms

The mechanism of SCAD is the formation of intramural hematoma at the border between the arterial media and adventitia, with subsequent intimal tears in some patients. An intimal tear may serve to decompress the false lumen, which may improve flow in the true arterial lumen (Fig. 28.3). This is different from iatrogenic coronary dissection, which originates after damage to the intima. It remains unclear whether SCAD may also originate from an intimal tear, but the consistent location of the intramural hematoma at the media-adventitia border and frequent observation of intramural hematoma in the absence of an intimal tear on pathology and on intracoronary imaging suggests otherwise. The mechanism ultimately seems to result from vascular fragility, which may be compounded by increased arterial shear stress. The association with fibromuscular dysplasia and triggering by physical and emotional stressors support this hypothesis. Genetic variants that predispose to SCAD have recently been described, including a variant expected to decrease the expression of tissue factors, and mutations in genes related to extracellular matrix function such as integrins, collagen, and metallopeptidases.[6] However, familial SCAD is rare, and it remains unclear what exactly underlies the association between fibromuscular dysplasia and SCAD.

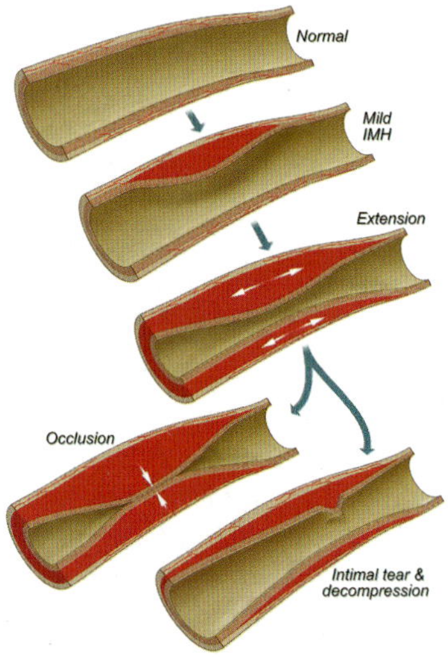

FIG. 28.3 Mechanisms of SCAD. SCAD begins with the development of an intramural hematoma (IMH), which progresses to severely narrow or occlude the vascular lumen. In some cases, there is intimal tear, which decompresses the IMH but leads to a double-lumen appearance. (From Hayes SN, Tweet MS, Adlam D, et al. Spontaneous coronary artery dissection: JACC state-of-the-art review. *J Am Coll Cardiol*. 2020;76(8):961–984. *https://doi.org/10.1016/j.jacc.2020.05.084*.)

Histopathologic examination of arteries affected by SCAD frequently reveals a mixed inflammatory infiltrate with the notable presence of eosinophils.[7] Eosinophils contain several proteins that have the potential to weaken arterial walls, and eosinophils are known to promote angiogenesis in relation to inflammation, which could relate to vascular fragility. Eosinophilic inflammation could be reactive in nature but is not observed in cases of iatrogenic dissection. The absence of an association with allergic reactions or disorders, or with eosinophilia, limits understanding of why eosinophils may be present in these arteries and how they may contribute to pathogenesis.

Making the Diagnosis

Careful review of coronary angiography is necessary to make the diagnosis of SCAD. There are three main angiographic patterns (Fig. 28.4). Type 1 SCAD, which accounts for 29% of cases, resembles iatrogenic coronary dissection, and is diagnosed based on the presence of a double lumen, a line between two lumens, often in a spiral pattern, or contrast staining within the arterial wall.[8,9] Type 2 SCAD is the most common pattern (60% of SCAD), diagnosed based on a long stenosis that does not (type 2a) or does (type 2b) reach the terminus of the vessel. Key to the identification of type 2 SCAD is the recognition of abrupt tapering of the artery, which may also affect branch vessels. It is helpful to survey the entire vasculature to ensure that all territories are perfused by adequately sized vessels; when an area appears to be served by only a small or short artery, particularly in a young patient or a woman, look carefully for SCAD. Administration of an adequate amount of intracoronary nitroglycerin is necessary to differentiate SCAD from coronary artery spasm. Type 3 SCAD is defined as a focal stenosis and may resemble atherosclerosis. Given that most focal stenoses are attributed to atherosclerosis, it seems likely that type 3 SCAD is particularly underdiagnosed, reported to account for 11% of cases of SCAD.[9] Thus intracoronary imaging to determine whether stenosis is due to intramural hematoma or plaque should be considered in patients who fit the demographic profile of SCAD and who have focal stenosis in one artery with otherwise normal vessels. This is important because percutaneous coronary intervention (PCI) is generally avoided in SCAD (see Role of revascularization in SCAD), due to increased risk combined with a high likelihood of spontaneous resolution. However, once SCAD is strongly suspected based on the angiographic appearance (e.g., type 2b angiographic profile), intracoronary wire placement and imaging should be avoided because of the risk of propagation of intramural hematoma. Again, SCAD is usually an angiographic diagnosis.

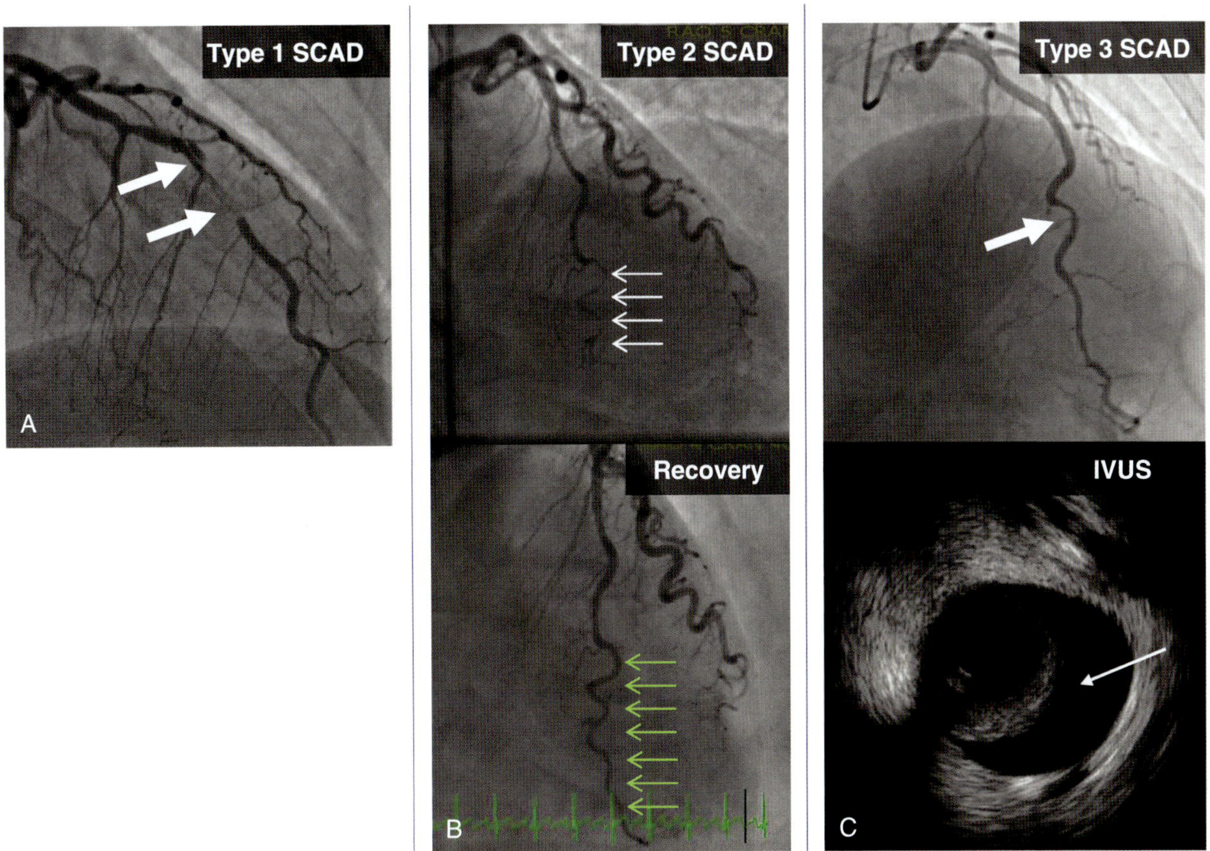

FIG. 28.4 Angiographic examples of SCAD subtypes. (A) Type 1 SCAD of the LAD is shown. Type 1 SCAD is characterized by a double lumen appearance (*proximal white arrow*), with a dissection flap leading to a subtotal occlusion of the vessel (*distal white arrow*). (B) Type 2b SCAD of the LAD coronary artery is shown. This is characterized by an abrupt change in the contour and caliber of the vessel (*white arrows*). There is also a narrowing of the vessel more proximally that may represent intramural hematoma as well. Repeat angiography performed to evaluate recurrent chest pain demonstrated a normal LAD appearance, with the vessel reaching the apex. (C) Type 3 SCAD of the LAD. Type 3. SCAD is characterized by a tubular area of narrowing (*white arrow*) that mimics atherosclerotic cardiovascular disease. The angiogram alone is not diagnostic, but intravascular ultrasound (IVUS) demonstrated an intramural hematoma compressing the true lumen, confirming the diagnosis of SCAD.

The most commonly affected coronary artery segment is the distal left anterior descending (LAD), followed by obtuse marginal branches, the mid-LAD, and the posterior descending artery. Multiple vessels are involved in 9%–23% of cases.[9] Tortuous coronary arteries are often observed in patients with SCAD and may be a clue to the diagnosis. Dissection may also occur at a site of myocardial bridging.

CT coronary angiography has more limited resolution than invasive coronary angiography, particularly in the more distal vessels which are often affected by SCAD, and cannot be considered a first-line imaging test at this time.[10] However, CT coronary angiography may be helpful in cases with more proximal stenosis to identify atherosclerosis at other sites when the diagnosis of SCAD remains unclear after angiographic review (e.g., type 3 appearance), and in follow-up to document healing.[10]

Role of Revascularization in Spontaneous Coronary Artery Dissection

The natural history of SCAD involves healing of the affected vessel in a few days to a few weeks. When repeat angiography has been performed, 95% of patients have improvement or resolution of the angiographic appearance.[2] Some have persistent dissection over years, however. The initial success rate of PCI is lower than in typical MI, only 54%, but the most important goal is reestablishment of normal or at least improved flow in the vessel, which can be achieved in 84%–90%.[11,12] The main complications of PCI include hematoma propagation, which can require placement of multiple stents; side branch occlusion; persistent distal dissection; and in rare cases, inadvertent stent placement in the false lumen with vessel closure. Even with conservative case selection, improved techniques, and a focus on flow restoration, emergency CABG may be needed in up to 8%–13% of SCAD patients undergoing PCI.[12]

Coronary artery bypass grafting may be associated with better initial success rates than PCI but graft failure is common, in approximately 30%, likely due to healing of the infarct artery with competitive flow.[13] Vein grafts may be considered preferentially when CABG is needed for patients with SCAD, with eventual healing of the infarct artery in mind, and because the traditional arterial bypass conduits may also be affected by fibromuscular dysplasia or vascular fragility.

Accordingly, American and European society statements and clinical practice guidelines suggest a conservative management strategy when possible, with PCI or CABG reserved for patients with ongoing ischemia,

TABLE 28.1 Key Differences Between Secondary Prevention Evidence and Recommendations for MI-CAD and MI Due to SCAD

MEDICAL THERAPY	MI DUE TO ATHEROSCLEROTIC CORONARY ARTERY DISEASE	MI DUE TO SCAD
Antiplatelet therapy	Yes, dual antiplatelet therapy preferred in the first 3–12 months, then single antiplatelet therapy indefinitely	Role is uncertain
Statin	Yes, lifelong	No – nonatherosclerotic mechanism (primary prevention statin OK)
Beta blockade	Yes, at least 2 years or indefinitely with reduced LVEF	Role is uncertain–pending clinical trials, consider strongly in patients with hypertension
Renin-angiotensin-aldosterone blockade	Yes	Yes, if EF is <40%; otherwise uncertain
Cardiac rehabilitation	Yes	Yes

hemodynamic instability, or perhaps left main dissection, recognizing that no clinical trials comparing revascularization to conservative management have been performed.[13,5] When PCI is necessary, long stents are recommended to avoid stent edges landing in an area with intramural hematoma (e.g., 5–10 mm extra in either direction). Additional techniques, such as a three-stent technique using short stents at the proximal and distal edges of the dissection before stenting the main body of the dissection, and the use of a cutting balloon for fenestration, may also be considered to minimize the potential for arterial injury and hematoma propagation.[14] Finally, approaches that minimize manipulation of the vessel may be desirable in some cases, such as direct stenting or balloon angioplasty without coronary stent placement, even with a suboptimal angiographic result.

Prognosis and Need for Prolonged In-Hospital Monitoring

The adverse prognosis of SCAD contrasts with the favorable risk profile of affected patients. The most common event for SCAD survivors is recurrent MI due to SCAD, which occurs in approximately 3%–7% of patients per year.[2,9] Recurrent SCAD nearly always affects a different arterial segment than the initial event. Therefore, recurrent stenosis in the same segment should prompt reconsideration of the diagnosis of coronary artery spasm as an alternative to SCAD. Additional major adverse cardiovascular events (MACE) occur at a rate of approximately 1% per year.[9] Survival is 94%–99% at 10 years.

In the reperfusion era, hospital stays for MI patients have become very short due to definitive treatment with coronary stenting and the availability of effective antithrombotic and antiatherosclerotic therapies. However, SCAD patients are often managed conservatively and healing may take weeks, leading to residual early in-hospital risk of hematoma propagation (2%) causing recurrent MI (4%), and of ventricular arrhythmias (4%) and hemodynamic instability (2%).[9] Urgent revascularization is performed in 4%–16% of cases.[9] Thus, a relatively longer initial in-hospital observation period may be appropriate for SCAD patients.

Postdischarge Treatment

The best secondary prevention medication regimen for patients with SCAD remains unknown and is the subject of ongoing clinical investigation. At present only limited observational data are available. Current approaches to the medical treatment of SCAD versus MI-CAD are shown in Table 28.1. Given that the mechanism of SCAD is bleeding rather than thrombosis, it is uncertain whether patients with SCAD who are not treated with PCI should receive any antiplatelet therapy, and if so, at what intensity or duration. True lumen thrombus is very rarely observed at autopsy or on intracoronary imaging.[7] In the past, dual antiplatelet therapy was often prescribed to conservatively managed patients, but this may change, based on recently published observational data indicating that dual antiplatelet therapy is associated with excess risk of MACE, and as clinical trials are conducted.[15] Statins are not typically needed in patients with SCAD unless there is a separate primary prevention indication.

Beta blockade is theoretically appealing as a method to reduce vascular shear stress and possibly reduce SCAD recurrence. Earlier reports from the Vancouver SCAD registry found that selection for treatment with beta blockade was associated with a marked reduction in the risk of SCAD recurrence, but the multicenter Canadian SCAD registry did not find a lower risk with beta blockade, perhaps related to changing practice patterns.[9] The young and otherwise healthy patients affected by SCAD frequently have low or normal blood pressure and may be bothered by side effects of beta blockade such as fatigue, depression, and weight gain. Thus, a clinical trial testing a strategy of beta blockade is needed. Until such trials are available, beta blockade should be strongly considered when there is hypertension in association with SCAD, and according to the clinician and patient preference otherwise. If the left ventricular ejection fraction (LVEF) is reduced, usual recommendations for neurohormonal blockade and SGLT2 inhibition apply.

Cardiac rehabilitation improves the quality of life in patients with SCAD.[16] Tailored exercise regimens in SCAD patients include avoidance of heavy lifting since Valsalva maneuvers have been reported to precipitate SCAD. A weight limit may be applied, or patients may simply be counseled to avoid lifting weights heavy enough to require them to strain to lift. In general, it seems wise to avoid activities that hold the potential to trigger SCAD (e.g., boot camp, endurance training, weightlifting).

Implantable cardioverter-defibrillator therapy for secondary prevention of sudden cardiac arrest in the setting of SCAD is warranted, and some authors recommend consideration of ICD placement even when cardiac arrest occurs in the first few hours of the event, in contrast to the guidance in MI-CAD patients.[17,18] This is considered because (1) the recurrence rate of SCAD is relatively high, (2) there is no known effective therapy, and (3) the patient may be presumed to have a predisposition to ventricular arrhythmia should SCAD recur based on this history. This is another area for future investigation.

Post-Spontaneous Coronary Artery Dissection Chest Pain

Post-MI chest pain is very common after SCAD, occurring in about half of patients and prompting an ER visit in 21%.[9] The mechanism is unclear. Chest pain concerning recurrent MI should be evaluated with repeat angiography with consideration of PCI as needed. CT coronary angiography may be considered if the original dissection was in a segment large enough to be visualized on CT. Often, extension or recurrent SCAD can be ruled out, but exertional and/or nonexertional pain persists. Emerging studies have shown a high prevalence of coronary microvascular dysfunction (CMD) in this setting, approximately 70%.[19] The finding that coronary flow reserve reduction and elevation of the index of microcirculatory resistance are similar in the infarct artery and noninfarct vessels suggests that CMD is not a direct result of the dissection event, but it is not clear what arteriopathy would predispose to both SCAD and CMD. Though this chest pain sometimes responds to nitrates or calcium channel blockers, one study of 10 patients found none had inducible coronary artery spasm.[20] At present, treatment of post-SCAD chest pain consists of therapeutic trials of various antianginal agents.

Summary – Spontaneous Coronary Artery Dissection

SCAD causes MI and sudden cardiac death in patients who are predominantly young and female. SCAD is due to intramural hematoma, not atherosclerosis or thrombosis. Inflammation including eosinophils is often present on histopathologic examination. The diagnosis is nearly always made angiographically based on either a long area of stenosis in a patient with otherwise normal arteries or, less commonly, a double-lumen appearance indicative of a dissection flap. Familiarity with angiographic patterns is of paramount importance in making the diagnosis. Occasionally, intracoronary imaging may be considered when SCAD is suspected but cannot be confirmed angiographically; routine intracoronary imaging is not recommended in patients with suspected SCAD on the grounds of safety. Association with extra-coronary fibromuscular dysplasia is common. Management is usually conservative, with revascularization reserved for patients with hemodynamic instability or ongoing ischemia. Healing of the affected artery occurs in nearly all patients in days to weeks. Repeat angiography is not necessary to document healing. When revascularization is needed, the technical approach should be tailored to the diagnosis and propensity for increased risk of complications. The role of antiplatelet therapy and beta blockade remains uncertain. Post-MI chest pain is common in SCAD patients and may be due to CMD in some patients.

MYOCARDIAL INFARCTION WITH NONOBSTRUCTIVE CORONARY ARTERIES

Overview of MINOCA

MINOCA is defined as myocardial infarction (MI) meeting the universal definition with less than 50% stenosis in all major epicardial vessels at angiography and without an apparent alternate cause of the clinical presentation (Box 28.1).[21] MINOCA occurs in 6%–8% of MI cases overall. The term is relatively new, coined in 2013. The development of uniform terminology has been a major advance in the field, giving patients and physicians a diagnosis and serving as a reminder that patients with MINOCA are considered to have MI. The latter point is important given that patients with MINOCA were inappropriately reassured in earlier years, often told they did not have a heart attack, when in fact there is an increased risk of cardiovascular events after a MINOCA event, and the pathophysiology is often similar to MI with obstructive CAD (MI-CAD). However, the term is inherently awkward, defining the diagnosis by what it is not rather than what it is. Moreover, the terms "obstructive" and "nonobstructive" have by convention centered on a stenosis threshold of 50%, when it is well known that (1) myonecrosis at rest occurs only with extremely low coronary blood flow, (2) lesions causing more than 50% stenosis may not limit flow based on physiologic testing such as fractional flow reserve, and (3) lesions causing less than 50% stenosis may not permit adequate increases in flow in response to stress. In general, MI occurs at rest, and the ability to augment coronary flow in response to stress may be irrelevant. In addition, the appearance of the coronary arteries at the time of testing may be different than it would have been if the arteries could have been imaged in the moments when myocardial

BOX 28.1 Definition of MINOCA[21]

The diagnosis of MINOCA is made in patients with acute myocardial infarction that fulfills the following criteria:

- Acute myocardial infarction (modified from the "Fourth Universal Definition of Myocardial Infarction" Criteria):
    - Detection of a rise or fall of cTn with at least 1 value above the 99th percentile upper reference limit AND
    - Corroborative clinical evidence of infarction evidenced by at least 1 of the following:
        - Symptoms of myocardial ischemia
        - New ischemic electrocardiographic changes
        - Development of pathological Q waves
        - Imaging evidence of new loss of viable myocardium or new regional wall motion abnormality in a pattern consistent with an ischemic cause
        - Identification of a coronary thrombus by angiography or autopsy
- Nonobstructive coronary arteries on angiography:
    - Defined as the absence of obstructive disease on angiography (i.e., no coronary artery stenosis ≥50%) in any major epicardial vessel
    - This includes patients with:
        - Normal coronary arteries (no angiographic stenosis)
        - Mild luminal irregularities (angiographic stenosis <30% stenoses)
        - Moderate coronary atherosclerotic lesions (stenoses >30% but <50%)
- No specific alternate diagnosis for the clinical presentation:
    - Alternate diagnoses include but are not limited to nonischemic causes such as sepsis, pulmonary embolism, and myocarditis

necrosis occurred in a MINOCA patient; for example, coronary artery spasm may cause transient coronary occlusion that is not evident by the time of angiography.

A key principle in the evaluation and management of a patient with suspected MINOCA is that the underlying cause of the presentation should be considered with additional imaging used to understand mechanisms, and patients should be treated according to the final diagnosis of the underlying cause. This is an extension of the differential diagnosis and management of other patients with elevated troponin as recommended in the Universal Definition of MI.[22] For example, when troponin is stably elevated, chronic myocardial injury from structural heart disease should be suspected. When there is a troponin rise and fall with symptoms, this may be due to acute myocardial injury without coronary ischemia, such as pulmonary embolism, acute heart failure, or clinically evident myocarditis. When a troponin rise and fall is due to acute ischemia, this may be due to unstable atherosclerotic plaque with thrombosis, but may instead be due to entities categorized as type 2 MI such as coronary artery spasm, SCAD, or supply-demand mismatch such as with sustained tachyarrhythmia, profound anemia, etc. Some patients with suspected MINOCA will not have any identifiable underlying cause, either because a full multimodality imaging evaluation is not performed or because test results are normal. These patients are still considered to have a diagnosis of MINOCA.

In the case of a patient meeting the criteria for MINOCA, the primary diagnostic task is to differentiate vascular causes from alternate, nonischemic causes of the presentation such as myocarditis, takotsubo syndrome or other nonischemic cardiomyopathy, or even pulmonary embolism. Once a nonischemic cause has been ruled out, the secondary diagnostic goal is to determine which vascular cause or causes underlies the presentation. Multimodality imaging is often needed to accomplish these goals.

Treatment is presently directed at the underlying cause when one is identified.[21,23] This is based on observational data and expert opinion, by extension from the treatment of related disorders such as MI-CAD and vasospastic angina. Clinical trials of treatment have yet to be completed. Challenges to the conduct of clinical trials in MINOCA patients include the low prevalence of MINOCA among MI patients, heterogeneity of underlying causes and an event rate that, while high enough to be concerning, would require a large sample size to achieve adequate power to detect a clinically important difference between treatment groups on clinical outcomes.[24] Several clinical trials are ongoing, using intermediate endpoints such as quality of life or biomarkers (Clinicaltrials.gov NCT05198791 and NCT05122780).

Epidemiology of Myocardial Infarction With Nonobstructive Coronary Arteries

MINOCA can be diagnosed in approximately 6%–8% of patients with spontaneous MI who are referred for coronary angiography, with approximately 65,000 MINOCA presentations in the United States each year.[25,26] The incidence of MINOCA is three times higher among females than males, affecting 10.5% of women and 3.4% of men with MI and without established CAD. Racial and ethnic variation has also been reported, with MINOCA more commonly reported in Black patients than those of White race or Hispanic ethnicity. Patients with MINOCA tend to be younger than those with MI due to obstructive atherosclerosis. Traditional cardiovascular risk factors, such as diabetes mellitus, dyslipidemia, or tobacco use, are less common in patients presenting with MINOCA than those with MI-CAD; however, nearly three quarters of patients with MINOCA have at least one cardiovascular risk factor. Most patients with MINOCA present with non-ST-segment elevation MI (NSTEMI), but when present, ST-segment elevations are associated with an increased risk of in-hospital mortality (as is ST depression).[27] Peak cardiac troponin concentrations tend to be lower than those in patients with MI-CAD, but large infarctions may occur in patients with MINOCA.

Prognosis of Myocardial Infarction With Nonobstructive Coronary Arteries

The short-term prognosis of patients with MINOCA is favorable compared to those with MI-CAD, but it is hardly reassuring.[1,26] Just as in patients with MI-CAD, MINOCA can cause cardiogenic shock, ventricular arrhythmias, mechanical complications of MI such as ventricular rupture, and some patients may not even survive to hospital evaluation; among prehospital cardiovascular deaths with histologic evidence of acute MI at autopsy, a substantial minority of decedents had nonobstructive coronary arteries. Among those who survive clinical evaluation, in-hospital mortality associated with MINOCA is approximately 1%, with a composite of in-hospital death, heart failure, cardiogenic shock, or reinfarction, in 5%.

Clinicians should follow patients with MINOCA closely after discharge. Overall, 1-year mortality after MINOCA is approximately 2%–5% and MACE occurs in nearly 10%.[28,29] A recent systematic review reported an annualized long-term mortality rate of 2.2% in patients with MINOCA.[26] At 4-year follow-up, MACE occurred in nearly 25% of individuals of all ages with MINOCA in the large SWEDEHART registry. Among older adults age ≥65, the risks of adverse outcomes are substantially higher, with nearly 12% mortality and 19% incidence of MACE reported at 1-year follow up.[29] The largest meta-analysis of outcomes, including approximately 30,000 patients with MINOCA, found a 1-year rate of death, recurrent MI, or heart failure of 9.6%.[26] Women with MI have a higher prevalence of MINOCA than men, but women and men with MINOCA have similar outcomes.[30]

Risk prediction to identify patients with MINOCA who are most likely to have late events remains challenging. Factors associated with MACE in patients with MINOCA tend to be similar to those in patients with MI-CAD, including older age, diabetes mellitus, ST-segment elevations on ECG, higher peak troponin, reduced LVEF, tobacco use, and history of stroke, peripheral artery disease, renal dysfunction, and chronic lung disease. Despite these similarities, the performance of standard clinical risk calculators, such as the Global Registry of Acute Coronary Events (GRACE) 2.0 risk score, is inferior among patients with MINOCA compared with MI-CAD and provides only modest accuracy for the prediction of death or MI at 1 year (c-statistic 0.685).[31] This may reflect the heterogeneous vascular mechanisms of MINOCA, which could theoretically each confer a different long-term prognosis. Improved risk stratification tools for patients discharged with MINOCA are needed.

Pathogenesis of Myocardial Infarction With Nonobstructive Coronary Arteries and Diagnostic Approaches

The potential mechanisms of MINOCA include vascular culprit lesions, collectively termed atherosclerotic plaque disruption (i.e., plaque rupture or plaque erosion), coronary thromboembolism, coronary artery spasm, and rarely, SCAD (Fig. 28.5). Patients with a provisional diagnosis of MINOCA may instead prove to have underlying acute myocarditis, takotsubo syndrome, or nonischemic cardiomyopathy, with the diagnosis only apparent after further testing. Once one of these alternate diagnoses has been established, patients are no longer considered to have MINOCA. Diagnostic testing in MINOCA typically includes electrocardiography, echocardiography, invasive coronary angiography, and cardiac magnetic resonance imaging (CMR); intracoronary imaging can provide important insights into atherosclerotic pathologies and SCAD, while coronary reactivity testing can identify coronary spasm.

Atherosclerotic Plaque Rupture and Erosion

Based on intracoronary imaging studies, a coronary culprit lesion is responsible for approximately half of MINOCA events.[1,32–35] Plaque rupture, a disruption of the thin intimal cap overlying a plaque, leads to extrusion of thrombogenic contents of the lipid-rich necrotic core into the bloodstream, promoting local thrombus formation. When thrombus forms on denuded endothelium overlying a fibrous plaque, rather than lipidic plaque, the process is termed plaque erosion. Each of these thrombotic processes can lead to transient coronary occlusion, distal embolization, or both, and cause biochemical and pathologic evidence of MI. However, at the time of invasive coronary angiography, thrombus may no longer be apparent due to a small residual volume of thrombus at the rupture site, either because of intrinsic thrombolytic activity, or due to embolization or migration of thrombus into small branch vessels that are not angiographically apparent. In cases of plaque rupture, depending on the duration of time between the initial event and cardiac catheterization, intracoronary imaging may reveal culprit plaques across the stages of healing, including intraplaque hemorrhage, and layered plaques.[36] Intraplaque hemorrhage and layered plaque are also observed at autopsy in cases of MI causing sudden cardiac death and are associated with increased risk of MACE when detected in other settings.[36–38]

Intracoronary imaging reveals substantial differences in plaque morphology between MINOCA and MI-CAD.[36] In general, culprit lesions in patients with MINOCA occur in smaller plaques and exhibit more subtle atherosclerotic pathologies than matched with MI in the setting of obstructive atherosclerosis. Atherosclerotic culprit lesions in MINOCA are less likely to have thin-cap fibroatheroma with plaque rupture or plaque erosion and are more likely to be characterized by intraplaque hemorrhage or layered plaque in various stages of healing. Furthermore, patients with MINOCA and plaque rupture tend to have smaller cavities and lower thrombus burden than patients with MI-CAD.[36] These findings often require careful review of intracoronary imaging to determine the culprit lesion that may guide subsequent treatment.

Intravascular imaging with OCT or IVUS permits identification of atherosclerotic and thrombotic mechanisms of MINOCA that are not evident by coronary angiography.

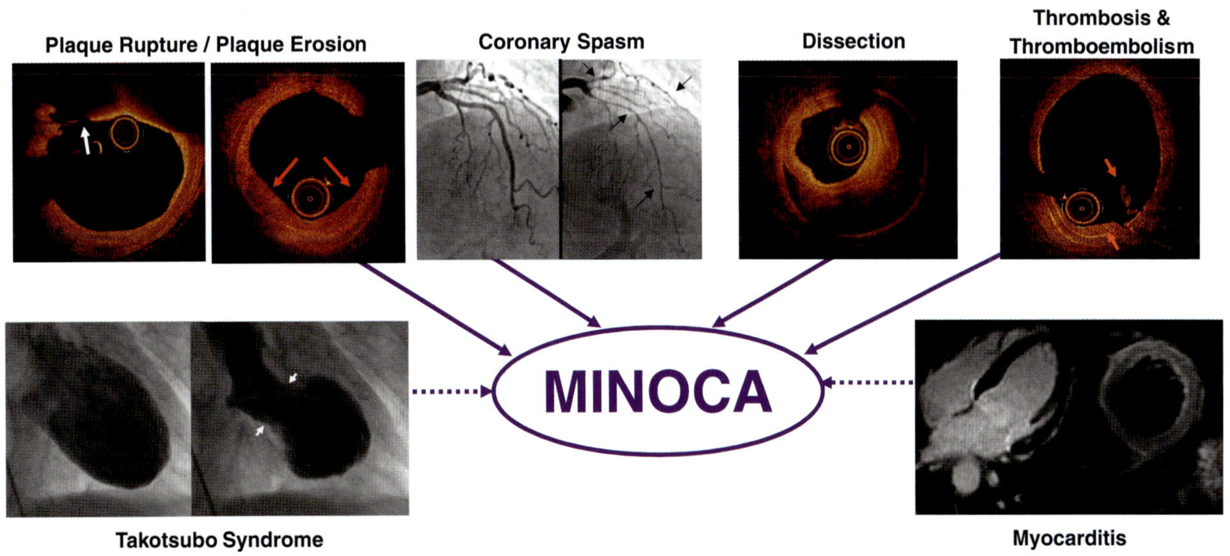

FIG. 28.5 Common mechanisms of MINOCA. Provisional diagnoses of MINOCA may be caused by atherosclerotic plaque disruption (i.e., plaque rupture or plaque erosion), coronary thrombosis or thromboembolism, coronary artery spasm, and rarely, spontaneous coronary artery dissection. Patients with a provisional diagnosis of MINOCA may also have an alternate mimicking condition (*dotted lines*), including myocarditis, takotsubo syndrome, or nonischemic cardiomyopathy. *(From Reynolds HR, Smilowitz NR. Myocardial infarction with nonobstructive coronary arteries. Annu Rev Med. 2023;74:171–188. https://doi.org/10.1146/annurev-med-042921-111727.* [This figure is licensed under a Creative Commons Attribution 4.0 International License, which permits unrestricted use, distribution, and reproduction in any medium, provided the original author and source are credited. No permissions are needed.]*)*

IVUS, which utilizes ultrasound to generate intravascular images, is widely available but has suboptimal resolution for identification of plaque disruption, particularly plaque erosion. OCT, which relies on light to generate images of the vessel lumen, requires clearance of the blood pool with contrast but generates imaging with far higher resolution than IVUS. In a prospective, multicenter study using multivessel OCT imaging performed at the time of index angiography for MINOCA, a vascular culprit lesion was identified in 46% of cases.[32] Unfortunately, the angiogram is inadequate to determine which coronary vessel(s) to image, and 30% of OCT-detected culprit lesions were identified in patients with normal coronary angiograms. This happens because plaques harboring culprit lesions in MINOCA are often small. Furthermore, the culprit vessel cannot be reliably identified from electrocardiography or echocardiography, likely because of variation in coronary anatomy (e.g., the left anterior descending artery may serve at least part of the inferior wall). In fact, electrocardiographic ST-depressions and T wave inversions were associated with the correct culprit coronary vessel in only 60% and 84% of cases of MI-CAD, respectively. In a study of 114 NSTEMI patients who underwent invasive coronary angiography and blinded CMR imaging, the infarct-related artery could not be identified in 37% of cases by angiography alone. Among those patients in whom an infarct-related artery could be identified, the infarct vessel as determined by CMR was discordant in 14% of cases.[39] Yet another 13% of patients diagnosed as NSTEMI had a CMR evidence of a non-MI pathology, such as myocarditis. Hence, given difficulties determining culprit vessels in MINOCA (and NSTEMI in general), intracoronary imaging of multiple vessels is necessary to ensure maximal diagnostic yield to identify the relevant atherosclerotic culprit lesion or lesions.

CT coronary angiography is highly sensitive for the detection of atherosclerosis but does not have the resolution needed to identify luminal thrombus or plaque rupture. Thus, while normal CT coronary angiography rules out an atherosclerotic culprit lesion, the presence of atherosclerosis does not inform whether there was a coronary culprit lesion responsible for MINOCA.

Coronary Thrombus or Embolism

Thromboembolism in the absence of plaque rupture or erosion is a cause of MINOCA, present in a minority of cases in intracoronary imaging studies.[1,32–35] Coronary emboli can originate from the left atrial appendage or left atrium in the setting of atrial fibrillation or other supraventricular arrhythmias, in the LV in the setting of dysfunction or noncompaction, or there may be paradoxical embolization of venous thrombosis through a patent foramen ovale or atrial septal defect. Thrombi are sometimes observed on intracoronary imaging without any evidence of a source. This may occur in patients receiving hormone therapy for contraception or treatment of uterine bleeding, or in cases of inherited thrombophilia. Some emboli may lead to a large vessel occlusion and a diagnosis of MI-CAD. Less well recognized is that distal embolization may occur into small branch vessels that cannot be recognized angiographically, either due to flush occlusion of a larger branch or vessel size that is below the resolution of angiography. If thromboembolism is detected by intravascular imaging without an apparent source, the patient has MINOCA due to thrombus.

Coronary Artery Spasm and Provocation Testing

Coronary artery spasm is a well-recognized cause of MINOCA that should be particularly suspected when there is prior history of episodic chest pain at rest, especially chest pain at night or in the early morning.[40] It must be recognized that most patients with MINOCA who prove to have coronary spasms based on provocative testing do not have ST-segment elevation on the electrocardiogram, even during ischemic symptoms. The true prevalence of coronary spasm is uncertain because provocative testing is not employed routinely. Prior series have reported spasms in 25%–70% of patients with MINOCA, with variability based on the patient population studied, coronary anatomy, the method of testing, and definitions of coronary spasm.[34,40–43] Establishing a diagnosis of coronary spasm is important because it impacts prognosis and treatment selection. In a series of 80 patients with MINOCA undergoing coronary provocation testing, spasm was associated with a higher risk of long-term mortality than patients without this diagnosis, and epicardial spasm was associated with poorer outcomes than microvascular spasm.[41] In a series of 437 patients with STEMI and successful reperfusion therapy who underwent provocation testing approximately 10 to 15 days after MI onset with evidence of coronary spasm, the use of a calcium channel blocker was associated with a significant reduction in the risk of death or MI or unstable angina (HR: 0.21, 95% CI, 0.08–0.55) in the years that followed the MI.

Coronary spasm is typically diagnosed based on acetylcholine coronary provocation testing, recognizing that spasm provoked in the laboratory may not reflect the status of the vessels at the time of MI. When specific testing has not been performed, a presumptive diagnosis of coronary artery spasm can be made when there is evidence of infarction or myocardial edema in a coronary territory on CMR in a patient without a coronary culprit lesion. The absence of a culprit lesion can be documented based on normal CT coronary angiogram or three-vessel intracoronary imaging. Invasive coronary angiography is not adequate to rule out a coronary culprit lesion in the case of MINOCA. Thus, coronary spasm often remains in the differential diagnosis of MINOCA after multimodality imaging.

An example of abnormal acetylcholine provocation testing in a patient with a history of MINOCA is shown in Fig. 28.6. When administered directly into the coronary arteries, acetylcholine acts to cause endothelium-dependent, nitric oxide-mediated vasodilation, along with vascular smooth muscle-mediated vasoconstriction. A normal response to acetylcholine is vasodilation or mild vasoconstriction. In patients with a propensity for epicardial coronary spasm, the vasoconstrictive response to acetylcholine predominates, and lumen narrowing of ≥90% that severely limits coronary blood flow can be observed by coronary angiography. Microvascular coronary spasm is a disorder characterized by ischemic symptoms and electrocardiographic changes without evidence of epicardial

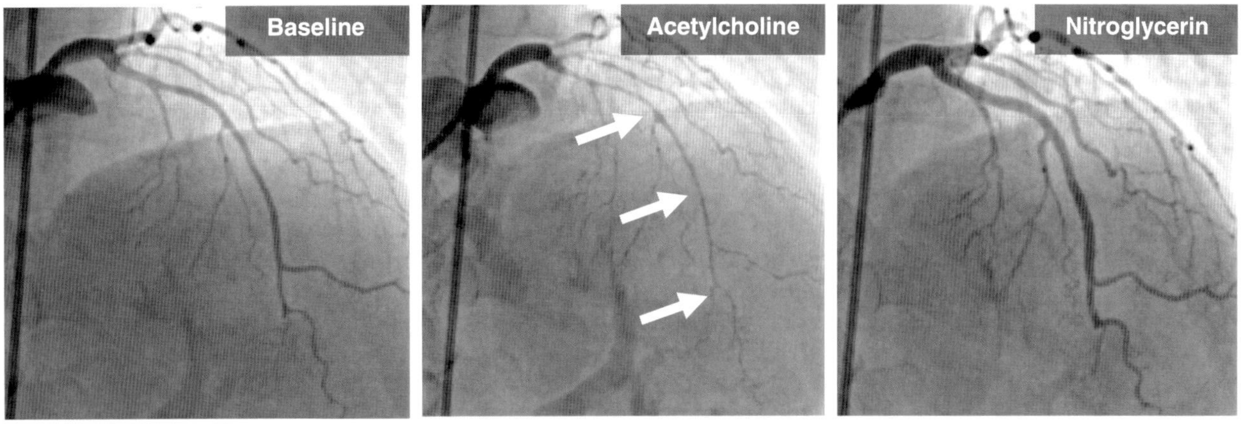

FIG. 28.6 Acetylcholine coronary reactivity testing for spasm. At baseline, mild narrowing of the LAD is seen. After intracoronary injection of acetylcholine, there is a severe diffuse coronary spasm of the LAD, associated with chest pain and ECG changes. The spasm is fully reversed by intracoronary nitroglycerin.

coronary spasm. Intracoronary acetylcholine provocation testing is performed with sequential intracoronary boluses of escalating doses of acetylcholine until coronary spasm is observed. When it occurs, epicardial coronary spasm may be focal or diffuse. Spasm is frequently observed within intramyocardial segments of patients with angiographic evidence of myocardial bridging. In fact, in a small series of 34 patients with MINOCA with angiographically apparent myocardial bridges who underwent acetylcholine provocation testing, coronary spasm occurred in the vast majority (88%) of cases.[44]

Coronary provocation testing has not been routinely integrated into the contemporary workflow of the management of MINOCA due to issues with drug availability in the cardiac catheterization laboratory. Concerns about safety of testing are unfounded; none of the studies investigating spasm testing in MINOCA patients reported any cardiovascular event related to testing, and a recent meta-analysis of 16 studies reporting outcomes of intracoronary acetylcholine in 12,585 patients (772 with MI) demonstrated that major complications of death, MI, or ventricular arrhythmia occurred in only 0.5% of patients, with minor complications (notably paroxysmal AF or transient bradycardia) in 3.3%.[45,46]

Provocation testing for spasms should be considered when patients have a history of episodic, nitrate-responsive chest discomfort or recurrent episodes of MINOCA. Testing may be appropriate at the time of index angiography in selected patients with MINOCA, including those with recurrent MINOCA and those with relatively lower levels of cardiac troponin elevation, hemodynamically stable patients without ventricular arrhythmias, patients with preserved EF, and those with a right dominant coronary circulation. In other patients in whom the mechanism of MINOCA is uncertain but who are at elevated risk for possible complications at the time of MI presentation, coronary reactivity testing may be performed electively at a later date.

Coronary Microvascular Disease

Pathologies of the coronary microcirculation have been postulated as potential mediators of MINOCA. This could be due to episodic increased resistance of the microcirculation, that is of microvascular spasm, or as failure to vasodilate microvascular arterioles in the setting of increases in myocardial oxygen demand. In a small study, coronary flow velocity ratios with endothelial-independent vasodilators were more abnormal in patients with MINOCA during hospitalization and one month later than age and sex-matched controls with noncardiac chest pain.[47] Unfortunately, it is difficult to assign causality of CMD in MINOCA. Post-MI abnormalities of microvascular function might simply be a result of myocardial edema, with the inciting ischemic event caused by another vascular mechanism (i.e., epicardial spasm or atherosclerotic plaque rupture). In patients with MI-CAD and STEMI, for example, the index of microcirculatory resistance (IMR) is commonly abnormal post MI.[48] Though CMD is undoubtedly a key prognostic indicator for survival after MI, the abnormal IMR is not attributed as an inciting cause of STEMI. Still, additional research into CMD in MINOCA is warranted to determine contributions to MINOCA pathophysiology and subsequent outcomes.

The Central Role of Cardiac MRI in Evaluation: Exclusion of MINOCA Mimics

Mimics of MI may be indistinguishable from MINOCA in terms of presentation with chest discomfort and elevations in troponin concentrations, and may be misclassified as MINOCA without additional imaging. Myocarditis, takotsubo syndrome, hypertrophic or nonischemic cardiomyopathy, and pulmonary embolism are some of the most common MINOCA mimics. MINOCA mimics appear to be particularly likely in cases of ST-elevation MINOCA, based on a consecutive series of all STEMI activations in the US Midwest region.[49] There should be a high index of suspicion for these diagnoses at the time of initial evaluation, and it is essential that testing is done to exclude these alternative diagnoses. CMR plays a key role in identifying patients with nonischemic mimics of MINOCA.[5] Earlier CMR in relation to the onset of ischemic symptoms results in a higher likelihood of identifying an abnormality, such as within 7–14 days, but later imaging, even after 30 days, is also frequently diagnostic.[50]

Myocarditis, which is characterized by an abnormal troponin and may be accompanied by chest discomfort, is present in up to 33% of patients assigned a provisional diagnosis of MINOCA.[32,50–52] Patients with angiographically normal coronary arteries were more likely to have myocarditis than those with mild, nonobstructive CAD, and younger patients and men had a higher prevalence than women and older adults. Takotsubo syndrome is characterized by reversible LV systolic dysfunction that tends to occur in postmenopausal women and is often preceded by an intense physical or emotional stressor. Patients typically present with chest pain, abnormal troponin concentrations, and ischemic ECG changes, but LV wall motion abnormalities in takotsubo syndrome are typically out of proportion to the peak troponin concentrations. Pulmonary embolism (PE), a potentially life-threatening alternate diagnosis that can cause ischemic symptoms and elevated troponin concentrations, must also be considered in all patients with a provisional diagnosis of MINOCA. In patients in whom pulmonary embolism might be clinically suspected, D-dimer measurement with or without CT pulmonary angiography should be assessed. However, in a series of 100 patients with MINOCA who underwent routine CT pulmonary angiography, none had PE. Once a diagnosis of myocarditis, takotsubo syndrome, or PE is established to explain the clinical presentation, this diagnosis supersedes any prior provisional MINOCA designation.

Suggested Approach to Testing to Identify an Underlying Cause of MINOCA

A stepwise approach to the diagnostic evaluation of patients with MINOCA is shown in Fig. 28.7. The evaluation begins with patients who meet the Universal Definition of MI and have no 50% or greater stenosis on coronary angiography; a brief reconsideration of alternate causes of the presentation should be entertained. It is not necessary to exclude all other potential diagnoses in order to make the diagnosis of MINOCA, however. The physician should keep in mind that the presence of a concurrent illness that has the potential to lead to elevated troponin does not rule out the diagnosis of MINOCA. For example, sepsis can lead to troponin elevation without MI, but it is also the case that patients with infection, or even sepsis, may have a concurrent MI event, which could be MINOCA. This is true whether or not there is severe CAD. When considering whether the clinical syndrome is most compatible with MI or acute myocardial injury,[22] providers should take into account the severity of the concurrent illness, the degree of troponin elevation, associated ECG changes, and any LV wall motion abnormalities.

The approach to diagnosis should proceed with a review of the electrocardiogram to identify any ST-segment elevations that might provide insights into the regional extent of myocardial injury. Echocardiography should be reviewed for new wall motion abnormalities that may indicate the areas of recent myocardial damage. Coronary angiography should be carefully studied for evidence of SCAD, thrombus, flush occlusions of side branches, distal embolization, or any other angiographic coronary abnormalities that might provide insight into the mechanism of MI.

After the coronary angiogram itself, CMR is the next most important test. CMR is critical to exclude potential mimics, such as myocarditis (Fig. 28.8). The presence of infarction or an area of regional edema on CMR indicates there was a vascular cause of the suspected MINOCA presentation and confirms that MI is the diagnosis. It must be recognized that areas of infarction on CMR may be quite small, as may be seen with embolic events. These small areas of late gadolinium enhancement are sometimes missed, so a comparison of late gadolinium enhancement sequences with cine CMR imaging sequences is particularly useful. Attention should also be paid to areas of myocardial edema within the coronary territory that are not associated with late gadolinium enhancement. These are thought to represent early myocardial injury in relation to a transiently occlusive or nonocclusive vascular event.

Meets Universal MI Definition with no Obstructive CAD?	o Rise and fall of cTn >99th percentile + ischemic signs / symptoms or new regional wall motion abnormality or perfusion defect
Is there an alternate cause of the presentation rather than MI?	o Sepsis o Pulmonary Embolism o Cardiac Contusion o Non-ischemic myocardial injury
Could something have been missed at angiography?	o Review angiography carefully for: o Obstructive CAD (≥50% lesion on angiography) o Occult thrombosis o SCAD (dissection)
Is it really MINOCA?	o Cardiac MRI to evaluate for MINOCA mimics: o Myocarditis o Takotsubo syndrome o Other cardiomyopathies (e.g., hypertrophic, dilated)
Why did this MINOCA happen?	o Cardiac MRI (patterns of LGE, regional edema) o Coronary vascular imaging (OCT, IVUS to search for culprit lesion) o Coronary functional assessment (test for spasm, microvascular disease)

FIG. 28.7 A stepwise approach to the diagnostic evaluation of patients with MINOCA.

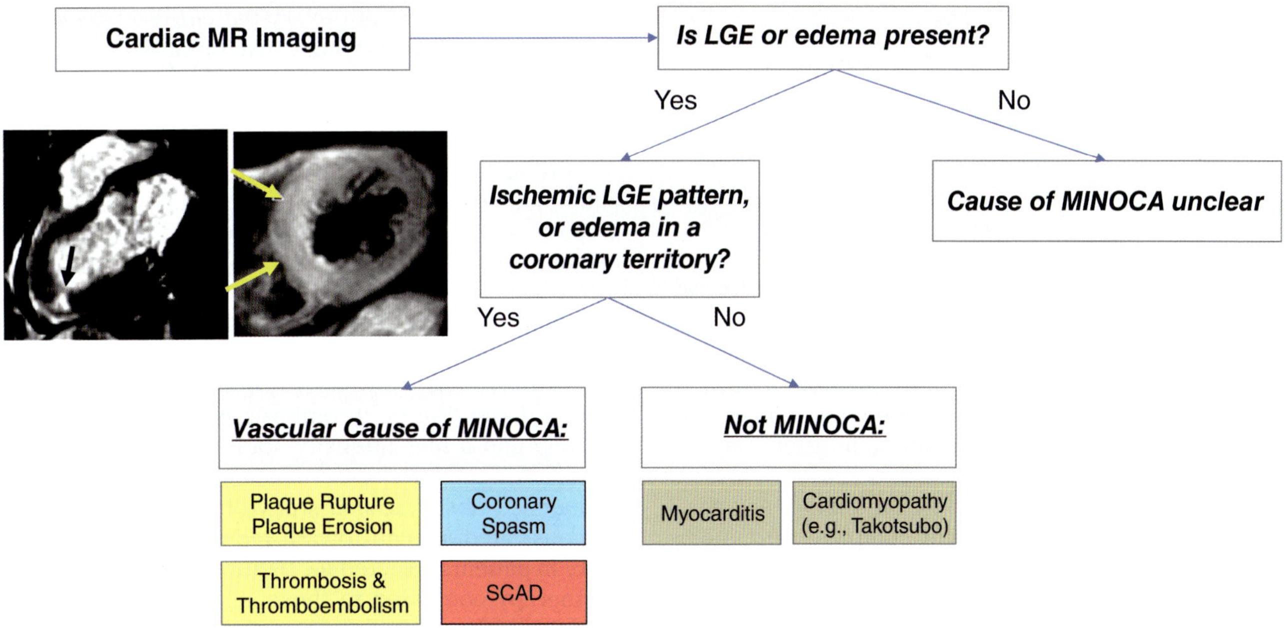

FIG. 28.8 Interpretation of CMR imaging to determine the mechanism of MINOCA. Sample CMR images show a small, transmural area of late gadolinium enhancement indicating infarction (*black arrow, left CMR panel*) and a different case in which there was no late gadolinium enhancement, but there was myocardial edema affecting the septum and anterior wall (*yellow arrows*), as noted based on increased T2 signal hyperintensity and thickening of the affected segments. When one of these ischemic findings, or a large area of infarction, is present, this shows the cause of MINOCA was vascular but does not indicate which vascular abnormality was the cause. When there is nonischemic LGE or characteristic wall motion abnormalities, myocarditis, takotsubo syndrome, or nonischemic cardiomyopathy will be diagnosed. When the CMR is normal, the cause of MINOCA is unclear.

However, the presence of LGE or myocardial edema in a coronary territory does not clarify which type of vascular compromise occurred. The possibilities include atherosclerotic plaque disruption, coronary artery spasm, thrombosis, or some combination of these.

Once alternate diagnoses to MI have been ruled out, the diagnostic evaluation turns to identifying an underlying cause of MINOCA. This is necessary whether the CMR shows an ischemic injury or infarction, or is normal. Normal CMR in MINOCA patients may reflect the limited sensitivity of magnetic resonance imaging or may reflect an injury that affected a broad area of myocardium with only small islands of necrosis that are too small to be visualized using current techniques.

When intracoronary imaging is available, intracoronary findings can be aligned with the results of CMR and echocardiography to determine the culprit vessel and associated mechanisms of infarction. Intracoronary imaging is recommended by ESC guidelines for ACS in general when the culprit lesion is unclear, and the culprit lesion is by definition unclear in MINOCA. Intracoronary imaging is also recommended to be considered in cases of MINOCA by ESC and AHA.[5,53] However, MINOCA studies demonstrate that identification of the vessel with a culprit lesion (in the absence of previously performed CMR) is difficult, similar to NSTEMI in general. In most cases, at present, multivessel intravascular imaging is not done during the index coronary angiography, and therefore, comprehensive evaluation for occult atherosclerotic mechanisms of MINOCA will be incomplete. In such patients, the options are to treat presumptively as if there were a culprit lesion, with antiplatelet therapy and statin-based lipid-lowering therapy, or to refer the patient back to the catheterization laboratory for multivessel intracoronary imaging after CMR rules out myocarditis and other alternate diagnoses.

Provocative testing for coronary artery spasm may be done during the acute angiogram, particularly in cases of recurrent MINOCA where suspicion is high. If this was not already undertaken, it is our practice to consider provocative testing most strongly in patients with recurrent symptoms or with an infarction on CMR. Intracoronary imaging can also be performed during that test. If provocative testing is not performed, consideration should be given to empiric treatment with a calcium channel blocker if blood pressure permits.

Though it is tempting to assign a single vascular cause for simplicity, it is likely that many events are multifactorial. Plaque disruption typically does not occlude the vessel in MINOCA, because by definition plaque is too small to compromise the lumen. Thus, superimposed thrombosis and/or coronary artery spasm are required to result in a sufficient decrement in blood flow to cause myocardial necrosis. Coronary spasm may lead to infarction on its own, or in combination with plaque disruption and/or thrombosis. Thrombus may form on an intact or disrupted plaque, or form spontaneously. Thrombus has the potential to occlude the lumen and cause infarction at the original site of formation, though in this regard the paucity of thrombus noted in intracoronary imaging studies is of interest. This interplay of atherosclerosis, thrombosis, and coronary artery spasm is illustrated in Fig. 28.9.

It is well recognized that coronary artery spasm is more likely to occur in areas affected by atherosclerosis. Further, intracoronary imaging studies in patients with vasospastic angina, or MI or out-of-hospital cardiac arrest in association with positive provocative testing for coronary artery spasm have demonstrated plaque rupture or erosion in a substantial minority of cases at spasm sites, based on intracoronary OCT imaging. Further support for a multifactorial nature of vascular compromise in MINOCA

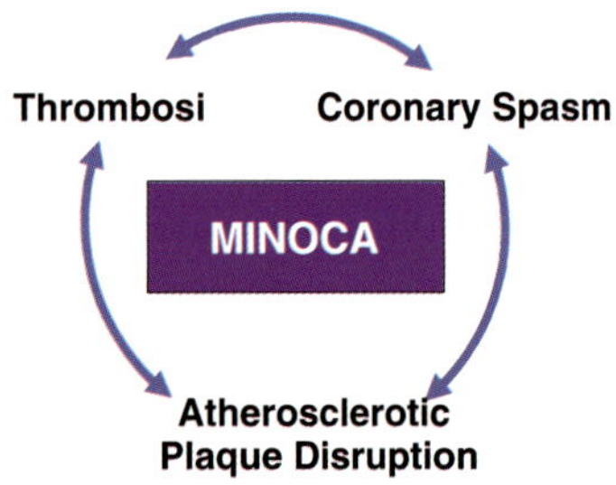

FIG. 28.9 Interplay between atherosclerotic plaque disruption, thrombosis, and coronary spasm in MINOCA.

patients is the fact that the territory of infarction or myocardial edema is often large on CMR when the angiographic appearance is nonobstructive. It can be inferred that the artery was temporarily severely narrowed with partial or complete relief of obstruction by the time of angiography. This can occur with transient complete thrombosis and subsequent thrombolysis, or with transient coronary artery spasm at the site of disrupted plaque. Alternatively, it remains possible that coronary artery spasm is an inciting event that leads to rupture, erosion, or thrombosis on a nonobstructive plaque. As with many aspects of MINOCA, the principle is generalizable to MI-CAD. For example, in MI-CAD, coronary artery spasm may occur at a site of plaque disruption and thrombosis, and the degree of vascular narrowing due to thrombus relative to plaque is variable from patient to patient.

Approach to the Management of Myocardial Infarction With Nonobstructive Coronary Arteries

The optimal long-term management of patients with MINOCA remains an area of great uncertainty. Ideally, treatment should be targeted to the underlying diagnosis (Fig. 28.10).[5,53] However, this approach has not been tested in clinical trials, and not every patient receives a specific diagnosis of the underlying cause of MINOCA. In comparison to MI-CAD, patients with MINOCA are less likely to receive medications for secondary prevention of MI at the time of discharge. Substantial heterogeneity in medication prescribing for patients with MINOCA indicates clinical equipoise regarding optimal care.[54] Clinical trials dedicated to secondary prevention after MINOCA are urgently needed.

When the Underlying Cause Is Known

Based on the evidence from trials of medical therapy for MI-CAD, patients with MINOCA due to atherosclerotic plaque disruption or thrombosis warrant antithrombotic therapy and a high-intensity statin. The intensity of antiplatelet therapy required is unclear. A large, propensity-matched observational study of patients with MINOCA demonstrated a trend toward reduction in all-cause mortality in patients selected for treatment with dual antiplatelet therapy compared to those selected for aspirin alone (HR: 0.75, 95% CI, 0.56–1.01) but no significant difference in major adverse cardiovascular events (HR: 0.90, 95% CI, 0.74–1.08). High-dose clopidogrel was associated with increased risk among MINOCA patients compared with regular dose in a posthoc analysis of the CURRENT-OASIS trial, but high-dose clopidogrel is rarely given in ACS in general.[55] At present, our practice is to give dual antiplatelet therapy for up to 12 months, followed by single antiplatelet therapy for life. The question has been raised of whether PCI with a stent or bioresorbable scaffold may reduce the risk of MACE in MINOCA patients; this is a potential area of clinical investigation.

Patients with MINOCA due to coronary spasms should receive a calcium channel blocker at hospital discharge for secondary prevention. Long-acting nitrates or a second calcium channel blocker are added for persistent symptoms. Antiplatelet therapy is recommended because it is not clear

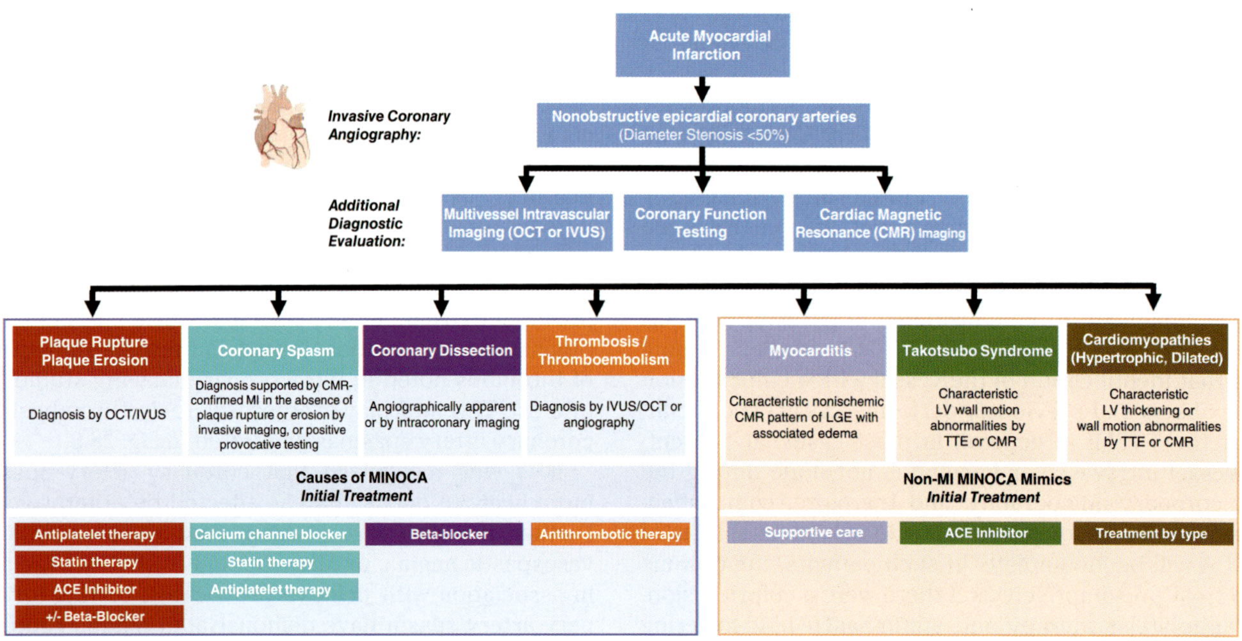

FIG. 28.10 Disease-specific approach to the management of patients with a provisional diagnosis of MINOCA. Treatment follows directly from the results of the diagnostic evaluation.

to what extent thrombosis may contribute to spasm-induced MI. Intracoronary thrombi have been observed on angioscopy in patients with vasospastic angina.[56]

Individuals with SCAD are typically treated with a beta blocker, though supportive evidence is limited to one observational study (see SCAD Treatment). Single or no antiplatelet therapy may be appropriate.

When the Underlying Cause Is Not Known

When the underlying cause of MINOCA is uncertain, European clinical practice guidelines for ACS recommend the same secondary prevention medications as for MI-CAD[23]; American guidelines stress the goal of finding an underlying cause and do not address this situation directly, though a scientific statement on MINOCA suggests treating for the most likely diagnoses, which are plaque disruption and spasm.[21,57]

Treatments That Are Not Specific to Underlying Cause of Myocardial Infarction With Nonobstructive Coronary Arteries

A single antiplatelet agent is given nearly universally to MINOCA patients, with consideration of dual antiplatelet therapy as above for patients with a confirmed or suspected coronary culprit lesion. Cardiac rehabilitation is recommended, as is done in general for MI patients.

Observational studies provide important insights into the optimal long-term treatment of patients with MINOCA. In a propensity-matched analysis of 9466 patients with MINOCA in the SWEDEHEART registry in which the underlying cause of MINOCA was not known, treatment with statins was associated with 23% (95% CI, 13%–32%) and 34% (95% CI, 23%–43%) lower rates of 4-year MACE and all-cause mortality, respectively. ACEi or angiotensin receptor blockers [ARB] were associated with an 18% (95% CI, 7%–23%) lower rate of 4-year MACE, and there was a trend toward a 13% lower all-cause mortality (95% CI, -2% to 24%). Selection for treatment with beta blockade was associated with a 19% lower all-cause mortality (95% CI, 1% to 34%) and a trend toward 14% lower MACE (95% CI, -1% to 26%). In the separate registry of 350 patients with MINOCA from the United Kingdom, ACEi at discharge was associated with 69% lower odds of death at 6 months, while no association was observed for beta blockers. A prospective multicenter registry from Korea also reported two-fold greater hazard of death at 2 years among patients who did not receive statins and ACEi/ARB at hospital discharge.[40] However, not all studies demonstrate a benefit of ACEi/ARB after MINOCA, and in a 621-patient Italian registry, beta blockers, but not ACEi, were associated with lower risk of long-term MACE.[58]

Although calcium channel blockers are reasonable at discharge for patients with a provisional diagnosis of MINOCA due to coronary spasm, observational studies have not yet demonstrated any reductions in future cardiovascular risk associated with these agents in MINOCA. Still, calcium channel blockers are often recommended empirically when the cause of MINOCA is not known, or when spasm testing has not been performed.

Ultimately, much of the current approach to care in patients with MINOCA relies on extrapolation of data from studies of patients with MI-CAD or common-sense approaches to targeted therapy based on the presumed underlying mechanism of infarction. Clinical trials are ongoing, and more are needed.

Myocardial Infarction With Nonobstructive Coronary Arteries Summary

MINOCA is common, associated with adverse outcomes, and may be caused by atherosclerotic plaque disruption, coronary thromboembolism, coronary artery spasm, occult SCAD, or a combination of mechanisms. Systematic, stepwise evaluation of patients with MINOCA with multimodality imaging can establish the etiology of MI or identify alternate diagnoses, such as myocarditis, takotsubo syndrome, or nonischemic cardiomyopathy. Once the mechanism of MINOCA has been determined, this can guide medical therapy for secondary prevention to reduce long-term cardiovascular risk.

UNSTABLE ANGINA

In selected patients presenting with ACS, normal concentrations of cardiac troponin will be measured at the time of the initial presentation, consistent with a diagnosis of unstable angina rather than MI. Coronary angiography in such cases may reveal the absence of obstructive CAD, posing a challenge to determine the cause of ischemic symptoms and the best medical therapy. In these cases, epicardial and microvascular coronary spasms, as previously described, should be considered in the differential diagnosis. CMD may also play a role in clinical symptoms. When appropriate clinical diagnostic testing is available, patients with unstable angina and no obstructive coronary arteries should undergo provocation testing for coronary spasm and assessment of the coronary microvasculature to determine the underlying etiology of symptoms and to guide subsequent medical therapy. CMD can be diagnosed invasively based on low CFR or high IMR. Noninvasive options for diagnosis include vasodilator stress positron emission tomography or quantitative single photon emission computed tomography; stress CMR is less well correlated with invasive measures but remains an option as well.[59,60]

Atherothrombotic etiologies of pain, such as plaque disruption, are far less likely to cause unstable angina in the absence of detectable myocardial injury and are generally not entertained in the differential diagnosis. The prevalence of unstable angina is likely to decrease over time as more hospitals transition from conventional to high-sensitivity cardiac troponin assays. High-sensitivity troponin assays are able to detect minute quantitates of myocardial injury, potentially reclassifying unstable angina with nonobstructive coronary arteries as MINOCA in many cases.

CONCLUSION

The management of the patient with ACS in the absence of obstructive atherosclerotic CAD requires consideration of a differential diagnosis including SCAD and MINOCA, keeping in mind that MINOCA in turn has its own differential diagnosis including atherosclerotic plaque disruption, thrombosis, and coronary artery spasm. It is of paramount importance to reinforce to the patient with MI not due to CAD that heart attack is the correct diagnosis because recurrent events and cardiovascular complications do occur. Additional imaging tests are usually needed to make the final diagnosis. Mimics of MI may ultimately be identified. Treatment is based on an extension of guidelines applicable to MI-CAD, with adaptation to the pathophysiology underlying the final diagnosis, when known. SCAD is caused by a unique pathophysiologic mechanism, with an intimal tear or subintimal hematoma leading to coronary narrowing, obstruction to myocardial blood flow, and MI. Thus most secondary prevention medications for MI-CAD are unnecessary or theoretically disadvantageous for SCAD patients. Clinical trials addressing the specifics of treatment and the utility of additional imaging tests are urgently needed.

CLASSIC REFERENCES

Collste O, Sorensson P, Frick M, et al. Myocardial infarction with normal coronary arteries is common and associated with normal findings on cardiovascular magnetic resonance imaging: results from the stockholm myocardial infarction with normal coronaries study. *J Intern Med*. 2013;273:189–196.

Deyama J, Nakamura T, Saito Y, et al. Effect of coronary artery spasm on long-term outcomes in survivors of acute myocardial infarction. *Int J Cardiol*. 2018;257:7–11. https://doi.org/10.1016/j.ijcard.2017.08.002.

Lindahl B, Baron T, Erlinge D, et al. Medical therapy for secondary prevention and long-term outcome in patients with myocardial infarction with nonobstructive coronary artery disease. *Circulation*. 2017;135:1481–1489.

Manfrini O, Morrell C, Das R, et al. Effects of angiotensin-converting enzyme inhibitors and beta blockers on clinical outcomes in patients with and without coronary artery obstructions at angiography (from a register-based cohort study on acute coronary syndromes). *Am J Cardiol*. 2014;113:1628–1633.

Shin ES, Ann SH, Singh GB, et al. OCT-defined morphological characteristics of coronary artery spasm sites in vasospastic angina. *JACC Cardiovasc Imaging*. 2015;8:1059–1067.

Smilowitz NR, Mahajan AM, Roe MT, et al. Mortality of myocardial infarction by sex, age, and obstructive coronary artery disease status in the ACTION registry-GWTG (Acute coronary treatment and intervention outcomes network registry-Get With the guidelines). *Circ Cardiovasc Qual Outcomes*. 2017;10:e003443.

Smilowitz NR, Sampson BA, Abrecht CR, et al. Women have less severe and extensive coronary atherosclerosis in fatal cases of ischemic heart disease: an autopsy study. Am Heart J. 2011;161:681–688.

REFERENCES

1. Zeng M, Zhao C, Bao X, et al. Clinical characteristics and prognosis of MINOCA caused by atherosclerotic and nonatherosclerotic mechanisms assessed by OCT. *JACC Cardiovasc Imaging*. 2023;16:521–532.
2. Hayes SN, Tweet MS, Adlam D, et al. Spontaneous coronary artery dissection: JACC state-of-the-art review. *J Am Coll Cardiol*. 2020;76:961–984.
3. Persu A, Lopez-Sublet M, Al-Hussaini A, et al. Prevalence and disease spectrum of extracoronary arterial abnormalities in spontaneous coronary artery dissection. *JAMA Cardiol*. 2022;7:159–166.
4. Chan N, Premawardhana D, Al-Hussaini A, et al. Pregnancy and spontaneous coronary artery dissection: lessons from survivors and nonsurvivors. *Circulation*. 2022;146:69–72.
5. Byrne RA, Rossello X, Coughlan JJ, et al. 2023 ESC guidelines for the management of acute coronary syndromes: developed by the task force on the management of acute coronary syndromes of the European Society of Cardiology (ESC). *Eur Heart J*. 2023;44(38):3720–3826.
6. Adlam D, Berrandou TE, Georges A, et al. Genome-wide association meta-analysis of spontaneous coronary artery dissection identifies risk variants and genes related to artery integrity and tissue-mediated coagulation. *Nat Genet*. 2023;55:964–972.
7. Jaspan VN, Rapkiewicz AV, Reynolds HR. The presence of thrombus in spontaneous coronary artery dissection: a systematic review of autopsy findings. *Am Heart J Plus*. 2022;15:100135.
8. Adlam D, Tweet MS, Gulati R, et al. Spontaneous coronary artery dissection: pitfalls of angiographic diagnosis and an approach to ambiguous cases. *JACC Cardiovasc Interv*. 2021;14:1743–1756.
9. Saw J, Starovoytov A, Aymong E, et al. Canadian spontaneous coronary artery dissection cohort study: 3-year outcomes. *J Am Coll Cardiol*. 2022;80:1585–1597.
10. Pergola V, Continisio S, Mantovani F, et al. Spontaneous coronary artery dissection: the emerging role of coronary computed tomography. *Eur Heart J Cardiovasc Imaging*. 2023;24:839–850.
11. Garcia-Guimaraes M, Fuertes-Ferre G, Jimenez-Valero S, et al. Characteristics, acute results, and prognostic impact of percutaneous coronary interventions in spontaneous coronary artery dissection (from the Prospective Spanish Registry on SCAD [SR-SCAD]). *Am J Cardiol*. 2022;171:177–178.
12. Lobo AS, Cantu SM, Sharkey SW, et al. Revascularization in patients with spontaneous coronary artery dissection and ST-segment elevation myocardial infarction. *J Am Coll Cardiol*. 2019;74:1290–1300.
13. Writing Committee M, Lawton JS, Tamis-Holland JE, et al. 2021 ACC/AHA/SCAI guideline for coronary artery revascularization: a report of the American College of Cardiology/American Heart Association joint committee on clinical practice guidelines. *J Am Coll Cardiol*. 2022;79:e21–e129.
14. Garcia-Guimaraes M, Bastante T, Antuna P, et al. Spontaneous coronary artery dissection: mechanisms, diagnosis and management. *Eur Cardiol*. 2020;15:1–8.
15. Cerrato E, Giacobbe F, Quadri G, et al. Antiplatelet therapy in patients with conservatively managed spontaneous coronary artery dissection from the multicentre DISCO registry. *Eur Heart J*. 2021;42:3161–3171.
16. Tweet MS, Olin JW, Bonikowske AR, et al. Physical activity and exercise in patients with spontaneous coronary artery dissection and fibromuscular dysplasia. *Eur Heart J*. 2021;42:3825–3828.
17. Scagliola R, Brunelli C, Balbi M. Implantable cardioverter defibrillator therapy for secondary prevention in spontaneous coronary artery dissection: to place or not to place? This is the matter. *Anatol J Cardiol*. 2020;23:240.
18. Garg J, Shah K, Shah S, et al. Implantable cardioverter-defibrillator in patients with spontaneous coronary artery dissection presenting with sudden cardiac arrest. *J Cardiovasc Electrophysiol*. 2021;32:2595–2600.
19. Sedlak T, Starovoytov A, Humphries K, Saw J. Coronary flow reserve in patients with prior spontaneous coronary artery dissection and recurrent angina. *J Am Heart Assoc*. 2020;9:e015834.
20. Waterbury TM, Tweet MS, Hayes SN, et al. Coronary endothelial function and spontaneous coronary artery dissection. *Eur Heart J Acute Cardiovasc Care*. 2020;9:90–95.
21. Tamis-Holland JE, Jneid H, Reynolds HR, et al. Contemporary diagnosis and management of patients with myocardial infarction in the absence of obstructive coronary artery disease: a scientific statement from the American Heart Association. *Circulation*. 2019;139:e891–e908.
22. Thygesen K, Alpert JS, Jaffe AS, et al. Fourth universal definition of myocardial infarction (2018). *Circulation*. 2018;138:e618–e651.
23. Collet JP, Thiele H, Barbato E, et al. 2020 ESC guidelines for the management of acute coronary syndromes in patients presenting without persistent ST-segment elevation. *Eur Heart J*. 2021;42:1289–1367.
24. Nordenskjold AM, Agewall S, Atar D, et al. Randomized evaluation of beta blocker and ACE-inhibitor/angiotensin receptor blocker treatment in patients with myocardial infarction with non-obstructive coronary arteries (MINOCA-BAT): rationale and design. *Am Heart J*. 2021;231:96–104.
25. Tsao CW, Aday AW, Almarzooq ZI, et al. Heart disease and stroke statistics-2023 update: a report from the American Heart Association. *Circulation*. 2023;147:e93–e621.
26. Pasupathy S, Lindahl B, Litwin P, et al. Survival in patients with suspected myocardial infarction with nonobstructive coronary arteries: a comprehensive systematic review and meta-analysis from the MINOCA global collaboration. *Circ Cardiovasc Qual Outcomes*. 2021;14:e007880.
27. Pelliccia F, Pasceri V, Niccoli G, et al. Predictors of mortality in myocardial infarction and nonobstructed coronary arteries: a systematic review and meta-regression. *Am J Med*. 2020;133:73–83.e4.
28. Williams MJA, Barr PR, Lee M, et al. Outcome after myocardial infarction without obstructive coronary artery disease. *Heart*. 2019;105:524–530.
29. Dreyer RP, Tavella R, Curtis JP, et al. Myocardial infarction with non-obstructive coronary arteries as compared with myocardial infarction and obstructive coronary disease: outcomes in a Medicare population. *Eur Heart J*. 2020;41:870–878.
30. Williams MGL, Dastidar A, Liang K, et al. Sex differences in patients with acute coronary syndromes and non-obstructive coronary arteries: Presentation and outcome. *Int J Cardiol*. 2023;372:15–22.
31. Eggers KM, Baron T, Hjort M, et al. GRACE 2.0 score for risk prediction in myocardial infarction with nonobstructive coronary arteries. *J Am Heart Assoc*. 2021;10:e021374.
32. Reynolds HR, Maehara A, Kwong RY, et al. Coronary optical coherence tomography and cardiac magnetic resonance imaging to determine underlying causes of myocardial infarction with nonobstructive coronary arteries in women. *Circulation*. 2021;143:624–640.
33. Taruya A, Tanaka A, Nishiguchi T, et al. Lesion characteristics and prognosis of acute coronary syndrome without angiographically significant coronary artery stenosis. *Eur Heart J Cardiovasc Imaging*. 2020;21:202–209.
34. Gerbaud E, Arabucki F, Nivet H, et al. OCT and CMR for the diagnosis of patients presenting with MINOCA and suspected epicardial causes. *JACC Cardiovasc Imaging*. 2020;13:2619–2631.
35. Opolski MP, Spiewak M, Marczak M, et al. Mechanisms of myocardial infarction in patients with nonobstructive coronary artery disease: results from the optical coherence tomography study. *JACC Cardiovasc Imaging*. 2019;12(11 Pt 1):2210–2221.
36. Usui E, Matsumura M, Smilowitz NR, et al. Coronary morphological features in women with non-ST-segment elevation MINOCA and MI-CAD as assessed by optical coherence tomography. *Eur Heart J Open*. 2022;2:oeac058.
37. Usui E, Matsumura M, Mintz GS, et al. Clinical outcomes of low-intensity area without attenuation and cholesterol crystals in non-culprit lesions assessed by optical coherence tomography. *Atherosclerosis*. 2021;332:41–47.
38. Holmstrom L, Juntunen S, Vahatalo J, et al. Plaque histology and myocardial disease in sudden coronary death: the Fingesture study. *Eur Heart J*. 2022;43:4923–4930.

39. Heitner JF, Senthilkumar A, Harrison JK, et al. Identifying the infarct-related artery in patients with non-ST-segment-elevation myocardial infarction. *Circ Cardiovasc Interv*. 2019;12:e007305.
40. Choo EH, Chang K, Lee KY, et al. Prognosis and predictors of mortality in patients suffering myocardial infarction with non-obstructive coronary arteries. *J Am Heart Assoc*. 2019;8:e011990.
41. Montone RA, Niccoli G, Fracassi F, et al. Patients with acute myocardial infarction and non-obstructive coronary arteries: safety and prognostic relevance of invasive coronary provocative tests. *Eur Heart J*. 2018;39:91–98.
42. Pirozzolo G, Seitz A, Athanasiadis A, et al. Microvascular spasm in non-ST-segment elevation myocardial infarction without culprit lesion (MINOCA). *Clin Res Cardiol*. 2020;109:246–254.
43. Camilli M, Russo M, Rinaldi R, et al. Air pollution and coronary vasomotor disorders in patients with myocardial ischemia and unobstructed coronary arteries. *J Am Coll Cardiol*. 2022;80:1818–1828.
44. Montone RA, Gurgoglione FL, Del Buono MG, et al. Interplay between myocardial bridging and coronary spasm in patients with myocardial ischemia and non-obstructive coronary arteries: pathogenic and prognostic implications. *J Am Heart Assoc*. 2021;10:e020535.
45. Takahashi T, Samuels BA, Li W, et al. Safety of provocative testing with intracoronary acetylcholine and implications for standard protocols. *J Am Coll Cardiol*. 2022;79:2367–2378.
46. Montone RA, Rinaldi R, Del Buono MG, et al. Safety and prognostic relevance of acetylcholine testing in patients with stable myocardial ischaemia or myocardial infarction and non-obstructive coronary arteries. *EuroIntervention*. 2022;18(8):e666–e676.
47. De Vita A, Manfredonia L, Lamendola P, et al. Coronary microvascular dysfunction in patients with acute coronary syndrome and no obstructive coronary artery disease. *Clin Res Cardiol*. 2019;108:1364–1370.
48. Maznyczka AM, Oldroyd KG, Greenwood JP, et al. Comparative significance of invasive measures of microvascular injury in acute myocardial infarction. *Circ Cardiovasc Interv*. 2020;13:e008505.
49. Quesada O, Yildiz M, Henry TD, et al. Mortality in ST-segment elevation myocardial infarction with nonobstructive coronary arteries and mimickers. *JAMA Netw Open*. 2023;18(8):ee2343402. doi:10.1001/jamanetworkopen.2023.43402.
50. Sorensson P, Ekenback C, Lundin M, et al. Early comprehensive cardiovascular magnetic resonance imaging in patients with myocardial infarction with nonobstructive coronary arteries. *JACC Cardiovasc Imaging*. 2021;14:1774–1783.
51. Williams MGL, Liang K, De Garate E, et al. Peak troponin and CMR to guide management in suspected ACS and nonobstructive coronary arteries. *JACC Cardiovasc Imaging*. 2022;15:1578–1587.
52. Hausvater A, Smilowitz NR, Li B, et al. Myocarditis in relation to angiographic findings in patients with provisional diagnoses of MINOCA. *JACC Cardiovasc Imaging*. 2020;13:1906–1913.
53. Tamis-Holland JE, Jneid H, Reynolds HR, et al. Contemporary diagnosis and management of patients with myocardial infarction in the absence of obstructive coronary artery disease: a scientific statement from the American Heart Association. *Circulation*. 2019;139:e891–e908.
54. Smilowitz NR, Dubner R, Hellkamp AS, et al. Variability of discharge medical therapy for secondary prevention among patients with myocardial infarction with non-obstructive coronary arteries (MINOCA) in the United States. *PLoS One*. 2021;16:e0255462.
55. Bossard M, Gao P, Boden W, et al. Antiplatelet therapy in patients with myocardial infarction without obstructive coronary artery disease. *Heart*. 2021;107:1739–1747.
56. Teragawa H, Orita Y, Oshita C, Uchimura Y. Intracoronary thrombogenicity in patients with vasospastic angina: an observation using coronary angioscopy. *Diagnostics (Basel)*. 2021;11:1632.
57. Gulati M, Levy PD, Mukherjee D, et al. 2021. AHA/ACC/ASE/CHEST/SAEM/SCCT/SCMR guideline for the evaluation and diagnosis of chest pain: a report of the American College of Cardiology/American Heart Association joint committee on clinical practice guidelines. *Circulation*. 2021;144:e368–e454.
58. Ciliberti G, Verdoia M, Merlo M, et al. Pharmacological therapy for the prevention of cardiovascular events in patients with myocardial infarction with non-obstructed coronary arteries (MINOCA): insights from a multicentre national registry. *Int J Cardiol*. 2021;327:9–14.
59. Schindler TH, Fearon WF, Pelletier-Galarneau M, et al. Myocardial perfusion PET for the detection and reporting of coronary microvascular dysfunction: a JACC: cardiovascular imaging expert panel statement. *JACC Cardiovasc Imaging*. 2023;16:536–548.
60. Zhang H, Caobelli F, Che W, et al. The prognostic value of CZT SPECT myocardial blood flow (MBF) quantification in patients with ischemia and no obstructive coronary artery disease (INOCA): a pilot study. *Eur J Nucl Med Mol Imaging*. 2023;50:1940–1953.

29 New Concepts in Cardiac Rehabilitation and Secondary Prevention After Acute Coronary Syndrome

ANN-DORTHE OLSEN ZWISLER AND ROD S. TAYLOR

INTRODUCTION

Contemporary evidence-based treatments for patients with acute coronary syndrome (ACS) have improved outcomes, with substantive reductions in mortality rates during the last decade. Nevertheless, patients who survive ACS remain at increased risk for recurrent events, rehospitalization, and death and also suffer from clinical symptoms and loss of physical, psychological, or social functioning after discharge that can lead to impaired health-related quality of life.[1]

The effectiveness and accessibility of cardiac rehabilitation (CR) and secondary prevention services after ACS have therefore never been more important, and therefore, there is a need for cardiologists to "re-engage" in CR and secondary prevention following ACS.[2]

In this chapter, we provide an overview of CR and secondary prevention. The key recent developments that we highlight are:

- Innovations in cardioprotective medication, especially the introduction of new class of SGLT2 inhibitors (gliflozins), glucagon-like peptide-1 receptor (GLP-1R), and developments in lipid-lowering drugs.
- During and following the COVID-19 pandemic, move towards remote models of CR that include home-based programs, digital support, and combination center and remote (hybrid) programs.

Given the rise in prevalence of multimorbidity and increasing complexity of cardiac disease, the need to increasingly focus on a personalized approach to patient management is growing.

DEFINITION OF CARDIAC REHABILITATION AND SECONDARY PREVENTION

CR [and secondary prevention] services are today defined as comprehensive, long-term programs. Although exercise training remains a cornerstone of intervention, current practice guidelines consistently recommend comprehensive programs. CR and secondary prevention should contain the necessary core components to optimize cardiovascular risk reduction, foster healthy behaviors and compliance with these behaviors, reduce disability, promote an active lifestyle to improve health-related quality of life, reduce rehospitalization, morbidity, and CVD mortality[3] (Fig. 29.1).

CR and secondary prevention services should begin in the inpatient setting for patients who have survived ACS and continue into the early-outpatient and late-outpatient phases of follow-up (Fig. 29.2). Effective services require close collaboration between patients, caregivers, and service providers. To ensure quality assurance, guidelines recommend[4–6] the involvement of a multidisciplinary team in the optimal delivery of CR programs.

Although in many countries this inpatient and early-outpatient care is covered by health care providers and insurers, the costs of late-outpatient or "maintenance" programs often need to be met by the patients themselves in home- or community-based settings.

EVIDENCE FOR CARDIAC REHABILITATION

Oldridge and colleagues published the first systematic reviews and meta-analyses of CR more than 30 years ago. The landmark JAMA review of 22 randomized controlled trials (RCTs) in 4347 post-myocardial infarction (MI) patients reported a pooled reduction in all-cause and cardiovascular mortality of 24%–25%, with exercise-based CR compared to a no-exercise control.

Since then a number of Cochrane meta-analysis and systematic reviews have been published with the latest update was conducted in 2021 and published in 2023.[7] The 2021 Cochrane Review includes 85 RCTs and 23,430 participants adding 22 additional trials since the 2016 update. Table 29.1 details a summary of the study and patient

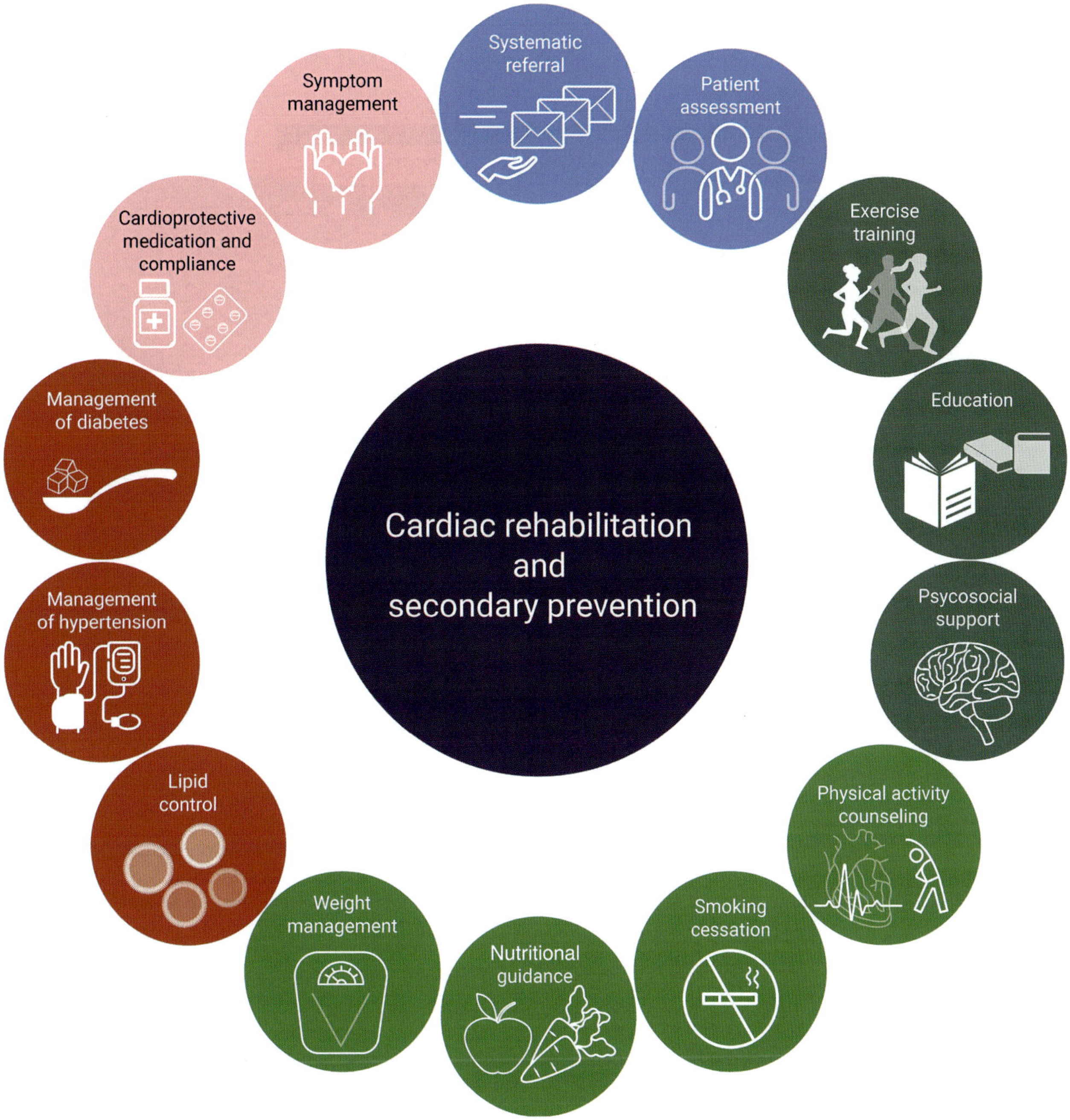

FIG. 29.1 Core components of cardiac rehabilitation and secondary prevention.

characteristics of the latest review. These trials comprised a third of the included patients, from a broader population more generalizable to the average patient than in previous reviews. There were slightly more women included than in the last review, but still <15% overall. Further 21 trials were from low- and middle-income countries, where the cardiovascular disease burden is greater and primary prevention and acute care are less accessed.[8]

The Cochrane Reviews support the conclusions of the previous versions that exercise-based CR provides important benefits to people with CHD overall and ACS in particular. The benefits are listed in Table 29.2 and include important reductions in the risk of all-cause hospitalization, along with associated health care costs, and improved health-related quality of life at up to 12 months' follow-up. Over longer-term follow-up (>12 months), benefits may also include a reduction in cardiovascular mortality and MI.[7]

A summary of the evolution of the Cochrane evidence base and findings over time are shown in Fig. 29.3, demonstrating the overwhelming body of evidence across several decades demonstrating the benefits of CR. This review indeed demonstrates the lifesaving impact of timely access to revascularization and other therapies, but that should not negate perceptions of the benefit of CR. CR supports patients in implementing all the secondary prevention strategies proven to prolong life which acute care providers recommend to their patients, in addition to optimizing patient's function (e.g., return to life roles) and psychosocial well-being. Through the repeated contact between

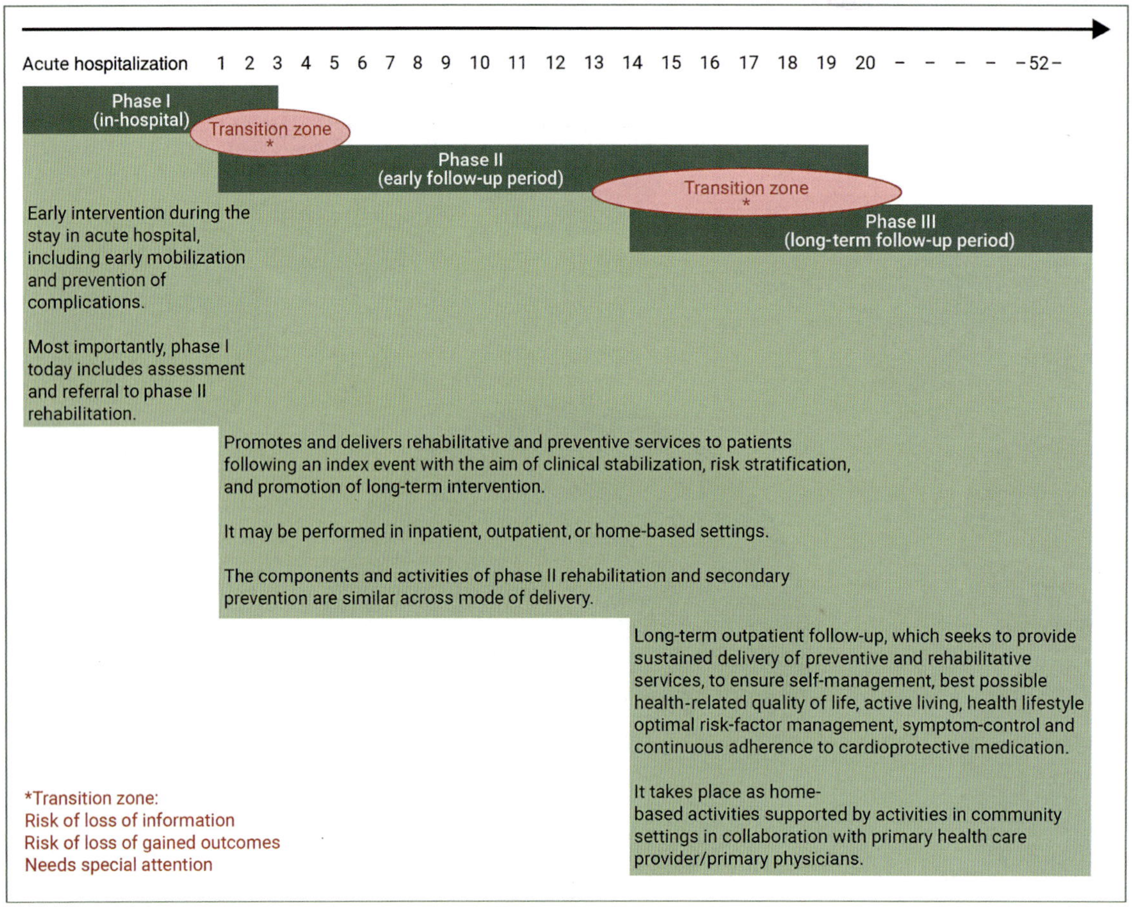

FIG. 29.2 The trajectory of cardiac rehabilitation and secondary prevention.

patients and the multidisciplinary team, patients are supported to implement and maintain the many lifestyle changes. Supporting patients in lifestyle changes including adherence to medications is time-consuming and labor-intensive and seems like a less active or aggressive approach, but the impact should not be minimized.[9]

COMPONENTS OF CR AND SECONDARY PREVENTION

Current American Heart Association, the American College of Cardiology, and the European Society of Cardiology guidelines endorse participation in CR and secondary prevention as key elements of standard post-ACS management as a level I grade A recommendation.[10,11]

The following section details the core components of CR and secondary prevention delivery based on international practice, policy, and guidelines statements published from 2019 onwards.[5,6]

Systematic Referral

Guidelines consistently recommend that eligible patients with ACS should be systematically referred to a comprehensive outpatient rehabilitation and secondary prevention program that includes an exercise component. This referral should take place either before hospital discharge or before first follow-up visit.[4–6]

Despite the substantive evidence for the benefits of such services, implementation, and patient enrollment in CR and secondary prevention programs remain poor across the globe. For example, a large observational US study in US Medicare Beneficiaries found that only one in four eligible patients participated in CR and marked disparities were observed.[12] This gap in delivery has been shown to be especially large in older patients, women, and members of ethnic minorities.[2,12] Potential barriers to referral to rehabilitation and prevention are complex but can be summarized at three levels—patient, clinician, and service level—Fig. 29.4. To ensure the opportunity for referral is not missed, especially clinicians need to be aware of these potential barriers.

Evidence from a Cochrane review published in 2019 shows that specific interventions may increase CR enrolment, adherence, and completion.[13] Some of these interventional approaches are presented later under the section "Innovative and Models of Rehabilitation and Prevention."

Patient Assessment and Tailored Planning

Formulation of an individually tailored, patient-specific plan for CR and secondary prevention should be based on a detailed risk assessment at discharge or as soon as possible after hospital admission and before initiation of the program. Table 29.3 details recommendations for patient risk assessment and clinical data collection.[6]

TABLE 29.1 Cochrane 2021 Review Summary of Study and Patient Characteristics

CATEGORY	NO. OF STUDIES (%) OR MEDIAN[a] (RANGE)
Study Characteristics	
Publication year	
1970–1979	2 (2%)
1980–1999	32 (38%)
2000–2019	44 (52%)
2020 onward	7 (8%)
Study continent	
Europe	48 (56%)
North America	13 (15%)
Asia	16 (19%)
Australia	5 (6%)
Other	3 (4%)
Low-middle-income countries	21 (25%)
Single center	61 (72%)
Sample size	137 (25–3959)
Duration of follow-up (weeks)	12 (6–228)
Population Characteristics	
Gender	
Males only	21 (25%)
Females only	1 (1%)
Both males and females	61 (72%)
Not reported	2 (2%)
Age (years)	56 (44–77)
Diagnosis	
Post MI only	40 (47%)
Revascularization only	14 (16%)
Angina only	5 (6%)
Mixed-CHD population	25 (29%)
Nonobstructive CHD	1 (1%)
Intervention Characteristics	
Intervention type	
Exercise-only programs	38 (45%)
Comprehensive programs	47 (56%)
Dose of intervention	
Duration	6 m (0.75–42)
Frequency	1–7 sessions/wk
Length	20–90 min/session
Intensity	• 50%–90% maximal/peak HR or HRR • 50%–95% VO2 max • Borg RPE 11–16
Setting	
Center-based only	40 (47%)
Combination center- and home-based	21 (25%)
Home-based only	21 (25%)
Not reported	3 (3%)
Comparator	
Usual/Standard care	50 (59%)
Usual care plus education, guidance, or advice about diet and exercise but no formal exercise training	24 (28%)
"No exercise"	8 (9%)
Other	3 (4%)

CHD, Coronary heart disease.
[a]Median of study means.
Adapted from Dibben G, Faulkner J, Oldridge N, et al. Exercise-based cardiac rehabilitation for coronary heart disease. *Cochrane Database Syst Rev.* 2021;11(11):CD001800.

Exercise Testing and Training

Symptom-limited exercise testing before participation in an exercise-based CR program is recommended.[6] Exercise test parameters should include assessment of heart rate and rhythm, signs, and symptoms, ST-segment changes, hemodynamics, perceived exertion, and exercise capacity. Based on this exercise test, patients can then be risk-stratified to select the appropriate level of supervision and monitoring required during their exercise-based rehabilitation program. When using these principles, exercise-based CR has been shown to be safe even for those patients with recent, complex, and/or multivessel PCI.[6]

Exercise training should be prescribed on an individualized approach after careful clinical evaluation, including risk stratification, behavioral characteristics, personal goals, and consideration of the patient's preferences. Exercise training should be regularly reviewed by the program team and modified if necessary. Current recommendations for exercise prescription are detailed in Table 29.4. Aerobic and resistance/strength training could be combined with flexibility training, balance training, and inspiratory muscle training.[6]

Education

Current CR and secondary prevention guidelines and policy statements[5,6] recommend education as part of post-ACS follow-up care. A Cochrane review from 2017 on patient education in the management of coronary heart disease found a positive impact on health-related quality of life, healthy behavior, and risk factor modification, which improves adherence to cardio-protective medications, as well as psychosocial support including vocational guidance and sexual functioning.

Several principles of behavior change and educational theories are helpful in improving the patient's motivation and ability to comprehend and digest a broad array of information. These principles (i.e., stages of change, self-efficacy concepts, outcome models, biofeedback) should be not regarded as mutually exclusive, but rather combined, depending on patients' needs and staff competencies.

Psychosocial Support

The relationship between psychosocial and cardiac health is complex, and both direct (e.g., psychological effects on immunologic function) and indirect (e.g., behaviorally mediated) mechanisms are thought to play a role. Consequently, patients may be offered a wide variety of psychological therapies to treat their depression, anxiety, stress, or maladaptive behaviors, and their overall psychological and cardiac health. Underpinning all psychosocial therapies for cardiac patients is some combination of the following four hypotheses: (1) that coronary heart disease and associated medical or surgical treatments may cause psychological distress; (2) that psychological symptoms may cause or exacerbate cardiac disease; (3) that unhealthy behaviors may be increased when people experience psychological distress; and (4) that psychological techniques may be useful in modifying risky

TABLE 29.2 Summary of Meta-Analysis of Effects of Exercise-Based Cardiac Rehabilitation for CHD on Clinical Event Outcomes 2021-Update (All Studies Longest Follow-Up)

OUTCOME	NO. OF PARTICIPANTS (NO. OF STUDIES)	NO. OF EVENTS/PARTICIPANTS INTERVENTION	COMPARATOR	RELATIVE RISK (WITH 95% CI)	STATISTICAL HETEROGENEITY[2]/ STATISTIC CHI-SQUARE TEST (WITH *P* VALUE)	GRADE/QUALITY OF EVIDENCE
All-cause mortality	16,829 (47)	919/8608	950/8221	0.96 (0.89–1.04)	0%	+ + + – Moderate[a]
CV mortality	7762 (26)	296/3997	382/3765	0.74 (0.64–0.86)***	0%	+ + + – Moderate[a]
Fatal and/or nonfatal MI	14,151 (39)	383/7181	437/6970	0.82 (0.70–0.96)*	9%	+ + + – Moderate[b]
CABG	5872 (29)	211/3028	215/2844	0.96 (0.80–1.15)	0%	+ + + + High
PCI	3878 (17)	171/1960	201/1918	0.84 (0.69–1.02)	0%	+ + + – Moderate[a]
All-cause hospitalization	7802 (21)	504/3958	593/3844	0.77 (0.67–0.89)**	32%	+ + + – Moderate[b]

CABG, Coronary artery bypass grafting; *CHD,* coronry heart disease; *CV,* cardiovascular; *GRADE,* grades of recommendation, assessment, development and evaluation (with plus or minus assigned for each of the four grading categories); *MI,* myocardial infarction; *PCI,* percutaneous coronary intervention.
[a]Downgraded by one level due to imprecision with a wide confidence interval.
[b]Downgraded by one level due to evidence of publication bias.
*$P < 0.05$, **$P < 0.01$, ***$P < 0.001$
Adapted from Dibben GO, Faulkner J, Oldridge N, et al. Exercise-based cardiac rehabilitation for coronary heart disease: a meta-analysis. *Eur Heart J.* 2023;44(6):452–469.

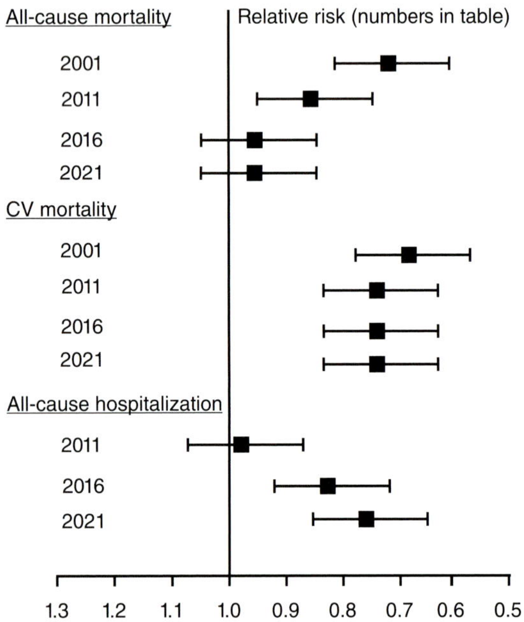

FIG. 29.3 Summary of meta-analysis of effects of exercise-based cardiac rehabilitation for CHD on clinical event outcomes across systematic reviews 2001–2021.

behaviors.[14] After myocardial infarction (MI) or ACS, the prevalence of depression is generally double that seen in the general populationH[15] which makes depression the most important psychosocial target in the clinical practice of cardiology. Depression and ischemic heart disease have a bidirectional relationship—that is, ischemic heart disease can cause depression, and depression is an independent risk factor for ischemic heart disease and its complications.

Depression among people with established ischemic heart disease is clinically important in that it is associated with worse medical outcomes including poorer health-related quality of life, greater morbidity and mortality, and higher use of routine and unscheduled health care.

The impact of psychological interventions for patients with coronary heart disease has been the subject of a Cochrane review.[14] The 2018 review included 35 RCTs comparing psychological interventions with usual care in 10,703 participants who were predominantly at low risk for adverse outcomes after an MI or PCI procedure. Psychological interventions led to a reduction in cardiovascular

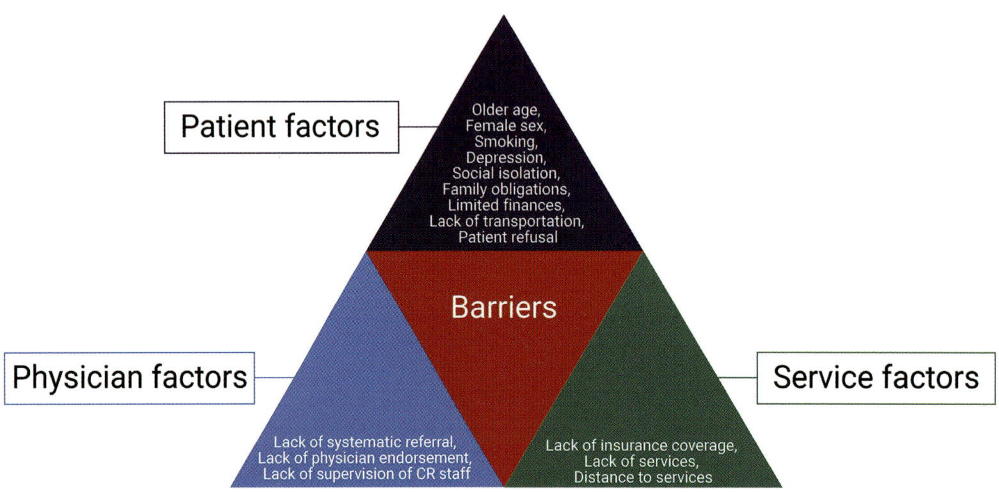

FIG. 29.4 Barriers to participation in cardiac rehabilitation and secondary prevention.

TABLE 29.3 Patient Risk Assessment and Clinical Data Collection Post-ACS as Part of Initiation of Cardiac Rehabilitation and Secondary Prevention

ASSESSMENT COMPONENT	DESCRIPTION
Clinical history	Screening for cardiovascular risk factors, comorbid conditions, and disabilities
Symptoms	Cardiovascular disease—NYHA functional class for dyspnea, Canadian Cardiovascular Society (CCS) class for symptoms of angina, Fontaine/Rutherford class for lower extremities peripheral arterial disease
Lifestyle	Initial assessment of physical activity level by history, smoking history, and dietary habits
Medication	Including dose, frequency, and side effects
Adherence	To medical regimen and self-monitoring (weight, BP, symptoms)
Psychosocial status	Initial assessment of psychological distress, family obligations, financial and vocational situation, social isolation, sexual functioning
Physical examination	General health status, body mass index (BMI), waist circumference, heart failure signs, cardiac and carotid murmurs, pulse, BP control, extremities for presence of arterial pulses and orthopedic pathology, neurological abnormalities
Ekectrocardiogram	Heart rate and rhythm, repolarization changes
Cardiac imaging	2D and Doppler echocardiography when appropriate—in particular, ventricular function, valvular heart disease, presence of effusion
Blood testing	For routine biochemical assay: including full blood count, electrolytes, renal and liver function, fasting blood glucose (HbA_{1C} if fasting blood glucose is elevated or with known diabetes), total cholesterol, LDL-C, HDL-C, triglycerides
Peak exercise capacity	Symptom-limited exercise testing, either on bicycle ergometer or on treadmill. If this is not feasible (e.g., because of recent surgery), submaximal exercise evaluation and/or six-minute walk test should be considered
Individual information and education as part of initial assessment and referral to cardiac rehabilitation and secondary prevention	Education on self-monitoring protocols (weight, blood pressure, warning symptoms, and signs of instability, e.g., angina, dyspnea) and self-management Clear, comprehensible information on the basic purpose of the CR program and the role of each component (including optimal medical therapy compliance)

BP, Blood pressure; *CR,* cardiac rehabilitation; *2D,* two-dimensional; *HbA_{1C}, A_{1C}* hemoglobin (glycosylated); *HDL-C,* high-density lipoprotein cholesterol; *LDL-C,* low-density lipoprotein cholesterol; *NYHA,* New York Heart Association.
Adapted from Ambrosetti M, Abreu A, Corra U, et al. Secondary prevention through comprehensive cardiovascular rehabilitation: from knowledge to implementation. 2020 update. A position paper from the secondary prevention and rehabilitation section of the European association of preventive cardiology. *Eur J Prev Cardiol.* 2021;28(5):460–495.

mortality (relative risk 0.79, 95% confidence interval [CI] 0.63–0.98), although no benefits were observed in terms of risk of total mortality, MI, or revascularization. Psychological interventions improved depressive symptoms (standardized mean difference -0.27, 95% CI -0.39 to -0.15), anxiety (standardized mean difference -0.24, 95% CI -0.38 to -0.09), and stress (standardized mean difference -0.56, 95% CI -0.88 to -0.24) compared with controls. While this review demonstrated that psychological intervention improved psychological symptoms and reduced cardiac mortality for people with CHD, there remains considerable uncertainty regarding the magnitude of these effects and the specific techniques most likely to benefit people with different presentations of CHD.[14]

Under the umbrella of psychosocial support, current guidelines also advocate the integration of vocational advice on return to work and advice on resuming normal sexual functioning (see Table 29.5). Most recently, reduction of environmental pollutants has been proposed as an important target for prevention of future cardiovascular disease.[16]

Comprehensive Risk Factor Management

As summarized in Tables 29.6 and 29.7, risk factor management is a pivotal part of comprehensive CR and secondary prevention.

Physical Activity Counseling

As described above, participation in exercise training is considered an important tool to increase long-term physical activity levels in post-ACS patients.[4–6] Regular physical activity is associated with a reduced risk of fatal and nonfatal coronary events in healthy people, persons with coronary risk factors, and cardiac patients over a wide age range. A sedentary lifestyle is one of the major risk factors for cardiovascular diseases. Engaging in regular physical activity is therefore suggested by guidelines as a very important nonpharmacologic component of risk factor control in primary as well as secondary prevention (see Table 29.4).

After ACS, a regimen of 30 to 60 minutes of moderate-intensity aerobic activity, such as brisk walking, at least 5 days and preferably 7 days per week, supplemented by an increase in daily lifestyle activity to improve cardiorespiratory fitness, should be encouraged. The basic goal is to move patients out of a "least-fit, least-active" and therefore high-risk status.

Smoking Cessation

Smoking is associated with an increased risk of all types of cardiovascular and coronary artery diseases. Smoking risk is primarily related to the amount of tobacco smoked daily and shows a clear dose-response relationship, with no lower limit for deleterious effects.[17]

Although the exact mechanisms by which smoking increases the risk of atherosclerotic disease are not fully understood, it is clear that smoking enhances both the development of atherosclerosis and the occurrence of superimposed thrombotic phenomena.[17] Stopping smoking after ACS is still considered one of the most effective preventive initiatives.

An updated Cochrane review from 2021 including 68 studies, and 80,702 participants included in cohort studies, and both cluster- and individually RCTs of at least 6 months' duration showed that smoking cessation is associated with a reduction of approximately one-third in the risk of recurrent cardiovascular disease in people who stop smoking at diagnosis. This association may be

TABLE 29.4 Exercise Prescription in ACS

	AEROBIC TRAINING	RESISTANCE/STRENGTH TRAINING
Frequency	At least 3 d/wk Preferable 6–7 d/wk	2 times/wk
Intensity	Moderate (i.e., 45%–59% of peak oxygen consumption, 50%–70% of peak (above the first ventilatory threshold), 55%–69% of peak heart rate, 40%–59% of heart rate reserve (to be calculated on top of rest HR), 4–6 METs, or 12/20–14/20 of the Borg scale) or moderate-to-high intensity for endurance continuous training. Higher intensities of exercise bouts for endurance high-intensity interval training according to the selected protocol. The "speech rule" (i.e., the respiratory rate should allow conversation) could be considered as an additional tool to control intensity when HR cannot be used	30%–70% of the 1-RM for the upper body and 40%–80% of 1-RM for lower body exercises, with 12–15 repetitions in one set
Time (duration)	At least 20–30 min (preferably 45–60 min) per session	
Type of exercise	Walking, jogging, cycling, swimming, rowing, stair climbing, elliptical trainers, and aerobic dancing	
Setting	Center-based, supervised homebased	Center-based, supervised homebased

Adapted from Ambrosetti M, Abreu A, Corra U, et al. Secondary prevention through comprehensive cardiovascular rehabilitation: from knowledge to implementation. 2020 update. A position paper from the secondary prevention and rehabilitation section of the European association of preventive cardiology. *Eur J Prev Cardiol*. 2021;28(5):460–495.

TABLE 29.5 Assessment, Clinical Interventions, and Expected Outcomes for Psychosocial Management and Vocational Advice After ACS

AREA OF INTEREST, WITH TREATMENT GOAL	EVALUATION AND ASSESSMENT	INTERVENTION	EXPECTED OUTCOMES
Psychosocial management • *Absence of clinically significant depression and anxiety;* • *Absence of other psychosocial problems*	Screen for psychological distress using interview and/or other standardized measurement tools (i.e., HADS, WHO5, HeartQol). Screen for substance abuse of alcohol and/or other psychotropic agents.	Offer individual and/or small group education and counseling on adjustment to heart disease, stress management, and health-related lifestyle change (e.g., profession, car driving, sexual activities), relaxation techniques. Whenever possible, offer spouses and other family members, domestic partners, and/or significant others access to information sessions. Teach and support self-help strategies and ways of obtaining effective social support. Provide vocational counseling in case of work-related stress. *Treatment of depression* in collaboration with mental health specialist and primary care provider with cognitive behavioral therapy as first choice.	Emotional well-being. Absence of clinically significant psychosocial problems and acquisition of stress management skills. Improved health-related quality of life.
Vocational advice • *Return to previous activities unless contraindications*	Before discharge, return to previous activities must be discussed with the patients and their partners and return to previous activities must be promoted, unless there is a medical contraindication. The presence of any barriers to return to work (RTW) after illness should be assessed.	All procedures to help patients to overcome barriers to RTW and thereby remain in, return to, or gain access to employment; e.g., retraining and capacity building, reasonable adjustments and control measures, disability awareness, condition management, and medical treatment.	Return to previous activities.
Sexual functioning • *Return to previous activities unless contraindicated*		Offer individual and/or small group education and counseling on sexual functioning and sexual activities. PDE5 inhibitor must be used with caution in patients using nitrates prn. And should be avoided when treated with prolonged nitrates or nicorandil because this can lead to low blood pressure.	Return to previous activities unless contraindicated.

Adapted from (A) Ambrosetti M, Abreu A, Corra U, et al. Secondary prevention through comprehensive cardiovascular rehabilitation: from knowledge to implementation. 2020 update. A position paper from the secondary prevention and rehabilitation section of the European association of preventive cardiology. *Eur J Prev Cardiol*. 2021;28(5):460–495. (B) Mehra VM, Gaalema DE, Pakosh M, Grace SL. Systematic review of cardiac rehabilitation guidelines: quality and scope. *Eur J Prev Cardiol*. 2020;27(9):912–928.

causal, based on the link between smoking cessation and restoration of endothelial and platelet function, where dysfunction of both can result in an increased likelihood of cardiovascular events.[18] Thus, the results from the review provide evidence that there is a decreased risk of secondary cardiovascular events in those who quit smoking compared with those who continue and that there is a suggested improvement in quality of life as a result of quitting smoking. Additional studies that account for confounding, such as the use of secondary prevention medication, would strengthen the evidence in this specific area.[18]

TABLE 29.6 Assessment, Clinical Interventions, and Expected Outcomes for Behavioral Interventions After ACS

AREA OF INTEREST, WITH TREATMENT GOALS[a]	EVALUATION/ ASSESSMENT	INTERVENTION	EXPECTED OUTCOMES
Physical activity counseling and exercise training • *Moderate aerobic activity,* 30 min/d, 5–7 days/wk; Higher intensities of exercise bouts each lasting > 10 min 2.5 h/wk • *Complementary resistance training,* 2 d/wk	Assess current physical activity level and determine domestic, occupational, and recreational needs. Assess readiness to change behavior, self-confidence, and barriers.	*Recommend* gradual increases in daily lifestyle activities over time, and how to incorporate it into daily routine and evenly spread throughout the week, i.e., minimum 5 d/wk. *Emphasize* sedentary lifestyle as risk factor and the benefits of physical activity: Any increase in activity has a positive health benefit. *Advise*: Individualize physical activity according to patient's age, past habits, comorbid conditions, preferences, and goals. *Reassure* regarding the safety of the recommended protocol. *Encourage* involvement in leisure activities that are enjoyable. *Forewarn*: Inform patients on the risk of relapses; education should underline how benefits may be achieved and the need for lifelong continuation. If physical activity interruption has occurred, physical, social, and psychological barriers should be explored, and alternative approaches suggested.	Increased participation physical activities. Improved psychosocial well-being. Prevention of disability. Improved aerobic fitness and body composition.
Smoking cessation • *Nonsmoker status*	Smoking status and use of other tobacco products Amount of smoking (per day) (number of years). Determine readiness to change; if ready, choose a date for quitting.	All smokers should be encouraged professionally to stop smoking all forms of tobacco permanently, and offered assistance from an evidence-based smoking cessation service. *Follow-up*: Referral to special programs and/or pharmacotherapy (including nicotine replacement) are recommended, as is a stepwise strategy for smoking cessation. Provide structured follow-up. Offer behavioral advice and group or individual counseling. *Consider nicotine replacement therapy,* combined with bupropion or varenicline if not contraindicated.	Long-term abstinence from smoking.
Nutritional counseling • *Heart-healthy diet*	Assess eating habits including daily caloric intake and dietary content of fat, saturated fat, sodium, and other nutrients. Adapt caloric intake to the expected consumption during phase II exercise training.	*Education* regarding dietary goals and how to attain them Healthy food choices: – Saturated fatty acids to account for <10% of total energy intake, through replacement by polyunsaturated fatty acids – Trans unsaturated fatty acids: as little as possible, preferably no intake from processed food, and <1% of total energy intake from natural origin – <5 g of salt per day – 30–45 g of fiber per day, preferably from wholegrain products – >200 g of fruit per day (2–3 servings) – >200 g of vegetables per day (2–3 servings) – Fish 1–2 times/wk, one of which to be oily – 30 g of unsalted nuts per day – Sugar-sweetened soft drinks and alcoholic beverages consumption must be discouraged – Consumption of alcoholic beverages should be limited to two glasses per day (20 g/d of alcohol) for men and one glass per day (10 g/d of alcohol) for women *Integrate* behavior-change models and compliance strategies into counseling sessions.	Patient understands basic principles of dietary content. Adherence to a healthy diet lowering CV risk.
Weight control management • *Body mass index (BMI)*: 18.5–24.9 kg/m^2 • *Waist circumference*: 80 cm in women, 94 cm in men	Measure weight, height, and waist circumference. Calculate BMI. Analysis of nutrition habits, calorie intake, and physical activity.	*Education:* provide behavioral and nutritional counseling with follow-up to monitor progress in achieving goals. *Weight reduction* by means of diet, exercise and behavior modification. It is recommended in obese patients (BMI ≥30 kg/m^2, or waist circumference ≥102 cm in men or ≥88 cm in women), and should be considered in overweight patients (BMI ≥ 25 kg/m^2, or waist circumference ≥94 cm in men or ≥80 cm in women), particularly if associated with multiple risk factors (such as hypertension, hypercholesterolemia, smoking and insulin resistance or diabetes).	– Among subjects with healthy weight, the maintenance of weight – Among overweight/obese patients, elaboration of an individualized strategy to reduce 5%–10% of body weight, and to modify associated risk factors – Where goal is not attained, consider referring patient to specialist in obesity/ endocrinologist – Consider use of GLP-1 agonists as part of weight-loss and to achieve reduction in cardiac events

Adapted from (A) Ambrosetti M, Abreu A, Corra U, et al. Secondary prevention through comprehensive cardiovascular rehabilitation: from knowledge to implementation. 2020 update. A position paper from the secondary prevention and rehabilitation section of the European association of preventive cardiology. *Eur J Prev Cardiol.* 2021;28(5):460–495. (B) Mehra VM, Gaalema DE, Pakosh M, Grace SL. Systematic review of cardiac rehabilitation guidelines: quality and scope. *Eur J Prev Cardiol.* 2020;27(9):912–928.

and with substantial disparities in referral, access, and participation.

Contemporary guidelines consistently recommend that patients with ACS should be offered CR and secondary prevention. Meta-analysis of RCTs shows that rehabilitation and prevention for post-ACS patients provide important health benefits that include reductions in the risk of cardiovascular mortality and rehospitalization and improvements in health-related quality of life. Despite the proven benefits of CR and secondary prevention services, only a minority of eligible ACS patients currently receive these services. While strategies to improve the delivery of services that include the expansion of home and technology-based programs are beginning to bear fruit, the capacity of current delivery models for rehabilitation and prevention services is insufficient to provide such services to all eligible patients. New delivery strategies are needed that will supplement traditional, center-based rehabilitation and prevention programs and expand the reach of these important services to meet the key challenges currently facing health care and rehabilitation and secondary prevention services including an aging population with high prevalence of frailty and multimorbidity.

CLASSIC REFERENCES

Oldridge NB, Guyatt GH, Fischer ME, Rimm AA. CR after myocardial infarction. Combined experience of randomized clinical trials. *JAMA*. 1988;260:945–950.

O'Connor GT, Buring JE, Yusuf S, et al. An overview of randomized trials of rehabilitation with exercise after myocardial infarction. *Circulation*. 1989;80:234–244.

Van Camp SP, Peterson RA. Cardiovascular complications of outpatient CR programs. *JAMA*. 1986;256:1160–1163.

Wenger N, Froelicher E, Smith L, et al. CR as secondary prevention. Agency for health care policy and research and national heart, lung, and blood institute. *Clin Pract Guidel Quick Ref Guide Clin*. 17:1995:1–23.

REFERENCES

1. Pocock S, Brieger DB, Owen R, et al. Health-related quality of life 1–3 years post-myocardial infarction: its impact on prognosis. *Open Heart*. 2021;8(1):1–11.
2. Beatty AL, Beckie TM, Dodson J, et al. A new era in cardiac rehabilitation delivery: research gaps, questions, strategies, and priorities. *Circulation*. 2023;147(3):254–266.
3. Redfern J, Gallagher R, O'Neil A, et al. Historical context of cardiac rehabilitation: learning from the past to move to the future. *Front Cardiovasc Med*. 2022;9:842567.
4. Visseren FLJ, Mach F, Smulders YM, et al. 2021 ESC guidelines on cardiovascular disease prevention in clinical practice. *Eur Heart J*. 2021;42(34):3227–3337.
5. Mehra VM, Gaalema DE, Pakosh M, Grace SL. Systematic review of cardiac rehabilitation guidelines: quality and scope. *Eur J Prev Cardiol*. 2020;27(9):912–928.
6. Ambrosetti M, Abreu A, Corra U, et al. Secondary prevention through comprehensive cardiovascular rehabilitation: from knowledge to implementation. 2020 update. A position paper from the secondary prevention and rehabilitation section of the European association of preventive cardiology. *Eur J Prev Cardiol*. 2021;28(5):460–495.
7. Dibben G, Faulkner J, Oldridge N, et al. Exercise-based cardiac rehabilitation for coronary heart disease. *Cochrane Database Syst Rev*. 2021;11(11):CD001800.
8. Pesah E, Turk-Adawi K, Supervia M, et al. Cardiac rehabilitation delivery in low/middle-income countries. *Heart*. 2019;105(23):1806–1812.
9. Grace SL. Evidence is indisputable that cardiac rehabilitation provides health benefits and event reduction: time for policy action. *Eur Heart J*. 2023;44(6):470–472.
10. Writing Committee M, Lawton JS, Tamis-Holland JE, et al. 2021 ACC/AHA/SCAI guideline for coronary artery revascularization: a report of the American College of Cardiology/American Heart Association joint committee on clinical practice guidelines. *J Am Coll Cardiol*. 2022;79(2):e21–e129.
11. Collet JP, Thiele H, Barbato E, et al. 2020 ESC Guidelines for the management of acute coronary syndromes in patients presenting without persistent ST-segment elevation. *Eur Heart J*. 2021;42(14):1289–1367.
12. Ritchey MD, Maresh S, McNeely J, et al. Tracking cardiac rehabilitation participation and completion among medicare beneficiaries to inform the efforts of a national initiative. *Circ Cardiovasc Qual Outcomes*. 2020;13(1):e005902.
13. Santiago de Araujo Pio C, Chaves GS, Davies P, Taylor RS, Grace SL. Interventions to promote patient utilisation of cardiac rehabilitation. *Cochrane Database Syst Rev*. 2019;2(2):CD007131.
14. Richards SH, Anderson L, Jenkinson CE, et al. Psychological interventions for coronary heart disease: cochrane systematic review and meta-analysis. *Eur J Prev Cardiol*. 2018;25(3):247–259.
15. Hare DL. Depression and cardiovascular disease. *Curr Opin Lipidol*. 2021;32(3):167–174.
16. Munzel T, Miller MR, Sorensen M, Lelieveld J, Daiber A, Rajagopalan S. Reduction of environmental pollutants for prevention of cardiovascular disease: it's time to act. *Eur Heart J*. 2020;41(41):3989–3997.
17. Ding N, Sang Y, Chen J, et al. Cigarette smoking, smoking cessation, and long-term risk of 3 major atherosclerotic diseases. *J Am Coll Cardiol*. 2019;74(4):498–507.
18. Wu AD, Lindson N, Hartmann-Boyce J, et al. Smoking cessation for secondary prevention of cardiovascular disease. *Cochrane Database Syst Rev*. 2022;8(8):CD014936.
19. Arnett DK, Blumenthal RS, Albert MA, et al. 2019 ACC/AHA guideline on the primary prevention of cardiovascular disease: a report of the American College of Cardiology/American Heart Association task force on clinical practice guidelines. *J Am Coll Cardiol*. 2019;74(10):e177–e232.
20. Dinu M, Pagliai G, Casini A, Sofi F. Mediterranean diet and multiple health outcomes: an umbrella review of meta-analyses of observational studies and randomised trials. *Eur J Clin Nutr*. 2018;72(1):30–43.
21. Williams B, Mancia G, Spiering W, et al. 2018 ESC/ESH guidelines for the management of arterial hypertension. *Eur Heart J*. 2018;39(33):3021–3104.
22. Whelton PK, Carey RM, Aronow WS, et al. 2017 ACC/AHA/AAPA/ABC/ACPM/AGS/APhA/ASH/ASPC/NMA/PCNA guideline for the prevention, detection, evaluation, and management of high blood pressure in adults: a report of the American College of Cardiology/American Heart Association task force on clinical practice guidelines. *J Am Coll Cardiol*. 2018;71(19):e127–e248.
23. Zhang W, Zhang S, Deng Y, et al. Trial of intensive blood-pressure control in older patients with hypertension. *N Engl J Med*. 2021;385(14):1268–1279.
24. Cholesterol Treatment Trialists C. Efficacy and safety of statin therapy in older people: a meta-analysis of individual participant data from 28 randomised controlled trials. *Lancet*. 2019;393(10170):407–415.
25. Gencer B, Marston NA, Im K, et al. Efficacy and safety of lowering LDL cholesterol in older patients: a systematic review and meta-analysis of randomised controlled trials. *Lancet*. 2020;396(10263):1637–1643.
26. Grundy SM, Stone NJ. 2018 American Heart Association/American College of Cardiology multisociety guideline on the management of blood cholesterol: primary prevention. *JAMA Cardiol*. 2019;4(5):488–489.
27. Mach F, Baigent C, Catapano AL, et al. 2019 ESC/EAS guidelines for the management of dyslipidaemias: lipid modification to reduce cardiovascular risk. *Eur Heart J*. 2020;41(1):111–188.
28. Writing C, Lloyd-Jones DM, Morris PB, et al. 2022 ACC expert consensus decision pathway on the role of nonstatin therapies for LDL-cholesterol lowering in the management of atherosclerotic cardiovascular disease risk: a report of the American College of Cardiology solution set oversight committee. *J Am Coll Cardiol*. 2022;80(14):1366–1418.
29. Cosentino F, Grant PJ, Aboyans V, et al. 2019 ESC guidelines on diabetes, pre-diabetes, and cardiovascular diseases developed in collaboration with the EASD. *Eur Heart J*. 2020;41(2):255–323.
30. Rosenzweig JL, Bakris GL, Berglund LF, et al. Primary prevention of ASCVD and T2DM in patients at metabolic risk: an endocrine society* clinical practice guideline. *J Clin Endocrinol Metab*. 2019;104(9):3939–3985.
31. ElSayed NA, Aleppo G, Aroda VR, et al. 9. Pharmacologic approaches to glycemic treatment: standards of care in diabetes-2023. *Diabetes Care*. 2023;46(Suppl 1):S140–S157.
32. Gadager BB, Tang LH, Ravn MB, et al. Benefits of cardiac rehabilitation following acute coronary syndrome for patients with and without diabetes: a systematic review and meta-analysis. *BMC Cardiovasc Disord*. 2022;22(1):295.
33. Kotseva K, De Backer G, De Bacquer D, et al. Lifestyle and impact on cardiovascular risk factor control in coronary patients across 27 countries: results from the European Society of Cardiology ESC-EORP EUROASPIRE V registry. *Eur J Prev Cardiol*. 2019;26(8):824–835.
34. Sandesara PB, Dhindsa D, Khambhati J, et al. Reconfiguring cardiac rehabilitation to achieve panvascular prevention: new care models for a new world. *Can J Cardiol*. 2018;34(10 Suppl 2):S231–S239.
35. Dibben GO, Faulkner J, Oldridge N, et al. Exercise-based cardiac rehabilitation for coronary heart disease: a meta-analysis. *Eur Heart J*. 2023;44(6):452–469.
36. Taylor RS, Long L, Mordi IR, et al. Exercise-based rehabilitation for heart failure: cochrane systematic review, meta-analysis, and trial sequential analysis. *JACC Heart Fail*. 2019;7(8):691–705.
37. McDonagh TA, Metra M, Adamo M, et al. 2021 ESC guidelines for the diagnosis and treatment of acute and chronic heart failure. *Eur Heart J*. 2021;42(36):3599–3726.
38. Heidenreich PA, Bozkurt B, Aguilar D, et al. 2022 AHA/ACC/HFSA guideline for the management of heart failure: a report of the American College of Cardiology/American Heart Association joint committee on clinical practice guidelines. *J Am Coll Cardiol*. 2022;79(17):e263–e421.
39. Taylor RS, Dalal HM, Zwisler AD. Cardiac rehabilitation for heart failure: "Cinderella" or evidence-based pillar of care? *Eur Heart J*. 2023;44(17):1511–1518.
40. Tegegne TK, Rawstorn JC, Nourse RA, Kibret KT, Ahmed KY, Maddison R. Effects of exercise-based cardiac rehabilitation delivery modes on exercise capacity and health-related quality of life in heart failure: a systematic review and network meta-analysis. *Open Heart*. 2022;9(1):e001949.
41. Buttery AK. Cardiac rehabilitation for frail older people. *Adv Exp Med Biol*. 2020;1216:131–147.
42. Vynckier P, Van Wilder L, Kotseva K, et al. Gender differences in health-related quality of life and psychological distress among coronary patients: does comorbidity matter? Results from the ESC EORP EUROASPIRE V registry. *Int J Cardiol*. 2023;371:452–459.
43. Buckley JP. The changing landscape of cardiac rehabilitation; from early mobilisation and reduced mortality to chronic multi-morbidity management. *Disabil Rehabil*. 2021;43(24):3515–3522.

44. Adlam D, Alfonso F, Maas A, Vrints C, Writing C. European Society of Cardiology, acute cardiovascular care association, SCAD study group: a position paper on spontaneous coronary artery dissection. *Eur Heart J*. 2018;39(36):3353–3368.
45. Hayes SN, Kim ESH, Saw J, et al. Spontaneous coronary artery dissection: current state of the science: a scientific statement from the American Heart Association. *Circulation*. 2018;137(19):e523–e557.
46. Neubeck L, McHale S, Ross M, MacGillivray S, Galbraith M, Hanson C. Spontaneous coronary artery dissection: a systematic review of physical and psychosocial recovery following discharge from hospital. *Eur J Cardiovasc Nurs*. 2022;21(7):665–676.
47. Samuel R, Alfadhel M, McAlister C, Nestelberger T, Saw J. Cardiac rehabilitation following coronary artery dissection: recommendations and patient considerations. *Expert Rev Cardiovasc Ther*. 2021;19(11):1005–1012.
48. Tweet MS, Olin JW, Bonikowske AR, Adlam D, Hayes SN. Physical activity and exercise in patients with spontaneous coronary artery dissection and fibromuscular dysplasia. *Eur Heart J*. 2021;42(37):3825–3828.
49. Thomas RJ, Balady G, Banka G, et al. 2018 ACC/AHA clinical performance and quality measures for cardiac rehabilitation: a report of the American College of Cardiology/American Heart Association task force on performance measures. *Circ Cardiovasc Qual Outcomes*. 2018;11(4):e000037.
50. Scherrenberg M, Wilhelm M, Hansen D, et al. The future is now: a call for action for cardiac telerehabilitation in the COVID-19 pandemic from the secondary prevention and rehabilitation section of the European association of preventive cardiology. *Eur J Prev Cardiol*. 2021;28(5):524–540.
51. Kluge HHP, Wickramasinghe K, Rippin HL, et al. Prevention and control of non-communicable diseases in the COVID-19 response. *Lancet*. 2020;395(10238):1678–1680.
52. Ghisi GLM, Xu Z, Liu X, et al. Impacts of the COVID-19 pandemic on cardiac rehabilitation delivery around the world. *Glob Heart*. 2021;16(1):43.
53. Thomas RJ, Beatty AL, Beckie TM, et al. Home-based cardiac rehabilitation: a scientific statement from the American association of cardiovascular and pulmonary rehabilitation, the American Heart Association, and the American College of Cardiology. *Circulation*. 2019;140(1):e69–e89.
54. Jin K, Khonsari S, Gallagher R, et al. Telehealth interventions for the secondary prevention of coronary heart disease: a systematic review and meta-analysis. *Eur J Cardiovasc Nurs*. 2019;18(4):260–271.

30 Tackling the Problem of Adverse Ventricular Remodeling After Myocardial Infarction

ANTONIO ABBATE AND MARCO G. DEL BUONO

INTRODUCTION

Improvement in the acute treatment of myocardial infarction (MI) has made it possible for many patients to survive an initial MI and be exposed to the risk of recurrent MI and/or of heart failure (HF). The acute ischemic and reperfusion myocardial injury (Chapter 24), as well as the acute hemodynamic effects of MI (Chapter 25) and the potential complications of MI (Chapter 26) are described elsewhere in this text (see also Chapter 13). The chronic consequences of MI leading to global structural and functional changes to the heart are summarized in a process known as "*adverse ventricular remodeling.*" The notation of "adverse" refers both to the disadvantageous changes from a hemodynamic standpoint as well as to the negative prognostic implications of the process. This chapter reviews the definition of ventricular remodeling, its macroscopic and microscopic characteristics, and the therapeutic approaches to mitigation of adverse remodeling. The role of stem cell therapy in MI is, however, treated separately (Chapter 22).

DEFINITION OF ADVERSE VENTRICULAR REMODELING

The definition of ventricular (or cardiac) remodeling refers to changes in size, shape, thickness, and elastance of the left and/or right ventricles involving both the infarcted and noninfarcted myocardial segments, and leading to impairment of regional/global systolic contractility and of diastolic function and HF-related morbidity and mortality (Table 30.1, Fig. 30.1). Quantitative evaluation of ventricular remodeling is used to predict clinical outcome, and the therapeutic effects of a drug or device intervention.

Larger infarct size, a greater extent of the initial wall motion abnormalities, and greater initial reduction in global systolic function are all independent predictors of adverse ventricular remodeling (Table 30.2). Ventricular dilatation, indeed, begets further dilatation. As such, in the pre-reperfusion era, adverse ventricular remodeling–defined as a significant increase in left ventricular (LV) end-diastolic volume (relative increase of at least 20%) or a reduction in LV ejection fraction (LVEF, decreasing to <45%)–was seen in more than half of MI survivors. The advent of reperfusion strategies has changed the treatment and revolutionized the natural history of MI (see Chapter 2 and Chapter 13). In the current reperfusion era with primary percutaneous coronary intervention, not only has acute in-hospital MI mortality significantly decreased, but the majority of MI survivors have preserved LV systolic function (at discharge and at 1-year follow-up), and, with this, the 1-year survival rate for MI survivors is generally excellent (>97%). Despite the marked improvement in survival, the incidence of HF after MI remains high.[1] This shifting incidence likely reflects multiple concurrent influences: (1) higher-risk patients with MI are surviving the acute MI yet remain at risk for HF; (2) patients presenting with MI are older than before, they may have survived a prior MI, they may have more comorbidities, and be at risk for preexisting HF; and (3) physicians may have improved recognition of HF symptoms. Of note, not all patients with HF after MI have systolic dysfunction. Indeed, the incidence and prevalence of HF with preserved LVEF (HFpEF), is rising, reflecting that impairment in diastolic function can occur independently of changes in global systolic function, and it is common in the general population, as well as in the post-MI population.[1]

TABLE 30.1 Structural and Functional Changes in Adverse Ventricular Remodeling

Infarct Segment	Edema Scar Formation Wall thinning → Aneurysm formation Hypokinesis→akinesis→dyskinesis
Border Zone Segment	Increase wall stress → Infarct Expansion Hypertrophy
Noninfarct Segments	Hyperkinesis Increased wall stress Hypertrophy
Global Dimensions	Eccentric Hypertrophy Dilatation
Systolic Function	Regional → global dysfunction
Diastolic Function	Impaired relaxation Elevated filling pressures
Dimensions and Function of the Atria	Atrial enlargement/dysfunction Atrial fibrillation
Valvular Function	Functional mitral regurgitation Functional tricuspidal regurgitation
Electrical Function	Conduction block (AV block, BB block) Increased automaticity Re-entry tachycardia Increased sympathetic tone Decreased parasympathetic tone
Systemic Vascular Function	Increase systemic vascular resistance Systemic venous hypertension Reduced venous capacitance
Pulmonary Vascular Function	Pulmonary venous congestion Postcapillary arterial hypertension Reactive precapillary arterial hypertension

AV, Atrioventricular; *BB*, bundle branch.

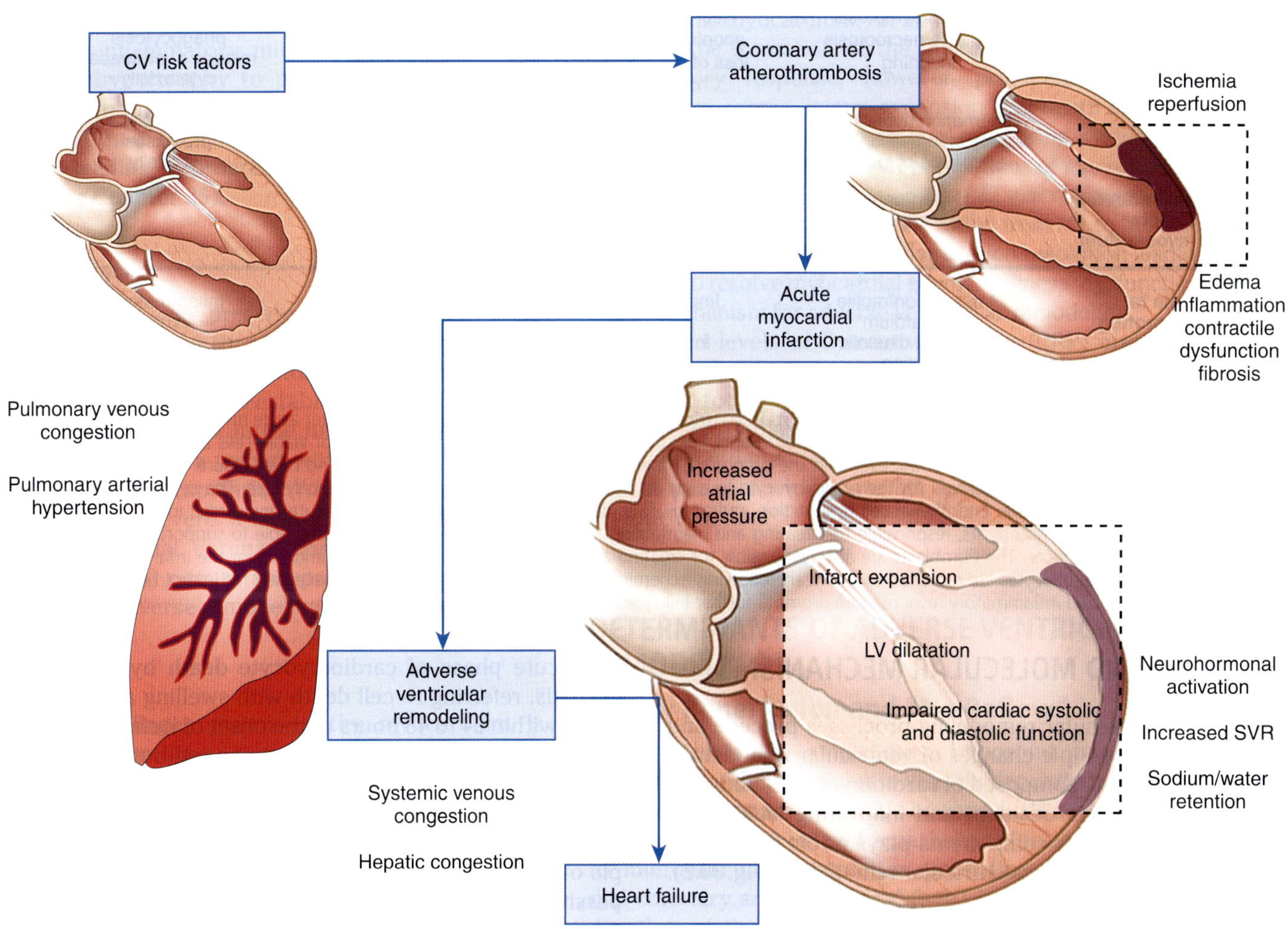

FIG. 30.1 Adverse ventricular remodeling after acute myocardial infarction. Acute coronary artery atherothrombosis is the most common cause of acute myocardial infarction (MI). The ensuing ischemia induces an acute injury to the myocardium and initiates an intense inflammatory response. The acute hemodynamic effects of MI are amplified by structural and functional changes in the infarct border zone and remote myocardium and by a systemic neurohormonal and inflammatory response. Impaired cardiac systolic and diastolic function and increased filling pressures with pulmonary and systemic venous congestion lead to the syndrome of heart failure. *CV*, Cardiovascular; *LV*, left ventricular; *SVR*, systemic vascular resistance.

stimulates ventricular dilatation. Markers of abnormal wall stress, that is, natriuretic peptides, hence predict adverse cardiac remodeling and HF after MI.

Neurohormonal Activation

The translation of results of preclinical studies of neurohormonal blockade to clinical trials in MI has been one of the greatest scientific and clinical successes in cardiology.[4] In experimental models, large unreperfused MI induces an intense activation of the renin-angiotensin-aldosterone and sympathetic adrenergic systems. During acute MI, as a consequence ischemia and injury, contractility drops and filling pressures rise, leading to a reduction in stroke volume and reflex vasoconstriction and tachycardia in the attempt to maintain an adequate perfusion of vital organs. While these mechanisms may be important for the immediate survival during large MI with hypotension, the very same mechanisms promote adverse ventricular remodeling and HF by favoring extension of the infarct size due to increased demand, infarct expansion due to increased wall stress, and compensatory eccentric hypertrophy in response to increased afterload (Fig. 30.6). The larger the infarct size and the initial hemodynamic compromise, the greater the neurohormonal activation and more likely is the progression toward adverse ventricular remodeling. As such, inhibitors of the renin-angiotensin-aldosterone system (RAAS inhibitors such as angiotensin-converting enzyme inhibitors [ACEi], angiotensin receptor blockers [ARB], aldosterone antagonists [AA], or angiotensin receptor neprilysin inhibitors [ARNI]) and beta-adrenergic receptor blockers—all tend to reduce the likelihood and severity of adverse ventricular remodeling and HF-related morbidity and mortality in high-risk MI (i.e., large MI, depressed LVEF, or HF symptoms).

Hibernating Myocardium

LV dysfunction in patients with coronary artery disease is often the consequence of an irreversible loss of viable myocardium following a large MI occasionally in combination with loss of contractility in ischemic, but still viable, myocardium (hibernating myocardium).[12] This condition is most commonly due to a chronically reduced blood flow in a region of myocardium supplied by a stenotic or a collateralized chronically occluded coronary artery. In the context of reduced blood flow, there is an adaptive response characterized by the downregulation of cardiac function and metabolism that serves the purpose of minimizing the occurrence of ischemia and preventing myocardial necrosis. The benefits

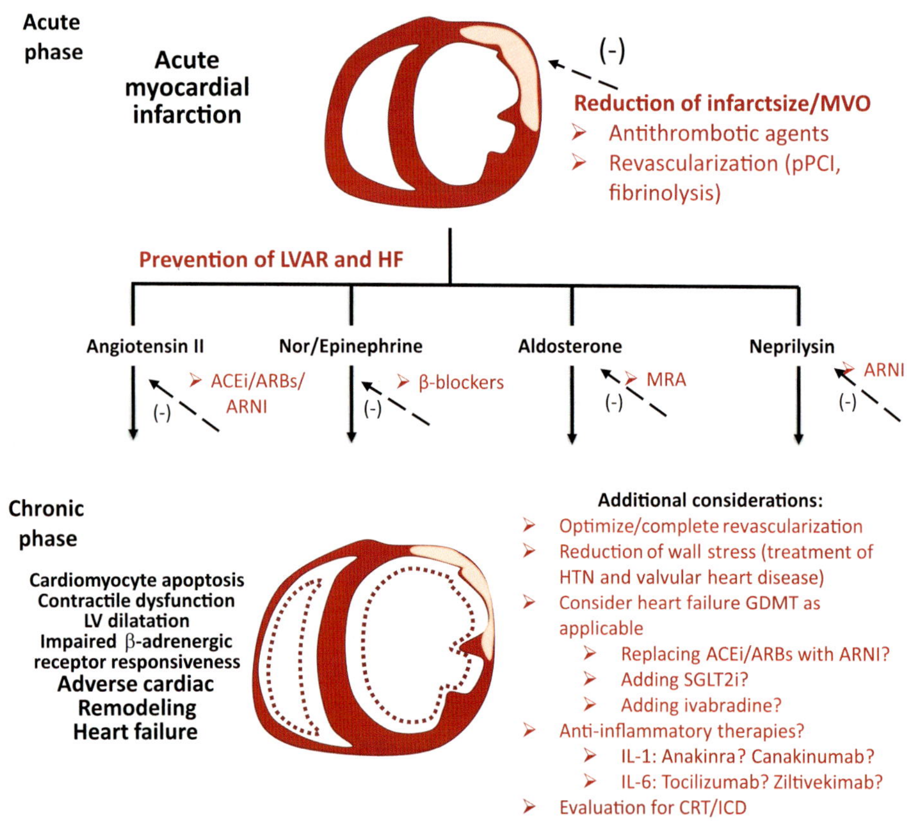

FIG. 30.6 Neurohormonal activation and ventricular remodeling. The initial tissue injury and the hemodynamic consequences initiate a systemic neurohormonal activation characterized by the activation of the renin-angiotensin-aldosterone and the neuroadrenergic sympathetic nervous systems. While these responses have been evolutionary conserved to preserve mean arterial pressure during hypotension, and thus may be, in part, necessary for the immediate survival in patients with acute cardiogenic shock, the same neurohormones promote the adverse ventricular remodeling and heart failure by directly promoting further cardiomyocyte loss and promoting increased cardiac stiffness, and indirectly by promoting sodium and water retention by the kidneys and increasing afterload acting on the systemic vascular resistance. Neurohormonal blockade in patients with acute myocardial infarction is shown to prevent adverse remodeling, prevent heart failure, and prolong survival. *ACE*, Angiotensin converting enzyme; *ARNI*, angiotensin receptor neprilysin inhibitor; *AT2*, angiotensin II; *CRT*, cardiac resynchronization therapy; *GDMT*, guideline-directed medical therapy; *HF*, heart failure; *ICD*, implantable cardiac defibrillator; *IL-1*, Interleukin-1; *IL-6*, Interleukin-6; *LA*, left atrium; *LV*, left ventricle; *LVAR*, left ventricular adverse remodeling; *MVO*, microvascular obstruction; *MRA*, mineral receptor antagonist; *pPCI*, primary percutaneous coronary intervention; *SGLT2i*, sodium-glucose transporter 2 inhibitors.

of myocardial revascularization in patients with hibernating myocardium, ischemic cardiomyopathy, and HF with reduced EF (HFrEF) are discussed elsewhere.

Inflammation

Inflammatory biomarkers predict cardiac rupture, worse ventricular remodeling, HF, and death after MI, independent of other variables such as infarct size or LV systolic function, reflecting that overzealous inflammation promotes further injury and adverse remodeling (see Chapter 8). Toll-like and Nod-like receptors (TLR and NLR) and other sensors are essential to detect microbial infection, activate the inflammasome, and initiate the inflammatory response. The TLR and NLR receptors and the inflammasome are, however, also activated in sterile injury such as acute MI (see also Chapter 4).[2] In the absence of a microbial factor, the inflammatory response is often excessive and inappropriate to the degree of injury and becomes itself a mechanism of disease. Inflammation promotes death (by apoptosis or pyroptosis) in cardiomyocytes, impairs contractile function of the surviving cardiomyocytes, favors destruction of the interstitial tissue leading to reduced tensile strength of the myocardium, and impairs formation of a structured infarct scar (Fig. 30.7).

Cardiac Electrical and Neuroautonomic Remodeling

Parallel to the changes in structure, the electrical function of the cardiomyocyte is also altered and is considered to promote arrhythmias, known as electrical remodeling. Ventricular and atrial arrhythmias are significantly more common in patients with adverse remodeling and HF. The structural changes in heart, primarily dilatation and fibrosis, promote reentry and other arrhythmogenic mechanisms. The heart is innervated by the sympathetic and parasympathetic nervous systems. HF is characterized by an increase in sympathetic tone and a reduction in parasympathetic tone that further aggravates adverse remodeling and HF (see Chapter 28). Vagal nerve stimulation is emerging as a potential treatment against neuroautonomic remodeling.[13] The inflammatory cytokines released during acute injury and healing also promote arrhythmogenesis.

TACKLING ADVERSE VENTRICULAR REMODELING IN CLINICAL PRACTICE

Treatments that have shown to affect adverse ventricular remodeling also reduce late mortality related to MI. It is therefore standard of care to assess for ventricular

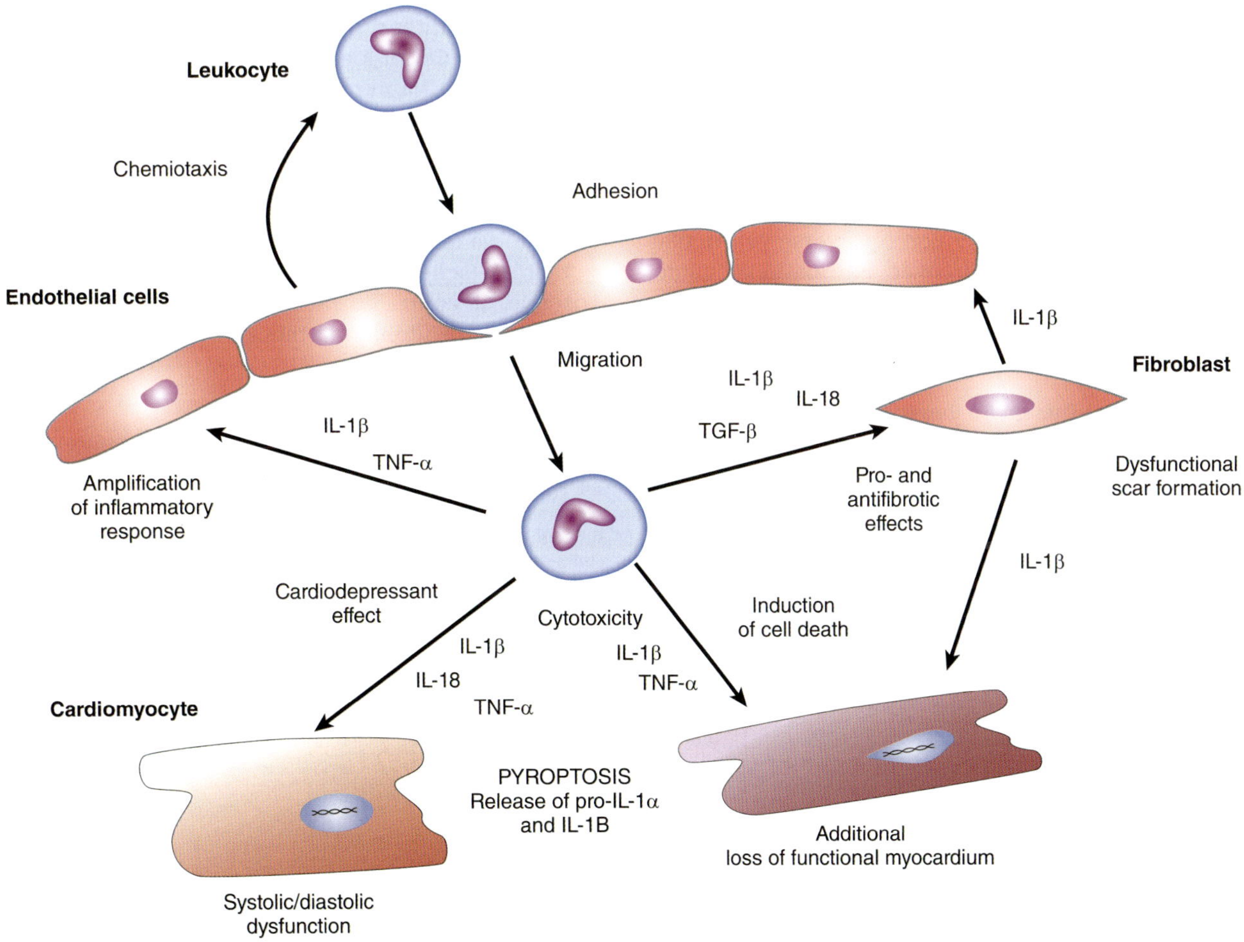

FIG. 30.7 Role of the leukocyte in the post-infarction inflammatory response. Leukocytes are recruited to the infarct area through the release of chemokines and the expression of adhesion molecules by the endothelial cells. Activated leukocytes amplify the inflammatory response and promote further myocardial injury and dysfunction through the release of pro-inflammatory cytokines (Interleukin-1β [IL-1β], Interleukin-18 [IL-18], Tumor Necrosis Factor-α [TNF-α], and Transforming Growth Factor-β [TGF-β]) and through direct cytotoxicity.

remodeling during the initial hospitalization in patients with acute MI and then again within 3–6 months to identify high-risk subjects (see Chapters 13 and 30).

Delayed Reperfusion and the "Open Artery Hypothesis"

The "open artery hypothesis" postulates that, compared with no reperfusion, delayed reperfusion of the infarct-related artery provides a benefit that is independent of infarct sparing and, at least in part, time-independent. This hypothesis was largely based on longitudinal analysis of reperfusion trials. The largest clinical trial randomizing >2000 patients who were asymptomatic 3 to 21 days after MI to PCI or medical therapy, however, failed to show any clinical advantage of late revascularization of a totally occluded artery. Smaller trials showed a reduction in final infarct size when PCI was performed between 13 and 48 hours. A meta-analysis of 5 studies, including an echocardiographic substudy of the largest trial, also showed a beneficial effect of late revascularization of a totally occluded artery on LV remodeling. The benefits of late revascularization were enhanced when the meta-analysis included studies enrolling also patients with significant yet nontotally occlusive disease of the infarct-related artery (Fig. 30.3). As such, late PCI in patients with STEMI should be considered only in patients presenting 13 to 48 hours after symptom onset, and in selected patients who are symptomatic with angina, heart failure, arrhythmias, or with evidence of myocardial viability after 48 hours.[11]

Guideline-Recommended Medical Therapy

Timely reperfusion during MI is the mainstay of therapy and the first step in mitigating infarct size and the likelihood of adverse remodeling. Adjunctive medical therapy is also indicated for the prevention of adverse ventricular remodeling (Table 30.3). Moreover, international guidelines recommend stratification of the patients with MI for the risk of HF.[14–16]

RAAS Inhibitors: Research in animals with MI has shown activation of systemic and regional activation of the renin-angiotensin system, and the benefits of ACEi. The benefits of remodeling and HF were reproduced in phase II and III clinical trials and contributed to a significant reduction in MI mortality in the pre-reperfusion era. However, the benefits accrued by the different RAAS inhibitors are largely limited to those patients already showing signs of adverse remodeling prior to initiation of therapy (i.e., LV systolic dysfunction or enlargement). Similar benefits were seen with ACEi, ARB, AA, and ARNI. Eplerenone reduced LV adverse remodeling and prevented major adverse cardiac events in patients with STEMI with reduced HFrEF or diabetes,[17] whereas spironolactone reduced mortality in patients with symptomatic HF with reduced EF and reduced hospitalizations in patients with HF with preserved EF. When compared with ramipril, sacubitril-valsartan was as effective, or more, in preventing adverse clinical outcomes in patients with large MI and high risk for HF[18] and showed additional beneficial effects on LV size and diastolic function.[19] Sacubitril-valsartan was also associated with favorable outcomes in patients with HF and preserved EF.[20]

With the advent of prompt reperfusion, infarct size tends to be smaller and the initial hemodynamic effects less pronounced. The efficacy of the RAAS inhibitors in asymptomatic patients with reperfused MI and preserved LV systolic function is not established, and thus treatment with RAAS inhibitors is recommended for those patients with MI and either reduced global systolic function, symptoms of HF, anterior location of ST-segment elevation MI, or diabetes (see Chapter 25).[14–16]

Beta-Blockers: Beta-adrenergic blockers are recommended to be started at low doses orally in all patients with MI, with particular emphasis on those with MI complicated by LVEF ≤40% and/or HF. Intravenous beta-blockers are generally reserved for patients with ongoing refractory ischemia, hypertension, or arrhythmias, in the absence of contraindications. Systematic use of higher doses of beta-adrenergic blockers early during MI is not

TABLE 30.3 Medical Therapy to Prevent or Treat Adverse Ventricular Remodeling

MEDICATION	RECOMMENDATIONS FOR PATIENTS WITH ACUTE MI (IN ABSENCE OF CONTRAINDICATIONS)
Beta-adrenergic receptor blocker(s)	• Oral beta-adrenergic receptor blockers in all patients without contraindications (Class IIa, LOE B) • Oral beta-adrenergic receptor blockers in patients with systolic dysfunction or HFrEF (LVEF <40%) (Class I, LOE A) • Intravenous beta-blockers at the time of presentation to patients with STEMI and no contraindications to their use who are hypertensive or have ongoing ischemia (Class IIa, LOE B)
Angiotensin-converting enzyme (ACE) inhibitor(s)	• All patients (Class IIa, LOE A) • Symptomatic heart failure, LV dysfunction (LVEF <40%), diabetes or anterior location (Class I, LOE A)
Angiotensin receptor blocker(s)	As an alternative to ACE inhibitor(s) (Class I, LOE B)
Angiotensin receptor neprylisin inhibitor (sacubitril/valsartan)	Preferred to ACE inhibitor(s) if: • Symptomatic heart failure and LVEF <40% (Class I, LOE A) • Symptomatic heart failure and LVEF ≥40% (Class II, LOE A)
Aldosterone antagonists (epleronone, finerenone and spironolactone)	In addition to ACE inhibitor(s) if LVEF <40% and: • Symptomatic heart failure (Class I, LOE B) • Diabetes mellitus (Class I, LOE B)
Sodium-glucose (co)transporter 2 (SGLT2) inhibitors (e.g., empagliflozin, dapagliflozin)	In addition to ACE inhibitor(s) and beta-adrenergic blockers: • Symptomatic heart failure, independent of LVEF (Class I, LOE B) • Diabetes mellitus (Class I, LOE B)

LOE, Level of evidence.

recommended as it increases the risk of hypotension and cardiogenic shock.

Sodium-glucose cotransporter 2 inhibitors (SGLT2i): Clinical data related to the use of SGLT2i in patients with MI is limited. SGLT2i significantly reduced the risk of HF hospitalization and cardiovascular death in patients with HF with both reduced and preserved EF. Pre-clinical and clinical data with SGLT2i show a favorable effect on cardiac remodeling.[21–23] In a small randomized clinical trial of empagliflozin initiated within 72 hours after an MI, empagliflozin led to a greater reduction in NTproBNP levels and improved LV remodeling and diastolic function compared to placebo.[22] Two larger randomized clinical trials (clinicaltrials.gov NCT04509674 and NCT04564742) are ongoing to evaluate the effects of SGLT2i on hard clinical outcomes in patients with MI who are at risk of developing HF.

Soluble Guanylate Cyclase Receptor Stimulator: Vericiguat, a novel soluble guanylate cyclase stimulator, reduced the incidence of cardiovascular death or hospitalization for HF in a population of high-risk patients with HFrEF who had recently been hospitalized or received intravenous diuretic therapy.[24] However, there are no clinical data related to the use of vericiguat in patients with MI.

ONGOING CLINICAL AND TRANSLATIONAL RESEARCH

Anti-Inflammatory Therapies

Despite a wealth of preclinical research, many therapeutic attempts aimed at reducing inflammation in acute MI during the past several decades have failed to translate to the clinical setting due to concerns related to impaired healing, increased risk of cardiac rupture, or lack of additional benefit in addition to standard therapies (Table 30.4). While there are no targeted anti-inflammatory therapies proven to prevent or treat adverse LV remodeling to date, the field is an object of intense research.[25]

Non-specific Anti-Inflammatory Agents

Steroids: The clinical trials of glucocorticoids in patients with MI have shown conflicting results. Early concerns regarding impaired infarct healing in the pre-reperfusion era are not supported by the more recent clinical trials, and it is either only seen in some subset of patients (i.e., long-term steroid use, first MI, transmural MI without reperfusion) or is more of a perceived rather than a real effect. However, glucocorticoids also have an effect on water retention, edema, hyperglycemia, and muscular atrophy. Therefore, current guidelines advise against the use of glucocorticoids in MI.

Nonsteroidal anti-inflammatory drugs (NSAID): Observational studies in MI in the pre-reperfusion era showed an association between NSAID use, worse clinical outcomes, and increased risk of ventricular rupture. NSAID also led to a significant increase in blood pressure values, reduced renal blood flow, increased platelet aggregation, and increased risk of gastrointestinal bleeding. Current clinical guidelines recommend against NSAID treatment, and actively recommend NSAID discontinuation at the time STEMI is indicated.

Inhibition of Targeted Inflammatory Processes

Leukocyte Adhesion and Migration

Clinical trials blocking the key integrins, such as CD11, CD18, and P-selectin, failed to show a clear improvement in infarct healing or clinical outcomes.25 A possible explanation for negative results observed with these agents is that the duration of ischemia observed in trials is longer than

TABLE 30.4 Overview of Clinical Trials with Anti-Inflammatory Therapies

INTERVENTION	PRECLINICAL RESEARCH	PHASE II CLINICAL TRIALS	PHASE III CLINICAL TRIALS	NOTES/COMMENTS
Colchicine	Favorable results in animal models of myocardial ischemia-reperfusion injury.	Phase II clinical trials, showed inconsistent efficacy in acute MI.	Phase III trials showed significant reduction in major adverse cardiac and cerebral events in recent MI and stable CAD.	Colchicine is clinically available for the treatment and acute and chronic inflammatory disease. Low-dose colchicine (0.5 mg once daily) may be considered to reduce cardiovascular risk (Class IIB, LOA A).
Glucorticoids (methylprednisolone, prednisone, hydrocortisone)	Mixed results depending on ischemic model and species used.	Conflicting results of the many phase II clinical trials.	No large phase III trial completed Meta-analysis of phase II trials shows no harm and a trend toward a small beneficial effect in terms of recurrent MI.	Glucocorticoids have many undesired effects such as sodium/ volume retention, hyperglycemia, impaired healing.
Integrin-targeted blockers (recombinant human antibody against CD18, Hu23F2G, inclacumab)	Favorable results in animal models of myocardial ischemia-reperfusion injury.	Phase II clinical trials, including between 394 and 544 patients each, showed no beneficial effects or effects inconsistent across endpoints.	None available.	None of these drugs are currently used in clinical practice.
Inhibitors of the complement cascade (pexelizumab)	Favorable results in animal models of myocardial ischemia-reperfusion injury.	Phase II clinical trial of pexelimumab failed to reduce infarct size but reduced 90-day mortality.	Phase III clinical failed to confirm the beneficial effects of pexelizumab.	Not approved for clinical practice.

TABLE 30.4 Overview of Clinical Trials with Anti-Inflammatory Therapies—Cont'd

INTERVENTION	PRECLINICAL RESEARCH	PHASE II CLINICAL TRIALS	PHASE III CLINICAL TRIALS	NOTES/COMMENTS
Interleukin-1 blockers (anakinra, canakinumab)	Favorable results in animal models of myocardial ischemia-reperfusion and of ischemic cardiomyopathy without reperfusion.	Three small studies with anakinra showed inhibition of the acute inflammatory response and reduction of heart failure-related events after ST-segment elevation MI. Canakinumab showed a significant reduction of CRP in stable patients with CAD.	Canakinuman significantly prevented major adverse cardiac events and heart failure-related events in patients with prior MI.	Anakinra and canakinumab are clinically available for the treatment of rheumatologic diseases. Anakinra is also used to treat severe COVID-19 pneumonia. Anakinra is also in the treatment of pericarditis refractory to colchicine. Neither anakinra nor canakinumab is approved for the treatment of MI.
Interleukin-6 blockers (tocilizumab, ziltevekimab)	Favorable results in animal models of myocardial ischemia-reperfusion.	A pilot study of tocilizumab showed a reduction in infarct size in patients with ST-segment elevation MI. Ziltevekimab showed a significant reduction of CRP in stable patients with CAD.	A phase III clinical trial of ziltevekimab in patients with established vascular disease is ongoing.	Tocilizumab is clinically available and clinically utilized across a wide range of rheumatologic diseases. Tocilizumab is also used to treat severe COVID-19 pneumonia. Ziltevekimab is not clinically available. Neither tocilizumab nor ziltevekimab are approved for the treatment of MI.
Nonsteroidal anti-inflammatory drugs - NSAIDs (diclofenac, ibuprofen, aspirin [high dose])	Mixed results depending on ischemic model and species used.	Conflicting results of the many phase II clinical trials.	None available.	NSAIDs increase risk of gastro-intestinal bleeding, increase blood pressure, and increase risk of thrombotic events.
Metalloproteinase inhibitors (PG-116800, doxycycline)	Favorable results in animal models of myocardial ischemia-reperfusion and of ischemic cardiomyopathy without reperfusion.	Doxycycline showed a significant improvement in ventricular remodeling vs. placebo at 6 months, in patients with ST-segment elevation MI and LVEF <40%.	None available.	Doxycycline is widely available and has an established safety profile.
p38 MAPK inhibitor (losmapimod)	Favorable results in animal models of myocardial ischemia-reperfusion.	A phase II study showed beneficial effects of losmapimod on inflammatory biomarkers in patients with non-ST-segment elevation MI undergoing PCI.	A phase III clinical trial of losmapimod in patients with ST-segment and non-ST-segement elevation MI showed no significant effect on major adverse events. In patients with ST-segment elevation MI, favorable effects on inflammatory biomarkers and NT-proBNP were seen ongoing.	Losmapimod is not clinically available.

LVEF, Left ventricular ejection fraction; *MI*, myocardial infarction.

that in experimental models of ischemia-reperfusion, leading to irreversible endothelial cell barrier damage and thus limiting the efficacy of the proposed intervention. Colchicine is a microtubule assembly inhibitor that interferes with the migration of leukocytes and with the formation of the inflammasome. A benefit of colchicine in limiting myocardial injury during MI has been seen in some, but not all, clinical studies. Long-term treatment with colchicine in patients with recent MI[26] or chronic ischemic heart disease,[27] on the other hand, significantly reduced the risk of major adverse cardiovascular events compared with placebo, mostly due to a reduction in recurrent MI or need for revascularization.[28]

Complement Cascade

Despite promising preclinical research with complement inhibitors, favorable safety/tolerability studies, and positive signals from phase II studies, the phase III clinical trials with complement cascade inhibitors, pexelizumab, failed to show the proposed clinical benefit.[25]

Cytokine-Targeted Therapies

More recent strategies aimed at selectively blocking cytokines acting upstream in the cascade rather than globally suppressing the response downstream have shown some promising results in preclinical research and pilot clinical trials.[27] IL-1β is an apical cytokine in the cascade, released at the site of injury following activation of the inflammasome and amplifying the local and systemic inflammatory response.[28] Three phase II clinical trials (VCU-ART studies) have shown acceptable safety/tolerability of IL-1 blockade with anakinra, recombinant IL-1 receptor antagonist, for 14 days during ST-segment elevation MI, associated with a significant reduction in acute inflammatory response and prevention of new-onset HF and HF-related hospitalizations.[29] The CANTOS trial, a large phase III secondary prevention clinical trial of IL-1β blockade with canakimumab in patients with prior MI showed a significant reduction in recurrent atherothrombotic events and in HF-related hospitalizations and deaths.[30]

IL-6 is a secondary cytokine synthesized and released by mononuclear cells in response to IL-1β and other stimuli, and responsible for the amplification of the inflammatory response (acute phase reaction) and increasing the thrombogenicity of the blood.[30] Tocilizumab, an antibody directed against the IL-6 receptor has shown to increase myocardial salvage in preclinical MI models and in phase II trials of patients with reperfused STEMI. A large phase III cardiovascular outcome trial is ongoing with ziltevekimab, an antibody against IL-6, and shown to significantly reduce CRP with an acceptable safety profile in a phase II trial.[31]

Tumor necrosis factor (TNF) is upregulated early in MI, promoting cardiac dysfunction. Blockade of the TNF-α system in experimental MI, however, led to conflicting results. A small clinical trial with etanercept, a TNF-α-blocker acting as a circulating trap, in 26 patients with acute MI showed reduced neutrophil count and plasma IL-6 concentrations at 24 hours but unexpectedly increased platelet-monocyte aggregation.[25] TNF blockers (etanercept and infliximab) have had disappointing results in patients with chronic HF, with a dose-dependent increase in adverse cardiac events. Therefore, TNF-blocking drugs are considered contraindicated in patients with or at risk of HF.[25]

Losmapimod

Losmapimod is a small molecule inhibiting p38 mitogen-activated protein kinase MAPK downstream of IL-1, IL-6, and other cytokines. In a large phase III trial including patients with MI, losmapimod failed to reduce major adverse cardiac events. A secondary analysis stratifying by type of MI showed that in patients with ST-segment elevation MI, losmapimod significantly attenuated the inflammatory response and lowered levels of NT-proBNP as compared to patients treated with placebo.[32]

Metalloproteinases

Preclinical research suggested that inhibition of metalloproteinases (MMPs) MMP-2 and -9 would lead to more favorable remodeling and prevent HF. Clinical trials with a targeted MMP inhibitor however failed to show benefits in a phase II clinical trial, whereas doxycycline, a tetracycline antimicrobial, which also inhibits MMP-2 and -9, was shown in phase II clinical trial to reduce ventricular dilation at 6 months in patients with ST-segment elevation MI and LV systolic dysfunction.[33]

Noncoding RNA

Noncoding RNAs play a role in regulating cardiac remodeling in HF and post-MI. miR-132 promotes the transition from acute inflammation to proliferating wound healing. The use of specific antisense inhibitors to silence miR-132, CDR132L, in vivo has demonstrated improvement in adverse myocardial remodeling in preclinical model. CDR132L was shown to be tolerated in phase I and is now being investigated in a phase II randomized, double-blind study involving patients with reduced LVEF (≤45%) following MI.[34]

Growth Factors

Despite a significant number of preclinical studies showing beneficial effects of erythropoietin (EPO) and derivatives, granulocyte colony-stimulating factor (G-CSF), and granulocyte monocyte colony-stimulating factor (GM-CSF), the results of clinical trials in patients in ST-segment elevation MI are not sufficient to justify their use in clinical practice (Table 30.5). To date, therefore, there are no targeted growth factor therapies proven to prevent or treat adverse LV remodeling in large randomized clinical trials.

TABLE 30.5 Overview of Clinical Trials with Growth Factors

INTERVENTION	PRECLINICAL RESEARCH	PHASE II CLINICAL TRIALS	PHASE III CLINICAL TRIALS	NOTES/COMMENTS
Erythropoietin (EPO)	Favorable results in animal models of myocardial ischemia-reperfusion and of ischemic cardiomyopathy without reperfusion.	Conflicting results of the phase II clinical trials.	Conflicting results of phase III clinical trials.	Concerns raised regarding thrombotic complications.
Granulocyte colony-stimulating factor (G-CSF)	Favorable results in animal models of myocardial ischemia-reperfusion and of ischemic cardiomyopathy without reperfusion.	Favorable results of multiple phase II clinical trials.	There have been no large phase III clinical trials. A meta-analysis of all studies showed no significant effects on clinical endpoints and a small potential benefit on ventricular remodeling.	G-CSF is clinically used to treat febrile neutropenia, and as an adjunct to cancer chemotherapy regimens.
Granulocyte monocyte colony-stimulating factor (GM-CSF)	Favorable results in animal models of myocardial ischemia-reperfusion and of ischemic cardiomyopathy without reperfusion.	One pilot clinical trial in patients with ST-segment elevation MI not eligible for early reperfusion showed promising results in terms of remodeling and outcomes.	None available.	GM-CSF is clinically used to treat febrile neutropenia and as an adjunct to cancer chemotherapy regimens.

MI, Myocardial infarction.

known as efferocytosis, can impair healing and function of the infarcted myocardium in mice.[26] This resident subset of mononuclear phagocytes exhibits functions that could contribute to myocardial healing by formation of granulation tissue and the extracellular matrix. In particular, this less inflammatory subset of mononuclear phagocytes has relatively less proteolytic potential, but it produces transforming growth factor-β (TGF-β), which is a strong stimulus to extracellular matrix gene expression and an inhibitor of inflammation. These reparative macrophages, which in mice arise from the "classical" pro-inflammatory Ly6c monocytes, also secrete angiogenic molecules such as vascular endothelial growth factor VEGF), a mediator implicated in neo-angiogenesis, a characteristic of granulation tissue (Table 32.2 and Fig. 32.4). [20] Integrins (e.g. α5) on the surface of macrophages can mediate crosstalk with the extracellular matrix mediated eliciting proangiogenic mediators such as VEGF A.[27] Fig. 32.5 depicts postulated functions of proinflammatory monocytes in the early phase of myocardial ischemic injury (see Fig. 32.5A) and the less inflammatory, reparative mononuclear phagocytes in the latter phase (see Fig. 32.5B). In mice, extreme hypercholesterolemia impairs healing of MI, which is likely related to a striking proinflammatory monocytosis.[25,28] Adaptive immunity may also modulate the function of mononuclear phagocytes in MI. Regulatory T cells, a subset that elaborates TGF-β, interleukin (IL)-10, and IL-13, can slant the macrophage population in experimental MI in mice toward a reparative/pro-resolving palette of functions that may foster healing and improve survival.[29]

Recruited Monocyte Origins in Myocardial Infarction

Because of the rapid appearance of monocytes recruited to the infarcting myocardium, joining the resident subset, further studies sought to delineate the origin of these cells. These investigations disclosed the existence in mice of a preformed pool of proinflammatory monocytes in the subcapsular region of the red pulp of the spleen.[30] Following coronary artery ligation, intravital microscopic and cell-tracking studies showed the traversal of these proinflammatory monocytes from the spleen to the infarcting myocardium. Thus, the spleen warehouses a set of monocytes poised to respond to tissue injury on an emergency basis. Subsequent studies indicated that in the mouse spleen, extramedullary hematopoiesis can furnish and replenish this pool of proinflammatory monocytes that provide "early responders" to acutely injured tissues such as the infarcting myocardium.[31]

Further investigation identified specific hematopoietic factors that regulate this extramedullary hematopoiesis. Retention of hematopoietic progenitors in the spleen rely on the interaction of VLA-4 with vascular cell adhesion molecule-1 (VCAM-1), which is expressed by CD169⁺ splenic macrophages. Ablation of these cells, or silencing of VCAM-1 using in vivo RNAi, leads to a loss of progenitor cells from the spleen.[32] In addition, post-MI splenic myelopoiesis depends on IL-1β. A subpopulation of B lymphocytes, known as innate response activator B cells, elaborate the hematopoietic growth factors, such as granulocyte-monocyte colony stimulating factor, that engender extramedullary hematopoiesis in the context

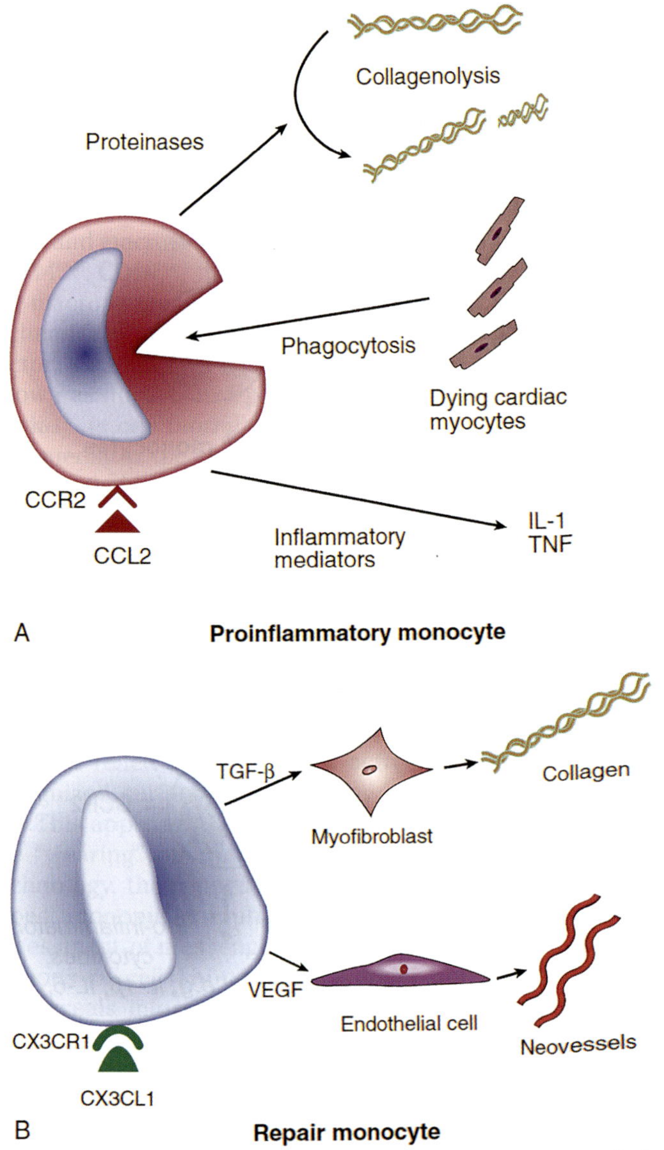

FIG. 32.5 Subtypes of mononuclear phagocytes exhibit distinct functional palettes in the infarcting myocardium. (A) A proinflammatory monocyte (marked by high levels of Ly-6c in mice and high levels of CD14 with low levels of CD16 in humans). These cells possess high phagocytic capacity that permits them to clear the debris of dead and dying cells, acting as a "demolition" crew following acute ischemic myocardial injury. These cells also produce hydrolytic enzymes at high concentrations that permit them to degrade macromolecules released by dead or dying cells and also to remodel the extracellular matrix to prepare the way for production of a provisional extracellular matrix, and ultimately, scar formation. **(B)** A less inflammatory monocyte characterized in particular by high concentrations of transforming growth factor (TGF-β), which is a potent stimulus to extracellular matrix synthesis needed for repair and scar formation. These less inflammatory cells also elaborate angiogenic mediators, such vascular endothelial growth factor (VEGF), that promote the formation of new microvessels. Fibrosis and microvascularization characterize granulation tissue, long recognized as part of the healing response of injured tissues. The appropriate balance between the proinflammatory and reparative subset of mononuclear phagocytes can influence both the structure and function of the myocardium following coronary occlusion and critically modulate the healing process. *IL*, Interleukin; *TNF*, tumor necrosis factor.

of atherosclerosis, and possibly in MI as well.[20] Cytokines unleashed during tissue injury (e.g., IL-1β) increase bone marrow hematopoietic stem cell proliferation after coronary artery ligation in mice by direct actions on hematopoietic cells and by modulating the microenvironment in

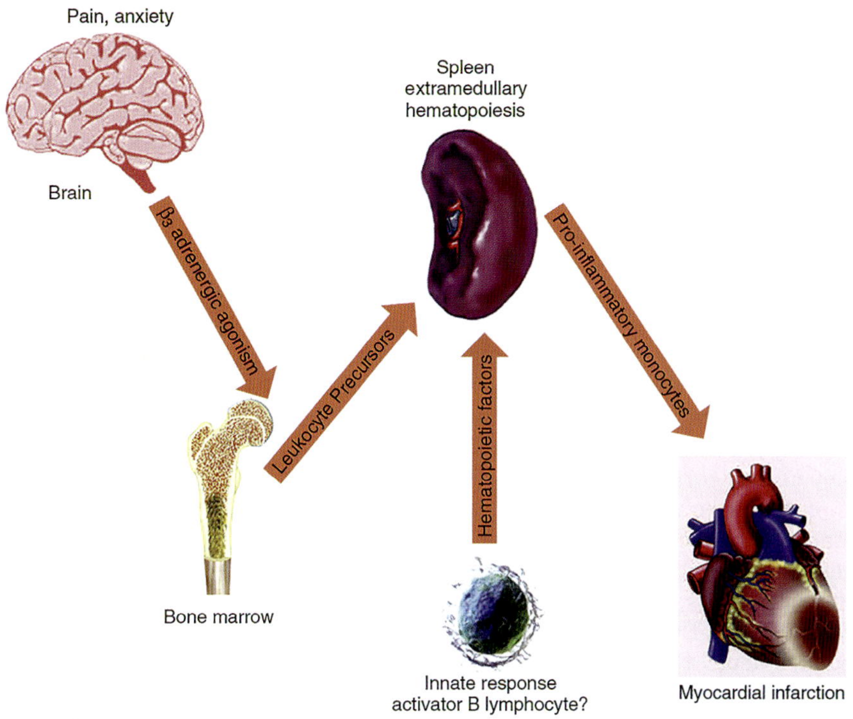

FIG. 32.6 Activation of extra cardiac organs following myocardial infarction: a cardio-spleno-neuro-medullary network. Coronary ligation elicits a hyperadrenergic state caused by activation of the sympathetic nervous system in response to pain and hemodynamic alterations. β3-adrenergic signaling can mobilize myeloid precursor cells from a bone marrow niche to the spleen where they can multiply in response to hematopoietic growth factors, some of which arise from innate response activator B cells. The spleen, in an angiotensin II–dependent manner in mice, can rapidly mobilize proinflammatory monocytes from a preformed pool to migrate to injured tissues (e.g., the infarcting myocardium) and engage in a first phase of tissue remodeling that may help to restore homeostasis. The myeloid precursor cells mobilized from bone marrow provide the precursors of mature leukocytes in the spleen where they undergo expansion by extramedullary hematopoiesis. Hematopoietic growth factors that promote the expansion of leukocyte populations may derive in part from innate response activator B cells.

the bone marrow niche.[33] Myeloid precursor cells that bear the chemokine receptor CCR2 appear to be pivotal to the development of macrophages in mouse MI that participate in tissue healing and influence the development of heart failure post-MI.[34]

Efforts to unravel further layers of the control of emergency leukopoiesis following coronary artery ligation in mice focused on the recruitment of precursors of the myeloid cells from niches in the bone marrow. The proinflammatory cytokine IL-6, produced by endothelial cells in the bone marrow niche can boost hematopoiesis.[35] IL-6, downstream from IL-1, rises as part of the inflammatory response to tissue injury during MI. Activation of the sympathetic nervous system following coronary artery occlusion can spur mobilization of these progenitors of myeloid cells from the bone marrow.[36] The results implicated β_3 adrenergic activation of bone marrow niche cells as a stimulus that activates these precursors of leukocytes found in the myocardium during ischemic injury and the bone marrow. These studies elucidated a novel neuro-splenic-myocardial axis that operates during MI in mice (Fig. 32.6).

"Cardiosplenic" Axis in Humans

Do these observations in mice relate to MI in humans? Although indirect, preliminary observations support the translatability of these concepts derived from mouse experiments to humans who sustain an MI.[37] The spleens of MI patients contain more cells bearing markers of myeloid precursors (C-kit positive) that also manifest markers of mitosis (Ki67).[36] These observations indicate increased extramedullary hematopoiesis in the spleen of humans who have experienced MI. Humans hospitalized for acute MI who received treatment with β-adrenergic blocking agents before their event (in a nonrandomized allocation) had lower total leukocyte and monocyte counts in peripheral blood in a post hoc analysis. This observation, although subject to several types of confounding factors, supports a link between β-adrenergic signaling and leukocyte biology in humans.[36]

Studies of psychological stress produced experimentally both in mice and in medical residents subjected to emotional stress because of rotations in intensive care units showed increased peripheral leukocyte counts, and in the case of mice, leukopoiesis.[38] Human observations support the operation of a "cardiosplenic" axis in patients who experienced an acute MI.[39] During MI, macrophage metabolism can shift towards increased glycolysis, consuming glucose.[40] Using uptake of the glucose analog fluorodeoxyglucose-18 (^{18}F-FDG) can serve as a clinically applicable marker of inflammatory activation, reflecting this metabolic shift. Patients (n = 22) with an ACS and an equal number of sex-matched control subjects without ACS, but who had atherosclerotic disease, underwent positron emission tomography scanning to assess ^{18}F-FDG uptake. The spleens of ACS patients displayed a statistically significant increase in the ^{18}F-FDG signal compared with the control subjects (P = .03). These results corroborated the concept of altered splenic metabolic activity in patients with ACS. These investigators further retrospectively studied a cohort of approximately 500 patients who underwent ^{18}F-FDG imaging for various clinical indications. The investigators dichotomized this cohort into those who had splenic uptake of ^{18}F-FDG above or below the median. The analysis showed a striking and statistically significant increase in cardiovascular events in individuals who exhibited ^{18}F-FDG uptake above the median ($P = .002$). In this cohort, which was followed up for cardiovascular events, the ^{18}F-FDG uptake in various arteries correlated well with splenic uptake of ^{18}F-FDG. These findings supported the relationship between metabolic activity in the spleen and in arteries. These results, taken together, indicated an altered metabolism associated with macrophage activation, or perhaps even monocyte production, in the spleens of patients with ACS. They further corroborated the potential clinical implications of metabolic activity in the spleen of ACS patients. Further analyses indicated that messenger RNAs that encode several inflammation-related genes in the peripheral leukocytes of patients with ACS correlated significantly with the uptake of ^{18}F-FDG in the spleen. The patients with above-median splenic ^{18}F-FDG uptake had significantly more cardiovascular events during follow-up in a post hoc analysis.

This ensemble of results supports the notion that MI elicits a systemic inflammatory response and can alter functions of remote organs (e.g., the spleen) that participate in the regulation of inflammation and immunity. The interruption of renin-angiotensin signaling by administration of angiotensin-converting enzyme inhibitors limits the recruitment of proinflammatory monocytes from the spleen to the infarcting myocardium in mice.[41] Thus, the observations that support the operation of a cardiosplenic axis in humans provide novel insight into the mechanisms by which existing therapies might modify MI. Similarly, some of the benefits observed in survivors of MI because of the administration of β-adrenergic blocking agents might result from modulation of leukopoiesis and the flux of inflammatory cells, as indicated by the animal experiments.

Areas of Ongoing Investigation

This blossoming of new knowledge regarding the roles of leukocytes in the healing of MI and previously unsuspected links between the central nervous system, the bone marrow, the spleen, and the ischemic myocardium represents a panel of new potential therapeutic targets for modifying outcomes after MI beyond restoration of blood flow or interventions to reduce the oxygen requirements of the myocardium. Initial forays into modifying the functions of leukocytes using nanoparticles that target receptors involved in recruiting proinflammatory subsets of leukocytes (the chemokine receptor CCR2) provide experimental validation of the concept that targeting leukocyte functions following MI might mitigate ischemic injury.[41]

Myocardial Infarction Begets Myocardial Infarction

We know that recurrent MIs cluster in the first months following an index acute coronary syndrome. Experimental work has shed some mechanistic insight into this well documented clinical observation. MI in mice stimulates hematopoiesis that can augment recruitment of inflammatory leukocytes to existing atherosclerotic plaques boosting their local inflammatory activity and thus predisposing to plague disruption and another acute coronary syndrome.[36] Moreover, evidence is emerging that "trained" immunity may operate following MI. Bone marrow transfer experiments in mice support the concept that epigenetic changes wrought by an initial MI can augment atherosclerosis again predisposing to a recurrent event.[42] Interrupting sympathetic nervous system signaling can mute these responses to an initial acute coronary syndrome.

SUMMARY

In contrast to the venerable recognition of angina pectoris, the elucidation of the relationship between acute MI and coronary artery disease came about only a century ago. The initial fatalistic view that MI immediately produced irreversible injury gave way to an era of a more nuanced understanding of the pathophysiology of MI that has transformed clinical care by use of pharmacologic and mechanical interventions, most of which target improvements in the balance of oxygen supply and demand.

We have now entered a new area of understanding of the biological responses of the myocardium itself, and particularly the inflammatory cells, which are predominantly myeloid cells that populate the evolving infarct and likely critically influence the extent of tissue injury and the quantity and quality of myocardial healing. Harnessing these novel insights in the development of new therapies may help improve further outcomes in patients who have survived MIs.[37] In particular, because of advances in revascularization strategies and management of arrhythmias, more patients survive MIs. Yet, chronic impairment of ventricular function promotes the development of heart failure caused by ischemic cardiomyopathy. Perhaps manipulation of the inflammatory response during acute MI could help forestall the development of left ventricular dysfunction that fuels the growing epidemic of heart failure confronted by contemporary cardiology.

ACKNOWLEDGMENT

The authors thank Drs. R. N. Mitchell and A.J. Connolly for permission to adapt Fig. 12.13 and Table 12.5 from Chapter 12 of *Pathologic Basis of Disease* (10th Edition).

CLASSIC REFERENCES

Braunwald E. Thirteenth Bowditch lecture. The determinants of myocardial oxygen consumption. *Physiologist*. 1969;12:65–93.

Fye WB. *Classic papers on coronary thrombosis and myocardial infarction*. Birmingham, AL: The Classics of Cardiology Library; 1991.

Heberden W: *Commentaries on the history and cure of diseases*, London, 1802, Printed for T. Payne, Mews-Gate.

Herrick J. Certain clinical features of sudden obstruction of the coronary arteries. *Transactions of the American Association of Physicians*. 1912;27:100–116.

Herrick JB. *A Short History of Cardiology*. Springfield, MA: Charles C. Thomas; 1942.

Leibowitz J. *The history of coronary heart disease*. Berkeley, CA: University of California Press; 1970.

Levine SA. *Coronary thrombosis: its various clinical features*. Baltimore: The Williams & Wilkins Company; 1929.

Obrastzow WP, Straschesko ND. Zur Kenntnis der Thrombose der Koronararterien des Herzens. *Z Klin Med*. 1910;71:116–132.

Warren J. Remarks on angina pectoris. *New England Journal of Medicine and Surgery*. 1812;1:1–11.

REFERENCES

1. Roberts W. Editorial: Coronary thrombosis and fatal myocardial ischemia. *Circulation*. 1974;49(1):1–3.
2. Braunwald E. 50th anniversary historical article. Myocardial oxygen consumption: the quest for its determinants and some clinical fallout. *J Am Coll Cardiol*. 1999;34(5):1365–1368.
3. Braunwald E, Epstein SE, Glick G, Wechsler AS, Braunwald NS. Relief of angina pectoris by electrical stimulation of the carotid-sinus nerves. *New England Journal of Medicine*. 1967;277(24):1278–1283. doi:10.1056/NEJM196712142772402.
4. Black J. Nobel lecture in physiology or medicine–1988. Drugs from emasculated hormones: the principle of syntopic antagonism. *Vitro Cellular And Developmental Biology*. 1989;25(4):311–320.
5. Braunwald E, Maroko PR, Libby P. Reduction of Infarct Size Following Coronary Occlusion. *Circulation Research*. 1974/09/01;1974 35(3_supplement):III-192–III-201. doi:10.1161/res.35.3_supplement.iii-192 .
6. Maroko P, Libby P, Ginks W, et al. Coronary artery reperfusion: I. Early effects on local myocardial function and the extent of myocardial necrosis. *J Clin Invest*. 1972;51:2710–2717.
7. Pfeffer MA, Pfeffer JM. Ventricular enlargement and reduced survival after myocardial infarction. *Circulation*. 1987;75(5 Pt 2):IV93–7.
8. Pfeffer JM, Pfeffer MA, Braunwald E. Influence of chronic captopril therapy on the infarcted left ventricle of the rat. *Circ Res*. 1985;57(1):84–95.
9. Libby P. Pathogenesis of Atherothrombotic Events: From Lumen to Lesion and Beyond. *Circulation*. 2024;150(16):1217–1219. doi:10.1161/CIRCULATIONAHA.124.070087 2024/10/15.
10. Falk E, Nakano M, Bentzon JF, Finn AV, Virmani R. Update on acute coronary syndromes: the pathologists' view. *European Heart Journal*. 2013;34(10):719–728. doi:10.1093/eurheartj/ehs411 ehs411 [pii].
11. Libby P. Mechanisms of acute coronary syndromes and their implications for therapy. *New England Journal of Medicine*. 2013;369(21):2004–2013.
12. Mallory GK, White PD, Salcedo-Salgar J. The speed of healing of mycardial infarction: A study of the patholigic anatomy in seventy-two cases. *Am Heart J*. 1939;18(6):647–671.
13. Kroop IG, Shackman NH. The C-reactive protein determination as an index of myocardial necrosis in coronary artery disease. *American Journal Of Medicine*. 1957;22(1):90–98.
14. Simpson PJ, Todd 3rd RF, Fantone JC, Mickelson JK, Griffin JD, Lucchesi BR. Reduction of experimental canine myocardial reperfusion injury by a monoclonal antibody (anti-Mo1, anti-CD11b) that inhibits leukocyte adhesion. *J Clin Invest*. 1988;81(2):624–629. doi:10.1172/JCI113364.
15. Swirski FK, Nahrendorf M. Leukocyte behavior in atherosclerosis, myocardial infarction, and heart failure. *Science*. 11 2013;339(6116):161–166. doi:10.1126/science.1230719.
16. Lavine K, Amrute J, Luo X, et al. Targeting Immune-Fibroblast Crosstalk in Myocardial Infarction and Cardiac Fibrosis. *Research Square Platform LLC*;. 2023.
17. Weber C, Zernecke A, Libby P. The multifaceted contributions of leukocyte subsets to atherosclerosis: lessons from mouse models. *Nat Rev Immunol*. 2008;8:802–815.
18. Libby P, Nahrendorf M, Pittet MJ, Swirski FK. Diversity of denizens of the atherosclerotic plaque: not all monocytes are created equal. *Circulation*. 2008;117:3168–3170.
19. Libby P, Hansson GK, Lichtman AH. Immune effector mechanisms implicated in atherosclerosis: from mice to humans. *Immunity*. 2013;38(6):1092–1104.
20. Hilgendorf I, Gerhardt LMS, Tan TC, et al. Ly-6C Monocytes Depend on Nr4a1 to Balance Both Inflammatory and Reparative Phases in the Infarcted Myocardium. *Circulation Research*. 2014-05-09 2014;114(10):1611–1622. doi:10.1161/circresaha.114.303204 .
21. Bajpai G, Bredemeyer A, Li W, et al. Tissue Resident CCR2– and CCR2+ Cardiac Macrophages Differentially Orchestrate Monocyte Recruitment and Fate Specification Following Myocardial Injury. *Circulation Research*. 2019;124(2):263–278. doi:10.1161/circresaha.118.314028 2019-01-18.
22. Zaman R, Epelman S. Resident cardiac macrophages: Heterogeneity and function in health and disease. *Immunity*. 13 2022;55(9):1549–1563. doi:10.1016/j.immuni.2022.08.009.
23. Bajpai G, Schneider C, Wong N, et al. The human heart contains distinct macrophage subsets with divergent origins and functions. *Nat Med*. 2018;doi:10.1038/s41591-018-0059-x.
24. Li W, Hsiao H-M, Higashikubo R, et al. Heart-resident CCR2+ macrophages promote neutrophil extravasation through TLR9/MyD88/CXCL5 signaling. *JCI Insight*. 2016-08-04 2016;1(12). doi:10.1172/jci.insight.87315 .
25. Nahrendorf M, Swirski FK, Aikawa E, et al. The healing myocardium sequentially mobilizes two monocyte subsets with divergent and complementary functions. *J Exp Med*. Nov 26 2007;204(12):3037–3047.
26. Wan E, Yeap XY, Dehn S, et al. Enhanced efferocytosis of apoptotic cardiomyocytes through myeloid-epithelial-reproductive tyrosine kinase links acute inflammation resolution to cardiac repair after infarction. *Circ Res*. Sep 27 2013;113(8):1004–1012. doi:10.1161/CIRCRESAHA.113.301198.
27. Li R, Chen B, Kubota A, et al. Protective effects of macrophage-specific integrin α5 in myocardial infarction are associated with accentuated angiogenesis. *Nature communications*. 2023;14(1):7555. doi:10.1038/s41467-023-43369-x.
28. Panizzi P, Swirski FK, Figueiredo JL, et al. Impaired infarct healing in atherosclerotic mice with Ly-6Chi monocytosis. *J Am Coll Cardiol*. 2010;55(15):1629–1638.
29. Wang Y, Wang C, Shen L, Xu D. The Role of Regulatory T Cells in Heart Repair After Myocardial Infarction. *J Cardiovasc Transl Res*. 2023;16(3):590–597. doi:10.1007/s12265-022-10290-5.
30. Swirski FK, Nahrendorf M, Wildgruber M, et al. Identification of splenic reservoir monocytes and their deployment to inflammatory sites. *Science*. 2009;325(5940):612–616.
31. Leuschner F, Rauch PJ, Ueno T, et al. Rapid monocyte kinetics in acute myocardial infarction are sustained by extramedullary monocytopoiesis. *J Exp Med*. 2012;209(1):123–137. doi:10.1084/jem.20111009 jem.20111009 [pii].
32. Dutta P, Hoyer FF, Grigoryeva LS, et al. Macrophages retain hematopoietic stem cells in the spleen via VCAM-1. *J Exp Med*. Apr 6 2015;212(4):497–512. doi:10.1084/jem.20141642.
33. Sager HB, Heidt T, Hulsmans M, et al. Targeting Interleukin-1beta Reduces Leukocyte Production After Acute Myocardial Infarction. *Circulation*. Nov 17 2015;132(20):1880–1890. doi:10.1161/circulationaha.115.016160.
34. Dutta P, Sager HB, Stengel KR, et al. Myocardial Infarction Activates CCR2(+) Hematopoietic Stem and Progenitor Cells. *Cell stem cell*. May 7 2015;16(5):477–487. doi:10.1016/j.stem.2015.04.008.
35. Rohde D, Vandoorne K, Lee I-H, et al. Bone marrow endothelial dysfunction promotes myeloid cell expansion in cardiovascular disease. *Nature Cardiovascular Research*. 2022-01-01 2022;1(1):28–44. doi:10.1038/s44161-021-00002-8 .
36. Dutta P, Courties G, Wei Y, et al. Myocardial infarction accelerates atherosclerosis. *Nature*. 2012;487(7407):325–329.
37. Hinterdobler J, Schott Simin, Jin H, et al. Acute mental stress drives vascular inflammation and promotes plaque destabilization in mouse atherosclerosis. *European Heart Journal*. 2021-10-14 2021;42(39):4077–4088. doi:10.1093/eurheartj/ehab371 .
38. Heidt T, Sager HB, Courties G, et al. Chronic variable stress activates hematopoietic stem cells. *Nat Med*. 22 2014;doi:10.1038/nm.3589.
39. Emami H, Singh P, MacNabb M, et al. Splenic metabolic activity predicts risk of future cardiovascular events: demonstration of a cardiosplenic axis in humans. *JACC Cardiovasc Imaging*. 2015;8(2):121–130. doi:10.1016/j.jcmg.2014.10.009.
40. Thorp EB. Cardiac macrophages and emerging roles for their metabolism after myocardial infarction. *Journal of Clinical Investigation*. 2023;133(18). doi:10.1172/jci171953 2023-09-15.
41. Leuschner F, Courties G, Dutta P, et al. Silencing of CCR2 in myocarditis. *European Heart Journal*. 2015;36(23):1478–1488. doi:10.1093/eurheartj/ehu225.
42. Dong Z, Hou L, Luo W, et al. Myocardial infarction drives trained immunity of monocytes, accelerating atherosclerosis. *European Heart Journal*. 2024-03-01 2024;45(9):669–684. doi:10.1093/eurheartj/ehad787 .

Index

Note: Page numbers followed by "*f*" indicate figures, "*t*" indicate tables, and "*b*" indicate boxes.